Cosmetic Surgery of the Asian Face

Second Edition

Thieme

Cosmetic Surgery of the Asian Face
Second Edition

John A. McCurdy, Jr., M.D., F.A.C.S.
Assistant Professor
Department of Surgery
John A. Burns School of Medicine
University of Hawaii
Honolulu, Hawaii

Samuel M. Lam, M.D.
Director
Lam Facial Plastics,
Lam Facial Plastic Surgery Center,
Lam Institute for Hair Restoration
Willow Bend Wellness Center
Plano, Texas

Thieme
New York • Stuttgart

Thieme Medical Publishers, Inc.
333 Seventh Ave.
New York, NY 10001

Consulting Editor: Esther Gumpert
Associate Editor: J. Owen Zurhellen IV
Vice President, Production and Electronic Publishing: Anne T. Vinnicombe
Production Editor: Print Matters, Inc.
Marketing Director: Phyllis Gold
Sales Manager: Ross Lumpkin
Chief Financial Officer: Peter van Woerden
President: Brian D. Scanlan
Compositor: Thomson Press
Printer: Everbest

Library of Congress Cataloging-in-Publication Data

McCurdy, John A. Jr.
  Cosmetic surgery of the Asian face / John A. McCurdy, Jr., Samuel Lam. — 2nd ed.
    p. cm.
  Includes bibliographical references and index.
  ISBN 1-58890-218-8 (US) — ISBN 3-13-747602-X (GTV)
  1. Face—Surgery.   2. Asians—Surgery.   3. Surgery, Plastic. I. Lam,
Samuel M. II. Title.
  RD119.5.F33M37 2005
  617.5'20592'08995—dc22
                              2005041782

Important note: Medical knowledge is ever-changing. As new research and clinical experience broaden our knowledge, changes in treatment and drug therapy may be required. The authors and editors of the material herein have consulted sources believed to be reliable in their efforts to provide information that is complete and in accord with the standards accepted at the time of publication. However, in view of the possibility of human error by the authors, editors, or publisher of the work herein or changes in medical knowledge, neither the authors, editors, or publisher, nor any other party who has been involved in the preparation of this work, warrants that the information contained herein is in every respect accurate or complete, and they are not responsible for any errors or omissions or for the results obtained from use of such information. Readers are encouraged to confirm the information contained herein with other sources. For example, readers are advised to check the product information sheet included in the package of each drug they plan to administer to be certain that the information contained in this publication is accurate and that changes have not been made in the recommended dose or in the contraindications for administration. This recommendation is of particular importance in connection with new or infrequently used drugs.

Some of the product names, patents, and registered designs referred to in this book are in fact registered trademarks or proprietary names even though specific reference to this fact is not always made in the text. Therefore, the appearance of a name without designation as proprietary is not to be construed as a representation by the publisher that it is in the public domain.

Printed in China

5 4 3 2 1

TMP ISBN 1-58890-218-8
GTV ISBN 3 13 747602 X

Dedication

To Leonard L. Hays, M.D., who "recruited" me into his fledgling residency program, provided the fertile environment and encouragement so important to the development of a facial plastic surgeon, and served as a personal example of the persistence and inner strength necessary to successfully cope with petty interspecialty and interpersonal rivalries that so often complicate the practice of cosmetic surgery.

Also, to my loyal office staff of 20-plus years, Dorothy, Barbara, and Kathy, as well as my two children, John Andrew and Elizabeth, who shepherded and supported me through difficult times, somehow managing to keep me on a relatively even keel.

Lastly, to my wife Kayoko, and son John Inoru, who continue motivating me to persevere and achieve.

To all of you, and to many more unmentioned, I am grateful.

John A. McCurdy, Jr.

To Ed Williams, my friend, colleague, and mentor.

Samuel M. Lam

Contents

DVD Contents

Disk One

Marking the Eyelid: Design and Planning

Double-Eyelid Blepharoplasty: The Full-Incision Approach

Revision Double-Eyelid Blepharoplasty: Making the Eyelid Crease Smaller

Disk Two

Lower Skin–Muscle Blepharoplasty

Nasal Implant Selection

Alloplastic Augmentation Rhinoplasty

Alar-Base Reduction

Gore-Tex Insertion and Liposuction of Nasolabial Folds

Cheek Lift

Preface

The first edition of *Cosmetic Surgery of the Asian Face*, published in 1990, was a monograph, commissioned by the American Academy of Facial Plastic and Reconstructive Surgery. It represented a compendium of techniques, developed during 15 years of personal experience, that had yielded the greatest versatility and reliability for me in achieving positive aesthetic results for the Asian patient. Fifteen years have passed since the publication of that monograph, and during the interim, there has been a natural evolution in my techniques as well as an explosion in the volume of cosmetic surgical procedures performed for the Asian face. This situation may be attributed to numerous factors. Perhaps the most important of these are the changing immigration patterns in the Western world and the increasing affluence of Asian populations. Even as the popularity of Asian facial cosmetic surgery has increased, the desires of the average patient requesting surgical intervention have also undergone a dramatic metamorphosis. In contemporary practice, cosmetic procedures seldom represent requests for "westernization" of the face. Most patients desire relatively conservative changes that improve facial balance and harmony while maintaining ethnic identity. It is my distinct impression that patient dissatisfaction following procedures performed by Western surgeons is often related to overly aggressive surgery, whereas unhappiness following surgery performed in Asia is more likely to be related to an overly conservative approach.

It was apparent that a need existed for an updated edition of this volume, and in spring of 2002, Dr. Lam approached me regarding development of a second edition. We agreed to collaborate and decided upon a two-section format. The first section is an expansion of my personal techniques, now representing 30 years of experience. The second section discusses variations of the basic surgical procedures available for modification of the eyelids, forehead and brow, nose, cheeks, and neck, as well as other ancillary cosmetic techniques. Dr. Lam has supplemented his personal experiences with a compendium of surgical techniques that he has experienced during visits with surgeons in Asia as well as the West.

In addition to expanding and updating descriptions of the basic techniques that I currently employ, I have added a new section discussing the cultural and psychological differences between Asians and Caucasians that substantially affect the relationship between the surgeon and the patient. Careful, precise pre- and postoperative communication equals, or exceeds, the importance of actual surgical technique in achieving satisfactory results. The Western surgeon must understand that Asian cultures differ substantially from those of the West, and that these differences exert significant influence on patients' perceptions about surgery (and about the surgeon), surgical expectations, and behavior during the postoperative period. Indeed, among the questions most commonly asked during my lectures on Asian cosmetic surgery are those related to understanding and coping with the postoperative behavior of Asian patients.

My section of the book is liberally infused with personal philosophy that I hope will be beneficial in understanding the processes by which my preferred techniques evolved and crystallized over the years. Even though, in my hands, the techniques that I describe yield the best results, experience has taught me that, in most cases, there are several alternative methods that produce equally good results in the hands of other surgeons. In this regard, two statements made by Dr. Jack Anderson, one of the founders of the American Academy of Facial Plastic and Reconstructive Surgery, are indelibly etched in my mind. When asked why he steadfastly pursued one technique of rhinoplasty, apparently ignoring alternative methods, Dr. Anderson replied, "I'm not stupid; I wouldn't use this technique if it didn't work," but followed this statement with the charge "There is a better way; find it."

Another aphorism applicable to those of us who are rather entrenched in our ways crosses my mind. There are two kinds of fools; the first says, "Things turn out better if they are performed the way they always have been." The second says, "This method is new; therefore, it must be better!" The truth usually lies somewhere in between; and in this regard, I am extremely pleased that Dr. Lam has researched and gained personal experience in numerous alternative methods, allowing him to collaborate in presenting a more balanced view of current concepts of cosmetic surgery of the Asian face.

It occurs to me that surgery is similar to athletic performance in that two surgeons using the same techniques often achieve different results. This observation is analogous to the one that students of golf, for instance, being of equal ability and having equal perseverance, and being taught by the same competent professional, will, because of personal idiosyncrasies that are difficult to define objectively, play the game differently. It is wise to recall this metaphor when wondering why one cannot produce results identical to those of a particular surgeon even when following precisely the techniques that he or she has described.

It is my hope that surgeons of all levels of experience and expertise will be able to extract information from the insights and approaches described in this volume that will be of benefit in meeting future surgical challenges.

John A. McCurdy, Jr., M.D., F.A.C.S.

Preface

Fifteen years have transpired since the first edition of this book. During the intervening years, many new procedures have arisen in the world of Asian facial cosmetic surgery, including facial implants, skeletal surgery, and brow-lifting techniques, to name only a few. Despite these advances, no authoritative textbook has been published on Asian facial aesthetic surgery in the English language since the first edition appeared over a decade ago. This book strives to fill that void and to be significantly more comprehensive than the prior edition.

This book really constitutes an entirely new venture in its ambition and scope. Dr. McCurdy's technique has evolved since the publication of the first edition, and these new modifications and refinements are elaborated in the first half of the book. The second half of the book is completely new and represents alternative surgical strategies that differ from Dr. McCurdy's techniques. For instance, the suture and partial-incision techniques for "double-eyelid" creation are described in detail so that the reader can understand the mechanics of these operations that differ from the senior author's full-incision method. The second half of the book also delves into entirely new subject matter not covered in the first half of the book, for example, skeletal surgery, dimple fabrication, and injectable agents. As part of the research for this project, many months were spent abroad in Asia interviewing and observing prominent surgeons to procure their knowledge and experience. In addition, leading practitioners of Asian facial plastic surgery in the West have been invited to describe their techniques. Only techniques that have proven their validity from extensive operative experience were considered worthy of inclusion. Clinical photographs that substantiate the surgical result are present throughout the text, with proper credit given to the respective surgeon.

After carefully reviewing the first edition, the authors decided that the clarity of the book would be further enhanced by lavish full-color photography that would demonstrate the principal surgical procedures in a stepwise fashion, as the first edition was printed exclusively in black and white. Therefore, all the photographs were meticulously chosen for their illustrative purposes in support of the text. However, despite the benefits of a printed book as an instructional tool, the authors realized the limitations of this medium. Therefore, two full-length DVDs have been included to bridge this educational gap and to provide the most insightful method by which a surgeon can digest the presented material and thereby feel comfortable in recreating the described techniques in the operative theater. The value of this second edition of *Cosmetic Surgery of the Asian Face* lies in its being both a printed manual and a video tutorial—both formats complement each other and provide the most comprehensive knowledge possible. In the video series, separate sequences are dedicated to a systematic method of upper-eyelid marking for the double-eyelid procedure as well as to proper selection and individual carving of the nasal implant.

The world has rapidly become smaller with globalization. Asian emigrants have scattered abroad and reside as much in the Western hemisphere as in the Far East. Miscegenation has become more frequent, and ethnic divides have been breached through cultural, economic, and social exchange. The newfound wealth of many Asians has led to a dramatic explosion in Asian cosmetic surgery, as disposable income climbs. Cultural biases against cosmetic surgery in Asia are also relaxing, with a greater acceptance of cosmetic surgery there than ever before. The Western surgeon cannot afford to ignore the Asian patient today. Further, trying to use Occidental surgical techniques on the Asian face may often be a precarious exercise, as many experienced Western techniques fail to provide the intended aesthetic objective or, worse yet, ends with a disastrous outcome. "Westernization" procedures that were popular two decades ago have now been replaced by more understated surgical endeavors in which the essential ethnic identity is not violated. Correction of this problem has been addressed both in the text and in the DVD video format. Using Western aesthetic values for Asian surgery should be discouraged, as this does not take into consideration the cultural sensitivity of the Asian and may render the Asian face unnatural and foreign. This book hopes to bridge the gap between the Orient and the Occident so that the best of both worlds can be brought together.

Samuel M. Lam, M.D.

Special Thanks

The authors would like to thank the following physicians, surgeons, and practitioners for sharing their expertise and perspective on their unique contributions to the field of Asian cosmetic surgery.

Ki-Young Ahn, M.D., Ph.D.
Director and Professor
Department of Plastic and Reconstructive Surgery
Daegu Catholic University Hospital
Daegu, South Korea

Edward W. Chang, M.D., D.D.S.
Director of Facial Plastic Surgery Education
Department of Otolaryngology–Head and Neck Surgery
Columbia University Medical Center
New York, New York

Nabil Fanous, M.D.
Director of Facial Plastic Surgery Fellowship Program
Associate Professor
Department of Otolaryngology–Head and Neck Surgery
McGill University
Montreal, Quebec, Canada

Patricia Shibley-Gauthier
President
Canadian Micro-pigmentation Centre
Mississauga, Ontario, Canada

Don-Hak Jung, M.D.
Private Practice
Seoul, South Korea

Yong-Ha Kim, M.D., Ph.D.
Associate Professor
Department of Plastic and Reconstructive Surgery
Yeungnam University School of Medicine
Daegu, South Korea

Young-Kyoon Kim, M.D.
Private Practice
Bucheon, South Korea

Jung Bock Lee, M.D.
Private Practice
Chairman Emeritus
Department of Dermatology
Yonsei University College of Medicine
Seoul, South Korea

Jung Soo Lee, M.D.
Private Practice
Seoul, South Korea

Shin Kyu Lee, M.D.
Private Practice
Seoul, South Korea

Yukio Shirakabe, M.D.
Private Practice
Tokyo, Japan

Tetsuo Shu, M.D.
Private Practice
Tokyo, Japan

Tomoyuki Takahashi, M.D.
Private Practice
Tokyo, Japan

Joseph K. Wong, M.D., F.R.C.S.C.
Director, Head and Neck–Facial Plastic Surgery Program
Division Head, Otolaryngology–Head and Neck Surgery
Department of Surgery
Credit Valley Hospital
Peel Regional Cancer Centre Ontario
Mississauga, Ontario, Canada

Constance Yam, M.D.
Private Practice
Hong Kong

Cosmetic Surgery of the Asian Face

Second Edition

Section I

General Considerations and Basic Techniques

John A. McCurdy, Jr., M.D.

1

Understanding the Asian Patient

I have had the good fortune of practicing facial plastic surgery in Hawaii since 1976. The composition of my practice has mirrored the ethnic makeup of Hawaii with ~70% Asian and 30% Caucasian. Thus, I have gained considerable experience in cosmetic surgery of the Asian face. As every surgeon who has experience in Asian cosmetic surgery knows, there are considerable differences as compared with a cosmetic surgical practice emphasizing Western patients. These differences are not merely anatomic. In fact, the psychological aspects of Asian cosmetic surgery provide a greater challenge than mastery of the surgical techniques themselves.

Cultural and psychological factors often prove more complex and cannot be underestimated. It is sometimes difficult for many Western surgeons to understand exactly the Asian patient's needs, which is why much of this surgery is increasingly performed by Asian-American surgeons.

To understand the Asian patient, it is crucial to take into consideration the cultural and sociological particularities.

◆ Anatomic Considerations

The Mongoloid branch of mankind, easily the largest race of our species, originated in eastern Asia and later migrated to areas both contiguous and distant, including Indochina and the Indian subcontinent, Malaysia, Polynesia, Melanesia, and Micronesia, as well as North and South America (i.e., Eskimos and North and South American indigenous peoples, aka "Indians"). Because of the wide geographical diffusion, the physical characteristics of this race show a tremendous variation, as do, for example, the many ethnic subdivisions of the Caucasian race.

Westerners tend to possess a stereotyped conception of the physical traits of Asians: yellow skin pigmentation; straight, coarse black hair; a flat face with high malar eminences; a broad, flat nose; and narrow, slitlike eyes with a characteristic epicanthal fold. Although the stereotype may be loosely applied to the eastern Asian group of people (i.e., Chinese, Koreans, and Japanese), the aesthetic surgeon should appreciate that considerable individual variation exists in all of these physical traits. For example, ~40% of East Asians originating from the more northerly latitudes have a straight or convex nasal dorsum.

Similar variations exist in other Asian subgroups. In general, however, individuals originating from southern Asia tend to have more deeply pigmented skin, exhibit greater flattening and concavity of the nasal dorsum, and display a more westernized eyelid configuration (i.e., a more clearly defined superior palpebral fold, although generally smaller and less well defined than Caucasians, and absent or rudimentary epicanthal fold as compared with the features of northern Asians). The lips of southern Asians tend to be more voluminous than individuals originating from northern Asia.

From the point of view of the aesthetic surgeon, the physical diversity of the Asian population notwithstanding, certain facial features do form a reasonably distinct basis for surgical intervention and justify specialized study of surgical techniques that consistently and reliably produce good aesthetic results in the Asian face. These facial features typically include the following traits:

1. The upper eyelid, characterized by an absent or poorly defined superior palpebral fold, abundant periorbital fat, and an epicanthal fold of varying configuration and size

3

2. A small, flat nose with poor lobular definition

3. Prominent, wide malar eminences, the zygomatic prominence often being associated with a relative hollowness of the temporal fossa, particularly in the aging patient

4. A tendency toward hypoplasia of the midfacial skeleton with maxillary retrusion and anterior inclination of the maxillary incisors

My observations suggest that microgenia is somewhat more common in Asians than in Caucasians. Many Koreans exhibit prominence of the mandibular angle at times accentuated by masseteric hypertrophy.

◆ Skin Color and Texture

Whereas the classic Western stereotype of Asian skin being yellowish in coloration is not without considerable biological justification, there is actually wide variation in color and texture of the skin in individuals of this race. Generally, skin pigmentation is darker in Asians originating from southern latitudes, and this is consistent with the observation that skin color, as well as other biological traits, evolved as an adaptation to the climatic environment. Approximately 75% of individuals who originate from the northern and central latitudes of eastern Asia (i.e., northern Chinese, Koreans, and Japanese) have light-colored, somewhat milky skin pigmentation; the remainder exhibit varying degrees of brownish coloration. The yellowish hue of Asian skin is largely a consequence of the number and distribution of melanin granules rather than of variations in lipoproteins or other biochemical components of the skin.

A wide variation in skin texture and thickness exists among East Asians, the dermis being thicker and more fibrous in individuals with darker pigmentation. The skin of lightly pigmented Asians, however, tends to demonstrate greater density than that of pale-skinned Caucasians. This greater collagen density is manifested in a tendency toward a more vigorous fibroplastic response during wound healing, which may result in prolonged hyperemia during scar maturation and an increased incidence of hypertrophic scarring as well as occasional keloid formation. Such prolonged hyperemia of incisions tends to occur even in lightly pigmented Asians.

Increases in dermal thickness may account for a substantially lower incidence of fine wrinkles in both darker and more lightly pigmented Asians than in comparably pigmented Caucasians. This may account for the myth that the Asian face ages more slowly than the Caucasian face. Actually, a considerable number of fair-skinned Asians do develop fine wrinkles as aging progresses. Aging is associated with a substantially greater incidence of pigmented dermatosis (lentigines, actinic keratoses, seborrheic keratoses, etc.) as compared with Caucasian skin. In general, however, skin malignancies of all types are considerably less common in the Asian face than in the Caucasian face.

In many Asians, accumulation and/or ptosis of fat, particularly in the jowls, nasolabial mound, buccal area, and submental region, appears to be more marked than noted in Caucasians of comparable age, necessitating special attention in planning facial rejuvenation procedures. In other patients, particularly Koreans, facial aging is accompanied by atrophy of fat in the buccal region and temporal fossa.

Although wide variations in sebaceous activity are apparent among Asians, the dry skin that frequently plagues aging Caucasians is less common (except in the external auditory canal, where dry, flaky cerumen is a distinctive East Asian trait). Whereas acne is reasonably common among Asians living in hot, humid environments, severe acne resulting in dermal destruction and subsequent scarring is less common in East Asians than Caucasians.

◆ Cultural and Psychological Considerations

In spite of the significant influence of the Western world on modern Asia, the tremendous differences between Western and Asian cultures soon become obvious to Westerners who associate with native East Asians. Although these differences become less defined in the generations descended from immigrant populations, certain powerful cultural influences persist, and these often influence attitudes concerning (or behavioral reactions following) cosmetic surgery. The basic appreciation of these cultural factors is therefore helpful in providing insight into the psychological makeup of the various Asian nationalities and enables the aesthetic surgeon to communicate more effectively with, and respond more appropriately to, the desires and concerns of Asian patients. It is important to recognize that, although all humans experience the same feelings, desires, and emotions, cultural influences determine to a large extent how these feelings are expressed.

All traditional Asian societies are male-dominated, and the traditional woman's duty is to be supportive, comforting, beautiful, and alluring. The quest for beauty and youth, and attempts to delay its demise, often puts individuals under enormous pressure. Among the basic foundations of Asian cultures are strong beliefs in fate, destiny, and the importance of luck (both good and bad) in daily affairs. Certain maxims or "folklorish" superstitions (as evidenced by sayings or proverbs) may be applied to important situations and challenges encountered in daily life. These powerful beliefs, many of which are derived from Buddhism, Daoism, and Shinto, affect attitudes concerning behavioral reactions following cosmetic surgery. Subconscious guilt regarding cosmetic surgery (indicating disrespect of parents) may be operative, especially in younger individuals, and result in withdrawal ("hiding") that robs the patient of emotional support that would be beneficial during the healing process. This guilt, as well as the obsession with youth and beauty, renders patients susceptible to unflattering comments from friends or family during the healing period.

Traditional Asian cultures have a tendency to place great significance on physiognomy, that is, the relationship of physical traits and characteristics to behavior and personality as well as to prospects for success in business, friendship, marriage, and other relationships. These beliefs, coupled with the strong cultural appreciation for symmetry and harmony and attention to detail characteristic of all Asian cultures, often translate into excessive postoperative concern and worry that precipitates what may seem to be inappropriate, or even irrational, complaints and requests for early revision surgery.

In traditional Asian society, substantial respect exists for physicians and other professionals. In such societies, it is often considered disrespectful to question the opinion of such professionals, a fact that may impair effective communication about the patient's desires preoperatively and concerns postoperatively. This description of traditional Asian society and beliefs notwithstanding, it is important to be cognizant of substantial differences between traditional and contemporary Asia. A social and cultural metamorphosis is accelerating with the increasing influence of Western culture, urbanization, and affluence. Although still formidable, traditional values and beliefs are eroding as Western materialism and hedonism mesmerize the populace. Modern Asian women are declaring their independence and, in increasing numbers, straying from traditional values. Young Asian women tend to be stylish, carefree, independent, and often seemingly self-indulgent. During my 29-year experience, I have noted that young Asian-Americans are virtually indistinguishable from their American counterparts in terms of behavior, mannerisms, speech patterns, and so on. Although young patients do seem to be less obsessive about cosmetic surgery, mothers of young women (or men) generally do not demonstrate such patience, which may lead to a lack of communication.

◆ Ethnic Differences

Although many of the cultural nuances discussed in the previous section are common to most of the Asian societies, each ethnic group shares certain behavioral traits

Table 1–1 Expressiveness Scale

Korean
Chinese
Vietnamese
Filipino
Thai
Japanese

and attitudes that, though not universal, tend to distinguish members of each nationality. Similar nuances, of course, exist with reference to various Caucasian nationalities, and indeed, it is helpful to distinguish regional differences between individuals of the same nationality in determining the most effective means of communication (i.e., all Americans recognize the differences in communicating with a New Yorker vs. a Texan, etc.). Asians love to talk about the behavioral characteristics of other Asian nationalities, and much of my understanding in this area has been gleaned from discussions of this topic with patients. To be able to facilitate effective communication between patient and surgeon, it is important to have some experience with the different Asian nationalities.

Rather than attempt to describe the variations between Asian nationalities, for purposes of this discussion, I have formulated what I term an expressiveness scale (Table **1–1**). In general, increases in expressiveness are associated with a greater tendency toward obsessive concern, unreasonable complaints, and requests for revision surgery during the early postoperative period that often surprise surgeons regardless of their experience with Asian patients. In keeping with the described differences between traditional and contemporary Asia, it is important to understand that this expressiveness scale is most applicable to native-born Asians and becomes less accurate and functional in subsequent generations.

However, it should be mentioned that the scale is based on my personal experience and not scientifically founded.

◆ Preoperative Considerations

In general, there are three prerequisites that a patient should meet prior to acceptance for cosmetic surgery:

1. A treatable "defect," that is, an aesthetic concern that is within the technical skills of the surgeon to "correct" with a reasonable expectation of a good result

2. Motivation for surgical correction that is reasonable and comes from within rather than being the desire of a loved one, parent, or other individual

3. Realistic expectations and an understanding that the goal of cosmetic surgery is improvement, not perfection

During the preoperative interview with an Asian patient, it should be understood that, generally speaking, requests for modification of the eyelids or nose are not requests for "westernization." Rather, contemporary Asian patients generally want improvement that matches their "Asian face" not conversion of ethnicity. The surgeon must be aware of the fact that effective communication may be impaired by several factors, including language barriers, respect for the physician that may stifle patient comments and questions, and an assumption on the part of the patient that a learned and competent surgeon knows exactly what is best for each face. Many Asian patients appear to be reserved and self-effacing, at least preoperatively. I have found that use of actual pre- and postoperative photographs in preoperative consultation is by far the most effective means of accurate and precise communication regarding patient desires for cosmetic transformation.

As much potential dissatisfaction postoperatively is related to asymmetry (especially of eyelids and nares/alae), it is critically important to stress and document preexisting asymmetry that may not be entirely correctable surgically. The surgeon must stress the limitations of cosmetic surgery and carefully discuss the required healing period. Expect price sensitivity during the preoperative evaluation. Remember that, as with all patients, Asians too hope for and actually expect perfection, that is, perfect symmetry, no residual wrinkles, and rapid convalescence with minimal edema or ecchymosis. The surgeon must accept the apparent futility of some aspects of these preoperative discussions but ensure that all essentials are well documented.

◆ Anesthesia Considerations

Asian patients tend to be sensitive to oral and parenteral medication, an observation that may relate to induction of the cytochrome p450 system. There is, however, no increased sensitivity to inhalational anesthetics, as these agents are excreted via the pulmonary system without metabolic breakdown.

When performing surgery under local anesthesia, temporary sedation with propofol prior to anesthetic injection is beneficial. Patient's anxiety concerning surgery under local anesthesia is greatly relieved when they awaken from this temporary sedation and learn

that the local anesthesia has already been injected. Most will relate to their friends the fact that surgery was actually painless (as the surgeon promised), and this is certainly beneficial in terms of patient referrals.

Inhalational anesthesia or conscious sedation administered by an anesthesiologist/anesthetist is recommended for large local anesthetic infiltrations (e.g., rhytidectomy). Dexamethasone (6–8 mg) is used for all general anesthesia/conscious sedation cases because, in addition to possibly reducing postoperative edema (a contention that is admittedly anecdotal), it is a potent and long-lasting antiemetic at this dosage level.

Use of freshly mixed local anesthetic/epinephrine solutions (as opposed to commercially available premixed solutions) yields superior hemostasis, decreasing operative time as well as postoperative edema. I use an epinephrine concentration of 1:50,000 (0.2 cc epinephrine 1:1000 per 10 cc plain local anesthetic) for eyelid and nasal surgery and a concentration of 1:100,000 (0.1 cc epinephrine 1:1000 per 10 cc plain local anesthetic) for other procedures. Buffering of the local anesthetic is currently in vogue, but any potential benefit of diminished discomfort during injection is outweighed by its detrimental effect on intraoperative hemostasis.

◆ Postoperative Considerations

Patient's behavior postoperatively is often in stark contrast to their preoperative demeanor and may be difficult and challenging for the surgeon. As ethnic tendencies toward expressivity increase, the surgeon may be faced with various degrees of impatience (I tell patients that doctors' customers are called patients because they must be patient). Consistent with the expressiveness scale (excessive) what often seems to be obsessive, concern and preoccupation with the healing process, as well as intolerance of minor imperfections that may precipitate passionate requests or demands for early revision surgery, tends to be the norm. As previously noted, some younger patients experience some degree of guilt about undergoing cosmetic surgery. This may result in withdrawal, robbing the patient of needed emotional support. The surgeon must be aware that, during the early postoperative period, patients are often subjected to unflattering (perhaps precipitated by envy or jealousy) comments of friends and family. Awareness of this potential allows the surgeon to warn the patient of such possibilities and to ensure that both the surgeon and his or her staff pay extra attention to such patients.

In general, a compassionate, understanding, nondictatorial demeanor, infused with light humor as appropriate in each individual case, is usually the most successful approach to postoperative management of the Asian patient. However, surgeons should react firmly and authoritatively to irrational or inappropriate behavior. Doing something (e.g., local massage, creams, dilute triamcinolone injections) is often helpful in placating an impatient patient. The surgeon must resist demands for inappropriate revision. In my practice, I do not charge for most revision procedures, as assessing an additional charge for what the patient perceives as a "mistake" by the surgeon is particularly aggravating to the patient. Attempts to convince the patient that a small residual defect is not the result of a surgical mistake generally prove to be futile and only serve to further antagonize the patient.

Postoperative pain is rarely an issue. In spite of the complaints and professions of unhappiness, litigation is rare in dealing with Asian patients.

Most Asians are extraordinarily comfortable talking to both friends and strangers about cosmetic surgery. Patients often make unsolicited comments about other patients' appearances while in the waiting room. In my practice, I take this fact into consideration in arranging appointment schedules.

◆ Conclusion

Cosmetic surgery of the Asian face is both a challenging and fascinating endeavor. A large part of the challenge is an effort to understand cultural and psychological differences that translate to behavior that is sometimes difficult for non-Asians to comprehend. I hope that the previous discussion will be of assistance in formulating an effective approach to the Asian patient.

2

Asian Blepharoplasty

Blepharoplasty is undoubtedly the most complex aspect of Asian cosmetic surgery, as the eyes are the single most distinguishing feature of the Asian face, and several surgical variations are available. Although most attention, deservedly, has been directed toward upper blepharoplasty, surgery of the lower eyelid is also worthy of special consideration.

◆ Upper Blepharoplasty

Upper blepharoplasty is the most commonly requested cosmetic operation by Asian patients, and because of the large Asian population now residing in the West, it is important that aesthetic surgeons have a working knowledge of techniques available for this procedure. Although, strictly speaking, upper blepharoplasty in the Asian is a variation of standard upper blepharoplasty as performed in the Caucasian patient, important anatomic differences that characterize the Asian eyelid warrant intensive description and study of possible surgical options. This is a challenging procedure that requires focused preoperative planning and meticulous attention to intraoperative detail if consistent aesthetic results are to be achieved.

One of the major differences between Asian blepharoplasty and standard upper blepharoplasty in the Caucasian is the flexibility in sculpturing upper-eyelid configuration offered by relatively subtle variations in surgical technique. Differences in the level of the palpebral fold and depth of the palpebral sulcus produce substantial effects on the appearance of the eyelid. Aesthetic surgeons who wish to become expert in this operation must possess a clear understanding of the interactions between the various factors that allow construction of upper eyelids that vary in size and shape.

The goal of this chapter is to provide more than a basic description of upper blepharoplasty in the Asian patient—a system for reliable construction of an upper lid of a specific size and shape and a system for staged modification of the epicanthal fold are presented. Gone are the days in which a surgeon could perform the same operation on every Asian upper eyelid; the ability to individualize each and every operation is essential to success in the contemporary environment. All surgeons owe their patients an opportunity to choose the type of eyelid transformation that they desire; patients should not be condemned to construction of the classic "westernized" eyelid that was the sine qua non of this procedure in earlier years.

The first step in the study of Asian upper blepharoplasty is to understand the Asian colloquialisms "single eyelid" and "double eyelid." At least 50% of East Asians demonstrate a single eyelid, so termed because in the absence of a superior palpebral fold, the upper lid drapes like a single, unruffled curtain from the supraorbital ridge to the eyelashes (Fig. **2–1**). Surgical creation of a palpebral furrow divides the single eyelid into two well-defined segments (pretarsal and preseptal), thus producing the "double eyelid" (Fig. **2–2**).

Although the popularity of upper blepharoplasty in Asia has undergone a quantum leap since the 1950s, it would be erroneous to assume that this popularity is solely related to Western influences in Asia. Asian cultures have long regarded the alert and bright-eyed look imparted by a double eyelid as aesthetically desirable, and the first surgical description of Asian upper blepharoplasty was published in Japan in the late

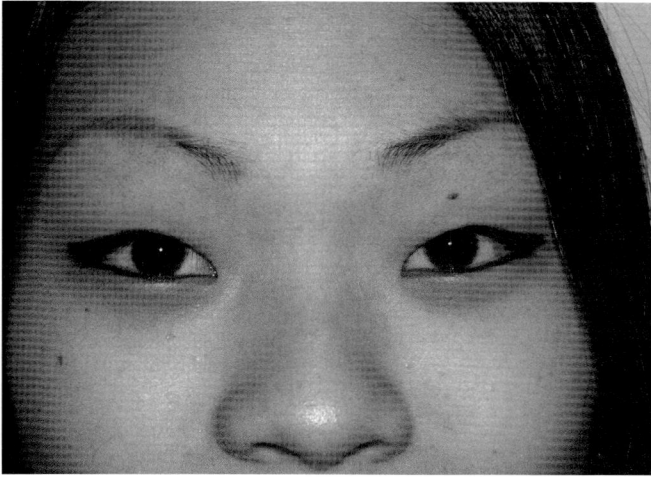

Figure 2–1 The single eyelid. In the absence of a superior palpebral fold, the lid hangs like an unruffled curtain from the supraorbital ridge.

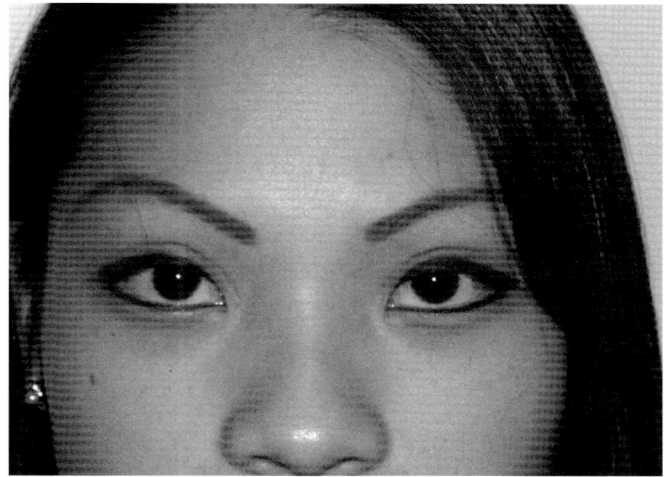

Figure 2–2 The double eyelid. Creation of a palpebral sulcus divides the lid into two well-defined (pretarsal and preseptal) segments.

19th century. The majority of Asians who have natural "double eyelids" exhibit a rudimentary or small fold associated with abundant periorbital fat and excess eyelid skin. Many of these individuals desire surgical enhancement of this lid configuration, and thus Asian upper blepharoplasty is not restricted to individuals demonstrating "single eyelids."

A third facet of Asian upper blepharoplasty is management of the aging lid in individuals who possess natural palpebral furrows or who have previously undergone "double lid" surgery.

Prior to proceeding further, it is of paramount importance to emphasize that the aesthetic surgeon must clearly understand that, at the present time, a patient's request for surgical modification of the eyelid is usually not a request for "westernization "of the eye. In actuality, the vast majority of contemporary Asian patients, particularly those who have been born in Western countries, wish to maintain the character of the upper lid, enhancing its natural beauty. Westernization requires reduction of lid fullness and creation of a large, deep-set upper lid by removing large amounts of skin and fat as well as effacement of the epicanthal fold. In contrast, contemporary Asian upper blepharoplasty is characterized by placement of incisions closer to the ciliary margin, resection of smaller amounts of skin and fat, and conservative manipulation of the epicanthus in patients who request modification of this structure. In my experience, westernization procedures have been requested with markedly decreased frequency during the past 20 years and are sought primarily by recent immigrants to the West. Significantly, patients who have undergone westernization procedures years ago often request surgery to create a more "natural" look that "matches"

the Asian face. As such surgery is fraught with difficulty, and the desired results are often impossible to fully achieve, it is incumbent on the surgeon to understand the desires of each patient regarding postsurgical eyelid appearance to avoid patient unhappiness by production of a result that may be difficult or impossible to modify satisfactorily.

Anatomic Considerations

A commonly accepted anatomic explanation of the difference between the single and double eyelid has formed the basis for Asian upper blepharoplasty in the past: In the double eyelid, filaments of the levator expansion penetrate the orbital septum and orbicularis muscle, attaching to the overlying dermis thus creating a superior palpebral fold when the lid is opened, dividing the upper lid into two distinct segments (Fig. **2–3**). In the single eyelid, these levator filaments, rather than penetrating the orbital septum and orbicularis muscle, terminate on the tarsal plate, and thus no palpebral fold is formed upon eyelid opening, the upper lid consisting of a single unit (Fig. **2–4**).

Although this description has proven to be useful in planning surgical procedures for creation or modification of the palpebral fold, such traditional teaching is an oversimplification. Contemporary anatomic studies have found no evidence of a direct attachment between levator filaments and the dermis, suggesting instead that filaments of the aponeurosis course inferiorly into the pretarsal segment of the eyelid, attaching to fibrous septa that course from tarsus to pretarsal skin (penetrating pretarsal orbicularis), thereby producing adherence between the pretarsal skin, orbicularis, and tarsus.

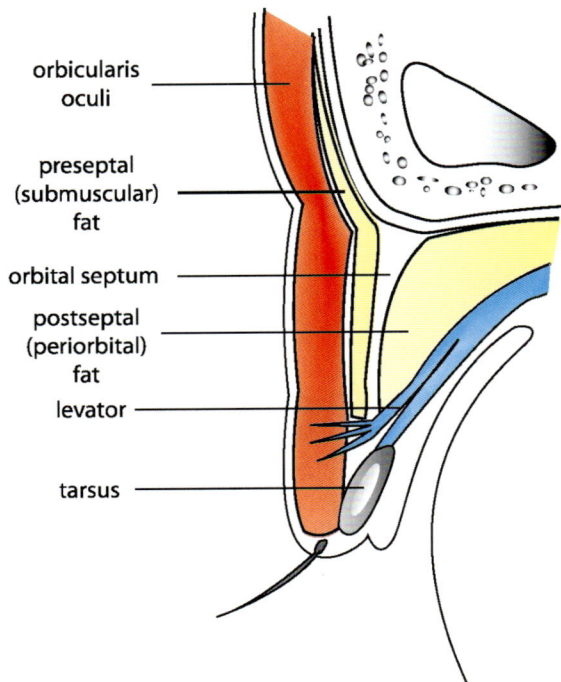

Figure 2–3 Anatomy of the Caucasian ("double eyelid") upper eyelid.

It is the adherence of these tissues that is responsible for creation of the superior palpebral fold, creating a boardlike pretarsal structure that elevates as a single unit upon levator contraction. The preseptal skin, in contrast, is nonadherent and thus relatively mobile. Levator contraction thus results in invagination of the

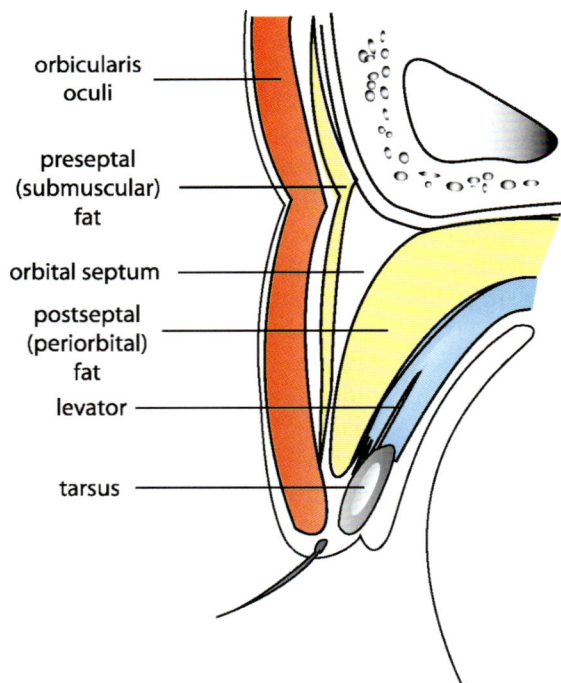

Figure 2–4 Anatomy of the Asian ("single eyelid") upper eyelid.

unified pretarsal unit beneath the mobile preseptal skin, creating a pretarsal fold. This description of the lid fold mechanism is consistent with the fact that in eyelids lacking a well-defined fold, the pretarsal skin is redundant because of an absence of attachments to pretarsal muscle and tarsal plate. Surgical procedures for creation of a superior palpebral furrow achieve this goal in spite of the fact that they were conceived based on the previously described anatomic oversimplification. Creation of an adhesion between the pretarsal dermis and levator aponeurosis or tarsus[1] effectively produces an adhesion at the point of fixation, thus creating the boardlike unit that invaginates beneath preseptal skin on levator contraction. A more stable adhesion can be formed by undermining pretarsal skin 1 to 2 mm inferiorly prior to fixation, a maneuver that I accomplish by excision of a strip of pretarsal orbicularis oculi muscle.

The anatomy of the periorbital fat compartment differs in the Asian upper lid as compared with the Caucasian lid (Figs. **2–3**, **2–4**). In both, the periorbital fat compartment is enclosed by the orbital septum, but in the Asian lid, because of the lack of preseptal adhesions, the periorbital fat compartment descends inferiorly, coursing a variable distance anterior to the tarsal plate. The more inferior location of periorbital fat and the increased amount of subcutaneous and suborbicularis fat are responsible for the characteristic puffiness of the "single" eyelid. In conjunction with redundant pretarsal skin, this fat abundance imparts an impression of diminished width of the palpebral fissure and occasionally produces a suggestion of ptosis (pseudoptosis orientalis). This wedge of fat descending anterior to the tarsal plate must be removed surgically to achieve fixation as it serves as a barrier between pretarsal skin and the lid opening mechanism.

A third difference between the Asian and Caucasian upper eyelid is the epicanthal fold, a structure that is present in ~90% of East Asians. There is substantial variation in the size and configuration of the epicanthus, and if large, this weblike structure blunts the medial canthus, obscures the lacrimal caruncle, and is associated with diminished length of the palpebral fissure as well as diminished intercanthal distance that produces an aesthetically undesirable widening of the nose. Surgical modification of the epicanthus is often a goal of Asian blepharoplasty even in cases in which westernization is not desired; some patients request this procedure to improve nasal aesthetics.

Preoperative Considerations

The desires of patients requesting double-eyelid surgery vary tremendously. Many patients request only creation or enhancement of a superior palpebral fold, wishing to retain other characteristics of the Asian lid, whereas others prefer more extensive transformation; the amount of skin and fat removed during surgery varies accordingly. In this regard, the ability to translate individual patient desires into an operation that reliably sculptures the upper eyelid to each patient's general specifications is a major asset for the aesthetic surgeon.

Preoperatively, patients are counseled that three basic decisions are necessary prior to surgery:

1. Eyelid size
2. Eyelid shape
3. Disposition of the epicanthal fold

As a starting point, eyelid size is arbitrarily characterized as small, medium, or large and eyelid shape as round or oval. Perhaps the best method of communication regarding eyelid size and shape involves examination of pre- and postoperative photographs that illustrate the basic sizes and shapes of eyelids (Figs. **2–5** to **2–10**). Another method of demonstrating eyelid size and shape is manipulation of the eyelid skin with a bent paper clip (or an instrument especially designed for this purpose available from Asian surgical supply companies) while the patient is looking into a mirror. Some patients bring photographs of magazine models to their consultations. Although it must be stressed that the surgeon cannot construct an eyelid to the patient's exact specifications, examination of these images in

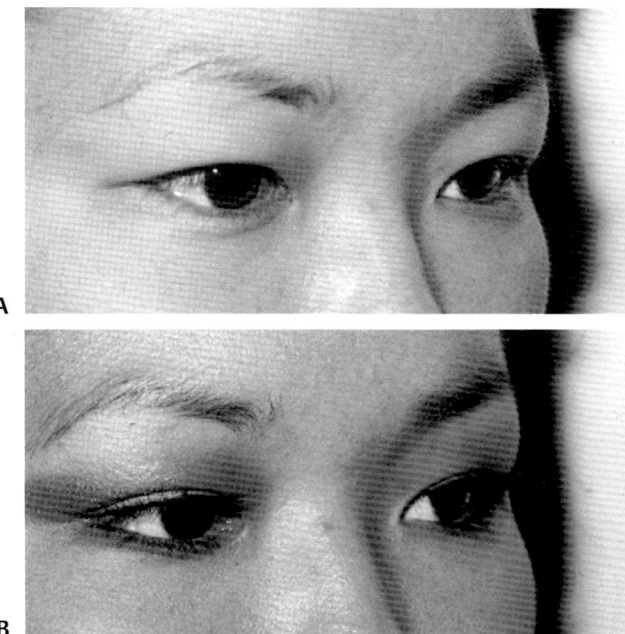

Figure 2–6 (A,B) Surgical creation of a small, oval double eyelid with an inside fold. The incision was placed 7 mm above the ciliary margin, and 3 mm of skin was excised. Note the rudimentary left double eyelid characterized by a shallow palpebral fold and pretarsal skin laxity with inferiorly oriented eyelashes. It would be unwise to operate only on the right eye in an attempt to match the left eyelid because a surgically created fold will not assume the characteristics of the rudimentary natural fold.

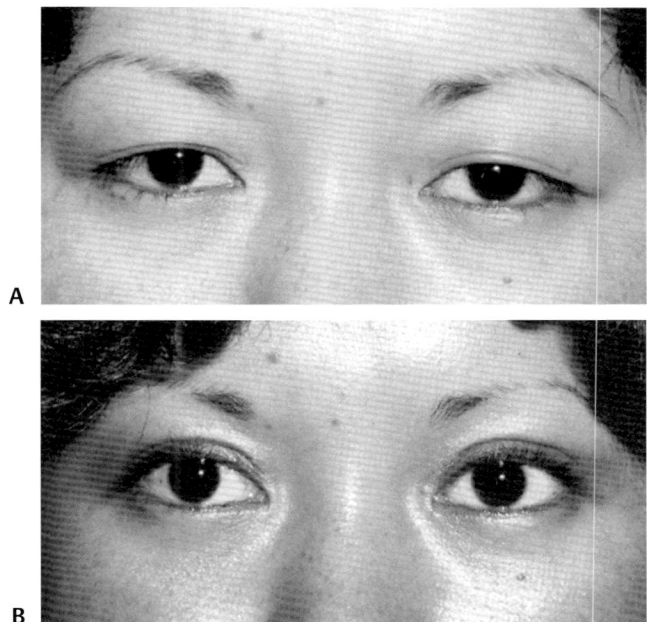

Figure 2–5 (A,B) Surgical creation of a small, round double eyelid with an inside fold. The incision was placed 6 mm above the ciliary margin, and 3 mm of skin was excised.

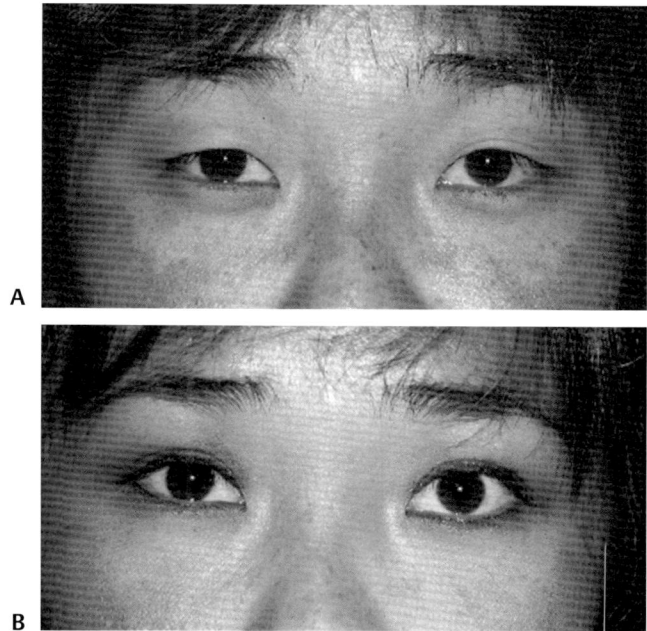

Figure 2–7 (A,B) Surgical creation of a medium, round double eyelid with an outside fold. The incision was placed 8 mm above the ciliary margin, and 50% of the maximum amount of skin that could be removed (as determined by forceps pinching) was actually removed. Note the rudimentary double eyelids for which the patient requested surgical enhancement.

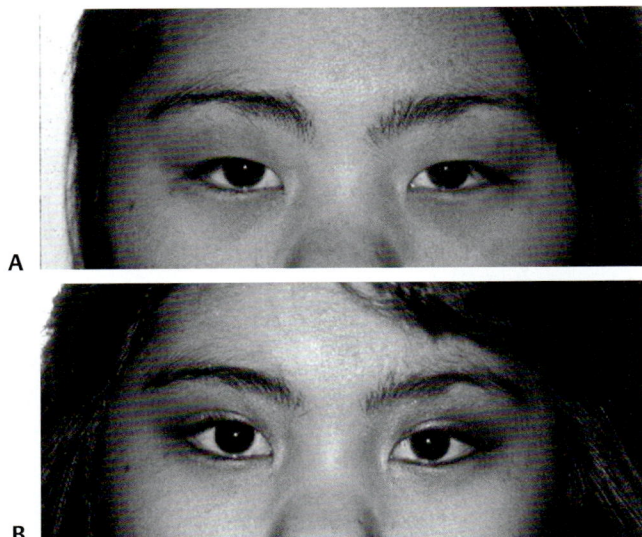

Figure 2–8   (A,B) Surgical creation of a medium, oval double eyelid with an inside fold. The incision was placed 8 mm above the ciliary margin, and 50% of the maximum amount of skin that could be removed (as determined by forceps pinching) was actually removed.

conjunction with actual pre- and postoperative photographs often facilitates determination of the general size and shape of eyelid that the patient desires.

In discussing modification of the epicanthal region, pre- and postoperative photographs are exceedingly helpful in demonstrating the difference between the so-called inside and outside fold (Fig. **2–11**) and enables a meaningful discussion of possible surgical variations.

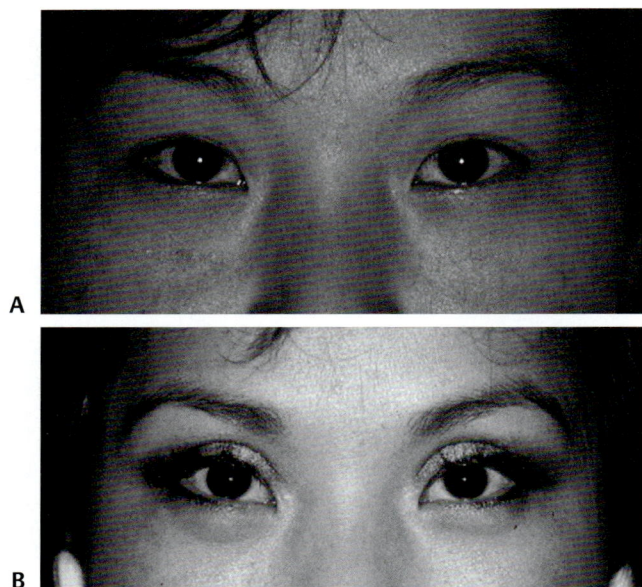

Figure 2–9   (A,B) Surgical creation of a large, round double eyelid with an outside fold. The incision was placed 9 mm above the ciliary margin, and the maximum amount of skin that could be removed as determined by pinching the skin with forceps, less 3 mm, was actually removed.

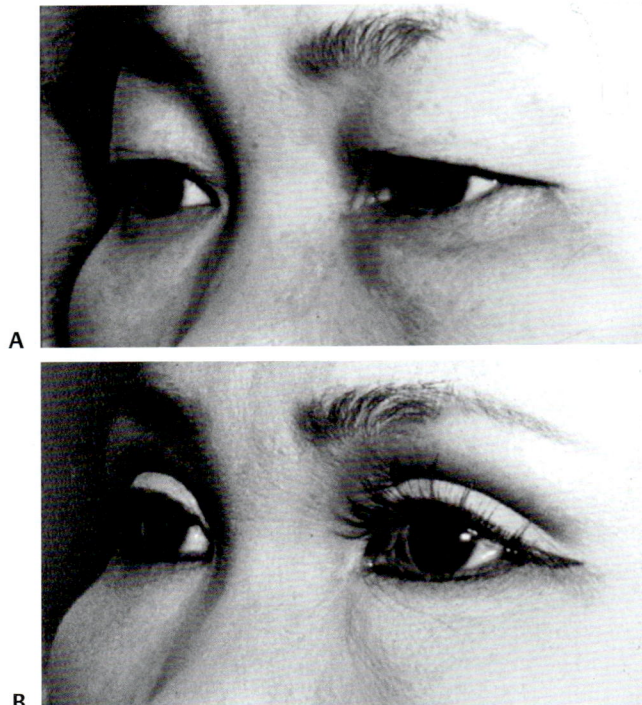

Figure 2–10   (A,B) Surgical creation of a large, oval double eyelid with an outside fold. The incision was placed 10 mm above the ciliary margin, and the maximum amount of skin that could be removed as determined by pinching the skin with forceps, less 3 mm, was actually removed.

Preoperative Planning

See DVD Disk One, Marking the Eyelid:
Design and Planning

Because postoperative asymmetry is by far the most common reason for patient dissatisfaction, the key to success in Asian upper blepharoplasty is to perform each and every step (from preoperative marking to final suturing) with the express goal of achieving eyelid symmetry. Two variables controlled by the surgeon determine the level or height of the superior palpebral fold that is

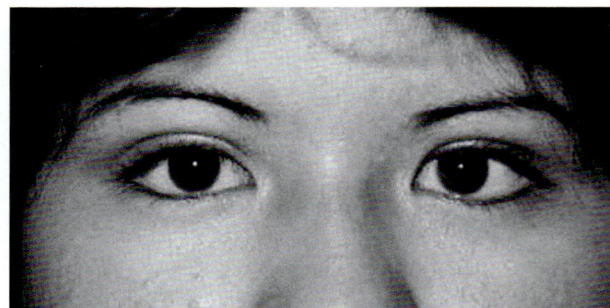

Figure 2–11   The left eye exhibits an outside fold (epicanthal effacement), and the right eye exhibits an inside fold (no epicanthal effacement).

eyelid size (small, medium, or large), the first being the distance from the ciliary margin at which the inferior lid incision is made. This level ranges from 6 to 10 mm above the ciliary margin, depending on the eyelid size desired. The second variable that determines eyelid size is the amount of preseptal skin that hoods over the surgically created palpebral fold and pretarsal skin post-operatively. In other words, pretarsal show determines actual lid size; as the amount of overhanging skin increases, pretarsal show decreases (and the lid appears smaller), and vice versa. It should be obvious that the amount of preseptal skin available to hood over pretarsal skin is determined by the amount of skin that is excised above the surgically created palpebral fold, a factor that is determined by the level of the superior incision.

Putting these two variables together allows creation of a formula or system, the utilization of which allows reliable construction of a small, medium, or large upper eyelid (Table **2–1**).

The shape of the eyelid can be controlled by the configuration of the inferior incision. To create an eyelid with an oval shape, the incision is drawn so that it is at approximately the same height (distance from the ciliary margin) at the lateral limbus as at the lateral canthus. If a round eyelid shape is desired, the lateral aspect of the incision is drawn so that it is ~2 mm more inferior at the level of the lateral canthus than at the level of the lateral limbus. In either case, the incision is then extended

Table 2–1   Guidelines for Determination of Eyelid Size

Size	Distance from Ciliary Margin (inferior incision)	Amount of Skin Excision (superior incision)
Small	6–7 mm	3 mm
Medium	8 mm	50% of maximum amount*
Large	9–10 mm	maximum amount − 3 mm*

*Maximum amount of skin that can be removed is determined by forceps pinching, as in standard blepharoplasty.

laterally as far as necessary so that it will fall in a lateral periorbital line, just as in Caucasian blepharoplasty.

The patient's desires regarding management of the epicanthal region determine the configuration of the medial aspect of the incision. If an inside fold is requested, the incision is drawn lateral to the existing epicanthus (Fig. **2–12A**). If an outside fold is desired, the incision terminates medial to the epicanthal web (Fig. **2–12B**). Many patients request a "compromise" fold, in which the lateral aspect of the epicanthus is effaced while the origin is preserved. In such cases, the medial aspect of the incision is placed so that it terminates on or near the epicanthal origin (Figs. **2–12C**, **2–13A,B**).

Proper preoperative markings are critical for achieving surgical success. Prior to marking the inferior

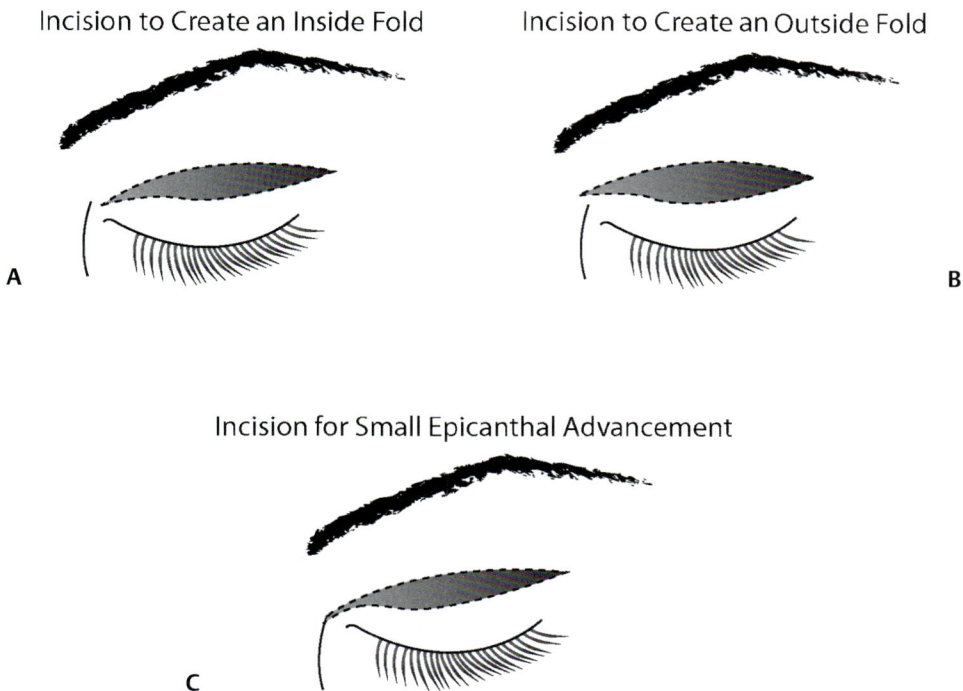

Incision to Create an Inside Fold   Incision to Create an Outside Fold

A

B

Incision for Small Epicanthal Advancement

C

Figure 2–12   **(A)** Incision used for creation of an inside fold. **(B)** Incision used for creation of an outside fold. **(C)** Incision used for creation of a fold terminating on the origin of a small epicanthus (compromise fold).

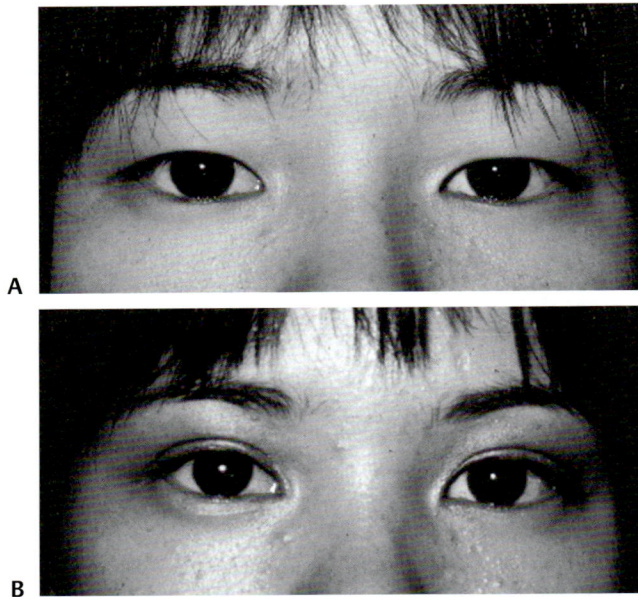

Figure 2–13   (A,B) Surgical creation of a medium, oval double eyelid with a compromise fold.

incision, it is extremely important to tense the lax pretarsal skin cephalically to the point of slight eyelash eversion. If this is not done, surgical fixation is likely to result in a palpebral furrow that is higher than planned or unattractive postoperative fullness of the pretarsal skin. A mark in the depression located just superior to the ciliary margin (placed at midpupillary level) assists in symmetrical marking of the inferior incision. The distance above the ciliary margin can be measured from this mark with a caliper or ruler.

Before marking the superior incision, the maximal amount of skin that can be excised is determined by pinching the skin with forceps and asking the patient to open and close the eyes as done in standard Caucasian blepharoplasty. The actual amount of skin to be removed, however, is determined by reference to the formula (Table **2–1**), and the superior incision is marked at this level. It is imperative to understand that, although the usual Asian eyelid exhibits considerable skin redundancy, and even in the teenage patient the maximum amount of skin that can be removed frequently exceeds 10 mm, a much more conservative skin excision (as indicated by the formula) is necessary in all patients except those who truly desire westernization. After determining its proper level, the superior incision is marked so that it parallels the inferior incision, tapering to join the inferior incision at its medial and lateral termini.

A third variable to be considered in preoperative planning is the amount of fat, primarily periorbital, that requires removal. Although of paramount importance in determining the depth of the palpebral sulcus, the extent

of lipectomy has a definite influence on lid size. As progressively larger amounts of fat are resected, increasing concavity is created into which preseptal skin invaginates, making less of this skin available to hood over the palpebral fold, thus increasing the amount of pretarsal show that determines eyelid size. For this reason, unless westernization of the eyelid is planned, fat removal in Asian blepharoplasty is more conservative than in Caucasians.

Anesthesia

Surgery is performed under local anesthesia (1% lidocaine or 0.5% bupivacaine freshly mixed with epinephrine (1:50,000) administered following intravenous sedation. Because the patient is asked to open and close the eyes at frequent intervals during placement of fixation sutures to evaluate symmetry, general anesthesia is not recommended. For the same reason, the level of sedation during surgery should be light. Diazepam and midazolam are best avoided, as both agents may interfere with voluntary lid opening. Use of intravenous methohexital or propofol just prior to infiltration of local anesthetic yields excellent results, as the patient is hypnotic and amnestic during anesthetic injection and sufficient residual sedation persists during surgery.

Operative Procedure

See DVD Disk One, Double-Eyelid Blepharoplasty: The Full-Incision Approach

A step-by-step description of the operative procedure follows:

1. Skin and underlying subcutaneous tissues are excised as marked, exposing the orbicularis muscle (Fig. **2–14**).
2. A 3 to 5 mm strip of orbicularis is excised above the level of the tarsal plate, exposing the orbital septum (Fig. **2–15**).

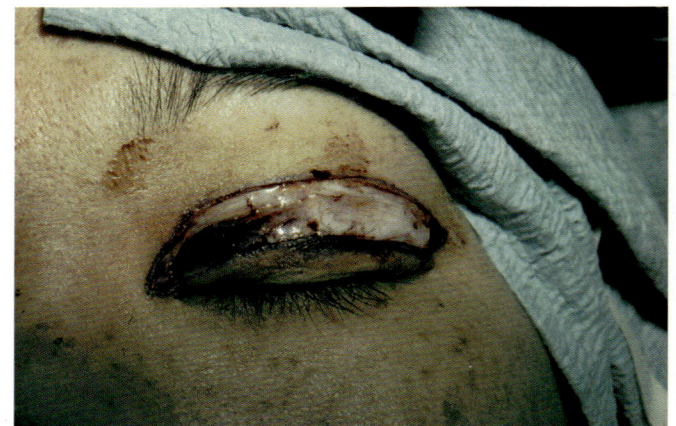

Figure 2–14   Skin is excised, exposing the orbicularis muscle.

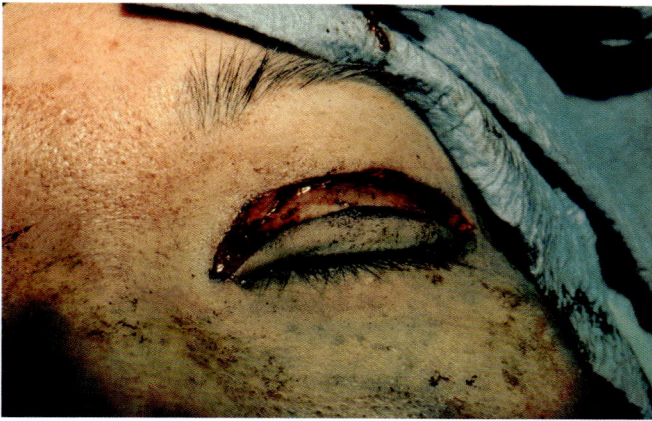

Figure 2–15 Following skin excision, a 3 to 5 mm strip of orbicularis is excised in the superior aspect of the wound, i.e., above the level of the tarsal plate, exposing the orbital septum. Incision of the orbital septum affords access to the periorbital fat and following lipectomy, the levator aponeurosis is identified. Care must be taken to avoid confusing the orbital septum with the levator aponeurosis.

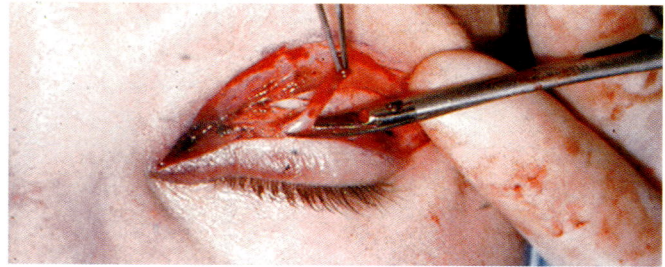

Figure 2–16 Following lipectomy and prior to placement of fixation sutures, a 2 to 3 mm strip of pretarsal orbicularis is removed at the level of the superior tarsal margin.

3. The orbital septum is incised, affording access to periorbital fat (Fig. **2–15**). In contrast to the thin, filmy septum that characterizes most Caucasian lids, in many Asian eyelids the orbital septum is relatively thick, having a glistening white appearance that can be confused with the levator aponeurosis. The inexperienced surgeon is even more likely to confuse the orbital septum with the levator aponeurosis in patients who exhibit substantial amounts of submuscular fat, creating the impression that this fat represents periorbital fat, and the glistening white layer posteriorly therefore must be the levator aponeurosis. The periorbital space should be entered as superiorly as possible to minimize the possibility of injuring the levator aponeurosis. The extent of lipectomy depends on the type of eyelid transformation planned. If a small double eyelid is the surgical goal, only sufficient fat to allow accurate identification of the tarsal plate/levator aponeurosis is removed. If a large westernized eyelid has been requested, removal of substantial amounts of fat in the central and lateral compartments is performed as in Caucasian blepharoplasty so that the levator expansion is completely cleared. Construction of a medium-sized lid dictates lipectomy between these extremes. In all cases, however (including westernization procedures), removal of fat in the medial compartment must be very conservative, as creation of a deep hollow in the medial aspect of the lid does not produce the aesthetically desirable effect that results from sculpturing this area in the Caucasian eyelid. Excessive fat removal medially

also predisposes to hypertrophic scarring in this area, as more tension on the skin closure results. In contrast, care must be taken to ensure that the point of fixation (tarsus/levator aponeurosis) is adequately cleared in the lateral aspect of the eyelid, as this is the most common area for early failure of a fixation suture resulting in localized fold loss or inadequacy. Even if a small double fold is to be constructed, the surgeon must ensure that periorbital fat and orbital septum, which is more substantial laterally, is adequately removed in the lateral aspect of the eyelid.

4. The wound has now been prepared for placement of fixation sutures, but prior to their placement, a 2 to 3 mm strip of pretarsal orbicularis is removed from beneath the skin at the level of the inferior skin incision (Fig. **2–16**). This maneuver is performed for two reasons: (1) the pretarsal skin is effectively undermined 2 to 3 mm providing a wider base for the adhesion creating the palpebral fold, and (2) this undermining allows more effective tightening of pretarsal skin during fixation, reducing post-operative laxity.

5. External fixation sutures of 5–0 nylon are then placed, sequentially incorporating the skin edge of the inferior incision, the levator aponeurosis/tarsus at the desired point of fixation, and the superior skin incision, each suture being tied externally (Fig. **2–17A**). In determining the point of fixation, the pretarsal skin is stretched cephalically just to the point of beginning eyelash eversion; having a constant reproducible end point is important in achieving eyelid symmetry. Buried internal fixation sutures (Fig. **2–17B**) of permanent or absorbable material incorporating only the inferior skin incision and levator/tarsus may be substituted for the "external" fixation sutures, but including the upper skin edge in the fixation process provides a major advantage as it enhances intraoperative determination of symmetry because the precise effect of hooding contributed by the preseptal skin is

External Fixation Suture

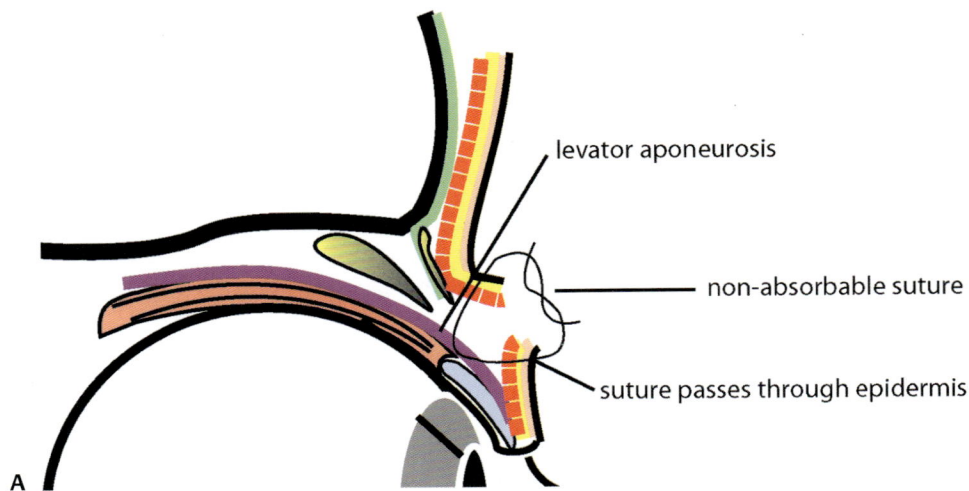

- levator aponeurosis
- non-absorbable suture
- suture passes through epidermis

A

Internal Fixation Suture

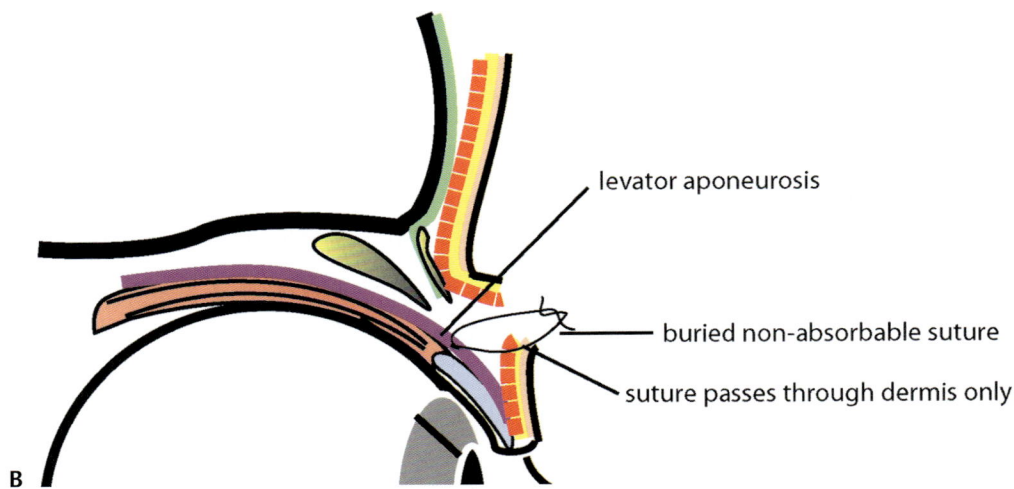

- levator aponeurosis
- buried non-absorbable suture
- suture passes through dermis only

B

Figure 2–17 **(A)** External fixation suture. **(B)** Internal fixation suture. External fixation sutures are preferred for reasons ascribed in the text.

more easily assessed. Three fixation sutures are routinely used, being placed (1) laterally at a point approximately half the distance between the lateral canthus and lateral limbus, (2) centrally at the mid-pupillary level, and (3) medially at the level of the medial limbus (Fig. **2–18A,B**). Assessment of symmetry is greatly enhanced if the sutures are placed sequentially in the right and left eyelids; that is, the lateral fixation suture is placed in the right upper lid, following which a matching lateral fixation suture is placed in the left lid. The patient is asked to open his or her eyes, and symmetry is assessed by inspection and direct measurement. If absolute symmetry is not present, one of the fixation sutures is removed and

replaced, allowing symmetry to be achieved. In a similar fashion, the middle fixation suture is placed in the right and then the left eyelid, following which symmetry is again assessed. The medial fixation sutures are then placed sequentially, and the lids are examined for symmetry. In many cases, one or two additional medial fixation sutures are placed following undermining of the pretarsal skin in this area to modify the epicanthal fold. Such medial advancement of the epicanthal fold by undermining and fixation sutures satisfies the desire of most contemporary patients with respect to epicanthoplasty. On occasion, however, more advanced techniques of epicanthal effacement described in a later section are used.

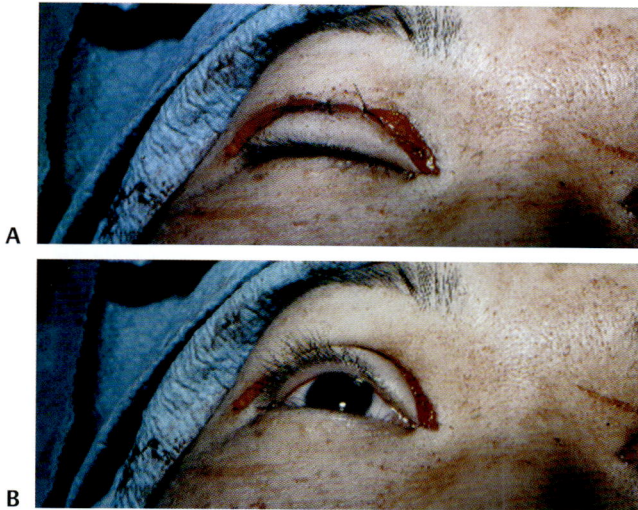

Figure 2–18   **(A)** Three (lateral, middle, and medial) fixation sutures have been placed. **(B)** The double eyelid is noted on lid opening following fixation suture placement.

6. The entire incision is then approximated with a running suture of 6–0 nylon. Use of absorbable suture material for skin closure often results in prolonged erythema of the incision and thus is not recommended. Many surgeons advocate the use of a running subcuticular suture for upper lid closure, but placement of such a suture places the fixation sutures at risk both intraoperatively and at the time of removal.

7. Following this, 0.2 cc of triamcinolone (10 mg per cc) is injected subcutaneously in the medial aspect of the wound. This area exhibits a biological predisposition for hypertrophic scar formation even in the absence of significant epicanthal modification, and prophylactic treatment with triamcinolone greatly reduces the incidence of induration and/or hypertrophic scarring in this region.

Special Considerations and Variations in Asian Upper Blepharoplasty

Preexisting Small Double Eyelid

A substantial number of Asian patients who request upper-lid blepharoplasty present with an existing double eyelid. Many of these individuals have small natural double lids, and others have undergone previous eyelid surgery but are unhappy with the size or shape of the surgically created lid. It is not uncommon for an Asian patient to exhibit a small unilateral double lid, having a typical single lid on the contralateral side. Surgeons should resist requests by such patients to perform surgery on the single eyelid only, as it is difficult to

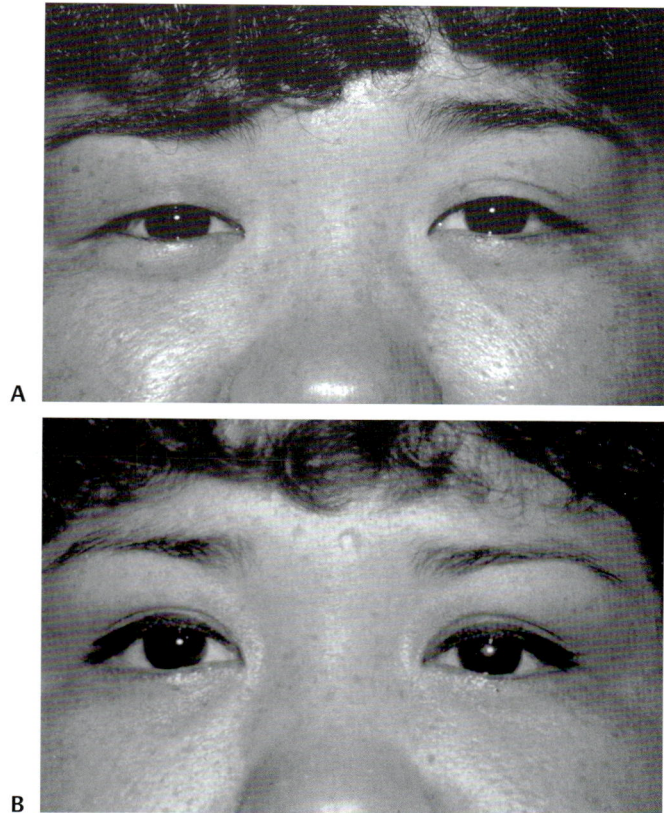

Figure 2–19   **(A,B)** Pre- and postoperative results in a patient with a preexisting unilateral double eyelid who underwent bilateral upper blepharoplasty rather than attempting unilateral surgery on the single eyelid only.

achieve symmetry in these cases unless bilateral surgery is performed (Fig. **2–19A,B**).

Regardless of the etiology of the problem, the goal of upper-lid blepharoplasty in this group is usually to enlarge the existing lid, deepen the sulcus, and/or change the shape of the lid from round to oval (or, rarely, from oval to round). Additional benefits of surgery include tightening of the preseptal skin and eversion of the eyelashes into a more aesthetically pleasing orientation. Upper blepharoplasty allows enhancement of lid aesthetics by enabling more effective use of cosmetics that provide transformation of the sad, tired appearance often imparted by small lids to a more "bright-eyed" look (Fig. **2–20A,B**).

The surgical procedure in such patients is conducted according to the guidelines described above, the level of the inferior incision and extent of skin removal depending on the eyelid size and shape desired. Of utmost importance, however, is the observation that in most natural double eyelids, the pretarsal skin exhibits considerable laxity, and thus the inferior incision must be placed inferior to the existing fold (the actual

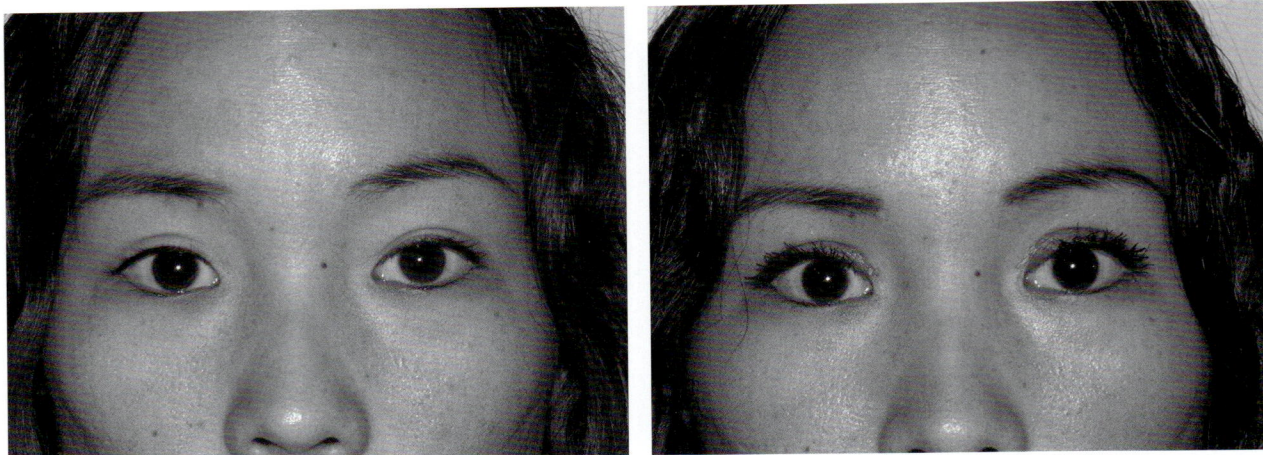

Figure 2–20   (A,B) Pre- and postoperative results in a patient with preexisting natural double eyelids who requested a larger upper eyelid with a more well-defined palpebral fold.

location being determined by cephalic traction on the eyelid skin as previously described).

The Aging Asian Eyelid

An increasing number of older Asian patients who have never undergone eyelid surgery are requesting blepharoplasty to combat dermatochalasis of the upper lid. Many of these patients do not desire a well-defined upper lid furrow and merely request removal of redundant overhanging skin. In such patients, the inferior incision is placed 5 to 6 mm above the ciliary margin, and ~3 mm less than the maximum amount of skin that can be resected (often in excess of 15 mm) is excised, following which the incision is closed without fixation sutures.

If a small double lid is requested, fixation sutures are placed 6 mm above the ciliary margin (generally requiring fixation to the tarsal plate instead of the levator aponeurosis) following removal of 75% of the determined maximum amount of skin, as contrasted with 2 to 3 mm skin removal for creation of a small lid in a young patient (Fig. **2–21A,B**). The surgeon must be

somewhat wary of the older patient who requests a large double eyelid, making absolutely certain that the patient appreciates the aesthetic consequences of this request prior to proceeding (Fig. **2–22A,B**). Remember, it is relatively easy to convert a small double lid into a larger lid, but it is almost impossible to make a large, westernized lid substantially smaller.

The ravages of aging affect eyelids that have previously undergone double eyelid surgery, and many of these patients seek surgical rejuvenation. Assuming the surgical fixation is intact and at a satisfactory position, it is used as the level for marking the inferior skin incision, and blepharoplasty proceeds in the same manner as a standard operation in the aging Caucasian upper lid (Fig. **2–23A,B**). In many such patients, however, the fixation is at a point that, following cephalic stretching of the skin, it would be located considerably higher that 10 mm above the ciliary margin (these individuals exhibit considerable laxity of the pretarsal skin). This condition requires that a new fixation be constructed inferior to the preexisting fixation, and preoperative markings are planned as described for a new double-eyelid operation. Care must be

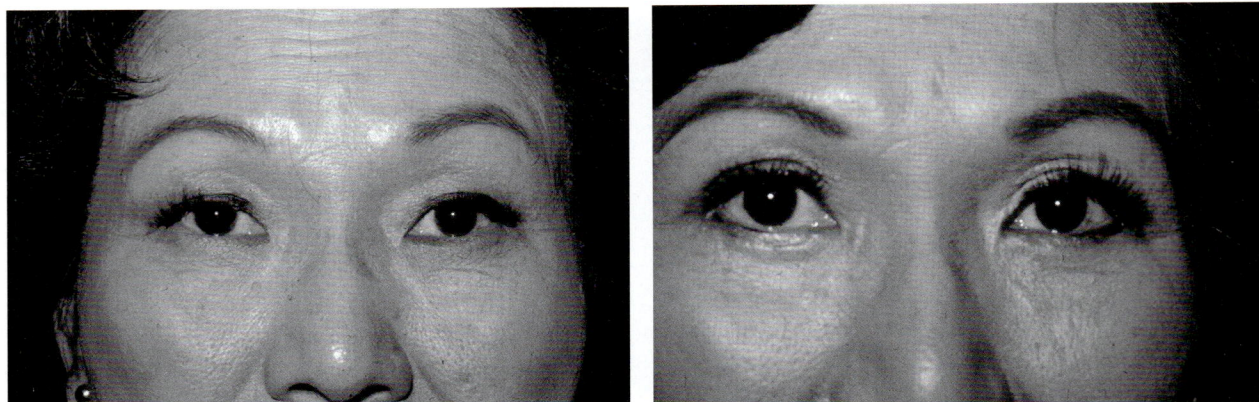

Figure 2–21   (A,B) Conservative upper blepharoplasty in an older Asian patient with dermatochalasis; no fixation sutures were used.

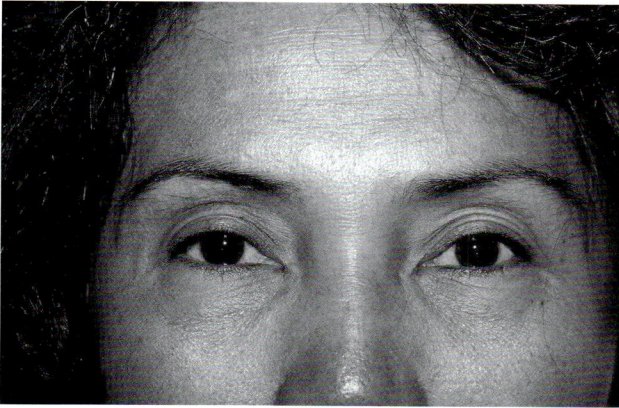

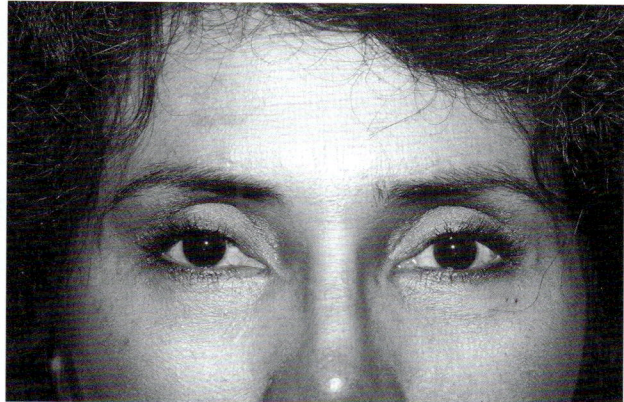

Figure 2–22 (A,B) Pre- and postoperative results in a patient with dermatochalasis who has undergone no previous eyelid surgery. As requested, a large, westernized eyelid was constructed.

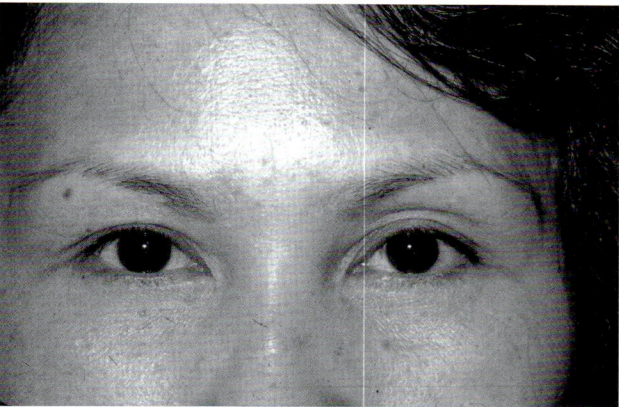

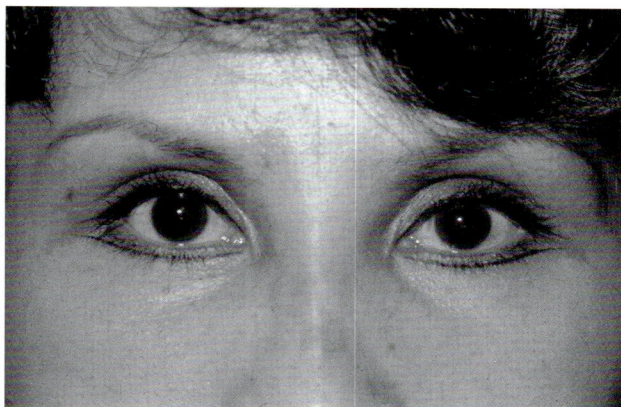

Figure 2–23 (A,B) Pre- and postoperative results of surgery performed without the use of fixation sutures in a patient in whom, following previous double eyelid surgery, the palpebral fold was at a level at which upper blepharoplasty for correction of dermatochalasis could be performed without alteration of the previously treated fold.

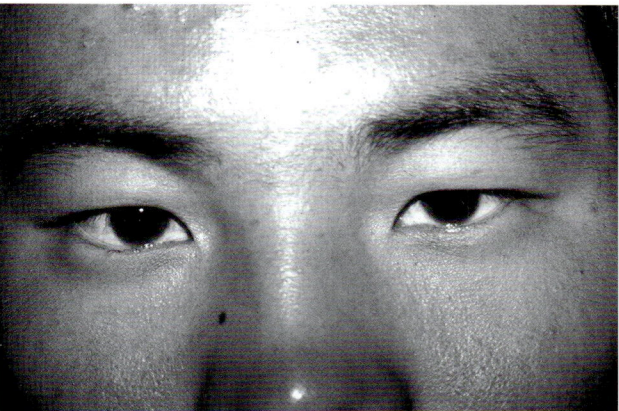

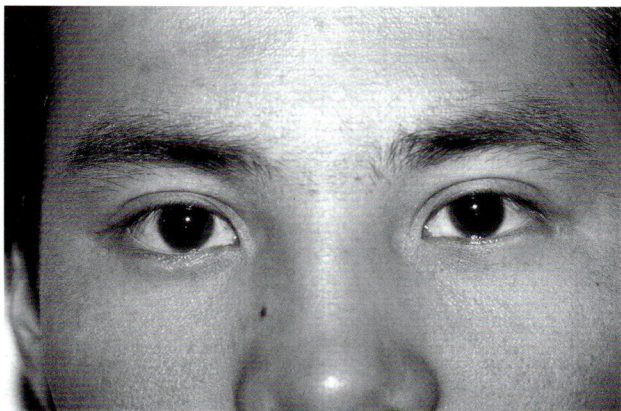

Figure 2–24 (A,B) A conservative double eyelid operation in a man.

taken to avoid levator injury during surgical excision of the old fixation.

Upper Blepharoplasty in Men

Although the percentage of men undergoing upper blepharoplasty is less than 5% of the total number of Asian blepharoplasty performed in my practice, an increasing number of men are requesting upper-lid surgery for formation of a double eyelid. As in older patients, such surgery generally should be conservative in scope, that is, creation of a small double eyelid (Fig. **2–24A,B**). Men who request a more radical transformation should be thoroughly counseled regarding

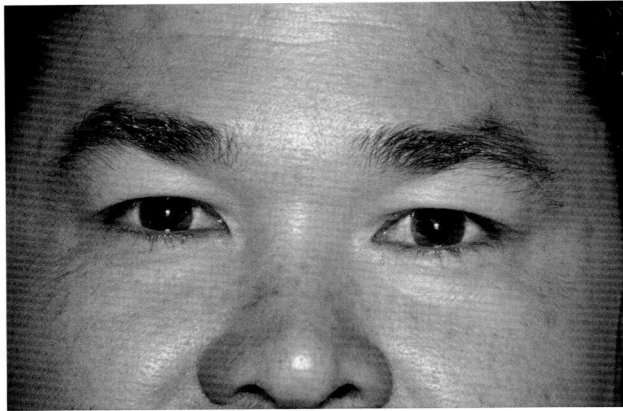

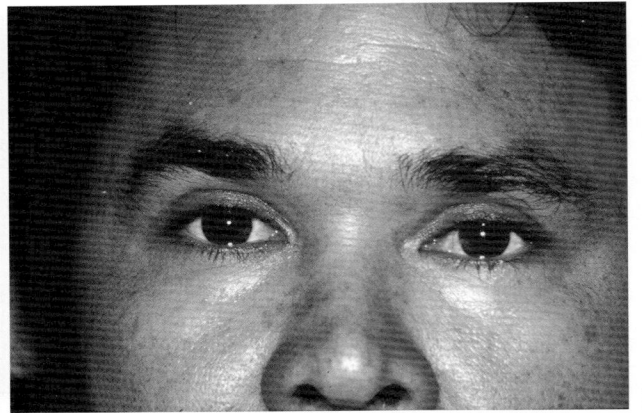

Figure 2–25   (A,B) Creation of a large, westernized eyelid in a man.

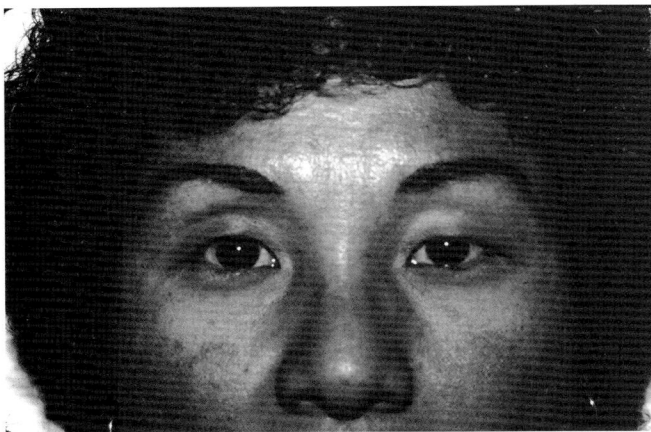

Figure 2–26   The "hollow" eye resulting from involution of periorbital fat, producing the illusion of a large double lid.

the aesthetic consequences of such a procedure (Fig. **2–25A,B**).

Many older men request removal of redundant skin without creation of a double lid, and the surgical technique in these cases is identical to that described above (i.e., the inferior incision being placed 5–6 mm above

the ciliary margin and ~75% of the determined maximal skin redundancy being removed). Postoperative edema is generally more troublesome in men as they are reluctant to use cosmetics for camouflage.

The "Hollow" Eye

A substantial number of Asian eyelids exhibit atrophy of periorbital fat, producing a "hollowed" or sunken appearance in the infrabrow region. Such atrophy or involution of periorbital fat tends to increase with advancing age but may begin in the early to mid-20s.

If a natural palpebral fold is not present, the hollowed appearance produces the illusion of a large double eyelid (Fig. **2–26**), while in the presence of a small palpebral furrow, a "triple eyelid" is often suggested (Fig. **2–27A,B**).

This type of eyelid presents certain challenges for the aesthetic surgeon. Perhaps the best plan of attack is to create a large double eyelid (Fig. **2–28A,B**), for if a small lid is fashioned, the triple-eyelid appearance described above may result (Figs. **2–26, 2–27**). Another approach is to explore the periorbital fat compartment, releasing

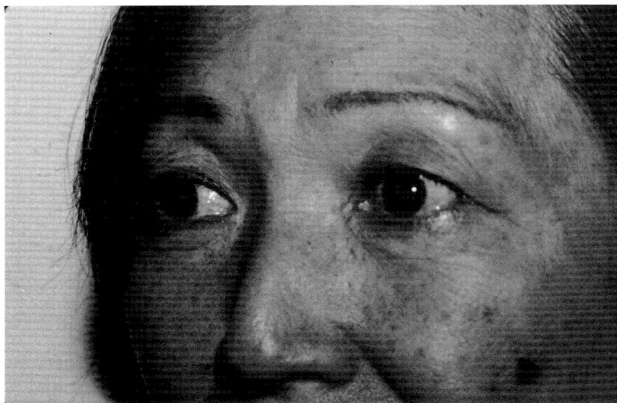

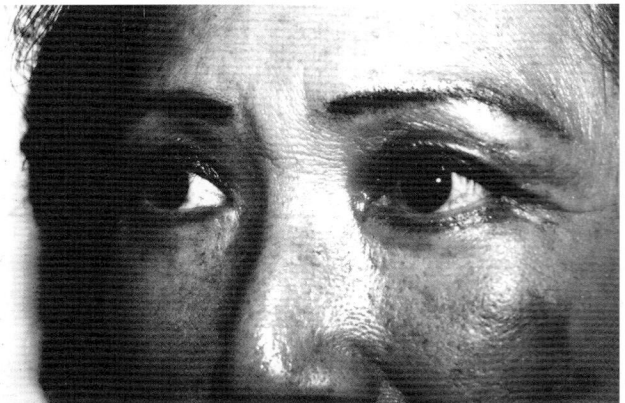

Figure 2–27   (A,B) The apparent "triple eyelid" following creation of a small palpebral fold in the "hollow" eye.

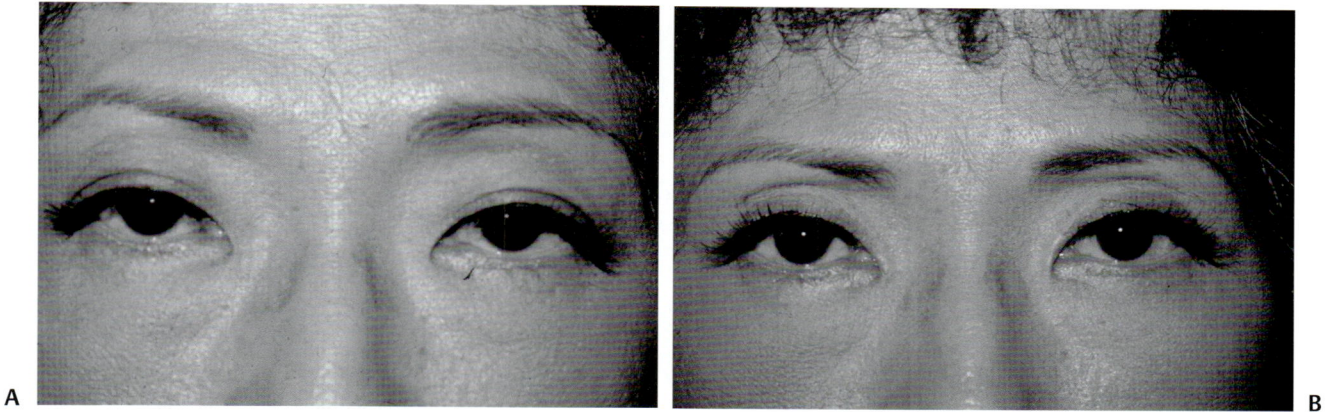

Figure 2–28 **(A,B)** Creation of a large double eyelid in the "hollow" eye.

fascial and orbital adhesions that may restrict the fat superiorly, attempting to encourage inferior descent of adipose tissue to fill the hollow. Although effective in an occasional case, this technique is often unsuccessful.

Historically, silicone "bag" prostheses were used in Asia to correct the "hollow" eye, but complications, including localized bulging secondary to capsular contracture around the prosthesis, as well as sensations of heaviness, ptosis, and ocular irritation, have relegated this technique to historical interest. Although fat grafting

may be unsuccessful, attempts to efface the hollow using fascia grafts may be more successful (Fig. **2–29A,B,C**). The precise correction and symmetry often demanded by Asian patients is difficult to achieve using this technique, however, and postoperative induration is often prolonged with the use of temporalis fascia. Therefore, if the patient will not accept a recommendation to create a large double eyelid, surgical intervention should be undertaken only with extreme caution, as there will be a high incidence of postoperative dissatisfaction.

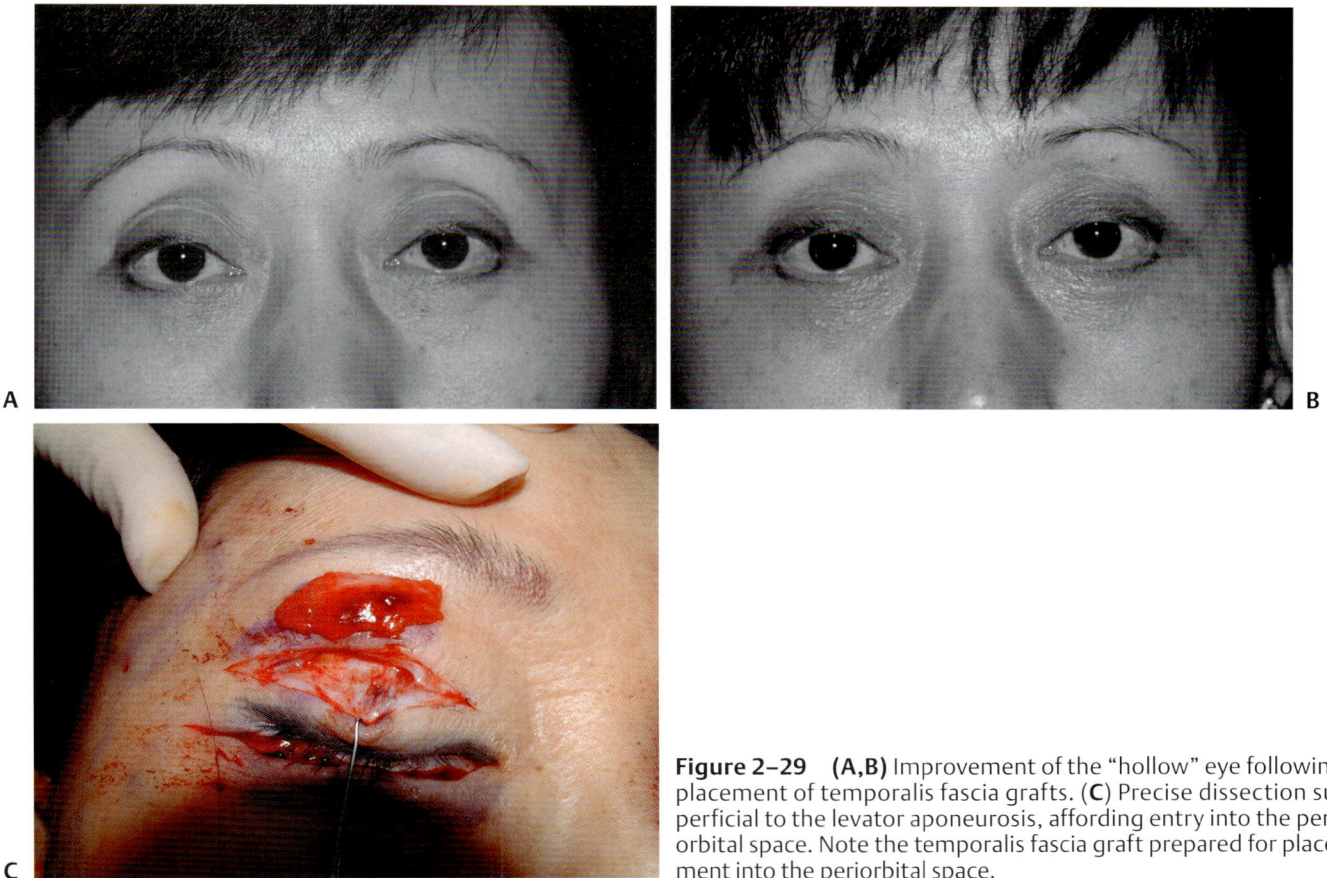

Figure 2–29 **(A,B)** Improvement of the "hollow" eye following placement of temporalis fascia grafts. (**C**) Precise dissection superficial to the levator aponeurosis, affording entry into the periorbital space. Note the temporalis fascia graft prepared for placement into the periorbital space.

Double-Eyelid Surgery Using Suture Techniques

A technique that allows formation of a double eyelid using sutures without a surgical incision enjoyed considerable popularity in Asia, but because of inherent limitations, it is becoming less popular. So-called partial-incision techniques are currently popular in Asia and are associated with a lower incidence of fold failure, but they do not allow the creative flexibility associated with the procedures planned using the formula described above.

The first step in the nonincision technique is marking the crease at the level of the superior margin of the tarsus. Local anesthetic is injected into this area, care being taken to avoid distortion of the tissues. The eyelid is then everted, and the conjunctiva just superior to the tarsus is infiltrated with anesthetic. A suture of 4–0 silk or polyethylene terephthalate (Mersilene, Ethicon, Somerville, NJ) is inserted through the skin at the midpupillary level, exiting on the conjunctival surface ~2 mm above the superior tarsal border. The suture is then reinserted through the conjunctiva, exiting through the skin at a point ~3 to 4 mm lateral to its initial entrance. This suture is then tied over a small rubber-band bolster. Three such sutures are placed along the proposed palpebral fold and remain in place for 10 to 12 days. This procedure creates an adhesion between the levator, orbicularis, and skin at the level of the superior tarsal margin (Fig. **2–30**).

A major limitation of this technique is the inability to sculpture precisely the size and shape of the double eyelid, as neither skin nor fat is removed. Modification of the epicanthus is not possible with this technique, and if an epicanthal fold exists, the crease must be placed so that it terminates lateral and inferior to the epicanthal origin (i.e., an inside fold).

Because the fold created by this technique is dependent upon a nonsurgical adhesion (i.e., a crush injury), it is more likely to be unreliable, falling out after a variable period of time.

The partial-incision technique offers another alternative to the full-incision method. I have been instructed personally in the partial-incision technique developed by Y. K. Kim, M.D., of Seoul, South Korea, and feel that it is an effective procedure in properly selected patients (generally younger individuals with relatively thin skin without excessive submuscular or periorbital fat). Flexibility in construction of eyelid size and shape, however, is not comparable to that of the full-incision technique as outlined by the formula in Table **2–1**, and this procedure does not readily permit epicanthal modification (Dr. Lam describes both the suture and partial-incision techniques in detail in Chapter 8.)

Postoperative Care

The early postblepharoplasty period is characterized by marked edema of the pretarsal portion of the eyelid as well as by variable degrees of blepharoptosis (Fig. **2–31**). The extent and duration of both edema and ptosis are directly related to the level of fixation, being more significant and longer lasting as surgically created lid size increases.

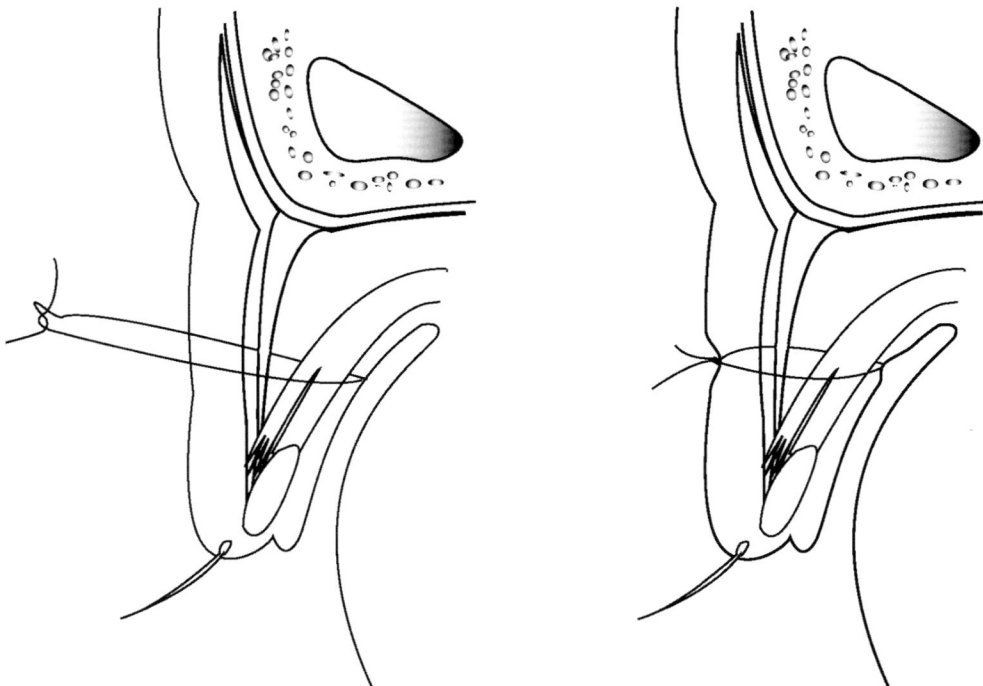

Figure 2–30   The suture technique for creation of a double eyelid.

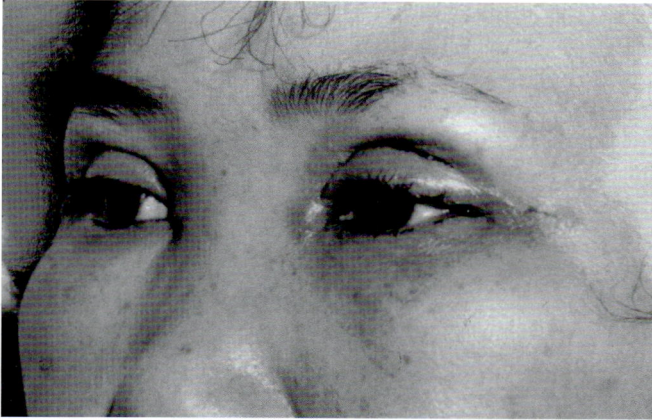

Figure 2–31 Typical edema of the pretarsal portion of the double eyelid. Note also the presence of ptosis secondary to the edema and fixation suture placement.

The running cutaneous sutures are removed on the second or third postoperative day, and the fixation sutures remain until the seventh postoperative day. Blepharoptosis is generally not objectionable following removal of the fixation sutures but occasionally causes concern because of asymmetry that results when one eyelid is somewhat more edematous than the other. Asian patients often exhibit a seemingly inappropriate concern with apparent imperfections during the early postoperative period, and it is helpful to explain that upper blepharoplasty is actually two separate operations, one on each eyelid, and thus different amounts of swelling are to be expected. The surgeon can also point out that the eyelid on the side on which the patient sleeps is often more edematous.

Slowly resolving asymmetric ptosis is often related to edema or hematoma of Müller's muscle. The surgeon must firmly resist inappropriate requests for early revision in such cases. In some patients, residual pretarsal edema may be detectable for as long as 6 months postoperatively, but in most cases, it is usually satisfactorily camouflaged by cosmetics following suture removal. Obviously, the lid appears to be larger than the final result during the edematous period. Anxious patients benefit from (and often request) constant reassurance that lid size will decrease as edema resolves.

Complications of Asian Upper Blepharoplasty

Complications of Asian upper blepharoplasty are the same as in all blepharoplasty procedures: bleeding, hematoma, unsatisfactory scar formation, and, rarely, infection or injury to structures in the operative field. Several postoperative concerns, however, are of special concern in Asian upper blepharoplasty and deserve further discussion.

Asymmetry

By far the most common source of dissatisfaction following Asian upper blepharoplasty is postoperative asymmetry of the eyelids, an occurrence that is occasionally a problem for even the most experienced surgeon. Postoperative asymmetry is more common when brow or eyelid asymmetry exists preoperatively, and each candidate for upper blepharoplasty must be evaluated carefully in this regard. Minimal ptosis (often unnoticed preoperatively) also predisposes to postoperative asymmetry. If preoperative asymmetry exists, it must be pointed out to the patient, with a firm explanation given that precise postoperative symmetry will be more difficult to achieve. Preoperative asymmetry, of course, must be documented carefully in the medical record as well as by preoperative photographs.

Strict adherence to certain technical aspects of this operation helps to minimize the incidence of postoperative asymmetry. The surgeon must understand that each and every step of planning and execution of this procedure is undertaken in a manner designed to create postoperative symmetry in eyelid size and shape:

1. During the preoperative evaluation, be alert for preoperative asymmetry of the brows and palpebral fissure size, width, and orientation. Carefully explain findings to the patient, and document them in the medical records and photographically.

2. The preoperative markings of the upper eyelid must be performed while the skin is stretched cephalically. The skin is tensed to the point at which the eyelashes just begin to evert, a checkpoint that will facilitate accurate and symmetrical placement of the preoperative markings bilaterally.

3. After completing the markings, recheck them using a ruler prior to anesthetic infiltration. On remeasuring the incision markings, it is surprising how often 1 mm of asymmetry is discovered, allowing appropriate correction before beginning the procedure.

4. Avoid excessive sedation during the operative procedure, as it often interferes with voluntary lid opening, making it more difficult to assess symmetry while placing fixation sutures.

5. Prolonged surgical time increases intraoperative edema, which may impair assessment of symmetry. Perhaps the most common cause of prolonged surgical time is intraoperative bleeding, the control of which also creates increased intraoperative edema. Mixing fresh adrenaline with plain, unbuffered anesthetic solution just prior to infiltration results in substantially less intraoperative bleeding than use of commercially prepared solution. Mixing 0.4 cc of epinephrine 1:1000 with 20 cc of plain

anesthetic solution creates a solution with an epinephrine concentration of 1:50,000; use of 0.2 cc of epinephrine 1:1000 with 20 cc of anesthetic solution creates a mixture with an epinephrine concentration of 1:100,000. Buffering of local anesthetic solution with sodium bicarbonate is not recommended, as this substance diminishes the hemostatic effects of epinephrine.

6. As described above, fixation sutures are placed in a constant sequence. After placing the initial fixation suture, usually at the lateralmost fixation point, the corresponding fixation suture is placed in the opposite eyelid, following which the height of both sutures above the ciliary margin is carefully measured. In placing fixation sutures, the pretarsal skin is stretched to the point where the eyelashes just begin to evert, a visual checkpoint also used in preoperative marking. An identical inspection and measurement routine is performed following placement of middle and then medial fixation sutures. If a difference of even 1 mm is noted on measuring the height of any fixation suture, the suture is immediately removed and replaced in a more accurate position.

7. For reasons previously described, use of external fixation sutures are more conducive to intraoperative assessment of symmetry than are internal fixation sutures.

If Asian upper blepharoplasty could be characterized by a single mantra, it would be "Measure, remeasure, then measure again!"

Management of Asymmetry/Palpebral Fold Loss

As discussed in the section on postoperative care, some early postoperative asymmetry of the eyelids is common, usually as a consequence of differential edema and minor degrees of ptosis that may temporarily follow fixation procedures. Although many patients are concerned—some excessively—the surgeon should explain the mechanism of this problem and refuse to consider revision surgery until the edema/ptosis has resolved completely. Occasionally, however, more marked eyelid asymmetry as a consequence of failure of one or more fixation sutures occurs and may deserve earlier correction. Partial loss of the palpebral fold may occur following accurate fixation because of excessive tension secondary to inadequate undermining of pretarsal skin, failure to clear pretarsal soft tissue around the point of fixation, misidentification of the levator aponeurosis, or premature removal of fixation sutures. Occasionally, the cause of fixation failure is the displacement of a suture secondary to excessive edema or hematoma. By far the most common location of fixation suture failure is laterally, and this is almost always related to inadequate clearing of soft

tissue from the point of fixation. As previously noted, the orbital septum thickens in this region and can be confused with the levator aponeurosis. Prior to placement of the lateral fixation sutures, the surgeon must inspect the point of fixation and ensure that the aponeurosis/tarsus in this area is devoid of overlying soft tissue.

Asymmetry resulting from fixation suture failure requires revision, and the timing of the revision procedure depends on the postoperative period in which failure is noted. If gross asymmetry or loss of the fold is noted during the first or second postoperative weeks, repair at 2 to 3 weeks should be considered before adhesions form that could complicate surgery. If loss of the fold is noted later in the postoperative period, it may be preferable to wait at least 3 months before attempting revision. The dissection is more hazardous in such cases and must proceed with caution to avoid inadvertent damage to the levator mechanism.

Surgical correction of lateral fixation suture failure is relatively simple. A 5 mm segment of the original incision is opened at the point of failure, the point of fixation on the levator aponeurosis or tarsus is identified and cleared of overlying soft tissue, and a single fixation suture of 5–0 nylon is placed without excision of skin (Fig. **2–32A–D**).

Retraction of the Upper Lid

One of the benefits of upper blepharoplasty in Asians is eversion of the eyelashes into a more aesthetically pleasing position that occurs as a consequence of tightening the pretarsal skin. On occasion, however, the eyelid margin is excessively everted, resulting in an unpleasing appearance postoperatively, and is generally caused by fixation suture placement too high on the levator aponeurosis. This complication can be avoided if, in placing the fixation sutures, the surgeon uses as a checkpoint the point at which the eyelashes just began to evert (prior to actual eversion of the ciliary margin) as a guide for suture placement and carefully engages the sutures so that eyelash eversion is bilaterally symmetrical. Slight lid retraction is not uncommon in the early postoperative period as a consequence of pretarsal edema, but such retraction always resolves spontaneously (Fig. **2–33**). If persistent retraction related to fixation suture placement occurs, correction involves reopening the wound, undermining pretarsal skin, and replacing fixation sutures at a lower level on the aponeurosis.

Excessive Fat Removal

To a large extent, the depth of the palpebral sulcus is controlled by varying the amount of periorbital fat removal. Regardless of the type of eyelid transformation planned, lipectomy must be particularly conservative in

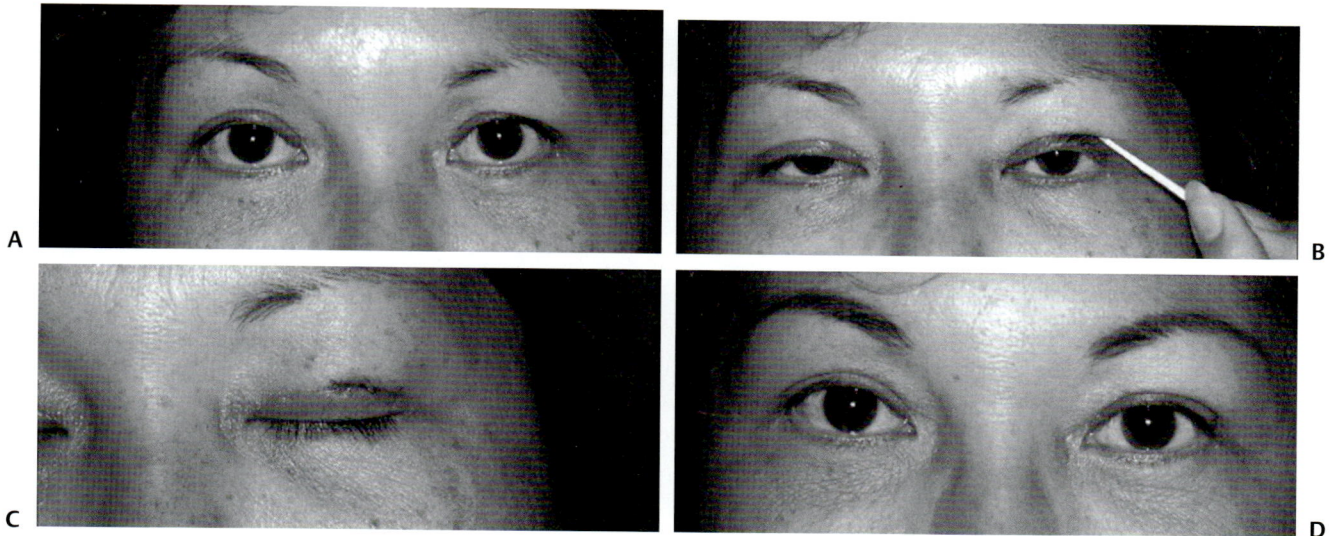

Figure 2–32 Correction of eyelid symmetry results from lateral fixation suture failure by revision of a small eyelid segment. **(A)** Preoperative skin redundancy and/or loss of fixation in the lateral aspect of the right upper lid. **(B)** determination of the point at which fixation must be achieved to restore symmetry. **(C)** Placement of one fixation suture at the determined point. The remaining incision is closed with a running suture of 6–0 nylon. **(D)** Postoperative results showing improved symmetry.

the medial aspect of the eyelid, even when westernization is planned. Excessive debulking in this area may produce an unattractive hollowness (Fig. **2–34**), the repair of which is difficult. Attempts at lipografting generally prove to be unsuccessful, as does rotation of orbicularis muscle flaps into the defect. Fascia grafts are a better choice, but prolonged induration is frequently a problem, and final results are seldom totally satisfactory. In rare cases in which a conservative approach to lipectomy in the medial fat compartment results in residual postoperative fullness in this area, it is far easier to remove a small additional amount of fat as a secondary procedure than to be confronted with the difficulties of placating an unhappy patient with postoperative hollowness in this area. Reduction of medial fat pad volume using electrocautery without actual excision is the procedure of choice in most patients requesting small or even medium-sized double eyelids. Remember that the approach to orbital fat in the lateral aspect of the eyelids is different; as stressed above, it is imperative that sufficient fat be removed in this area to

completely clear the point of fixation to minimize the incidence of postoperative fold failure.

Revision Surgery in Asian Blepharoplasty

See DVD Disk One, Revision Double-Eyelid, Blepharoplasty: Making the Eyelid Crease Smaller

By far the most common indication for revision blepharoplasty is asymmetry of the eyelids. In such cases, the surgeon must determine whether the patient is unhappy because one eyelid is too large or one eyelid is too small. Although this may seem to be a trivial matter, there is often indecision on the part of the patient, and the answer to this question must be certain prior to undertaking revision. In general, it is relatively easy to enlarge an eyelid but considerably more difficult (and in

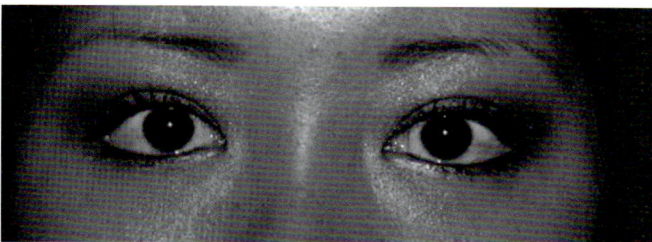

Figure 2–33 Mild retraction of the upper lid following blepharoplasty. Retraction of this extent usually resolves spontaneously.

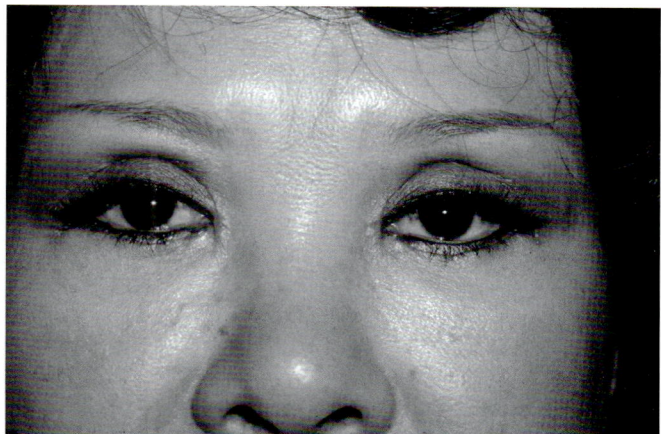

Figure 2–34 Deformity resulting from excessive periorbital lipectomy.

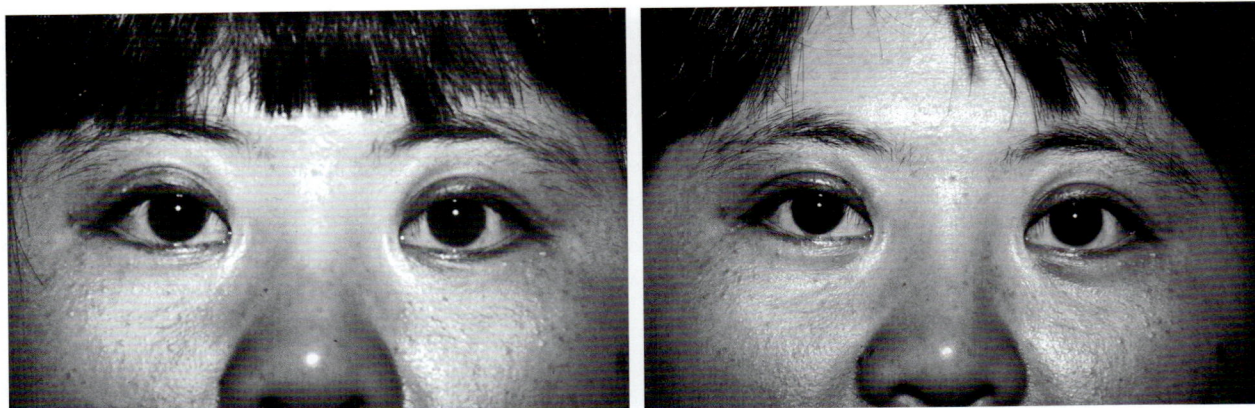

Figure 2–35   (A,B) Correction of eyelid asymmetry by reducing double-eyelid size.

some cases virtually impossible) to make a large eyelid smaller. An attempt to reduce eyelid size should be considered only in cases in which skin redundancy exists, as a lid can be made smaller only if the pretarsal incision can be placed closer to the ciliary margin. In these cases, the preexisting fold requires excision, and thus redundant skin above the original fold must be advanced inferiorly to allow closure of the defect (Fig. **2–35A,B**). Unfortunately, even if preoperative evaluation indicates that such a procedure is technically feasible, the actual results are often disappointing.

In contrast, enlarging the eyelid is a relatively straightforward procedure. In many cases the existing incision can be used, higher fixation being possible following undermining and advancement of the pretarsal skin. If necessary, however, a new incision can be made above the original scar to enable fixation at a more superior level. If this is necessary, pretarsal skin must be undermined to a level just inferior to the original incision. Depending on the desires of the patient, additional skin and/or fat may (or may not) be removed (Fig. **2–36A,B**).

When attempting revision of one upper eyelid, the patient must be informed that there can be no guarantee

of absolute symmetry. Indeed, because of postoperative edema, the ultimate result may not be apparent for 3 to 6 months. Fortunately, a large number of patients request revision surgery because they wish the size or shape of both lids to be modified; revision is generally successful in these circumstances, and the patient expresses fewer concerns about lack of symmetry during the healing period (Fig. **2–37A,B**).

The timing of revision surgery is discussed above (see eyelid asymmetry/fold loss), and revision for correction of other complications is described in conjunction with these situations.

In general, revision surgery is more common in Asian blepharoplasty than in Caucasian blepharoplasty, even experienced surgeons reporting a revision incidence approximating 10%. A large percentage of these revisions, however, are minor, consisting of replacement of one fixation suture through a 4 to 5 mm incision (Fig. **2–32A–D**).

Management of the Epicanthal Fold

Approximately 90% of Asian eyelids exhibit an epicanthal fold. The size of the fold, although showing wide

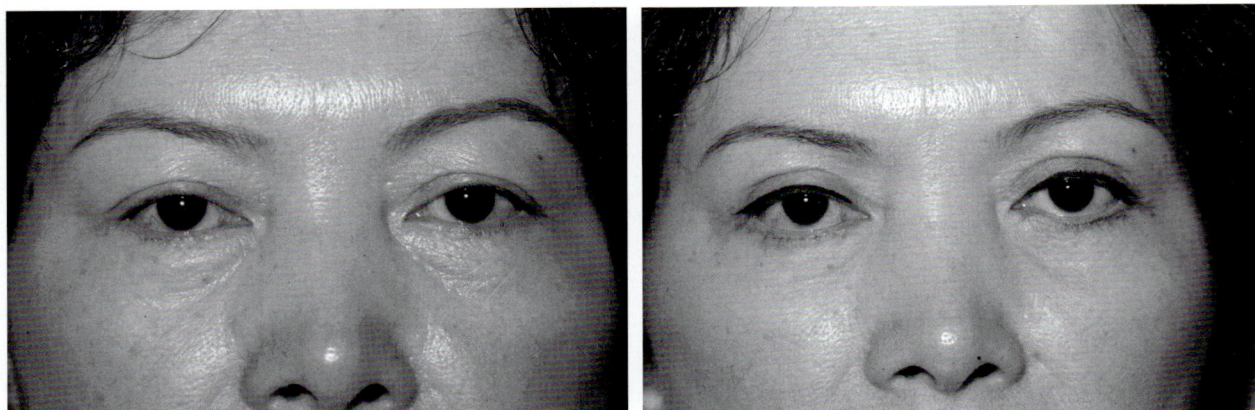

Figure 2–36   (A,B) Correction of eyelid asymmetry by creating a larger double eyelid.

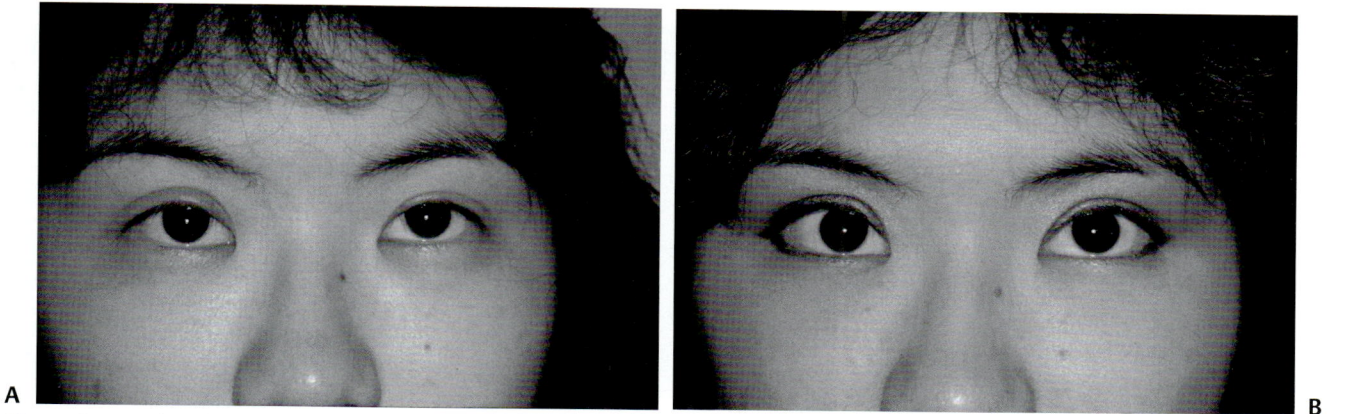

Figure 2–37 **(A,B)** Correction of asymmetry 6 months after the initial surgery. Both eyelids required revision to achieve symmetry.

individual variation, is usually relatively small, and surgical management rarely requires one of the complex procedures advocated for management of this condition in the Caucasian eyelid. A major reason for the relative ease in managing the Asian epicanthal fold is that, in contrast to the epicanthus encountered in Caucasians (usually congenital or traumatic in etiology), in which a vertical shortage of skin is problematic, the epicanthal fold in the Asian lid is usually associated with skin redundancy. Successful effacement of the fold is best conceptualized as an advancement procedure, the goal of which, in addition to modification of the fold itself, is elongation of the palpebral furrow in a medial direction (Fig. **2–38**). Further benefits of epicanthoplasty include the illusion of an increased intercanthal distance associated with apparent narrowing of the nasal bridge, the appearance of a wide nose being a concern of many individuals with prominent epicanthal folds.

In some patients, intervention in the epicanthal area is not required in conjunction with upper ble-

pharoplasty. Such patients are those who request an inside fold as well as those patients with a small fold in whom the surgical approach used to create the double eyelid results in sufficient medial advancement of the epicanthus to achieve effacement.

A major advantage of minimizing surgery in the epicanthal region is a reduction in the risk of hypertrophic scarring. This area exhibits a biological predisposition to hypertrophic scar formation, and even the most meticulously performed procedure may be complicated by an aesthetically unpleasant scar. Because of this risk, it is best to encourage patients who are uncertain if they really desire modification of the fold to defer epicanthoplasty at the time of primary surgery. If necessary, epicanthoplasty can be performed as a secondary procedure, but once performed, it is essentially impossible to reverse. Preoperatively, patients should be informed that effacement of the epicanthus tends to produce a more westernized appearance, whereas preservation or only slight modification of the fold preserves Asian characteristics.

Many surgeons, citing concerns about hypertrophic scarring, encourage patients not to undergo surgical modification of the epicanthus, suggesting such surgery invariably produces an unnatural look incompatible with the Asian face. This is an unfortunate attitude, however, because failure to modify the epicanthus deprives many eyes of their full aesthetic potential and, in many cases, is a source of patient unhappiness with an otherwise successful blepharoplasty. The flexibility in range of effacement possible using the procedures described below allows the aesthetic surgeon to select an operation that results in the modified epicanthus blending harmoniously with the rest of the lid and face.

Epicanthoplasty is perhaps the most misunderstood and confusing aspect of Asian blepharoplasty, but, as noted above, this procedure can be conceptually

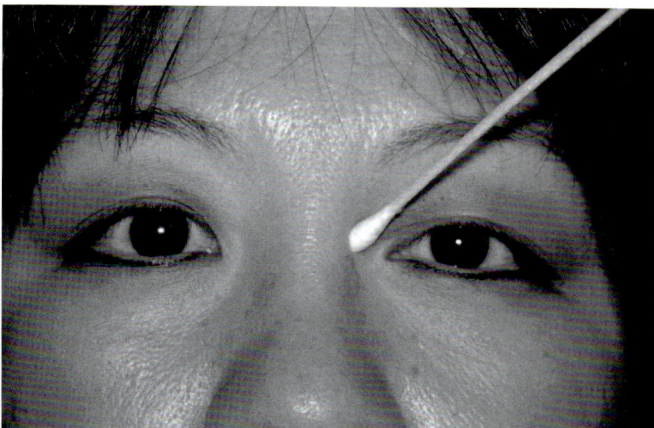

Figure 2–38 Medial displacement of the epicanthal skin with a cotton-tipped applicator showing effacement of the epicanthus by advancement of the skin in a medial direction.

simplified by regarding it as consisting of a medial advancement and/or excision of redundant tissue in the medial aspect of the upper eyelid. Technically, epicanthoplasty in conjunction with upper blepharoplasty is performed using one of three approaches depending on the size of the fold requiring modification. Each procedure is based on the general principle that effacement can be successfully accomplished by medial advancement of the existing fold.

Small Epicanthus: Advancement with Fixation Sutures

Advancement of a small epicanthus is performed in conjunction with the incision used for creation of the palpebral fold (Fig. **2–39A,B**). These incisions are extended to a point just medial to the origin of the epicanthus. The point of termination is frequently marked by a small naturally occurring depression or dimple. The pretarsal skin beneath the epicanthus is undermined to within 1 to 2 mm of the ciliary margin, and an underlying segment of pretarsal muscle is then excised. The lax skin is advanced medially and secured by placing one or two external fixation sutures. If a small "dog-ear" develops, it is excised in the direction of the skinfold, occasionally requiring

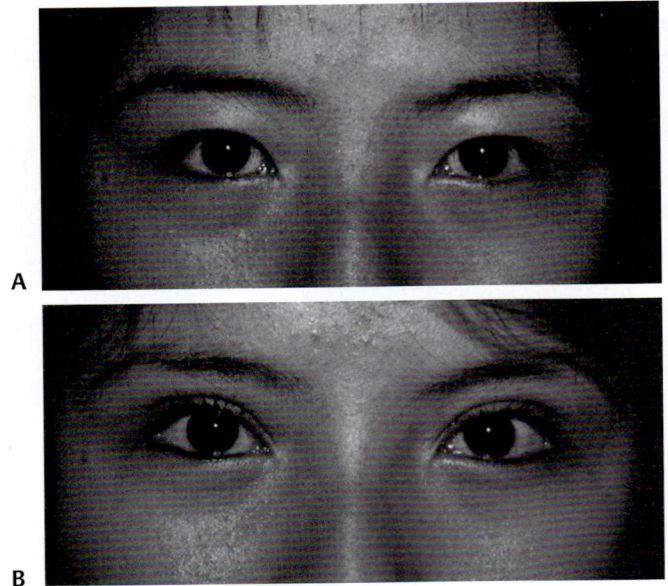

Figure 2–39 **(A,B)** Effacement of an epicanthal fold by advancement in conjunction with creation of an outside fold.

extension (i.e., a small back cut) on to the medial aspect of the lower eyelid if the epicanthal fold is large (Fig. **2–40A–H**).

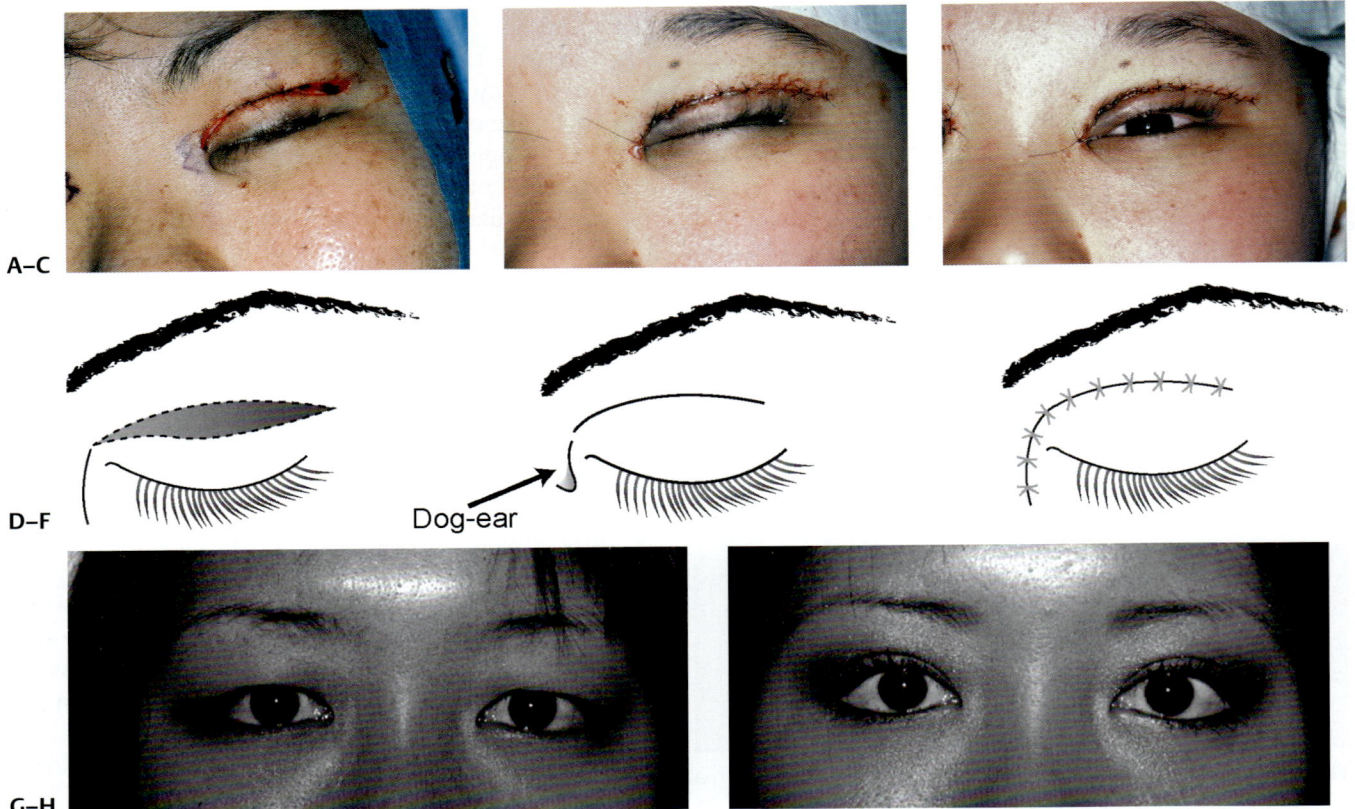

Figure 2–40 Effacement of a small epicanthus by medial fixation sutures combined with excision of a small "dog-ear." **(A–C)** Intraoperative, **(D–F)** schematic, **(G)** preoperative, and **(H)** postoperative views.

Medium Epicanthus: the Half Z-plasty

If a more substantial epicanthus requires additional advancement, the half Z-plasty procedure can be used (Fig. **2–41A–J**). The epicanthal fold is incised near the medial terminus of the palpebral wound, creating a triangular flap that is undermined and advanced nasally into a triangular defect created by a small medially oriented incision in the superomedial aspect of the wound. The resulting dog-ear is trimmed in the direction of the skin lines as described above.

Large Epicanthus: W-plasty Advancement

Effacement of a larger epicanthus may require greater medial advancement than is possible with the half Z-plasty technique. Such a fold often terminates on the medial aspect of the lower lid, necessitating advancement in this area as well. An excellent aesthetic result can be achieved by a W-plasty advancement procedure (Fig. **2–42A–J**) without resorting to the numerous techniques described for reconstruction of congenital or traumatic epicanthal "webs":

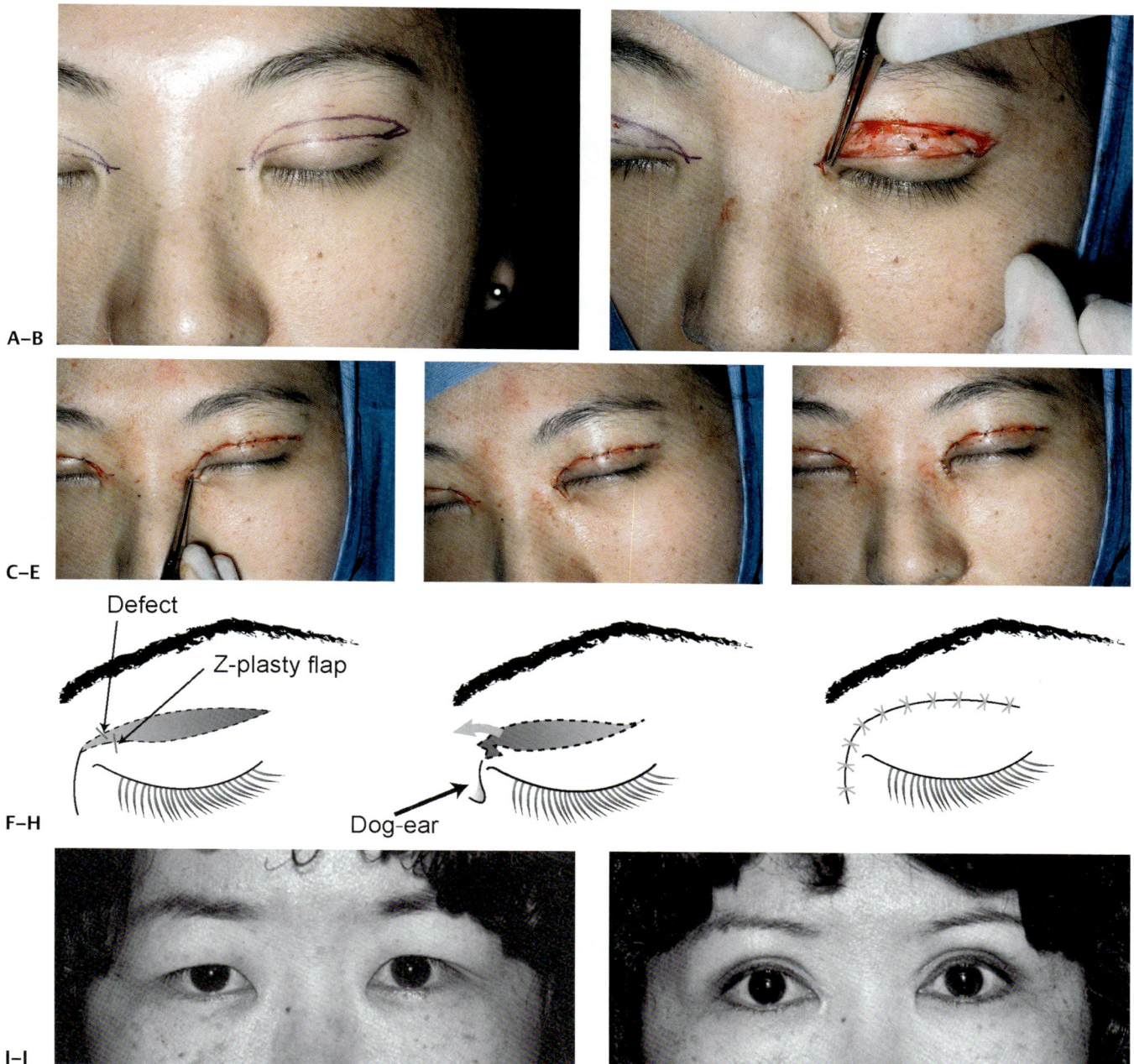

Figure 2–41   Effacement of the epicanthal fold using a half a Z-plasty, illustrating advancement of a triangular flap and subsequent trimming of a "dog-ear."(**A–E**) Introperative view. (**F–H**) Schematic illustrating the Z-plasty limbs and advancement of the created triangular flap into the medially created triangular defect followed by a "dog-ear" excision, if required. (**I**) Preoperative and (**J**) postoperative views.

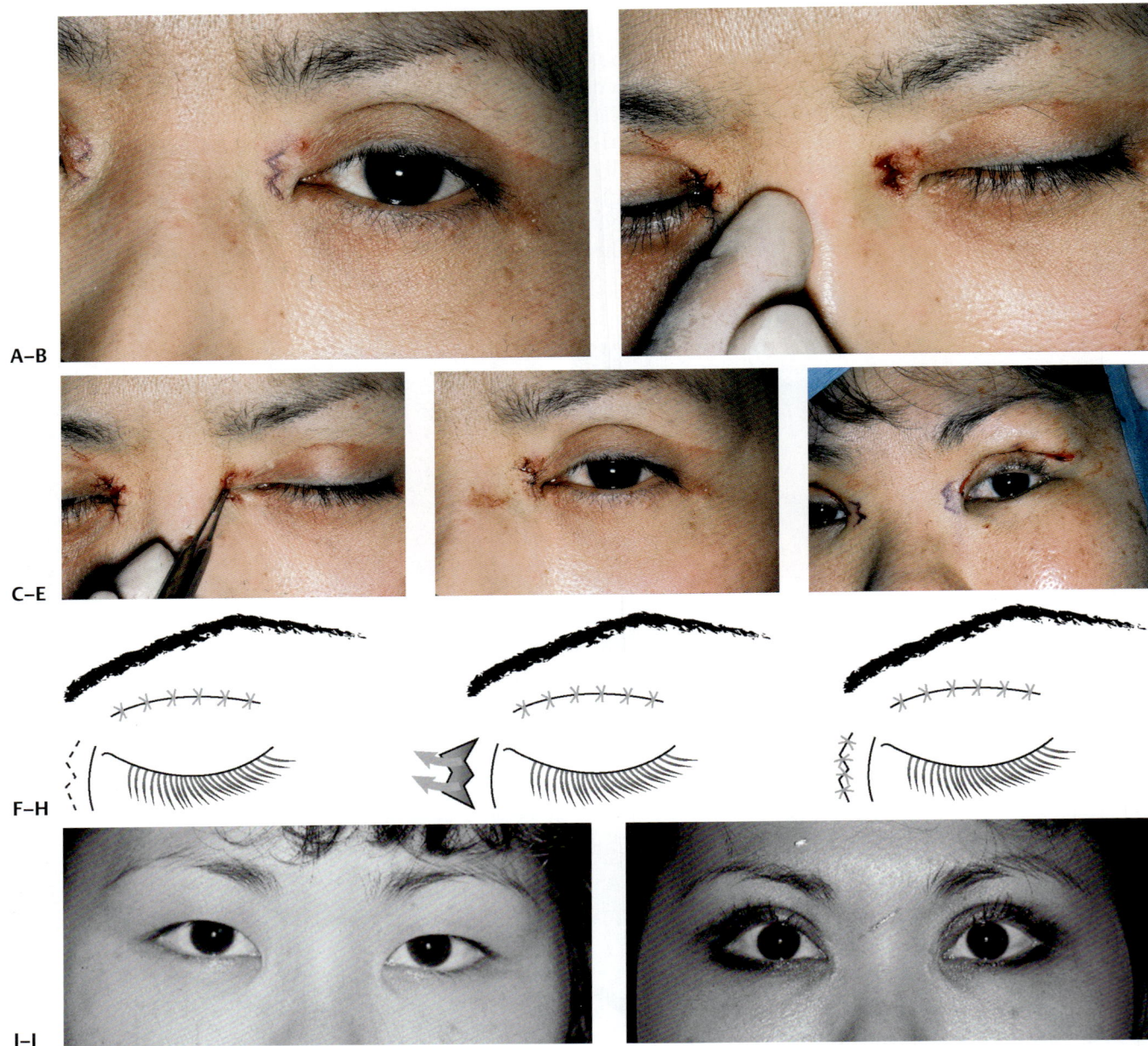

Figure 2–42   Epicanthoplasty using the W-plasty advancement procedure. **(A–E)** Intraoperative view. **(F–H)** Schematic illustrating creation and medial advancement of W-shaped flap. **(I)** Preoperative and **(J)** postoperative views.

1. The desired position of the palpebral fold terminus is marked, generally being a point ~2 mm medial to the desired position of the inner canthus. Two V-shaped flaps forming a *W* are outlined, the triangular flaps having their bases on the segments of the epicanthus located on the upper and lower lids.

2. The outlined *W* is incised, and the triangular flaps are undermined toward the inner canthus.

3. The skin medial to the apex of the *W* is incised toward the inner canthus, allowing advancement of the epicanthal fold medially.

4. The position of the palpebral fold terminus is established by suturing the skin at the end of the above

incision to the apex of the *W* (using 6–0 nylon), as illustrated in Fig. **2–41F**.

5. The undermined triangular flaps are then advanced medially, trimmed to fit precisely into the *W*, and sutured into place (using 6–0 nylon).

6. Sutures are removed in 5 to 7 days.

Complications of Epicanthoplasty

As previously stressed, even the most meticulously performed epicanthoplasty is often complicated by development of hypertrophic scars (Fig. **2–43**) regardless of the technique used. Because this problem is always

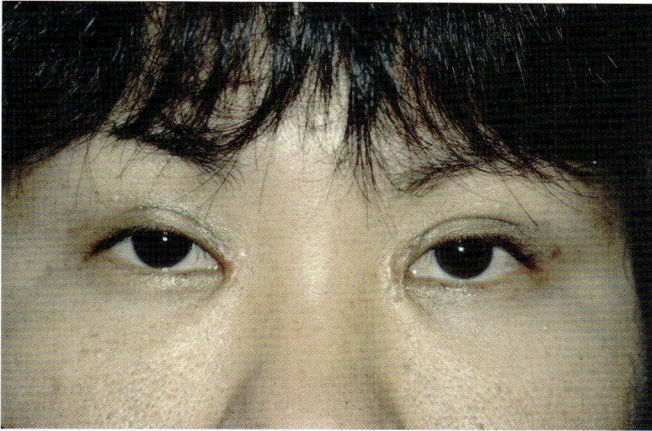

Figure 2–43 Hypertrophic scarring following surgery in the epicanthal region.

anticipated, intraoperative injection of triamcinolone (10 mg per cc) is utilized regardless of the type of epicanthoplasty employed. At the first sign of postoperative induration, aggressive treatment with topical and, if necessary, additional intralesional steroid is warranted.

Asymmetry is another potential complication. The surgeon should always inform patients about preexisting asymmetry of the eyelids, epicanthal region, and palpebral fissures, as they most often persist or become more apparent postoperatively. Patients must understand that differences in postoperative edema between the two eyes frequently translate into postoperative asymmetry, and that final judgment regarding symmetry may be unreliable for 6 months or more postoperatively.

Surgery of the Lateral Canthus

Occasionally, a patient requests elongation of the palpebral fissure to produce a longer, more oval-shaped eye. In general, requests for such surgery should be handled with caution, as the elongation afforded by existing techniques

is generally not sufficient to justify the risks of surgery (i.e., failure with recurrence of the original, or even a diminution of, the palpebral fissure length). If the patient insists, however, and is willing to risk undesirable scarring and the possibility of minimal improvement and/or recurrence, the following simple technique can be used:

1. The lateral canthus is incised, the incision traversing laterally a distance of 2 to 4 mm (Fig. **2–44A**).
2. Hemostasis is secured, following which the skin edges are sutured to the underlying conjunctiva using two or three sutures of 6–0 silk, in both upper and lower lids (Fig. **2–44B**).
3. The sutures are left in place for 1 week to allow adequate healing, thus minimizing the risk of recurrence.
4. The patient is instructed to apply triamcinolone cream, 0.1%, to the incision line three times a day for 2 weeks following suture removal.
5. The patient is also instructed in inferior and superior traction on the lower and upper lids, respectively, to distract the suture lines three or four times daily for 1 week postoperatively.

Postoperative results achieved with this technique are illustrated in Fig. **2–45A,B**.

Application of Asian Upper Blepharoplasty to Caucasian Eyelids

Upper blepharoplasty is generally considered to be an operation directed toward rejuvenation of the aging eyelid; however, aesthetic surgeons occasionally encounter young Caucasian women with puffiness of the upper lids secondary to fat protrusion and/or poor definition of the supratarsal fold, usually having a genetic basis (Fig. **2–46A,B**). This eyelid configuration imparts a sad, tired appearance that detracts from the expressive

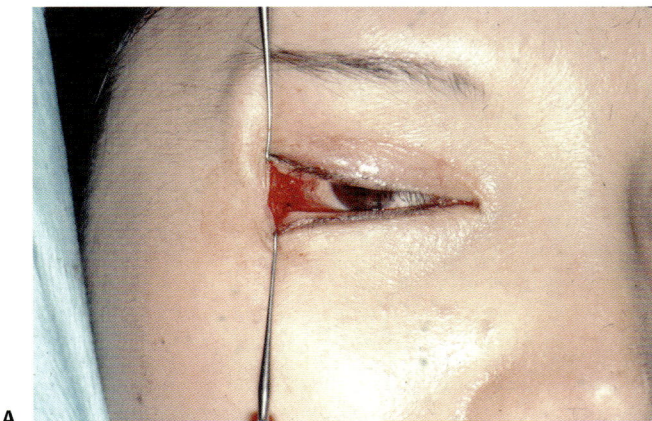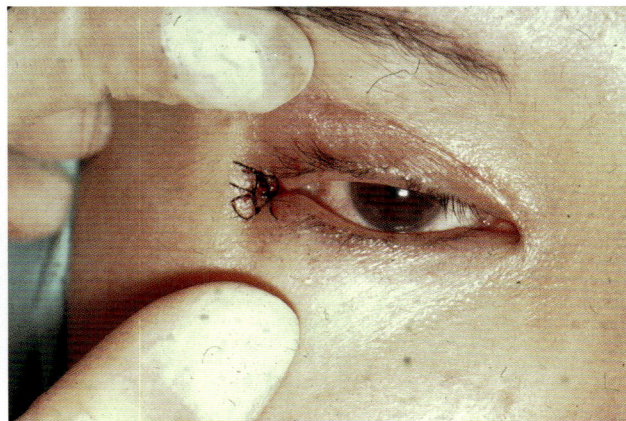

A   B

Figure 2–44 **(A)** An incision in the lateral canthus is made in preparation for lengthening of the palpebral fissure. **(B)** The skin edges and conjunctiva are approximated using two or three sutures of 6–0 silk in both upper- and lower-lid wounds.

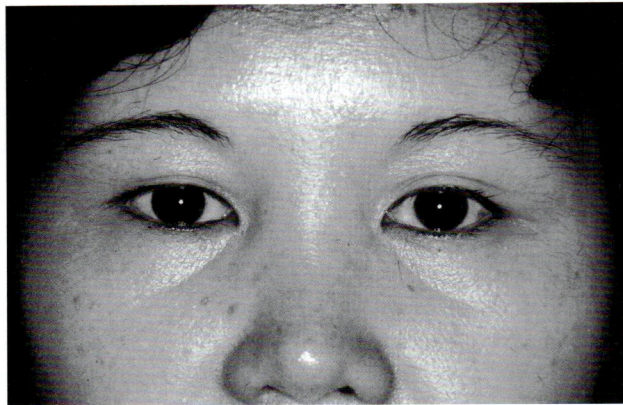

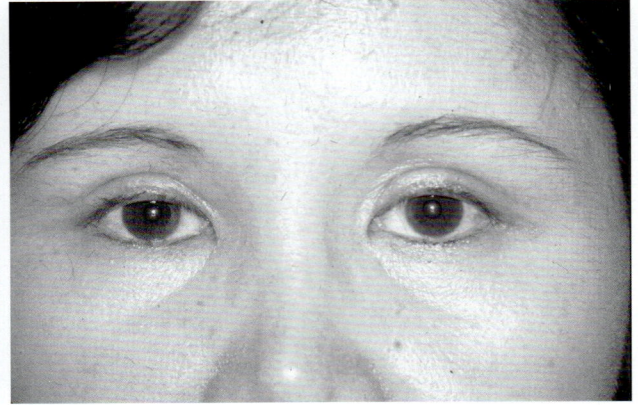

Figure 2–45 **(A,B)** Pre- and postoperative photographs illustrating result of lateral lengthening. (Upper blepharoplasty also was performed.)

potential of the eyelids and interferes with effective use of cosmetics. The condition is amenable to correction, using the techniques employed in the double-eyelid operation, and often produces a dramatic transformation of the periorbital region.

Although true absence of the superior palpebral fold is unusual in the Caucasian eye, the natural fold of young Caucasian women who are candidates for upper blepharoplasty is often lower (6–7 mm above the ciliary margin) and poorly defined. The eyelid skin is often thick in such patients. The procedure employed in most cases is virtually identical to that used for westernization of the Asian eyelid:

1. An incision is marked 9 to 10 mm above the ciliary margin.

2. The maximum amount of skin that can be safely excised is determined by pinching with a pair of forceps. To provide a margin of error, the upper incision is placed 2 mm below the point of maximal skin excision.

3. Skin and muscle are excised as described for the westernization procedure, but unlike the Asian eye, there is no hesitation to remove fat in the medial aspect of the eyelid. A strip of infrabrow fat is also often excised.

4. Undermining of the pretarsal skin to the level of the original fold is performed to enhance the appearance and tighten the pretarsal skin. It is seldom necessary to excise tissue in the pretarsal region to thin the eyelid, as it is occasionally performed in the Asian lid.

5. Three fixation sutures of 5–0 nylon are placed sequentially, as in the Asian eye, to enhance symmetry (Fig. **2–47**). In some cases, a medial fixation suture is unnecessary.

6. The wound is closed with a running suture of 6–0 nylon.

This procedure differs from the technique used in Asian lids in three aspects:

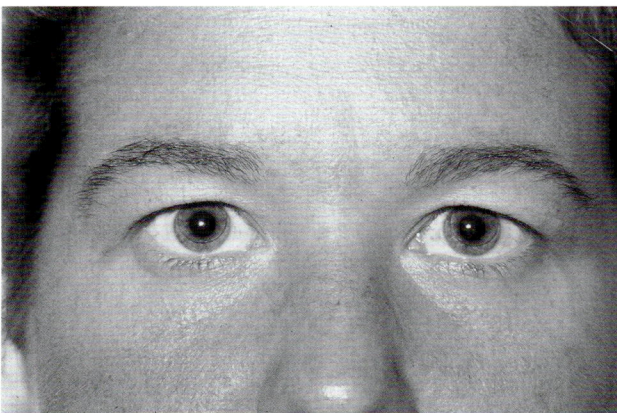

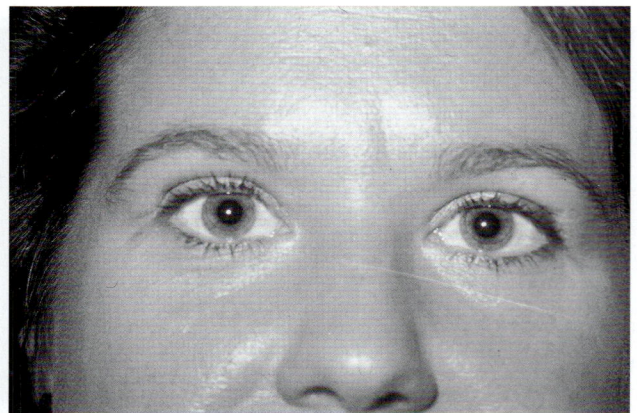

Figure 2–46 **(A,B)** Pre- and postoperative results of upper blepharoplasty in a young Caucasian woman with an Asian-like upper eyelid.

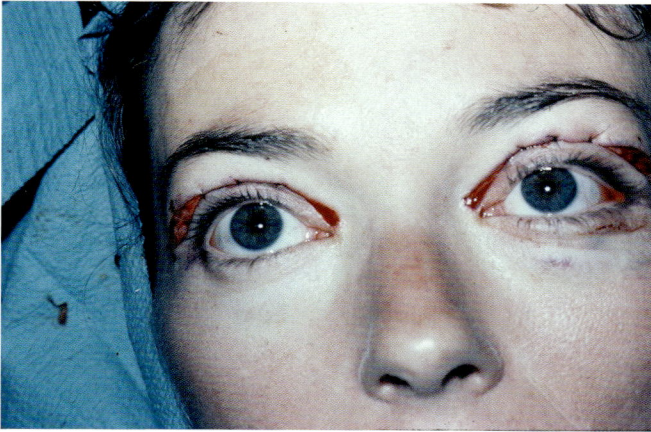

Figure 2–47 Placement of external fixation sutures in the left upper eyelid, producing a better definition of the palpebral fold than on the right, in which standard cutaneous sutures have been placed for demonstration purposes only.

1. Fat is removed more aggressively in the medial aspect of the lid as compared with the Asian eyelid.

2. Although the pretarsal skin is undermined (to the level of the original palpebral fold), no debulking of the pretarsal space is necessary.

3. Epicanthoplasty is seldom required in the Caucasian eye. Although fixation sutures may not be necessary in patients with a natural palpebral fold 9 to 10 mm above the ciliary margin, these sutures allow more exact sculpting of the superior palpebral fold and also encourage tightening of the pretarsal skin. Placement, however, must be precise to avoid troublesome asymmetry.

In many patients, aesthetically pleasing deepening of the palpebral sulcus can be enhanced by judicious removal of infrabrow fat.

Upper blepharoplasty should no longer be considered as an operation limited to rejuvenation of the aging Caucasian eyelid. The principles developed in surgery of the Asian eyelid can be applied to transformation of the young Caucasian upper eyelid, and an enlightened aesthetic surgeon can dramatically enhance its beauty and expressive potential (Figs. **2–46**, **2–48A,B**).

Conclusion

Upper blepharoplasty in the Asian eye is a challenging procedure requiring careful and considered preoperative preparation as well as meticulous attention to detail during the operative procedure. Anatomic differences as compared with the Caucasian eyelid must be appreciated and respected. This is a flexible operation that allows variations in the level of the palpebral fold, depth of the palpebral sulcus, and disposition of the epicanthus, all of which combine to allow significant aesthetic differences in the appearance of the surgically transformed eyelids. The preoperative desires of each patient regarding the type of eyelid transformation requested must be carefully elicited. At the present time, most patients desire retention of at least some Asian characteristics rather than frank westernization. Each patient should be allowed to scrutinize pre- and postoperative photographs of various types of double-eyelid procedures as an aid in selecting the type of eyelid desired.

Because postoperative asymmetry is the most frequent cause of dissatisfaction, it is especially important to note and document preexisting asymmetry and to execute every step in this operation with symmetry as a primary goal.

Although blepharoplasty in Asians is a variation of standard supratarsal fixation blepharoplasty, surgery of the Asian eyelid presents a unique and novel challenge even for the surgeon experienced in Caucasian blepharoplasty. As in other areas of cosmetic surgery, the best way to avoid unsatisfactory results is to identify potential problem situations preoperatively. In Asian blepharoplasty, these include preoperative asymmetry,

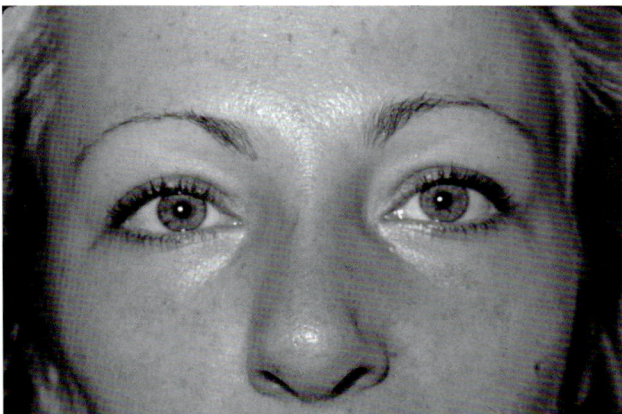
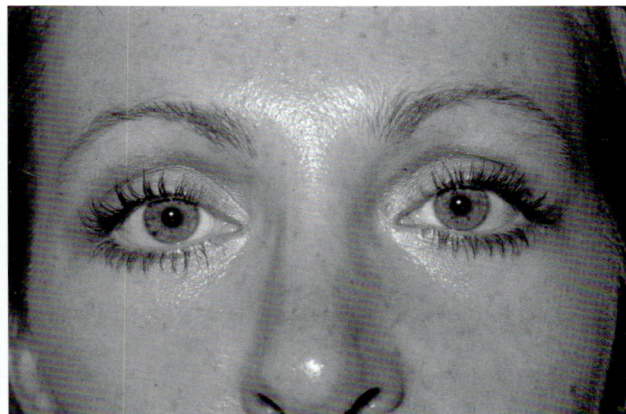

Figure 2–48 **(A,B)** Result achieved by application of Asian blepharoplasty in a young Caucasian woman.

patients who have undergone previous blepharoplasty, thick sebaceous skin, and the presence of a large epicanthal fold. Thorough understanding of anatomy, thoughtful and considered preoperative planning, and meticulous attention to detail during the operative procedure constitute a road map to success in Asian upper blepharoplasty.

◆ Lower Blepharoplasty in the Asian

For obvious reasons, discussions of blepharoplasty performed in the Asian patient concentrate on surgical modification of the upper eyelid. Although lower blepharoplasty is similar to that in the Caucasian eyelid, distinct differences in anatomy and in the pathophysiology of the aging process are noteworthy and translate into subtle differences in surgical technique. As with other procedures described in this text, I consider an important factor for success in lower blepharoplasty to be the mindset of the surgeon. As lower-lid malposition is by far the most common complication of this operation, the primary focus in lower blepharoplasty is preservation/reconstruction of lower-lid support. I present a five-point operative program, each and every step of which complements this focus on preservation of lower-lid position.

Anatomic Considerations

As in the upper eyelid, the Asian lower lid characteristically exhibits a considerable volume of periorbital fat that frequently results in a puffy, baggy appearance at a relatively early age. In addition to periorbital fat, in many patients, a considerable volume of fat is present in the submuscular plane (superficial to the orbital septum), contributing to eyelid puffiness. Although a wide spectrum exists, Asian lower eyelid skin tends to be thicker than Caucasian skin, and consequently, deeply etched rhytids extending laterally (i.e., "laugh lines" or crow's-feet) occur less frequently. Eccrine syringomas (Fig. **2–49**) are relatively common on the Asian lower-eyelid skin, and such patients must understand that these blemishes will not be eliminated by blepharoplasty and will require additional treatment should the patient desire their removal. Pigmented lesions (e.g., seborrheic keratoses, lentigos) are also common on the lower-lid skin in Asians.

The lower eyelids of Asian patients frequently exhibit hypertrophy of the orbicularis muscle, often producing an objectionable bulge in the infraciliary region even at a young age (Fig. **2–50**). Such patients must be counseled about the differences between eyelid puffiness caused by fat protrusion and orbicularis

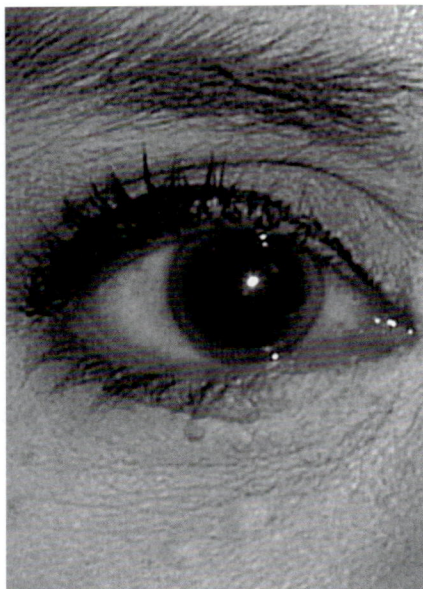

Figure 2–49   Eccrine syringomas on the lower eyelids.

hypertrophy, as well as the aesthetic limitations of partial muscle resection.

Lower-lid tone is generally more substantial in Asians than Caucasians, allowing somewhat more aggressive tissue resection. Although this increased skin tone offers some protection against lid retraction (scleral show) and ectropion, overzealous tissue excision will certainly produce these undesirable conditions.

An inferiorly directed extension of the upper-lid fold in the area lateral to the external canthus frequently necessitates modification of the lower-lid incision in order for lower blepharoplasty to avoid unsightly scarring. In Caucasian lower blepharoplasty, the lateral aspect of the incision is generally placed as horizontally as possible at the level of the external canthus. Such an

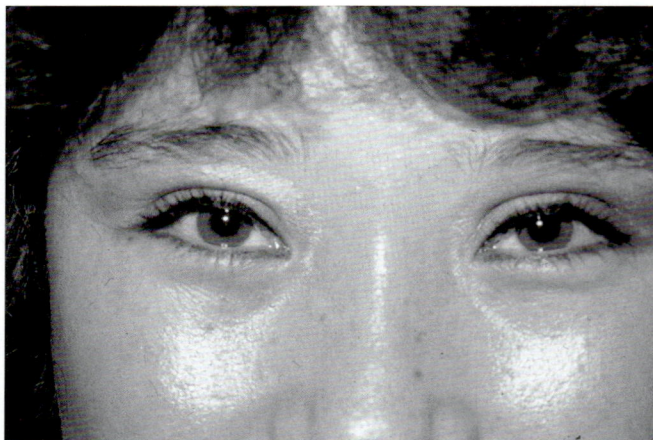

Figure 2–50   Hypertrophy of the orbicularis muscle producing a bulge in the infraciliary region.

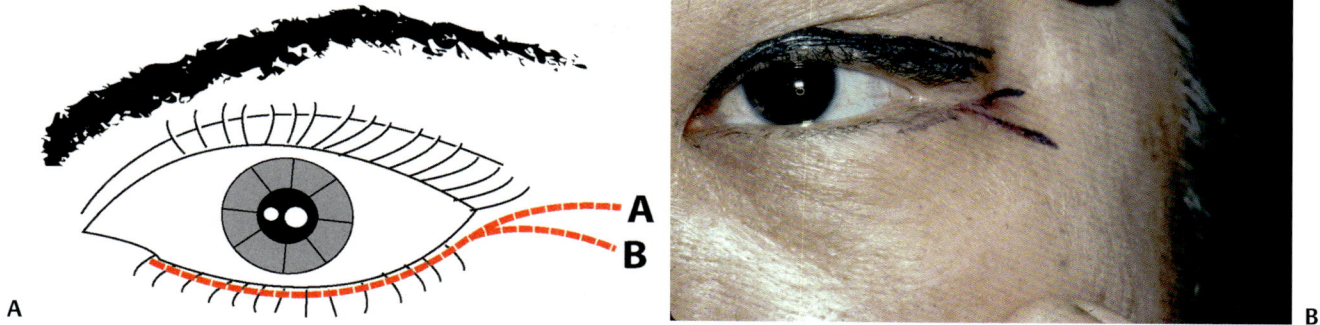

Figure 2–51   (A,B) Modification of the lateral aspect of the lower-eyelid incision necessitated by an inferiorly directed extension of the upper-lid fold. A more horizontal incision **(A)** is preferred to a more inferiorly oriented incision (option **B**). See text.

incision in the Asian lid, however, often violates this lateral extension of the upper lid; thus, the lateral incision must be modified in one of two ways (Fig. **2–51A,B**).

Selection of a Technique for Lower Blepharoplasty

To achieve maximum aesthetic improvement in lower blepharoplasty, the surgical plan must be directed toward all components of lower-eyelid "deformity"—skin, muscle, fat, and, occasionally (but rarely in the Asian lid), bone (infraorbital rim)—as determined by accurate preoperative analysis. Each patient who requests surgery manifests an individual problem in that the relative importance of skin, muscle, and fat correction varies from eyelid to eyelid. In my practice, the skin–muscle flap operation is the workhorse of lower blepharoplasty in that it provides excellent exposure for modification of all periorbital tissues and allows the procedure to proceed in a stepwise fashion in which every step contributes to the goal of maintaining lower-eyelid support.

Occasionally, older patients who manifest skin redundancy with minimal fat protrusion or orbicularis hypertrophy benefit from the skin flap procedure (fat being removed via muscle stab incisions). In some patients, orbicularis hypertrophy can be managed adequately by the skin flap operation. Younger patients whose main concern is fat protrusion without skin redundancy, or orbicularis hypertrophy, are best treated with the skin–muscle flap operation (preserving the pretarsal orbicularis during flap dissection), or by the transconjunctival approach. Caution, however, must be exercised in recommending transconjunctival blepharoplasty. Most Asian patients, regardless of age, are convinced that "too much skin" is a component of their problem, and thus are prone to dissatisfaction if the surgical result does not quite meet their expectations,

blaming their unhappiness on the fact that skin was not removed. A further disadvantage of the transconjunctival approach is that treatment of orbicularis hypertrophy is not possible. For these reasons, transconjunctival blepharoplasty is best preserved for the very young patient with absolutely no skin redundancy and minimal orbicularis hypertrophy, or for men whose only concern is "bags" resulting from fat protrusion. An occasional patient who has undergone blepharoplasty via an external approach and presents with residual fat protrusion is a candidate for the transconjunctival procedure.

I feel that the most important consideration in lower blepharoplasty is preservation and/or reinforcement of the anatomic support of the eyelid. Even the most experienced and accomplished surgeon must deal with the problem of lower lids whose posture in the immediate postoperative period is normal but relentlessly descends into a lower, aesthetically unappealing position as the healing process continues. Such lower lid malposition is commonly referred to as ectropion and is usually attributed to overzealous tissue excision. However, by far the most common cause of this situation is a process termed retraction, the pathologic basis of which is fibrosis in the plane of the middle lamella (orbital septum and capsulopalpebral fascia, generally also involving the posterior surface of the orbicularis oculi), resulting in scar contracture in this plane (vertical shortening) that overwhelms the often tenuous supporting structures of the lower eyelid that are so often compromised by the surgical procedure itself. Frank ectropion, in contrast, is related to shortening of the anterior lamella (skin and orbicularis oculi), resulting in eversion of the lid margin in addition to inferior displacement. Retraction and ectropion, of course, may coexist. Lower-eyelid retraction and ectropion are compared diagrammatically in Fig. **2–52**.

Lower-Eyelid Malposition

Pathogenesis of Lower-Eyelid Malposition

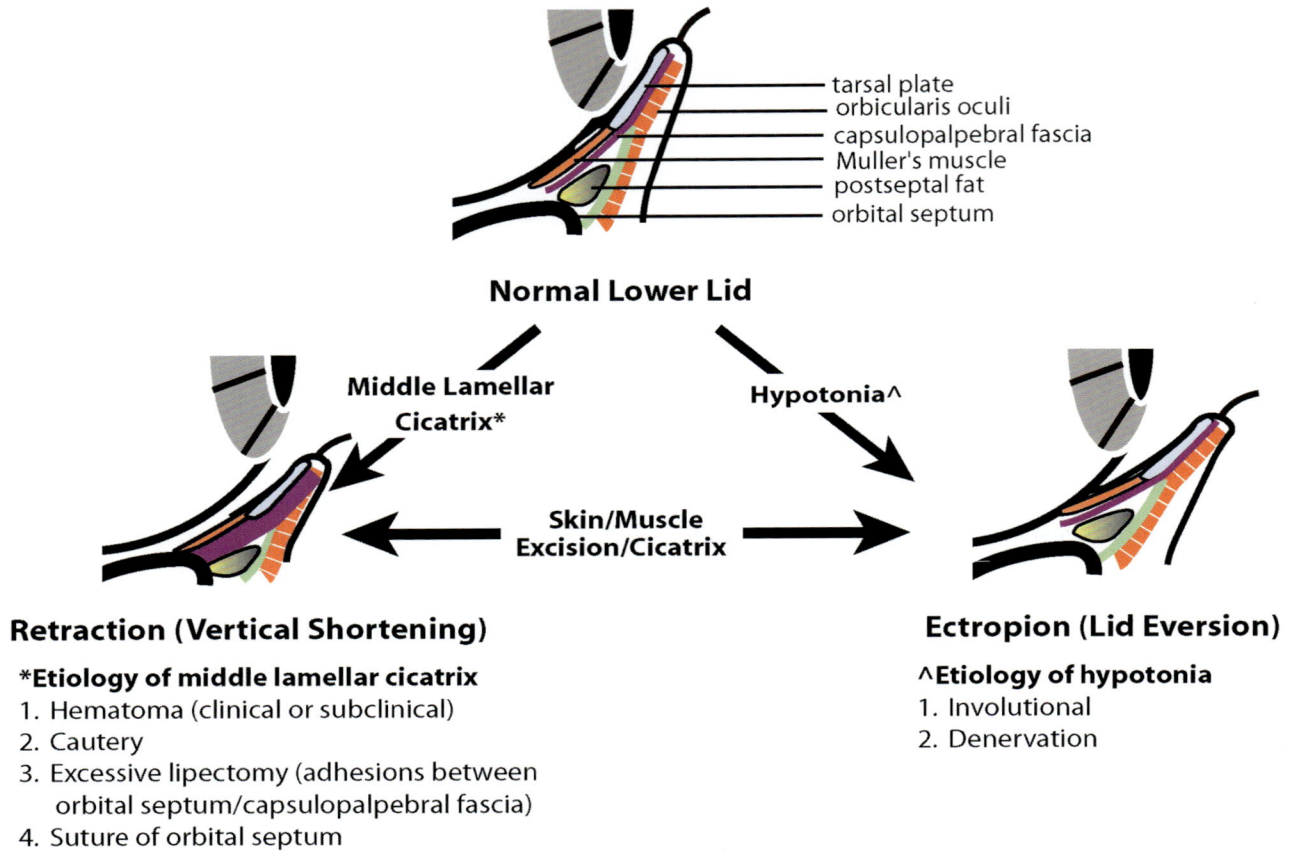

tarsal plate
orbicularis oculi
capsulopalpebral fascia
Muller's muscle
postseptal fat
orbital septum

Normal Lower Lid

Middle Lamellar Cicatrix*

Hypotonia^

Skin/Muscle Excision/Cicatrix

Retraction (Vertical Shortening)

*Etiology of middle lamellar cicatrix
1. Hematoma (clinical or subclinical)
2. Cautery
3. Excessive lipectomy (adhesions between orbital septum/capsulopalpebral fascia)
4. Suture of orbital septum

Ectropion (Lid Eversion)

^Etiology of hypotonia
1. Involutional
2. Denervation

Figure 2–52 A diagrammatical comparison of lower-lid malposition resulting from retraction and ectropion.

Dynamic Anatomy of Lower-Lid Support

Anatomic support of the lower eyelid consists of static and dynamic components. Static support is provided by the tarsal plate and associated medial and lateral canthal tendons, whereas the dynamic component consists of the pretarsal segment of the orbicularis muscle that is firmly adherent to the tarsal plate. The posture of the lower eyelid is determined by a balance between the supporting structures and the forces tending to displace the eyelid inferiorly, that is, gravitational and cicatricial forces subsequent to surgery or trauma (Fig. **2–53**). The static component of lid support is gradually attenuated by the aging process; the dynamic component is easily compromised during the skin–muscle flap operation.

The key to success in lower blepharoplasty is to preserve and/or reconstruct lid support during each and every lower-lid operation. A five-point operative plan is of value in achieving this goal and has proven to be a reliable method of reducing the incidence of postoperative lower-lid retraction.

Operative Technique

See DVD Disk Two, Lower Skin–Muscle Blepharoplasty

My five-point program for minimizing the incidence of lower-lid malposition is as follows:

1. The lateral extensions of the infraciliary incisions should be placed as horizontally as possible (preferably in a horizontal periorbital line) to minimize the tendency toward lateral canthal rounding and inferior displacement that may result as a consequence of the inevitable inferior migration of the scar during the postoperative period. A more inferiorly oriented

Opposing Forces on Lower-Eyelid Position

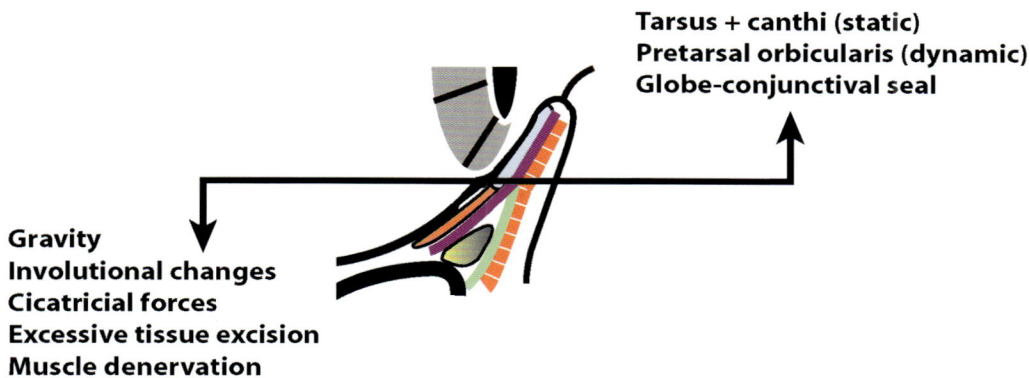

Tarsus + canthi (static)
Pretarsal orbicularis (dynamic)
Globe-conjunctival seal

Gravity
Involutional changes
Cicatricial forces
Excessive tissue excision
Muscle denervation

Figure 2–53 Opposing forces that determine lower-lid posture.

lateral extension is less resistant to the influences of such scar contracture than a horizontally placed incision. Because of the lateral extension of the upper lid mentioned previously, the lateral incision may require modification, as noted in Fig. **2–51**.

2. The pretarsal orbicularis of the lower eyelid is firmly adherent to the tarsal plate. In addition to contributing to the structural integrity of the lower lid, contraction of this muscle provides an element of dynamic support for the lid margin. Accordingly, a strip of pretarsal orbicularis should remain attached to the tarsal plate to help preserve the lid support necessary for maintaining normal lid posture postoperatively. This is accomplished by initially undermining the skin–muscle flap through the lateral portion of the incision. The infraciliary incision is then made in conjunction with scissors undermining of a skin flap for a distance of 3 to 4 mm inferior to the ciliary margin. The skin and muscle flaps are then connected at the base of the skin flap by incising the orbicularis muscle with a diagonally oriented scissors, thus preserving an adherent strip of pretarsal orbicularis on the tarsal plate (Fig. **2–54**). The orbicularis muscle may be thinned by resection of a portion of its anterior surface without disturbing its tarsal attachment if required for treatment of lower-lid deformity secondary to orbicularis hypertrophy. Following completion of the skin–muscle flap, the orbital septum, generally thin and filmy, is incised, allowing access to the periorbital fat. An appropriate amount of periorbital fat is then removed as in a standard Caucasian lower blepharoplasty, care being taken to ensure hemostasis, particularly following removal of medial fat.

3. When determining the amount of tissue to be resected from the skin–muscle flap, the flap is draped in a medial and superior direction as opposed to the

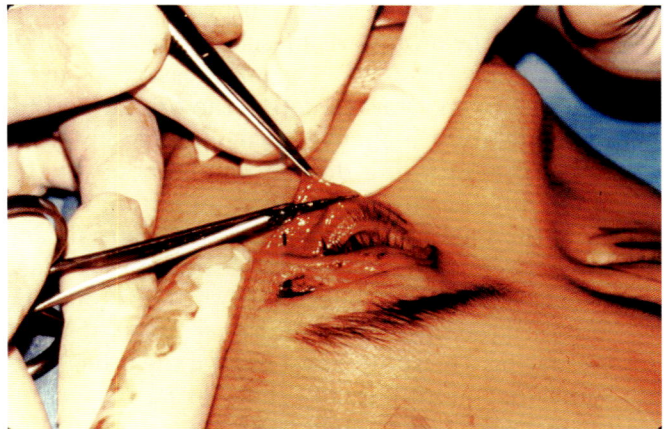

Figure 2–54 Connection of the skin–muscle flap and short infraciliary skin flap by incising the orbicularis muscle with diagonally oriented scissors.

lateral and superior draping generally practiced in lower blepharoplasty (Fig. **2–55**). This medial and superior draping offers several advantages, perhaps the most important of which is avoidance of concentrating tension in the lateral aspect of the eyelid. Such a concentration of tension may encourage inferior traction in the lateral canthal region, predisposing to shortening of the intercanthal distance that is associated with the so-called sad eye or hound dog look. This consideration is of particular importance in patients in whom the lateral canthal tendon and tarsal plate have been attenuated by the aging process.

Lateral traction on the lower-lid skin may also contribute to accentuation of lateral periorbital lines that may occur subsequent to lower blepharoplasty. An additional advantage of draping in the medial and superior direction is minimizing the length of the lateral incision as it is not necessary to "chase a dog-ear" laterally.

A

B

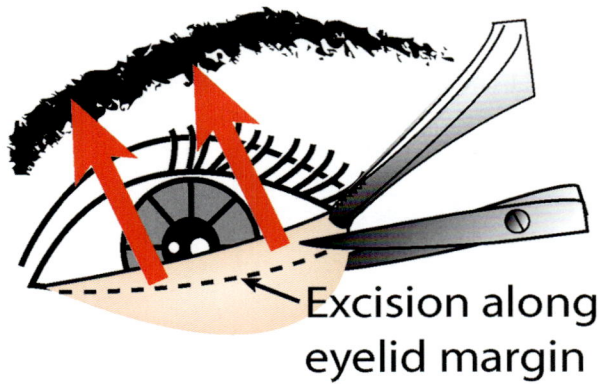

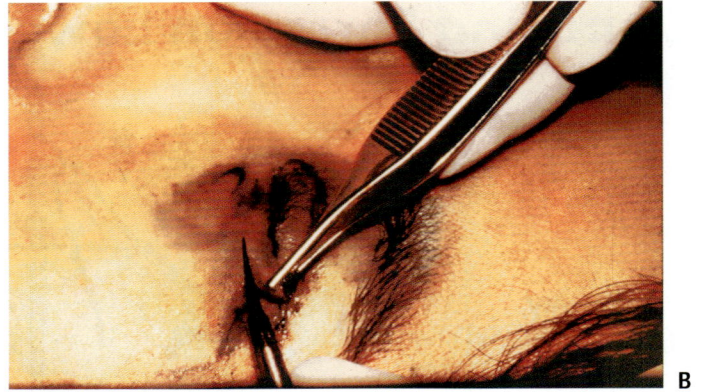

Figure 2–55   **(A,B)** The skin–muscle flap is draped in a medial and superior direction.

4. Before final skin suturing, a permanent suspension suture of 5–0 nylon is placed between the deep surface of the orbicularis muscle and lateral orbital periosteum (Fig. **2–56**). It is unnecessary to create a tunnel in an effort to define the orbital periosteum clearly, a maneuver that often accentuates the appearance of a dermal dimple beneath the site of muscle suspension. It is important to suspend the muscle at the level of the external canthus and to avoid excessive tension on the flap, which might lead to buckling of the tarsal plate or failure of the suspension suture secondary to muscle tearing. The suture must engage the orbicularis somewhat more laterally than initial inspection would suggest, as tightening the suspension suture following engagement of the periosteum pulls the flap medially.

Orbicularis suspension reinforces the static supporting sling of the lower lid and, like the buried septo-columellar suture advocated for support of the nasal tip during the critical postoperative healing phase, assists in resisting cicatricial forces that lead to displacement of the lower lid inferiorly during the healing period.

5. Finally, 0.2 mL of triamcinolone (10 mg per cc) is judiciously injected into the plane of the orbital septum before final skin closure (Fig. **2–57**). This has proven to be of considerable benefit in combating cicatricial forces and has not been associated with discernible complications attributable to steroid use (i.e., atrophy, telangiectasia). Use of steroids in this fashion results in a virtual absence of postoperative lower-lid induration that usually precedes the onset of clinical retraction. Perhaps the most powerful argument for the routine use of steroids in lower blepharoplasty relates to the observation that accumulation of small amounts of blood in the middle lamellar plane is probably the most frequent etiologic factor in lower-lid retraction: Even a minute amount of blood is a potent precipitator of fibrosis. Such accumulation of blood may develop following

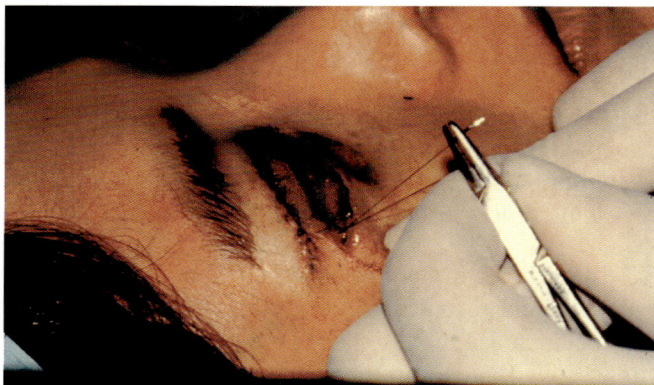

Figure 2–56   Suspension of the orbicularis muscle to the lateral orbital periosteum with a suture of 5–0 nylon.

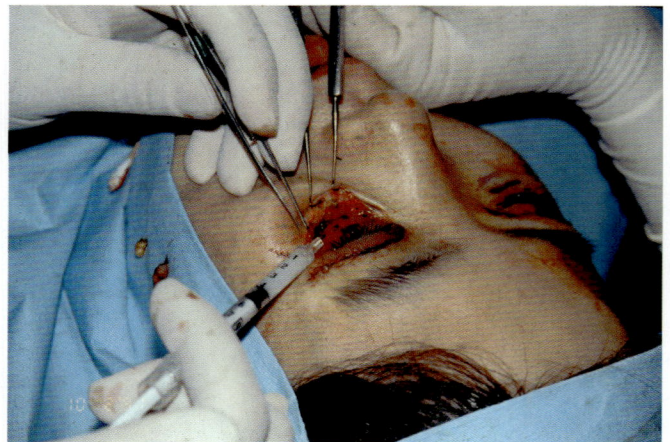

Figure 2–57   Injection of triacinolone (10 mg/cc) into the plane of the orbital septum.

meticulous intraoperative hemostasis. Thus, its occurrence is entirely unpredictable: this risk of a cicatricial process exerting inferiorly directed force on the healing lower eyelid provides justification for following the five-point operative program in each and every lower blepharoplasty.

Results of lower blepharoplasty using the techniques discussed are illustrated in Figs. **2–58** through **2–61**. A result achieved with transconjunctival blepharoplasty is illustrated in Fig. **2–62**.

Discussion

This five-point program is recommended for patients undergoing blepharoplasty who demonstrate no preoperative risk factors (Table **2–2**) predisposing to lower-lid malposition. Patients with preexisting lid laxity (a situation noted less frequently in Asians than in Caucasians) or those otherwise at risk for lower-lid malposition are candidates for other ancillary techniques (i.e., tarsal suspension, etc.) in conjunction with the blepharoplasty procedure.

A major thrust of this five-point operative program is mitigation of the effects of cicatricial forces (which are inevitable, but the clinical significance of which is unpredictable preoperatively) that occur during the healing process on the postoperative position of the lower eyelid.

The importance of fibrosis in the middle lamellar plane in the pathogenesis of postsurgical lower-lid retraction is supported by studies of lower-lid blepharoplasty in monkeys in which the effects of intentional overresection of skin and muscle were compared with those following intentional scarification in the plane of the orbital septum. Although most plastic surgeons and ophthalmologists who evaluated the monkeys following surgery attributed lower-lid malposition to excessive tissue resection, in fact intentional induction of fibrosis in the middle lamella was associated with a greater

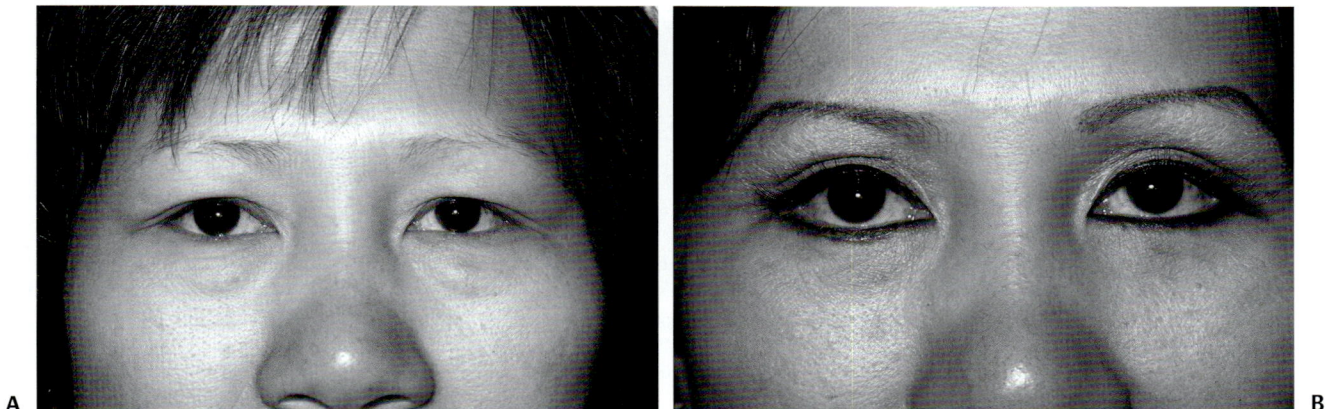

Figure 2–58   **(A,B)** Pre- and postoperative results of lower-lid blepharoplasty performed using a skin–muscle flap.

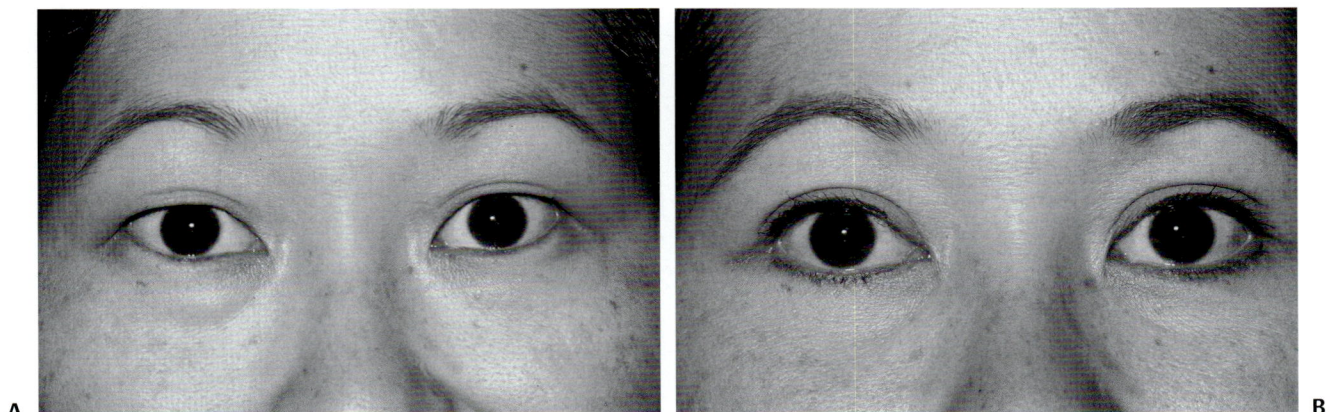

Figure 2–59   **(A,B)** Pre- and postoperative results of lower-lid blepharoplasty performed using a skin–muscle flap.

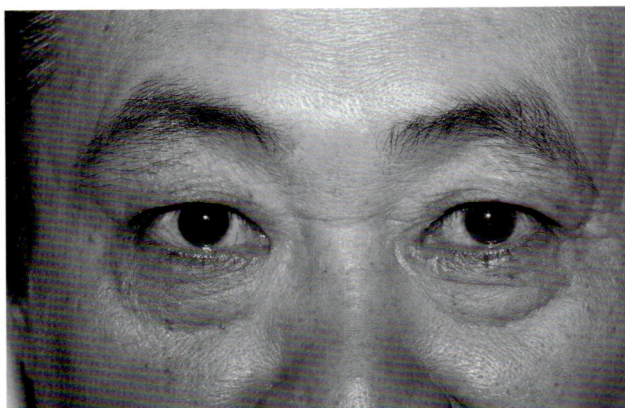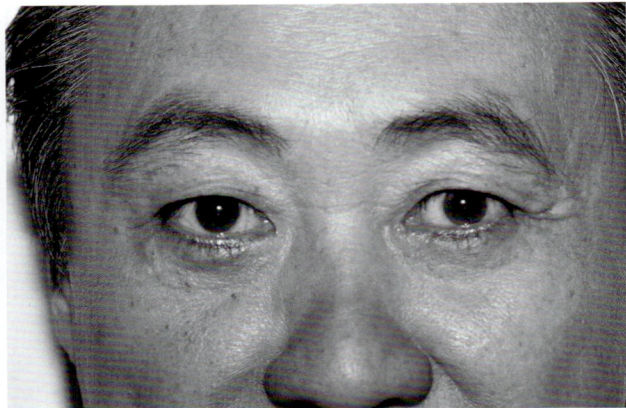

A   B

Figure 2–60   **(A,B)** Pre- and postoperative results of lower-lid blepharoplasty performed using a skin–muscle flap.

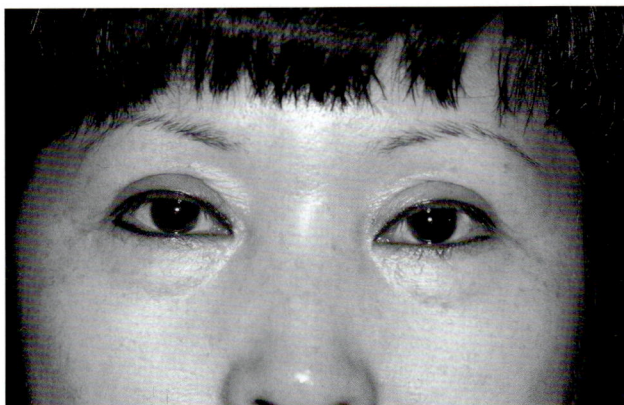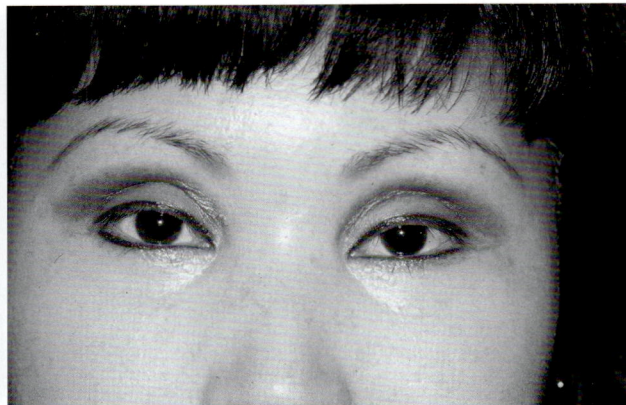

A   B

Figure 2–61   **(A,B)** Pre- and postoperative results of lower-lid blepharoplasty performed using a skin–muscle flap.

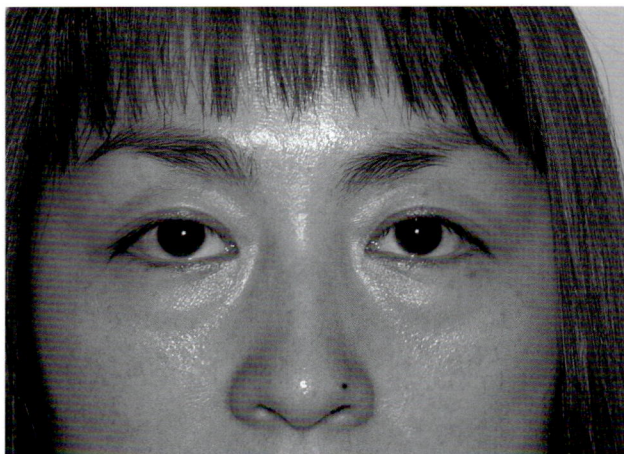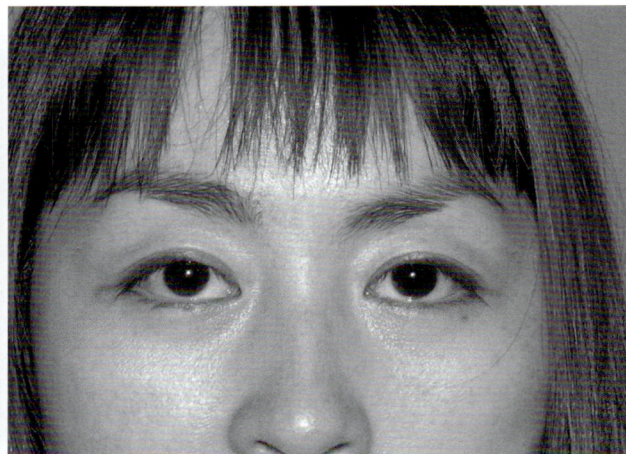

A   B

Figure 2–62   **(A,B)** Pre- and postoperative results of lower-lid blepharoplasty performed using a transconjunctival approach.

Table 2–2 Risk Factors for Lower-Lid Blepharoplasty

Prominence of globe
    Proptosis (relative or real)
    Exophthalmos
    Unilateral high myopia
Preexisting scleral show
    Congenital
    Acquired
Hypoplasia of maxilla (flat malar eminence)
Lower-lid laxity
    Previous blepharoplasty
    Males
    Females > 65 years

incidence of lower-lid malposition in this study. The observation that postoperative accumulation of even minimal amounts of blood in the middle lamellar plane is perhaps the most common cause of unanticipated fibrosis and subsequent lower-lid retraction cannot be overemphasized. This is the probable explanation for the occurrence of an expected lid retraction in patients with excellent preoperative lid support.

Although many patients who are predisposed to lower-lid malposition following blepharoplasty can be identified by noting certain risk factors during the preoperative evaluation (Table **2–2**), other patients who do not demonstrate such risks factors occasionally develop unexpected lid malposition postoperatively as the process of lid retraction (fibrosis in the plane of the middle lamella) inevitably occurs following skin–muscle flap blepharoplasty, but its extent, which determines the clinical significance of the process, is unpredictable. Use of the five-point operative program described has proven to be valuable in minimizing this undesirable situation.

The five-point operative program for minimizing the incidence of postoperative lower-lid malposition has been described in detail. The cardinal principles of this program are as follows:

1. Recognize the etiology of postblepharoplasty lower-lid malposition.

2. Preserve, when possible, the anatomic components of lower-lid support.

3. Reconstruct/reinforce these elements if they are attenuated or disrupted by surgery.

4. Combat the forces of contracture that inevitably occur postoperatively by judicious injection of triamcinolone in the middle lamellar plane.

Complications

Complications following lower blepharoplasty in the Asian are identical to those following this procedure when performed in the Caucasian eyelid. Although incipient hypertrophic scar formation may be slightly more common in the lateral extension of the infraciliary incision, local massage and occasional injection of triamcinolone provide a solution to this situation. The most debilitating complications of lower blepharoplasty, that is, lower lid retraction and/or ectropion, have been discussed in conjunction with operative techniques that minimize their occurrence. If these complications do develop, the response to standard methods of treatment has the same incidence of success as in the Caucasian lower eyelid.

◆ Conclusion

Although a thorough understanding of pertinent structural and functional anatomy as well as meticulous attention to detail are the keys to success in all facial plastic procedures, they are of particular importance in eyelid surgery, as a multitude of important structures having both aesthetic and functional significance are densely packed into a compact area. Surgical intervention in the eyelid region must be precise and deliberate if the beauty and expressiveness of the eyes are to be preserved or reconstructed, as well as enhanced.

Note

1. In discussions of fixation, I often use the term *levator aponeurosis/tarsus* when referring to the anatomic area in which fixation sutures are placed. Given the contemporary understanding of the mechanism of superior palpebral fold formation, it is apparent that fixation at any point inferior to the preseptal portion of the eyelid will result in creation of a double eyelid. In the Asian eye, the height of the superior tarsus is 5 to 6 mm, and thus tarsal fixation will necessarily produce a palpebral fold close to the ciliary margin. My personal preference (as the formula presented in Table **2–1** recommends that the inferior incision be placed 6–10 mm from the ciliary margin) is to use a supratarsal fixation (i.e., the point of fixation being on the levator aponeurosis). Nevertheless, it is conceptually important to understand that tarsal fixation can be used and, indeed, is recommended by some surgeons.

3

Asian Rhinoplasty

Although some Asian noses, most commonly in patients originating from the central and northern latitudes of Asia, benefit from the classic techniques employed in reduction rhinoplasty, the majority of such noses require an augmentation procedure to achieve maximum aesthetic benefit. The anatomy of these noses is characterized by a broad, flat dorsum with a shallow, depressed origin at the nasion (Fig. **3–1A**). The lobule is generally wide and often exhibits columellar retraction that may be accompanied by alar flaring. Although there are substantial individual variations, lobular skin tends to be thick and well endowed with abundant subcutaneous fibrofatty tissue. Tip projection is frequently deficient, and the lower lateral cartilages are usually thin and attenuated.

Augmentation rhinoplasty is extremely popular in East Asia and is requested with increasing frequency in North America and Europe, as well as in other areas with large Asian populations. Although it might be assumed that this is indicative of a desire for "westernization," it should be noted that in Asian cultures, a high, narrow nasal bridge is an aesthetically desirable feature. Few procedures in facial plastic surgery elicit the controversy that surrounds augmentation rhinoplasty in the Asian nose.

Regardless of whether a nose requires reduction or augmentation, the aesthetic goals of rhinoplasty are the same: creation of a strong, smooth dorsum exhibiting a prominent origin at the nasion but not competing with the tip as the leading point of the nasal profile (Fig. **3–1B**). Ideally, the lobule should be delicate and well defined, with definite columellar "show" and an oblique anteroposterior orientation of the nares. The nasolabial angle varies depending on the height of the individual patient. The characteristics of the ideal nasal lobule are the same regardless of ethnicity (Table **3–1**).

◆ General and Historical Considerations

In spite of the fact that there is agreement on the goals of Asian rhinoplasty, few procedures in facial plastic surgery elicit the controversy that surrounds augmentation rhinoplasty in the Asian nose, largely relating to the polarization of opinion regarding the choice of material best suited to achieve these objectives. This polarization generally follows geographical lines; Asian surgeons generally prefer alloplasts, particularly custom-crafted silicone implants, whereas Western surgeons tend to be more comfortable with augmentation procedures employing autogenous materials. Some academic Asian surgeons have begun to use autogenous materials for tip rhinoplasty (frequently in combination with silicone prosthesis for dorsal augmentation), often employing the external rhinoplasty approach. Although rank-and-file surgeons in the West tend to recognize the benefits of alloplasts, a strong academic bias against the use of alloplastic materials in any segment of the nose persists in Western countries. In the recent past, some influential surgeons have condemned silicone implants with the fervor of a Pentecostal preacher, admonishing that their use in the nose constitutes a cardinal sin of rhinoplasty, obviously ignoring the fact that long-term results using this material in the Asian nose have been excellent. As a result, few Western surgeons who advocate augmentation of the Asian nose with alloplasts have reported their results, and those who dare to submit such reports often assume a deferential, quasi-apologetic

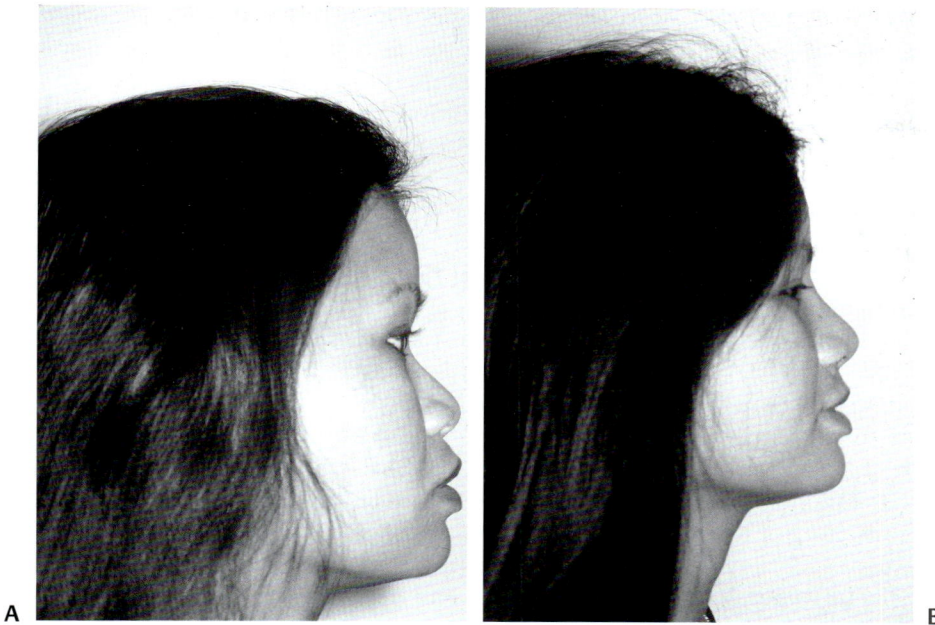

Figure 3–1   (A) The typical Asian nose demonstrating a relatively flat dorsum and sufficient tip projection. **(B)** Following augmentation rhinoplasty, both dorsum and tip show increased projection. Note the improvement in columellar "show" and the "double break" at the junction of the tip defining point and columella.

posture, fearful of being summarily crucified on the altar of fundamental dogma.

Thus, although augmentation with silicone implants remains the "bread and butter" of rhinoplasty in Asia, Western surgeons, historically at least, have forgone the tremendous advantages offered by this material. Recently enlightened surgeons suggest that, although alloplastic material may be satisfactory for augmentation of the dorsum, lobular modification is probably best performed using autogenous materials. Techniques of tip rhinoplasty that are highly successful in the

Caucasian nose are usually unsatisfactory in Asians because the attenuated lower lateral cartilages lack sufficient strength to accentuate tip projection and support, and the overlying skin and subcutaneous tissue are too thick to reflect sculpturing of the delicate cartilage. Thus, if tip projection is to be enhanced, the surgeon generally must reinforce or buttress lobular cartilage with cartilage grafts. Although such techniques often prove satisfactory for lobular enhancement alone, when accompanied by a dorsal alloplast, discontinuity between the dorsum and lobule is all too common, frequently being unapparent until final resolution of postoperative edema or later in the postoperative period. In contrast, continuity between the dorsum and lobule is a major advantage of L-shaped silicone prostheses.

My 27-year surgical experience in augmentation of the Asian nose has convinced me that the consistently superior aesthetics that can be achieved easily using silicone implants are rarely consistently matched by augmentation with other materials (Fig. **1A,B**). This experience, as well as my observation of results produced by other techniques, leads me to the conclusion that for augmentation of the Asian nose, the use of an L-shaped silicone implant is a procedure of choice. A primary goal of this chapter is to provide convincing evidence that this procedure is deserving of serious consideration and respect and is not inherently dangerous, when properly planned and executed, as Western dogma has purported.

Asian craftsmanship, renowned throughout the world, is characterized by pragmatic concern for function along with a keen eye for beauty and symmetry

Table 3–1   Aesthetic Features of the Ideal Nasal Tip

1. The tip should be the anteriormost point in the facial profile (i.e., higher than the dorsum) and accentuated by a slight supratip depression.

2. Dorsal projection from the anterior facial plane should be 30 to 40 degrees.

3. The nasolabial angle should be equal or greater than 90 degrees, depending on the sex and height of the patient.

   a. 90 to 100 degrees in males
   b. 100 to 120 degrees in females

4. The tip should approximate the shape of an equilateral triangle on basal view.

5. The nares should exhibit an oval configuration, with the long axis oriented anteromedially at 45 to 60 degrees.

6. The columella should parallel the alar rim at least 2 mm below the alar margin.

7. The columella should be convex and exhibit a "double break" at the junction of the lobule and columella

coupled with meticulous attention to detail. Augmentation rhinoplasty using silicone implants has been developed and refined by conscientious, experienced, and well-trained Asian surgeons. Irrational criticism of this material as inherently dangerous or unreliable is disrespectful to the accomplishments and experience of our Asian colleagues. Consider that (1) augmentation with silicone implants dwarfs the use of other materials in Asia and (2) the majority of complications following any cosmetic nasal operation, including augmentation with alloplastic prostheses, are related to technical or judgmental error.

The challenge in augmentation rhinoplasty employing silicone implants is the same as for all surgery: formulation of a surgical approach that minimizes potential problems. Such an approach to augmentation rhinoplasty rests upon a foundation consisting of three key pillars: (1) the surgical technique per se, (2) design and fabrication of the implant, and (3) postoperative follow-up enlisting the patient as a partner.

In planning a recent presentation for an Asian audience, it occurred to me that a fourth pillar of the foundation for success relates to the surgeon's conception of the operative goals. In the West, rhinoplasty is taught as a progressive series of steps, by far the most important of which is modification of the nasal lobule. Young surgeons are taught to first fix the position or projection of the tip and then alter the dorsum to complement tip position. Inadequate or excessive surgical manipulation of the lobule constitutes a virtual "kiss of death" for the entire rhinoplasty procedure. Surgery of the dorsum, in contrast, is relegated to the back burner, being virtually an afterthought, consisting of a mundane series of maneuvers that are relatively easy and forgiving of all but the most glaring of errors.

When, however, a Western surgeon conceives of augmentation of the Asian nose, his or her primary consideration is modification of the dorsum, lobular aesthetics playing a secondary role. Early versions of dorsal prostheses produced in the West provide graphic evidence of this observation. Attempts to refine and sculpture the lobule with conventional Western tip rhinoplasty techniques rarely bear fruit as a consequence of the anatomy of the Asian lower lateral cartilages, a fact that contributes to the relative neglect of this area.

I attribute whatever success I have achieved in performing and teaching augmentation rhinoplasty in the Asian nose largely to my persistence in retaining the Western concept of modification and enhancement of the lobule as a primary goal of this procedure, just as I do when performing reduction rhinoplasty.

A collateral benefit of this mindset is the additional margin of safety provided by virtue of the fact that the physical limitations of lobular augmentation are easily visualized intraoperatively if this area is the surgeon's primary focus. If the primary goal is dorsal augmentation, there is a temptation to "fit" the lobule to a more aggressively modified dorsum, a prescription for disaster, as lobular augmentation is the weak link of this procedure.

◆ A Personal Odyssey

A brief historical narrative describing the process by which my current approach to this operation developed may prove to be instructive.

During my residency training from 1973 to 1976, I operated on only an occasional Asian nose, for which augmentation involved autogenous cartilage (nasal septum and conchal cartilage). At times, complications of alloplastic augmentation were presented in our clinics, and we listened and believed admonitions against the use of alloplasts in the nose.

Between 1976 and 1979, I served at the Tripler Army Medical Center in Honolulu, Hawaii, and performed Asian augmentation rhinoplasties initially using autogenous cartilage; during the latter stages of this assignment, I began to use Mersilene mesh (polyethylene terephthalate) for augmentation of the nasal dorsum. Lobular sculpturing during this time was attempted using the basic techniques of tip surgery, but the results tended to be unimpressive. During this period, I developed a relatively large practice in Asian blepharoplasty, but this did not translate into an increased number of patients requesting nasal augmentation.

In 1979 I entered private practice and again utilized autogenous cartilage and Mersilene along with standard tip rhinoplasty techniques. Although my practice in Asian blepharoplasty blossomed, there was not, to my surprise, a concomitant increase in the number of patients requesting augmentation rhinoplasty. Prominent surgeons serving as panelists at national meetings during this time continued to equate the use of alloplastic material for augmentation of the nose with malpractice.

By 1981 it finally occurred to me that the reason my practice of augmentation rhinoplasty was stagnating was that my Asian patients were underwhelmed by the results that I achieved with the techniques that I used. Even though I was reasonably satisfied with the results, my patients, although rarely complaining overtly, did not share my enthusiasm. During my residency training and first 2 years of private practice, I had encountered numerous patients who had undergone previous augmentation with alloplastic material; most were very pleased with the results. I realized that if I were to be successful, that I must change my thinking and learn the safe and proper use of silicone prostheses for

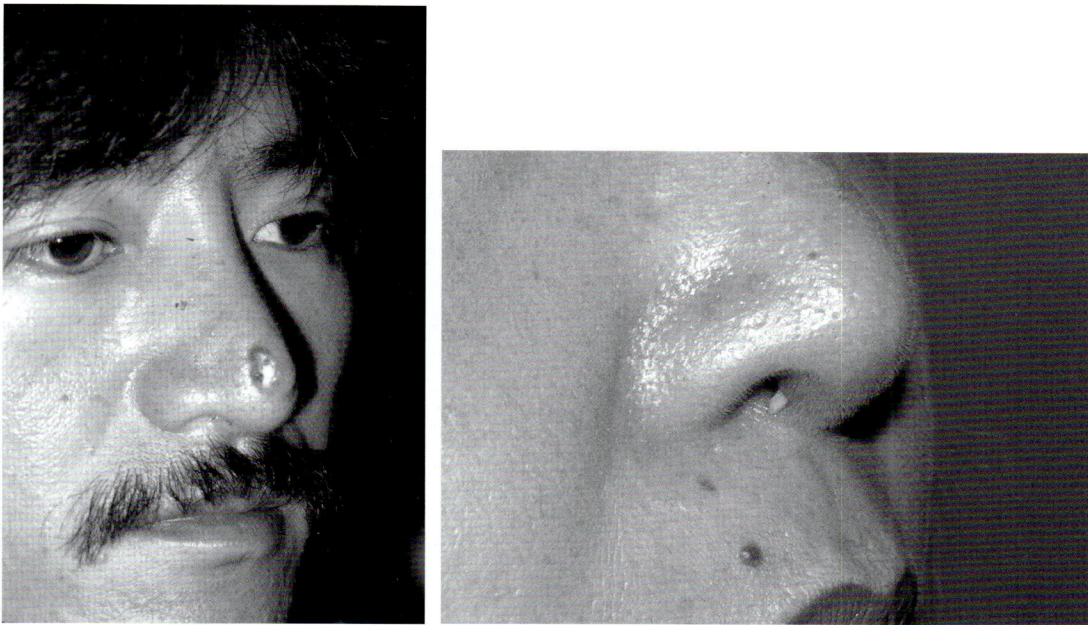

Figure 3–2 **(A)** Extrusion of a silicone prosthesis through the lobule. **(B)** Exposure of an implant via the columella.

augmentation rhinoplasty. My results did improve, and my practice of Asian augmentation rhinoplasty increased dramatically.

Looking back over this experience, I realize that the results achieved using autogenous cartilage and mesh were suboptimal because of the failure of standard techniques of lobular surgery to improve tip aesthetics. As I gained more experience with silicone prostheses, I realized that the ability of an L-shaped silicone prosthesis to sculpture the lobule as well as augment the dorsum in continuity with the lobule was the reason for improved aesthetic results, and that focusing on augmentation of the dorsum in the Asian nose rather than on improved lobular aesthetics led to inferior results. Use of an L-shaped prosthesis allowed for the shifting of my primary focus in augmentation rhinoplasty to enhancement of the lobule, just as it had for Caucasian rhinoplasty, relegating dorsal augmentation as a procedure that must complement, not overwhelm, lobular enhancement.

◆ Why Are Silicone Implants Held in Disrepute?

Before building the case for silicone implants as a procedure of choice in augmentation of the Asian nose, it is helpful to explore the reasons why silicone implants are held in such disrepute in the West. It is difficult to dispel the negative impressions engendered by photographs showing extrusion, most commonly in the lobular region, of alloplastic implants. In contemporary augmentation rhinoplasty, this situation is extremely rare. Most cases of implant exposure occur in the columella and are preceded by warning signs that allow early prophylactic intervention (Fig. **3–2A,B**).

The poor results of augmentation using a dorsal prosthesis fabricated by Western companies (Fig. **3–3**) have undoubtedly contributed to the poor impression of silicone implants. In addition, early Asian prostheses tended to be poorly designed, generally being excessive in size and constructed of firm elastomer. Another factor contributing to the notoriety of silicone implants has

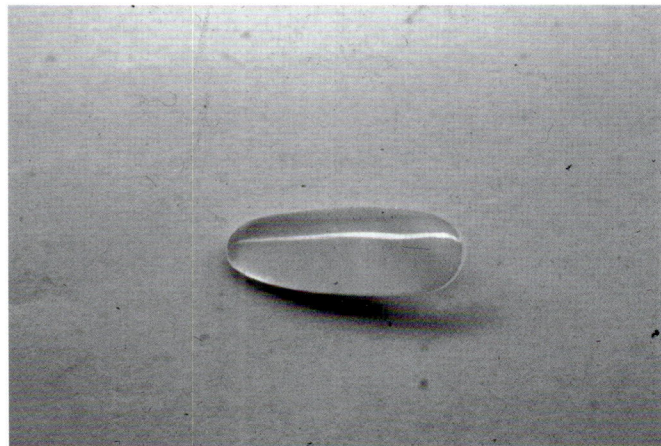

Figure 3–3 Dorsal silicone prosthesis manufactured in the West, circa 1978.

been the occasionally horrifying results of liquid silicone and paraffin injections, which, in the past, were common in Asia. It must be stressed that the reasons for historical disrepute are no longer valid because of advances in materials, surgical technique, and understanding of the dynamics of augmentation rhinoplasty.

◆ Choosing Prosthesis Material

All surgeons will agree that multiple factors are important in the choice of a material for augmentation rhinoplasty. Among these factors are the reliability, reproducibility, and precision of results, as well as the morbidity and complication rate, one measure of which is the incidence of revision surgery. Cost effectiveness is another consideration, as is patient satisfaction following augmentation. An L-shaped silicone prosthesis properly fabricated and placed with meticulous attention to technical detail rates an A+ in all of these categories.

◆ Formulating an Approach to Augmentation Rhinoplasty

Formulation of an approach to augmentation rhinoplasty employing silicone prostheses rests on four key pillars: (1) implant design, (2) surgical technique, (3) postoperative follow-up enlisting the patient as a postoperative partner, and (4) focusing on creation of superior lobular aesthetics rather than dorsal augmentation as the primary goal of the procedure. My goal is to present a detailed blueprint for planning and executing operations using an L-shaped silicone prosthesis.

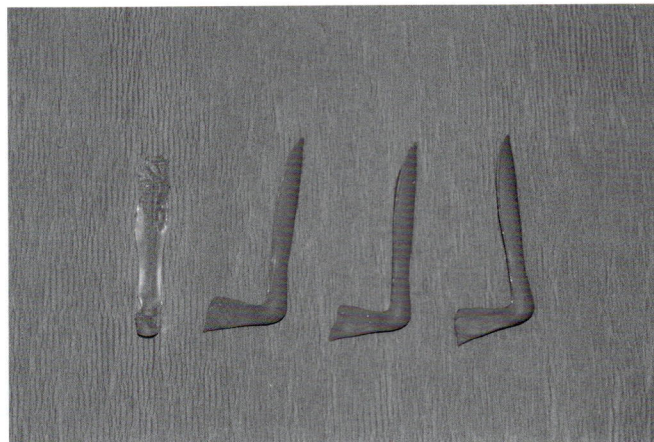

Figure 3–4   L-shaped silicone prostheses.

Implant Design

See DVD Disk Two, Nasal Implant Selection

The silicone implant that I designed (Table **3–2**) and currently use consists of three segments, each having distinct characteristics and functions: a dorsal component, a lobular component, and a columellar strut (Fig. **3–4**). All three components are made of soft silicone elastomer, of particular importance in that softness and flexibility (Fig. **3–5**) translate into diminished pressure at the tissue–prosthesis interface, resulting in less stress on the overlying skin. Historically, the first generation of silicone nasal implants designed in Asia were fabricated from hard elastomer and tended to be of excessive size, factors that contributed to complications, most notably implant exposure.

The soft, flexible dorsal component has a groove on its posterior surface that allows apposition to the dorsum. All edges are tapered to facilitate inconspicuous blending, thus minimizing prosthesis palpability or visibility.

Table 3–2   Design of L-shaped Silicone Implant

1. Dorsal component
  a. Soft, flexible: translates into decreased pressure at tissue–prosthesis interface
  b. Groove for apposition to dorsum
  c. Tapered edges to minimize palpability/visibility

2. Lobular component
  a. Soft, smooth
  b. Broad (not sharp or pointed)
  c. Projection 2 mm greater than that of dorsum
  d. Cantilever action

3. Columellar strut
  a. Inferior inclination to maximize columella sculpturing
  b. Broad, posterior flare for stabilization between caudal septum and columellar skin
  c. Soft, flexible

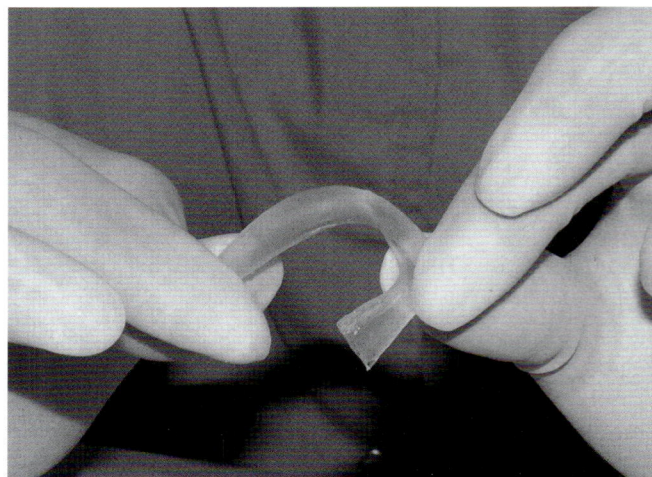

Figure 3–5   The flexibility of the soft L-shaped prosthesis is demonstrated.

The soft lobular component is smooth and broad (as opposed to narrow and pointed), a configuration designed to minimize and diffuse pressure on the overlying lobular skin. Anterior projection of the lobular component is 2 mm greater than that of the dorsal component. The final relative projection of these two components is adjusted on an individual basis by intraoperative sculpting of the prosthesis. Lobular projection is achieved by a cantilever mechanism of the combined dorsal and lobular components rather than by a tentpole mechanism involving the columellar strut.

The most misunderstood component of the L-shaped nasal implant is the columellar strut (Table **3–3**). Perhaps because surgeons who use struts of autogenous material teach that postoperative lobular position is a function of the thrusting action of these struts, it is assumed that the alloplastic strut functions in a similar manner. Utilization of the strut as a tent pole to increase tip projection, however, is a prescription for disaster.

In actuality, the columellar strut has two functions. First, it stabilizes the proximal (lobular) segment of the implant in the midline, thus providing resistance against displacement and malposition. Second, the strut allows sculpturing of the columella by displacing the characteristically retracted columella of the Asian nose inferiorly, thus increasing its show. An understanding of these two functions of the columellar strut allows the surgeon to resist any temptation to extend the strut the full length of the columella, thereby producing an undesirable "tent-pole" effect, because to perform its functions, the columella strut need extend only 50 to 75% of the columellar length.

In earlier years, I believed that a columellar strut fabricated from firm elastomer was best, as it could be relatively short and thin because of the resistance of the firm elastomer to deformation. This belief, however, proved to be erroneous because contraction of the fibrous capsule that naturally forms around the prosthesis often exerts a rotational force that occasionally results in displacement of the strut laterally. Pressure from such displacement may result in perforation in the vestibular aspect of the columella, that is, the site of the incision, by far the most common site of implant exposure. The rotational forces are less likely to be effectively transmitted to a columellar strut fabricated from soft elastomer because of the flexibility at the lobular-columellar junction of the implant. This flexibility, however, will result in superior displacement of the strut (by columellar tension) unless the strut has sufficient breadth to allow it to be wedged between the caudal septum and columellar skin/medial crura. Intraoperatively, the flared strut is carefully trimmed so that it fits gently between the medial crura and caudal septum at the most anterior point that allows aesthetically sufficient inferior displacement of the columella (producing columellar show). The inferior inclination (angulation) of the columellar strut with respect to the dorsal component assists in achieving this goal. Other commercially available nasal implants are constructed so that the columellar strut projects at a 90-degree angle from the dorsal component, a situation that renders the strut virtually useless in producing columellar show and reinforces the improper notion that the strut is of value for increasing tip projection.

It cannot be overemphasized that after final trimming, the columellar strut never extends posteriorly for a distance of greater than 75% of the length of the columella. Allowing the strut to contact the nasal spine and/or maxilla results in a "tent-pole" effect—an invitation to disaster in the form of implant extrusion secondary to pressure necrosis of the lobular skin. It cannot be stressed enough that the function of the strut is not to project the lobule; lobular projection is achieved by the cantilever effect of the rounded, slightly elevated lobular and contiguous dorsal segment in a fashion analogous to the cantilever action of bone grafts utilized for total nasal reconstruction.

Because of complaints that clear silicone implants may be visible through the nasal skin under bright indoor lighting, an implant of a neutral color (e.g., beige or flesh toned) should be considered, especially if the patient is fair complexioned.

Table 3–3 Functions of the Columellar Strut*

1. Midline stabilization of proximal implant
   a. Distal stabilization provided by groove for apposition to dorsum and periosteal growth around implant
2. Columellar sculpturing
   a. Inferior inclination of strut displaces columella, enhancing columellar "show."
   b. Posterior flare allows stabilization between the septum and columella.
   c. Flexibility combats rotational displacement by capsular contracture.

*The columellar strut does not project the tip in a tent-pole fashion; it does not extend to the nasal spine, extending only ~50% of the columellar length.

Surgical Technique

See DVD Disk Two, Alloplastic Augmentation Rhinoplasty

Preoperative Considerations

Of major importance in preoperative evaluation is detection of factors that may be relative or absolute contraindications to the use of alloplastic material. Such factors include thin nasal skin, the presence of a substantial dorsal convexity, and, importantly, an acute nasolabial angle (i.e., a "plunging" tip), a condition the correction of which is difficult to accomplish with an L-shaped implant. Another important "red flag" is diminished tissue elasticity, perhaps the most frequent cause of which is previous nasal surgery. All surgeons, particularly those who are inexperienced in the use of alloplasts, must realize that use of a silicone implant in such situations involves "pushing the envelope"—a judgmental factor that predisposes to unsatisfactory results and complications.

Interestingly, nasal obstruction resulting from septal deviation is extremely uncommon in the Asian patient requesting augmentation rhinoplasty. Obstruction as a consequence of turbinate dysfunction or hypertrophy, however, approximates the incidence of this condition in Caucasian patients.

It is of utmost importance that candidates for augmentation rhinoplasty completely and carefully communicate the specifics of the nasal transformation that is desired. Many Asian patients assume that the surgeon knows best and will automatically construct a nose to their exact specifications. If communication between patient and surgeon is unclear or imprecise, disappointment may ensue regarding matters such as dorsal height and contour, lobular configuration, and tip projection. It should be stressed to the patient that the surgeon cannot promise to construct a nose to exact specifications.

In previous times, most surgeons assumed that Asian patients requesting augmentation rhinoplasty desired as much enlargement as possible to achieve a Western look. In contemporary practice, however, most Asian patients do not desire westernization, but more subtle augmentation. A common request in 21st-century Asian rhinoplasty is "Please don't make my nose too high; I want it to match my Asian face!" This is a fortunate attitude in that the desire for conservative augmentation is a major ally in the quest for safety when using alloplastic materials. As emphasized previously, a focus on lobular aesthetics as the primary goal of the procedure reinforces intraoperative conservatism.

Surgical Approach

Augmentation rhinoplasty is most commonly performed under local anesthesia in an office operating suite or other outpatient facility. An oral cephalosporin or its equivalent is begun on the evening prior to surgery, and antibiotic prophylaxis is continued for 3 days postoperatively.

Preparation of the nasal vestibule is performed in the usual manner, and the vestibule is scrubbed with 5% povidone-iodine solution prior to sedation and local anesthetic infiltration.

1. Access to the dorsum and lobule is obtained via a marginal incision (i.e., an incision along the inferior

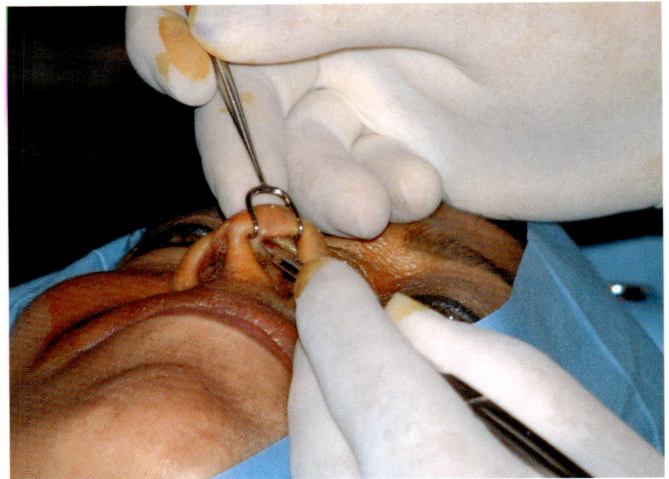

Figure 3–6   Access to the nasal lobule and dorsum is gained via a marginal incision.

border of the lower lateral cartilage, not a rim incision as recommended by many Asian surgeons) that extends into the superior half of the columella (Fig. **3–6**). Dissection of a precise subcutaneous midline pocket is facilitated by initiating the dissection via the columellar aspect of the incision (Fig. **3–7**). The lower lateral cartilages are freed from the lobular skin but are not otherwise modified, as the implant will rest on their anterior surfaces. Dissection of an ample pocket is performed in the lobular region, but the pocket becomes more glovelike (yet of sufficient volume to avoid tension) over the dorsum. There is a natural tendency for a right-handed surgeon to underdissect the lobular portion of the pocket on the right side (and vice versa for a left-handed surgeon); the surgeon must be aware of this situation and modify the dissection accordingly.

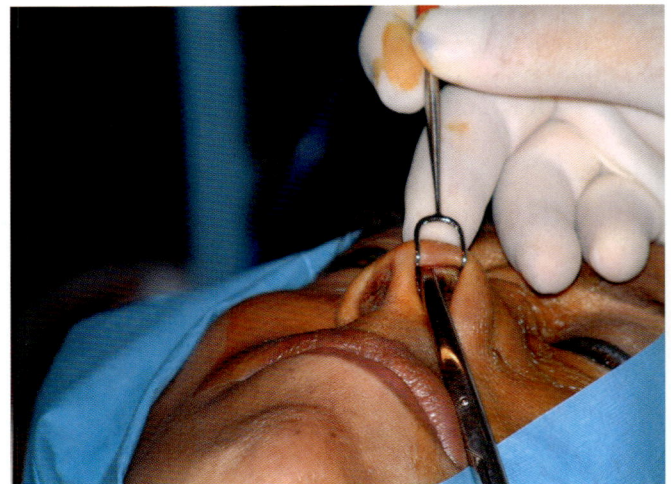

Figure 3–7   The dissection is initiated via the columellar aspect of the incision to ensure that pocket preparation is in the midline.

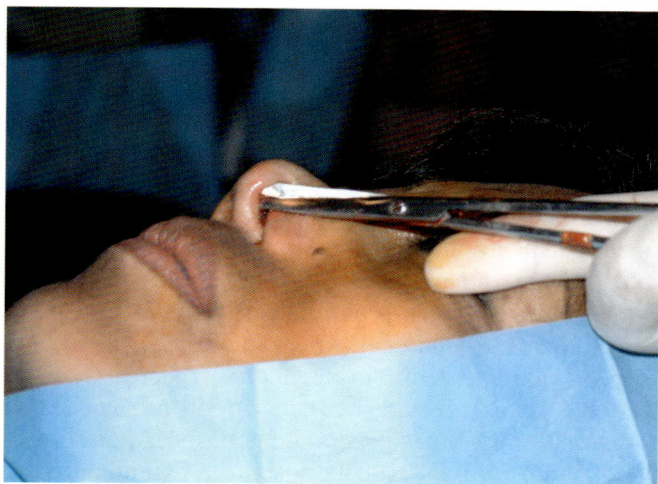

Figure 3–8 The scissors are rotated inferiorly to dissect a columellar pocket that is continuous with the dorsal pocket.

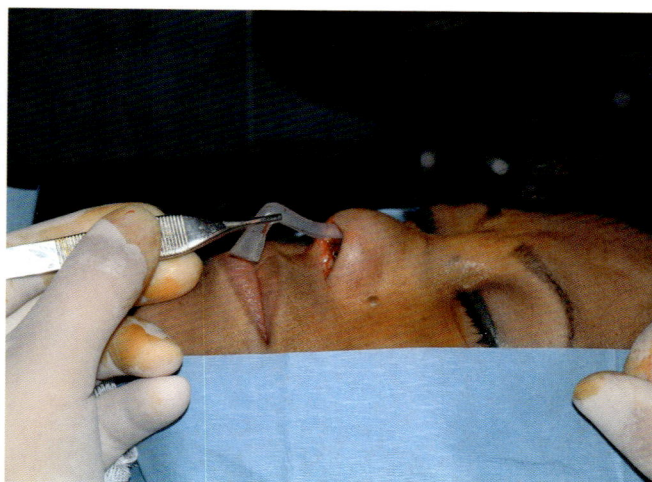

Figure 3–10 Insertion of the dorsal component of the prosthesis.

2. After undermining the skin of the lobule and dorsum, the tips of the scissors are directed into the columella, where a pocket continuous with the dorsal pocket is dissected between the medial crura for placement of the columellar segment of the prosthesis (Fig. **3–8**).

3. Following dissection of the subcutaneous pocket, the periosteum is shredded with a blunt scissors to encourage its growth around the implant, thus assisting in stabilization of the prosthesis (Fig. **3–9**).

4. After completing the pocket dissection, an L-shaped implant is inserted (Fig. **3–10**). The prosthesis is not premeasured but individually tailored at the time of surgery. This task is accomplished by observing the effect of the prosthesis, then removing it for sculpturing according to the requirements of each individual patient. Implant insertion, observation,

removal, and resculpturing are repeated as many times as is necessary to achieve the desired aesthetic result. During sculpturing, it is important to maintain the broad configuration of the lobular component, that is, avoid making it too narrow or pointed, and to taper the edges of the implant as needed, avoiding sharp projections.

The distal (glabellar) end of the prosthesis terminates at a point approximately halfway between the infrabrow and intercanthal lines and should be sculptured to blend inconspicuously with the nasion while preserving the nasofrontal angle.

If the surgeon experiences difficulty freeing both lower lateral cartilages via a single marginal incision, a corresponding incision should be made on the opposite side to facilitate proper pocket preparation required for symmetry of the implant in the lobular region. If resistance is encountered over the dorsum upon placement of the implant, the pocket is too small and should be enlarged to prevent tension on the nasal skin. If a small dorsal hump is present, it is generally easier to rasp the dorsum than to modify the implant to accommodate the hump.

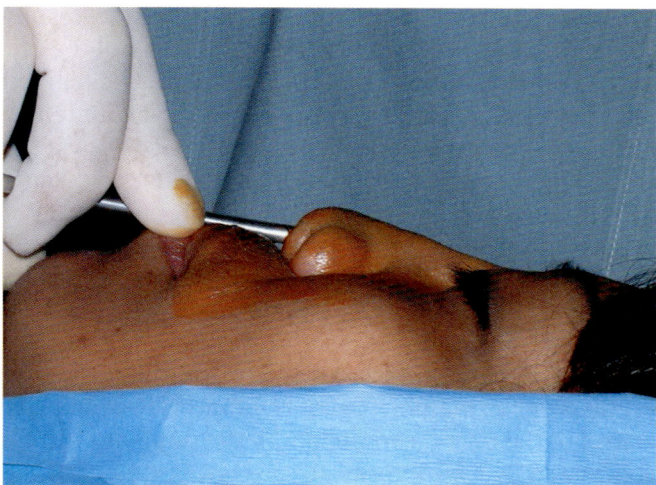

Figure 3–9 Blunt-tip scissors are used to shred the periosteum of the nasal dorsum.

5. Following placement of the dorsal and lobular components, the columellar strut is coaxed into the columellar portion of the pocket with forceps (Fig. **3–11**). The strut is trimmed prior to the first implant insertion, and further sculpturing is undertaken as required. Care must be taken to ensure that the strut does not contact the nasal spine or maxilla and that in producing columellar show, the columellar skin is under no tension.

6. The marginal incision is closed with two sutures of 5–0 chromic. Prior to suture placement, columellar

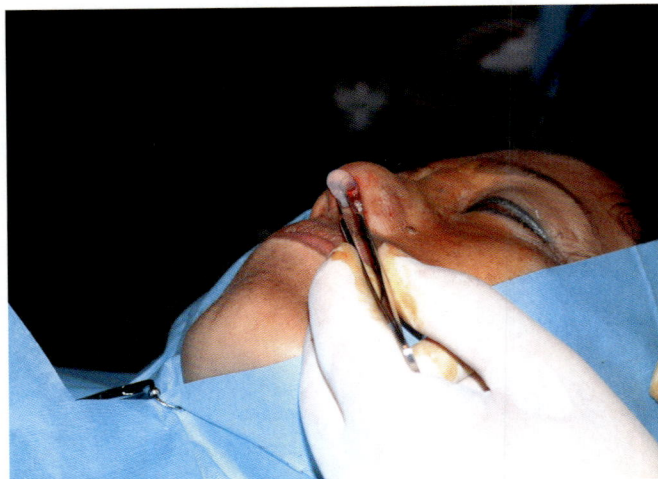

Figure 3–11   Insertion of the columellar strut using forceps.

tissue and the lobular portion of the flap are mobilized to ensure that the closure is free of tension. Antibiotic ointment is placed over the incision, and the nostril is occluded with a small piece of cotton that is removed on the first postoperative day. An external tape dressing is then applied and left in place for 5 to 7 days.

Pre- and postoperative photographs showing the results of augmentation rhinoplasty with L-shaped silicone prostheses are presented in Figs. **3–12** through **3–15**.

Ancillary Procedures

On occasion, a bulbous lobule may benefit from reduction in addition to placement of the nasal implant. Debulking is best performed via cartilage-splitting incisions prior to creation of the pocket for implant placement. Care is taken to preserve subcutaneous fibrofatty tissue on the skin under which the prosthesis will be placed, and the cartilage-splitting incisions are closed prior to initiation of the marginal incision for pocket creation.

Alar base reduction procedures are indicated in only 5 to 10% of my patients undergoing nasal augmentation. (A detailed discussion of this procedure is presented in a subsequent section.) The effect of the augmentation procedure on the lobule often renders what preoperatively may have appeared to be wide alae to be in harmony with the augmented nose.

Rarely, a patient benefits from lateral osteotomies in conjunction with nasal augmentation. If indicated, osteotomies are performed via a pyriform rim incision following implant placement and wound closure.

Complications

Long-term results of augmentation rhinoplasty in the Asian nose using silicone implants have been excellent

in spite of the admonitions of Western surgeons that alloplastic implants and the nasal dorsum are doomed to failure. In actuality, complications such as infection and displacement or extrusion of the implant are substantially lower than might be expected on the basis of experience with augmentation of the Caucasian nose with solid implants. The reason for increased tolerance of alloplastic implants in the Asian nose is unknown but may be related to a greater thickness of skin and subcutaneous tissue in this population as well as to the experience and technical expertise of the surgeon performing the operation. It has been suggested that the five soft tissue layers of the scalp (identified by the initialism SCALP [Skin, subCutaneous tissue, Aponeurosis salea, Loose areolar tissue, Periosteum]) extend onto the nasal bones and that all of these five tissue layers are more substantial in the Asian than in the Caucasian nose, providing protection and camouflage of alloplastic material. Most serious complications of augmentation rhinoplasty in the Asian nose are, in fact, a consequence of judgmental or technical error during surgery. A notable exception is infection that occurs late in the postoperative period.

Implant Malposition

Malposition of the prosthesis is the most common complication following augmentation rhinoplasty with alloplastic material (Fig. **3–16**). This generally occurs as a consequence of improper placement of the prosthesis because of imprecise pocket dissection. Although malposition is more common in the distal region of the implant, it can also occur in the lobular region. Symmetrical pocket preparation is technically more difficult in the lobular region (because of skin adherence to the lower lateral cartilages) than over the bony dorsum. Right-handed surgeons most commonly fail to perform adequate lobular undermining on the right side, resulting in displacement of the lobular component of the implant to the left, the converse being true for left-handed operators. Adequate pocket preparation is facilitated by beginning the dissection precisely in the midline via the columellar aspect of the marginal incision, displacing the superior aspect of the columella laterally with the scissor handles so as to ensure a midline position. Following preparation of the distal aspect of the pocket, care is taken to ensure that the lobular skin is elevated symmetrically over both lower lateral cartilages.

Maladaption of the implant to the nasal dorsum predisposes to malposition or asymmetry. The inferior aspect of the dorsal component of the implant must be concave so that it conforms to the convex surface of the dorsum. Incorporation of the columellar strut into a precise columellar pocket helps ensure that the prosthesis

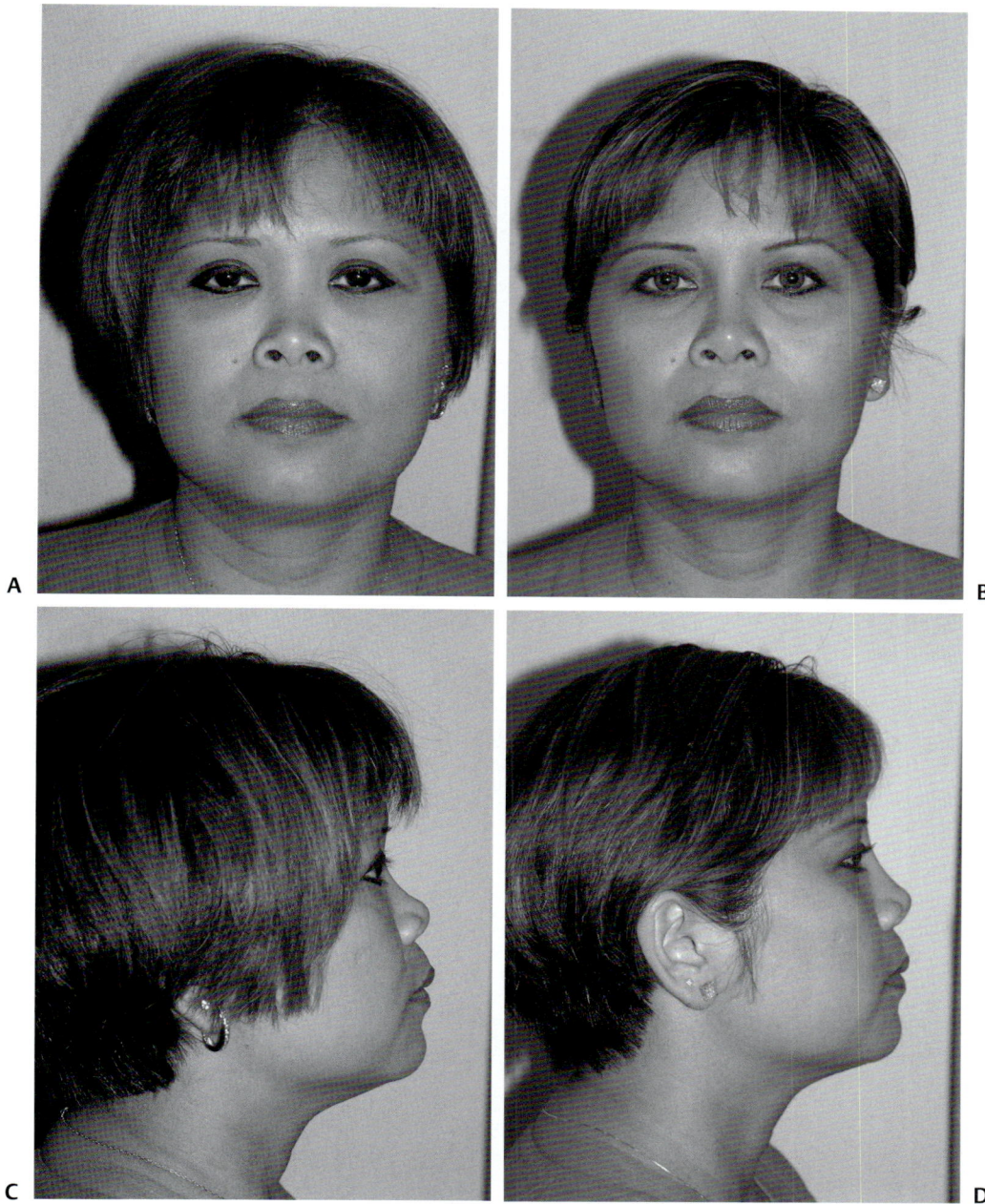

Figure 3–12   (A–D) Pre- and postoperative results of an augmentation rhinoplasty using an L-shaped silicone implant.

remains in the midline of the lobular region, stabilizing its proximal aspect.

Provision for adequate fixation of the implant lowers the incidence of malposition (as well as the incidence of late extrusion). Perhaps the most important aspect of distal prosthesis fixation is shredding of the periosteum, encouraging this tissue to encapsulate the implant during the healing process. A common misconception is that the skin undermining should only be sufficient to allow a glovelike adaptation of the skin over the implant. In actuality, skin undermining should be wide, ensuring an adequate pocket with no tension whatsoever on the

prosthesis. Thus, skin tension around the implant cannot provide accurate and predictable stabilization, notwithstanding the fact that allowing skin tension around an alloplastic prosthesis is contraindicated.

The combination of a concave posterior implant surface allowing adaptation of the prosthesis to the bony dorsum and subsequent periosteal fixation secures the implant distally, and placement of the columellar strut into an accurately dissected columellar pocket provides proximal stabilization. A popular misconception is that perforating the implant with multiple holes to allow tissue ingrowth improves stabilization. If periosteal

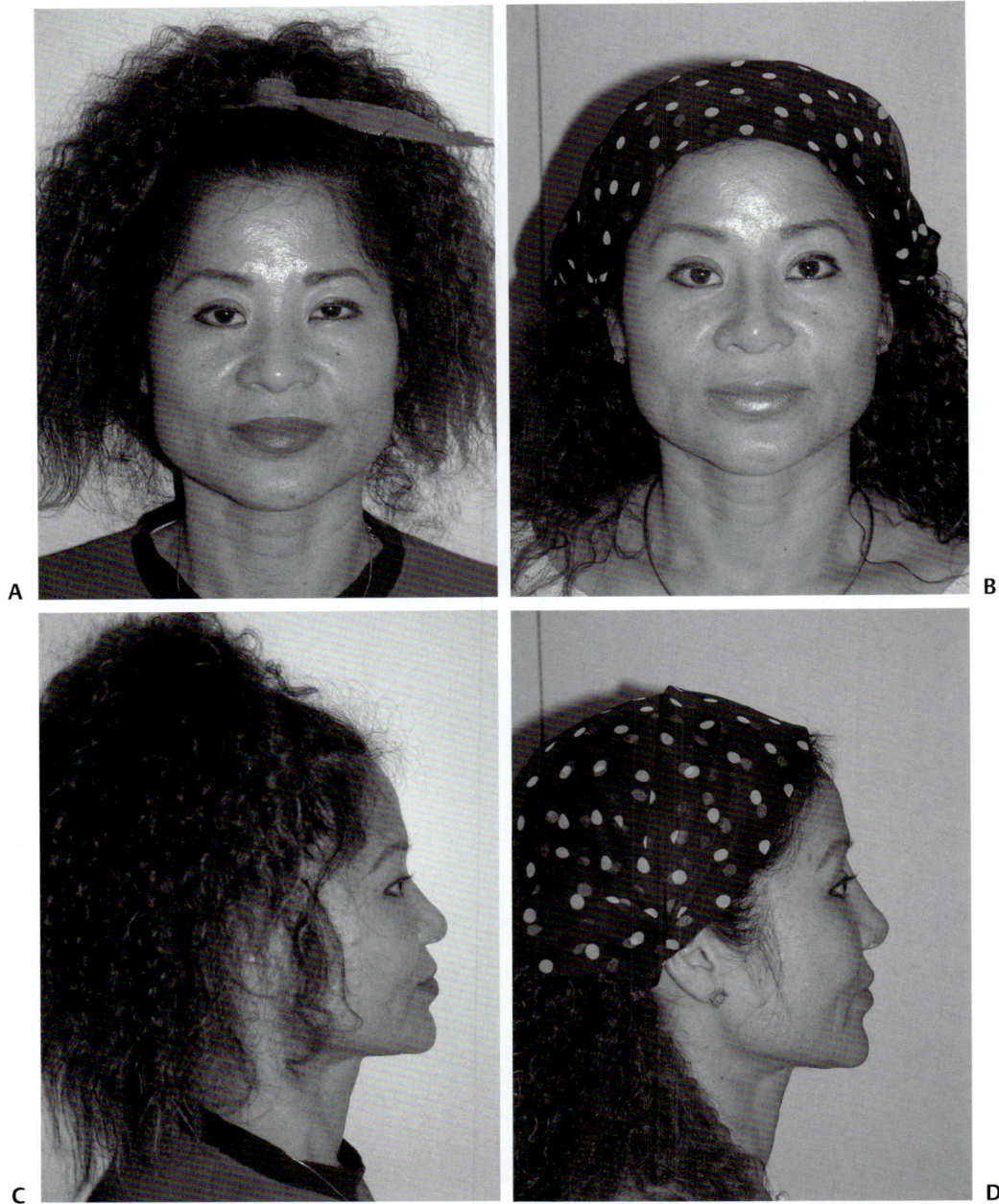

Figure 3–13   (A–D) Pre- and postoperative results of an augmentation rhinoplasty using an L-shaped silicone implant.

elevation is not also performed, the prosthesis may re-main mobile even following tissue ingrowth into the perforations. If proper periosteal shredding is per-formed, it is unnecessary to perforate the implant to en-sure stability.

Occasionally, despite apparently proper pocket preparation, slight asymmetry of the implant may occur in the early postoperative period. This situation may be a consequence of edema. Displacement occurring after resolution of acute edema may be related to prosthesis displacement by unequal scar contraction, as commonly occurs around chin implants.

If prosthesis malposition develops during the first several postoperative weeks, digital displacement maneuvers, perhaps combined with taping of the im-plant in the desired position, may serve to modify the capsular contracture process sufficiently to preserve midline position. If malposition persists, however, correction can only be effected by removal, pocket correction, and replacement of the implant.

Infection

Infection is a relatively infrequent occurrence follow-ing augmentation rhinoplasty, having an incidence

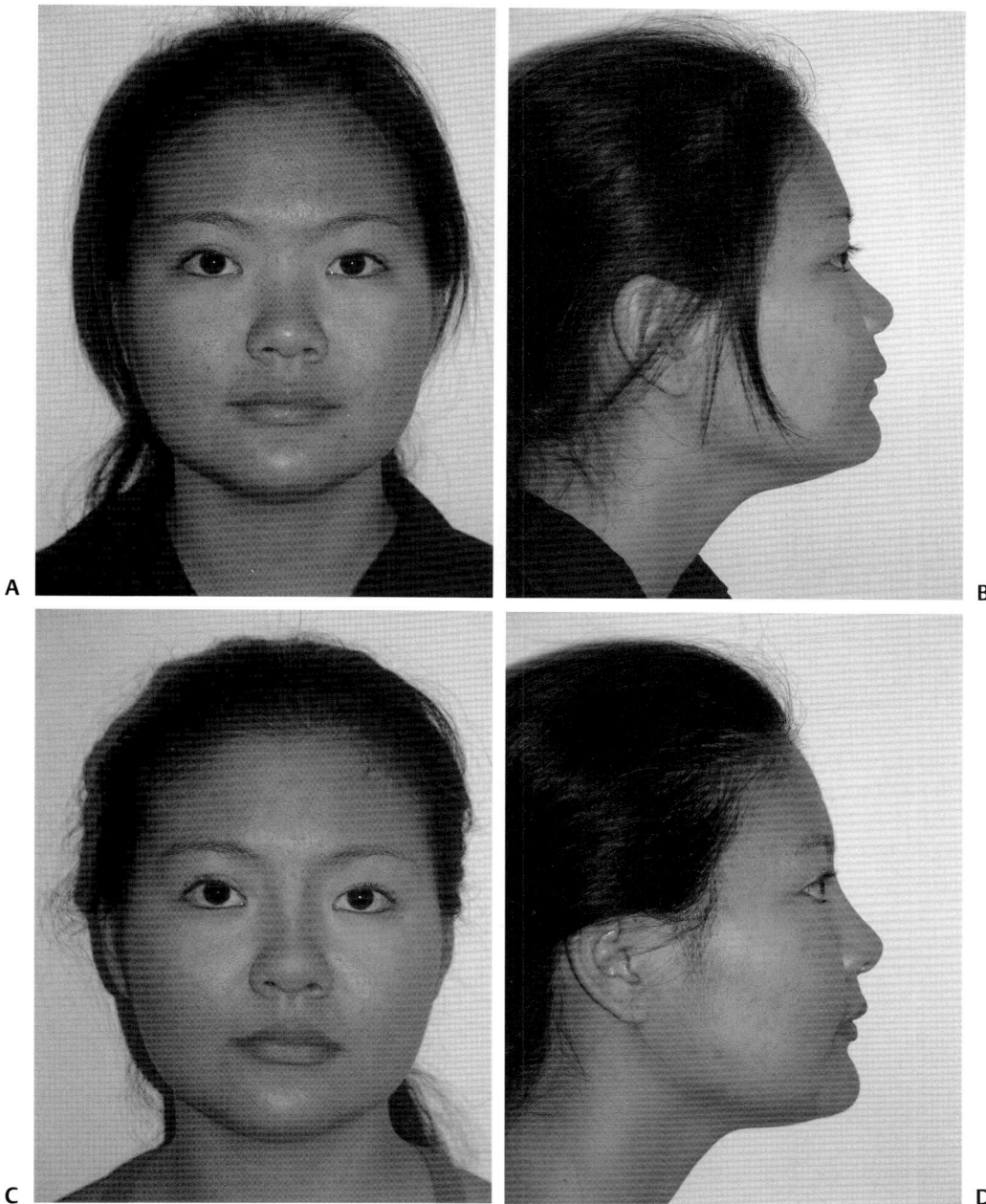

Figure 3–14 **(A–D)** Pre- and postoperative results of an augmentation rhinoplasty using an L-shaped silicone implant.

approximating 1 to 2%. To minimize the possibility of infection, routine use of prophylactic antibiotics, beginning 12 hours prior to surgery and continuing 72 hours thereafter, is recommended. Careful attention to the preparation of the nasal vestibule (i.e., trimming of the vibrissae and cleaning the vestibule and face with a surgical antiseptic prior to anesthetic infiltration) is of obvious importance. Irrigation of the pocket with povidone-iodine solution prior to implant placement may be of benefit. Meticulous closure of the nasal incision and application of antibiotic ointment or cream

to the incision site for 5 days postoperatively are routine.

Purulent infection requires immediate removal of the prosthesis (Fig. **3–17A,B**). If detected early in the stage of cellulitis, antibiotic therapy without implant removal is occasionally successful, but in most cases the prosthesis must be removed. Although purulence may appear to respond to antibiotic therapy, the infection generally remanifests itself within days of termination of antibiotic treatment, necessitating prosthesis removal. The infection then resolves rapidly, and replacement of the implant can be undertaken.

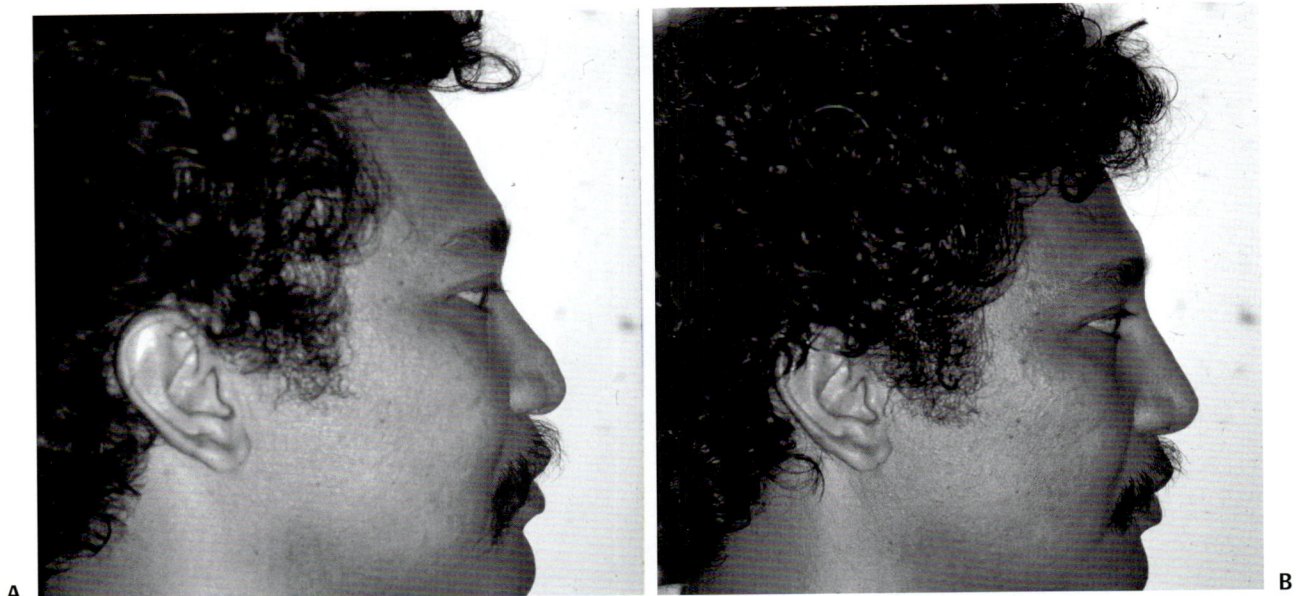

Figure 3–15 **(A,B)** Pre- and postoperative results of an augmentation rhinoplasty using an L-shaped silicone implant.

Although many surgeons recommend deferring revision surgery for 3 to 6 months, if the expanded skin in the lobular region is not supported within several weeks of implant removal, contraction will commence, often resulting in a surface dimple that is difficult to efface (Fig. **3–18**). In such cases, reaugmentation in the lobular region is best achieved with autogenous cartilage.

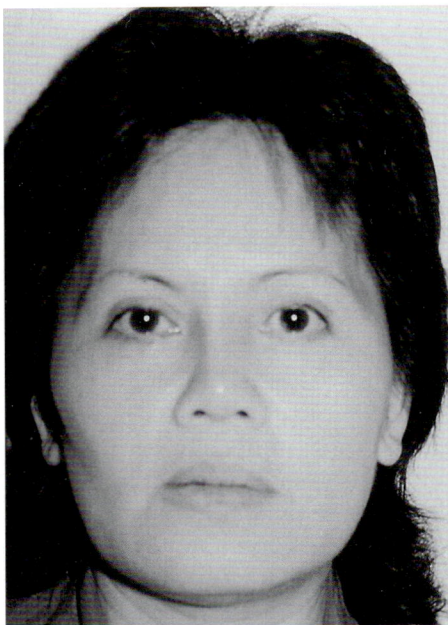

Figure 3–16 A "crooked" nose resulting from implant malposition.

Occasionally, infection of a nasal prosthesis develops months or years after surgery. The etiology of this condition is often difficult to determine, but it may be associated with antecedent skin or vestibular inflammation. Again, if the infectious process is detected at an early stage, prompt institution of antibiotic therapy may salvage the situation, but if abscess formation occurs, the implant must be removed and reaugmentation performed at a later time. Abscesses may occasionally appear in any area along the implant surface. If abscess formation occurs in the lobular region, a postremoval depressed scar (Fig. **3–18**) is likely to result. In such cases, it is important to perform reaugmentation as early as possible to minimize deformity caused by contraction of the injured dermis. Details of the reaugmentation procedure are discussed in this chapter.

Extrusion

Delayed extrusion is the most worrisome and devastating complication of alloplastic augmentation rhinoplasty in the Asian nose. The incidence of this complication is extremely low in contemporary practice (less than 1% in large series reported from both Korea and Japan), and is generally a consequence of technical or judgmental error. Perhaps the most common reason for delayed extrusion is excessive tension in the lobular region secondary to ill-conceived attempts to enhance tip projection with a columellar strut. Implant exposure is actually reduced by a properly prepared and

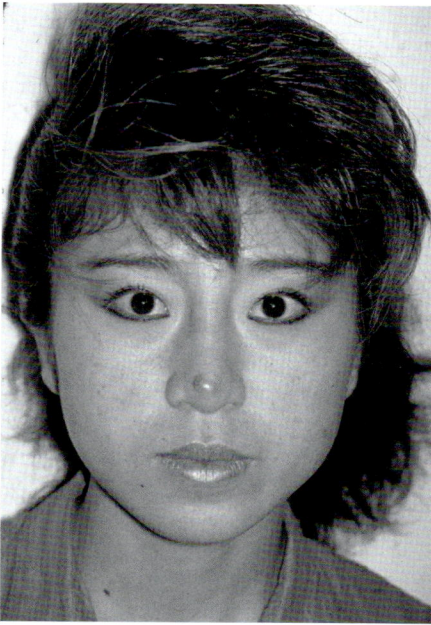

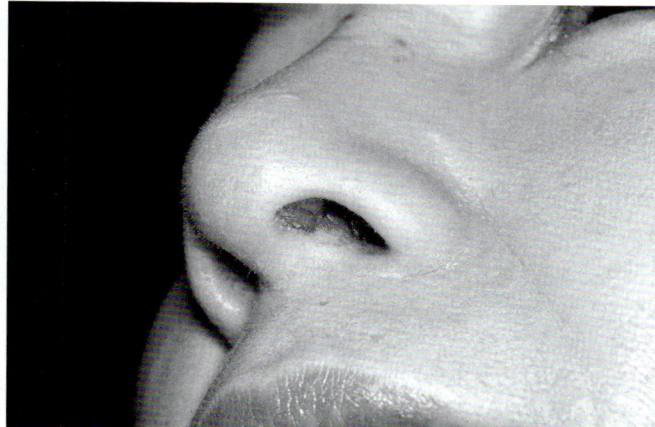

Figure 3–17   **(A)** An abscess formation around the silicone implant arising in the lobular region. **(B)** Abscess formation around the silicone prosthesis visible in the columellar region.

positioned columellar strut, as it reduces mobility of the proximal portion of the implant. By far the most common location of implant exposure is in the columellar region (Fig. **3–19**). This situation frequently can be corrected by removal of the offending portion of the strut without disturbing the remainder of the implant, assuming infection is not present.

Fortunately, most patients present to the surgeon when extrusion is impending, this stage being manifested by progressive thinning of the skin. As noted above, the most common location of impending implant extrusion in contemporary practice is in the columellar region. A common presentation of this phenomenon is development of a crust or granuloma in the region of the columellar scar (Fig. **3–20**), and removal of the strut without disturbing the remainder of the implant often solves a problem if infection is not present.

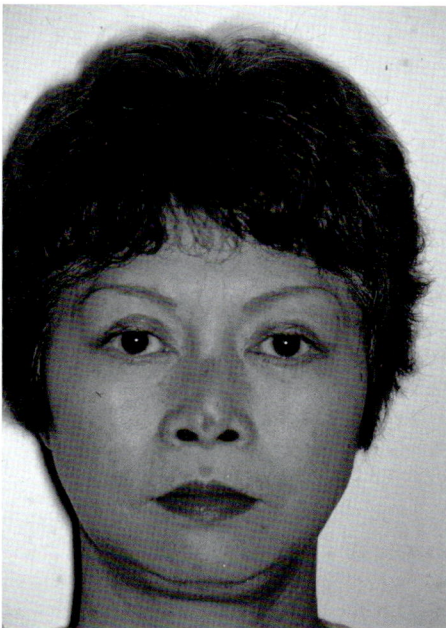

Figure 3–18   A depressed scar in the lobular region following removal of a silicone nasal prosthesis.

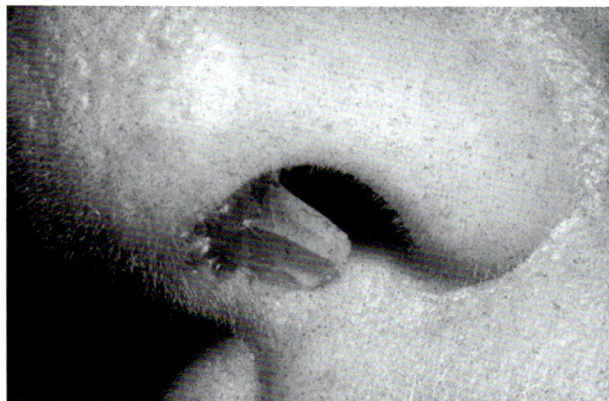

Figure 3–19   Prosthesis extrusion in the columella.

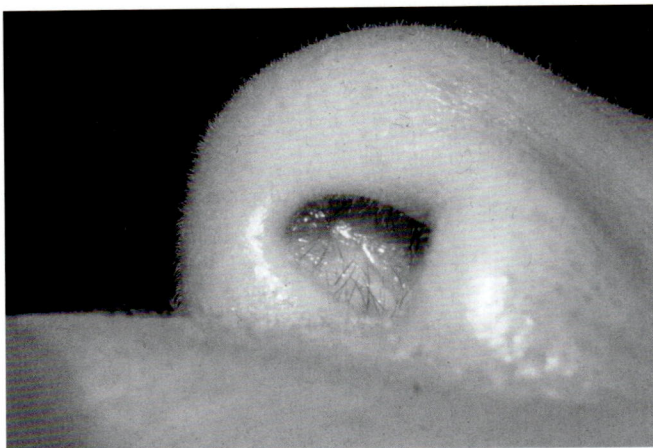

Figure 3–20 Impending columellar exposure indicated by granuloma formation and crusting.

If impending extrusion occurs at other locations and is recognized at an early stage, salvage of the implant can often be achieved by prompt removal. The implant is sculptured to a smaller size, a dermal or temporalis fascia (or crushed cartilage) graft is sutured over the lobular component, and the implant is replaced in the existing nasal pocket. Assuming that there is no evidence of infection, I do not recommend implant removal without immediate replacement in this situation. The prosthesis serves as the "new" nasal skeleton, and if it is removed, the thin skin often contracts over the lobular tip-defining point, producing a depression that is difficult to reconstruct.

Most commonly, extrusion is a consequence of a judgmental or technical error on the part of the surgeon, usually related to use of an implant that is too large (or too firm) or an attempt to increase tip projection with a thrusting type of columellar strut. Malacaption of the prosthesis to the nasal dorsum with resultant mobility of the implant secondary to inadequate fixation may predispose to delayed extrusion. The enemies of nasal augmentation with alloplasts are: (1) excessive prosthesis size and firmness, (2) implant mobility, and (3) utilization of a columellar strut in a "tent-pole" fashion.

One exception to the premise that implant extrusion is related to judgmental or technical error concerns that which occurs following a delayed infection. As mentioned previously, the etiology of infection around an implant occurring months to years after surgery is often difficult to determine. Thinning of the skin due to abscess formation along the implant requires prompt removal of the prosthesis.

Lysis of the depressor septia muscle has been advocated as a method for reducing tension on the nasal lobule, thus reducing the risk of skin thinning and implant extrusion.

Occasionally, for reasons that they are unable to explain, patients present with an actual protrusion of a portion of the implant through the nasal skin, and in such cases, prompt removal and subsequent reconstruction with autologous material is indicated.

Discoloration

Discoloration of the nasal skin is perhaps the most common adverse sequela of augmentation rhinoplasty using alloplastic materials. The etiology of this condition, which is most common in the lobular region, is unknown, but in most cases it is temperature related, being more visible during cold weather conditions. The most commonly noted discolorations are an amorphous red or bluish mottling, or telangiectatic change in the superficial dermis. These abnormalities appear to be more common if edema and ecchymosis during the early postoperative period have been more marked than usual. Treatment is generally frustrating, being expectant. In most cases, some improvement occurs with time, but in many patients, skin discoloration persists indefinitely. There is no association between this skin discoloration and subsequent infection or extrusion of the implant, and treatment is usually not necessary. In many cases, discoloration persists even if the prosthesis is removed. Occasionally, small telangiectasia respond to precise electrosurgical treatment, but for most patients the best approach is to camouflage the area with cosmetics.

Alar Asymmetry

Asymmetry of the nasal alae is occasionally noted following augmentation rhinoplasty with silicone prostheses. In many cases, such asymmetry existed preoperatively, and it is extremely important to point out such asymmetry to the patient prior to surgery and to document this situation photographically. Implant malposition may also result in asymmetry of the alae (Fig. **3–21**). This may be a consequence of implant malposition in the lobular region or simple displacement of the columellar strut toward one vestibule. In this case, the offending portion of the strut can be removed through a small columellar incision, solving the problem.

When the lobular aspect of the implant is malpositioned, however, treatment requires removal and repositioning of the prosthesis. The surgeon must endeavor to release skin in the proximal portion of the nose from the underlying nasal skeleton. Even if this is properly

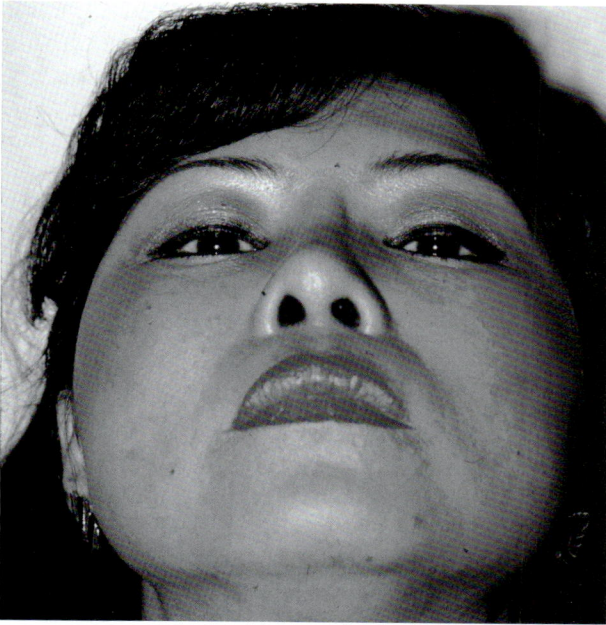

Figure 3–21   Alar asymmetry resulting from prosthesis malposition.

accomplished, subsequent scar contraction may sometimes produce recurrence of asymmetry.

Asymmetry may also result from improperly performed alar base surgery. In such cases, treatment consists of revision of the alar operation.

It is important that the surgeon never promise a patient with preexisting alar asymmetry that perfect symmetry can be restored with the operative procedure. Such patients should be reminded that facial asymmetry is common and that such minor imperfections do not detract from facial harmony and beauty.

Revision Rhinoplasty in the Augmented Nose

Although many of the complications noted above may necessitate revision rhinoplasty, by far the most common reason for revision surgery following augmentation of the Asian nose is patient dissatisfaction with the size or shape of the existing implant. The dorsal component of the implant may be either too wide or too narrow, or the dorsal profile may be too convex or too concave to satisfy the current desires of the patient. In many cases, the implant has been in place for years and shows no evidence of the impending complications just described. For such patients, dissatisfaction with the implant shape or size often reflects changing concepts of fashion or facial beauty.

If the surgeon agrees that reshaping the implant will enhance facial aesthetics, revision surgery may be undertaken with confidence. There is one important exception to this principle, however. The surgeon should proceed with extreme caution if the patient requests a larger implant or desires increased tip projection, as such intervention may predispose to extrusion of the larger prosthesis that would be required. Fortunately, most requests for changes in implant shape or size involve reduction in the size of the prosthesis, particularly modification of a straight or slightly convex dorsum to a more concave configuration (Fig. **3–22A,B**). Although

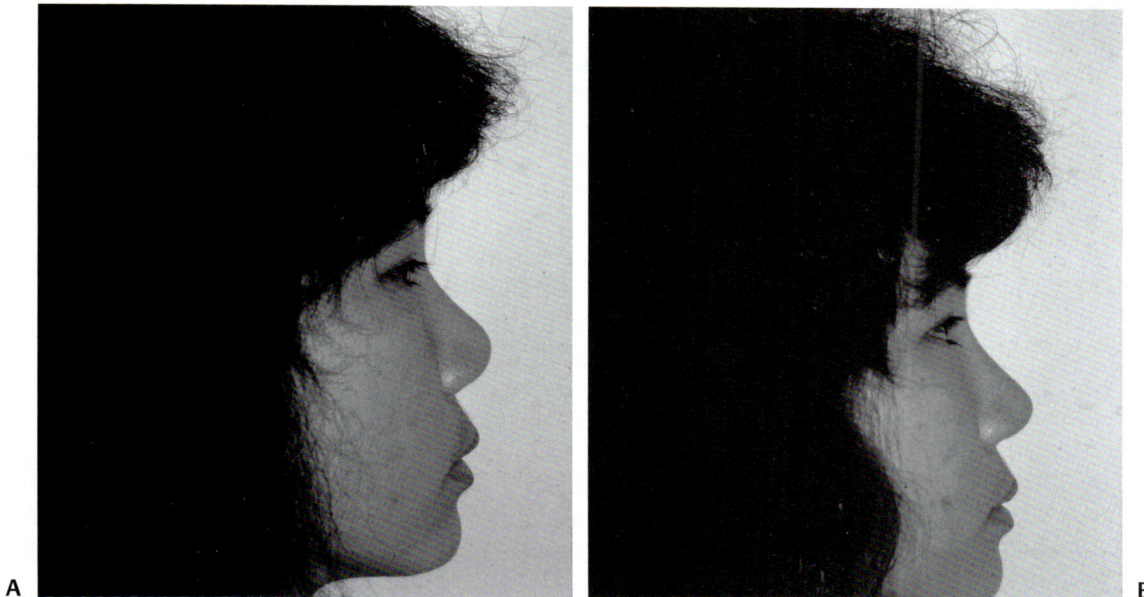

A   B

Figure 3–22   **(A,B)** Pre- and postoperative results of revision rhinoplasty by removing a silicone implant and replacing it with a new silicone prosthesis of a different configuration.

intervention of this type is usually successful, the patient should be informed that the risk of infection is higher in revision surgery as a consequence of diminished blood supply to the operative field.

Occasionally, a patient expresses dissatisfaction with nasal configuration in the early postoperative period and is persistent in demanding immediate revision. Assuming that the surgeon feels that it is technically feasible to construct a nose that more closely approximates the patient's desires, revision may be undertaken as early as 6 to 12 weeks, as tissues are more manageable during the period prior to the onset of more extensive fibrosis. As is the case with later revision surgery, the patient is counseled regarding the higher incidence of infection following secondary surgery and reminded that a nose cannot be sculptured to exact specifications.

Technical Details in Secondary Augmentation Rhinoplasty

The following technical details facilitate successful secondary nasal augmentation:

1. As the risk of infection is increased following revision surgery, the use of prophylactic antibiotics is important. The importance of meticulous preparation of the nasal vestibule is obvious, and it is beneficial to irrigate the pocket with an antiseptic solution such as povidone-iodine prior to implant placement.

2. If revision surgery is being undertaken because of asymmetry of the implant, bilateral vestibular incisions are often beneficial in facilitating symmetrical undermining of the pocket, particularly in the lobular region.

3. To ensure adequate fixation of the implant, it is important to remove the posterior aspect of the implant capsule and to shred the underlying periosteum with scissors to allow apposition of the implant directly onto bone, encouraging subsequent periosteal growth around the implant and thus producing adequate fixation.

4. If lobular skin is thin, it is wise to cover the lobular portion of the implant with dermis, fascia, or cartilage to protect and encourage thickening of the cutaneous cover.

5. As is the case in primary augmentation, it is important to avoid using a columellar strut to thrust the tip anteriorly. The functions of the columellar strut and admonitions regarding its use have been discussed earlier in this chapter.

6. In spite of reduced blood supply to the operative field in revision surgery, there is, paradoxically, an increased incidence of ecchymosis and hematoma around the implant because of impaired retraction of blood vessels supplying the preexisting capsule. Hematoma, of course, predisposes to infection, and thus it is important to drain any hematoma that forms. The most common site for hematoma formation in revision surgery is the nasion. Hematomas in this area are often satisfactorily treated by aspiration with an 18-gauge needle using aseptic technique during the early postoperative period.

◆ Conclusion

The major goals of rhinoplasty in the Asian nose include augmentation of the nasal dorsum in conjunction with enhancement and refinement of lobular configuration, a goal that must not be overlooked because of fixation on the obvious requirement for dorsal augmentation. Although various materials may be used to achieve these goals, individually sculptured solid silicone implants are the most commonly used prostheses worldwide.

Focusing on modification of the lobule as the primary goal, subsequently augmenting the dorsum to complement the modified lobule is an important concept that is often overlooked by surgeons, particularly by those practicing in the West. In addition to producing superior nasal aesthetics, this focus encourages a more conservative, and therefore inherently safer, augmentation procedure. The surgeon should realize that subtle enhancement often produces substantial aesthetic benefit. Conservatism is of utmost importance in attempts to enhance tip projection, as excessive tension on the lobular skin is a prime factor in delayed extrusion of alloplastic implants.

Use of a soft L-shaped silicone implant yields precise, accurate, and reproducible long-term results, with an incidence of complications and revision surgery comparable (or lower) to other modalities. There is no donor-site morbidity, and the cost effectiveness of this technique exceeds that of procedures that require harvest of graft material. Healing following augmentation with an L-shaped silicone implant is more rapid and less subject to the vagaries of wound healing and scar contracture. The technical simplicity of this procedure as compared with autogenous grafting levels the playing field, allowing excellent results when performed by surgeons of varying experience and technical sophistication.

It is important to understand that the reasons for the historical disrepute of nasal augmentation with silicone implants are no longer valid because of advances in materials, technique, and understanding of the dynamics of augmentation rhinoplasty.

Some surgeons currently advocate the use of cartilage grafts to enhance tip projection while using silicone implants for dorsal augmentation. Although my experience convinces me of the numerous advantages of L-shaped implants, I applaud the efforts of those surgeons who continue to seek the most advantageous use of autogenous materials in the Asian nose. Although recent reports suggest that long-term survival of cartilage grafts of the onlay type in the nose is excellent; the fate of columellar struts, subject to stresses of a different magnitude, may well be different. Is it significant that proponents of such techniques recommend overcorrection?

Unfortunately, there are no statistical data analyzing the long-term results of cosmetic autogenous nasal augmentation specifically with regard to patient satisfaction and incidence of revision surgery. It is obvious, however, that not all patients undergoing augmentation with autogenous material are satisfied with the immediate or long-term results and that reoperation is requested. An analysis of the reoperation rates of augmentation using alloplasts versus autogenous materials would constitute the best comparison of the relative merits of the two procedures.

When performing augmentation rhinoplasty with L-shaped silicone implants, the surgeon should be conservative in selecting the implant size, remembering that subtle enhancement often produces substantial aesthetic benefit.

Successful aesthetic rhinoplasty in the Asian nose requires knowledge of anatomic variables, appreciation of nasal aesthetics, thorough preoperative evaluation and counseling of the patient, and careful attention to detail in performing the operative procedure (Table **3–4**). Careful use of silicone implants in augmentation rhinoplasty offers the surgeon an opportunity to exploit his or her aesthetic senses to the fullest extent, enabling dramatic, long-lasting, and stable changes in nasal appearance with a technically simple operation. When such surgery is properly planned and executed, the incidence of complications remains low. Complications following this procedure are generally the result of technical errors and certainly not due to inherent deficiencies in the operation per se. In the final analysis, a thorough understanding of the basic principles and important safeguards when using such materials in the nose is essential for successful surgery.

◆ Reduction Rhinoplasty in the Asian Nose

General Considerations

Although the majority of rhinoplasties in Asian noses involve augmentation procedures, some patients present with large noses exhibiting a prominent dorsal hump. Asian surgeons often refer to this condition as "hump nose" and correctly note that in many of these noses, despite a dorsal hump, the nasion is low, often requiring a degree of augmentation following hump removal. Noses of this type are considerably more common in the northern and central areas of eastern Asia. Standard rhinoplasty techniques employed for the Caucasian nose form the basis for successful reduction rhinoplasty in Asian noses of this configuration. These techniques are well described elsewhere and will be only briefly reviewed here, emphasizing subtle differences that enhance aesthetic results in the Asian nose. A systematic appraisal of reduction rhinoplasty with or without augmentation can be found in management of the Japanese nose reviewed in Chapter 9.

A major portion of the success in reduction rhinoplasty is determined by the surgeon's ability to remodel the nasal lobule in an aesthetically pleasing fashion. It is important to remember that, although the configuration and projection of the tip may be satisfactory in the immediate postoperative period, it is not uncommon for undesirable changes in these parameters to occur during the ensuing 6 to 18 months, most commonly in the form of tip ptosis. When this condition is associated with supratip rounding, the classic "polly-beak" deformity results. Less common postoperative deformities include pinching, boxing, and asymmetry of the tip, cartilaginous irregularities, projections ("bossing"), and alar notching. To minimize the incidence of these deformities, the surgeon must be thoroughly familiar with the anatomic factors that support the nasal tip (Table **3–5**), as well as with the dynamics of tip rhinoplasty and postoperative healing in this region.

Surgical modification of the lobule, generally considered to be the most critical and demanding aspect of rhinoplasty surgery, is a particular challenge in the Asian patient. As in the Caucasian nose, inadequate,

Table 3–4 Safeguards for Successful Augmentation Rhinoplasty with L-shaped Silicone Prostheses

1. Do not thrust the nasal tip anteriorly with a columellar strut.
2. Remember that the columellar strut has two primary functions:
   a. Proximal stabilization of the implant in the midline
   b. Columellar sculpturing
3. Carve each implant individually according to the nasal anatomy anesthetic desires of each patient.
4. Ensure that there are no sharp surfaces on the implant.
5. Dissect an adequate pocket precisely in the midline, ensuring that there is no tension whatsoever on the implant.
6. Be conservative in selecting prosthesis size.
7. Use soft silicone elastomer for all components of the prosthesis.

Table 3–5 Anatomic Support of the Nasal Tip

1. Medial crura–caudal septum attachment
2. Lateral crura–sesmoid cartilage attachment
3. Interdomal ligament
4. Upper lateral cartilage–lower lateral cartilage aponeurosis

Source: Janeke JB, Wright WR. Arch Otolaryngol 1971;93:458

inappropriate, or excessive surgical manipulation of the lobule may produce unsightly results that overshadow an aesthetically pleasing modification of the cartilaginous and bony portions of the nose. Such postoperative deformities are often exceedingly difficult to correct; thus, optimum effort must be expended during the planning and execution of the primary procedure to offer the best chance of a satisfactory result.

The characteristic anatomy of the Asian lobule is a consequence of thick, lobular skin having a large complement of subcutaneous fibrofatty tissue superimposed over a cartilaginous skeleton characterized by lower lateral cartilages having a rounded (rather than horseshoe-shaped) configuration. In contrast to the Caucasian nose, the alar cartilages tend to be widely separated at the dome, often exhibiting fibrofatty tissue in the interdomal region.

Techniques of tip rhinoplasty involving modification of the lower lateral cartilages that are routinely successful in Caucasian noses are often unsatisfactory in the Asian nose because of attenuated lower lateral cartilages that are not sufficiently strong to accentuate tip projection and support. (Lobular refinement of noses that do not require increased tip support may demonstrate a satisfactory response to standard techniques of tip plasty.) If enhancement of tip projection is required, augmentation of the tip using cartilaginous onlay grafts or columellar struts is required to allow optimal dorsal reduction. An increasing number of surgeons rely on the external rhinoplasty approach for placement of such cartilaginous grafts. In some cases, use of a small L-shaped silicone implant instead of autogenous grafts following dorsal reduction produces excellent results.

As previously noted, it is not uncommon to debulk the lower lateral cartilages and lobular subdermal fibrofatty tissue in conjunction with placement of an L-shaped silicone prosthesis. In such cases, I prefer to place the implant via a marginal incision, and after closing this incision, proceed with lobular debulking with a cartilage-splitting incision.

The basic surgical approach to refine the Asian lobule consists of modification of the cartilaginous skeleton followed by debulking of the subcutaneous tissue to encourage optimum skin draping over the modified skeleton. In contrast to techniques that refine the lobule by subtotal excision of the lower lateral cartilages, the technique most applicable to the Asian nose involves preservation of these cartilages, modifying their configurations so that they serve as a firm foundation for support of the lobule. This usually involves removal of interdomal fibrofatty tissue, determination of the point at which a "new" dome is to be fashioned, scoring the lower lateral cartilages lateral to the position of the dome, and suturing the domes together with a mattress suture of 4–0 polyglycolic acid.

Because a substantial portion of lobular bulbosity in the Asian nose is a consequence of thick skin and abundant fibrofatty subcutaneous tissue, subcutaneous defatting is an essential component of this technique, enhancing the ability of the skin to conform to the new lobular skeleton. Although such debulking is avoided by many surgeons who fear postoperative skin dimpling, such irregularities are most unlikely because of the thick skin of the Asian lobule. On the contrary, destruction of the lobular skeleton by radical cartilage excision is more likely to result in postoperative deformity than is subcutaneous debulking. Preservation of at least a 3 to 4 mm rim of the caudal lateral crus minimizes the possibility of postoperative irregularities related to cartilage overresection.

In some cases, the columellar base may benefit from augmentation to modify an acute columellar-labial junction. Small alloplastic (soft silicone and expanded polytetrafluoroethylene [Gore-Tex]) or autogenous implants are appropriate for achieving this goal.

Alar-base reduction is occasionally indicated to maximize lobular aesthetics. This procedure is more common in patients originating from the southern Asian latitudes; my method of alar-base reduction is described in a subsequent section.

Surgical Technique

Modification of the Lobule

A lobule requiring minimal definition is approached using the cartilage-splitting incision, leaving at least a 4 mm caudal rim of lower lateral cartilage. Most Asian noses, however, benefit from more extensive modification of the configuration of the lower lateral cartilages as well as a greater degree of lobular defatting than can be achieved using the cartilage-splitting technique. The delivery technique, therefore, is the "workhorse" of lobular surgery in the Asian nose. Of utmost importance in lobular surgery is preservation and/or reconstruction of the anatomic components of tip support described by Janeke and Wright (Table **3–5**). The surgical approach is as follows:

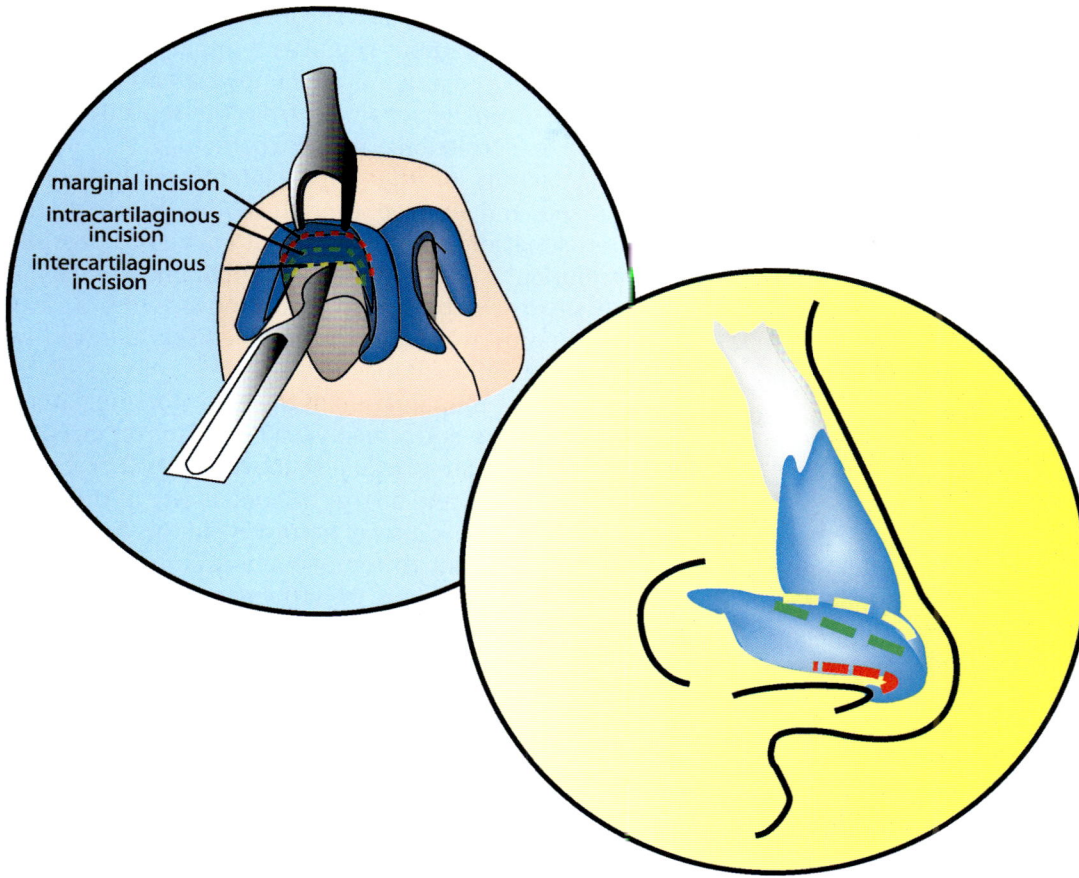

Figure 3–23   Incisions for lobular surgery.

1. Standard intercartilaginous incisions are made and extended into a modified transfixation incision. A full transfixation incision is not made to preserve the junction between the caudal septum and medial crura, a vital component of tip support (Table **3–5**).

2. Marginal incisions are made and extended into the columella (Fig. **3–23**).

3. The lower lateral cartilages are dissected from the lobular skin and delivered into the vestibule (Fig. **3–24**), where, under direct visualization, ~50% of the cephalic margins of the lower lateral cartilages are excised, preserving the underlying vestibular skin. Caudal rims of at least 4 mm in width are maintained.

4. The caudal remnants are scored at the dome, and the scoring is extended laterally to weaken the spring of the cartilage. If tip projection is to be enhanced, the scored cartilages are rotated medially, and a new dome is created by approximating the cartilages with a mattress suture of 4–0 polyglycolic acid. In addition to enhancing tip support, this maneuver re-creates the interdomal ligament, another important component of tip support.

5. The lobular region is carefully defatted using small dissecting scissors and forceps as the lobular skin is everted by an assistant.

6. Tip support is reinforced by placement of a buried suture of 4–0 clear nylon between the caudal septum and the medial crura (Fig. **3–25**). This suture is placed following modification of the cartilaginous and bony dorsum.

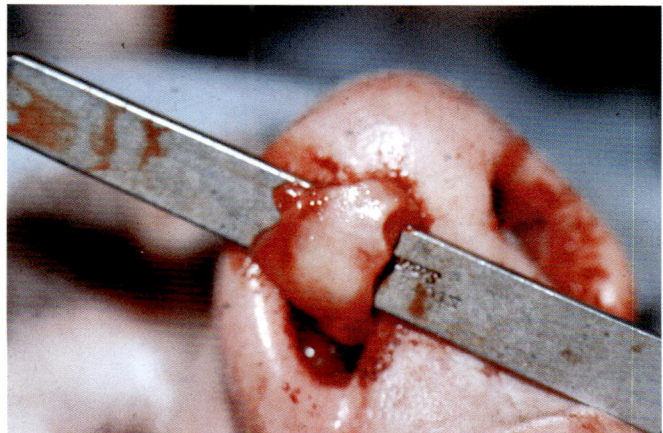

Figure 3–24   Delivery of the lower lateral cartilages into the nasal vestibule.

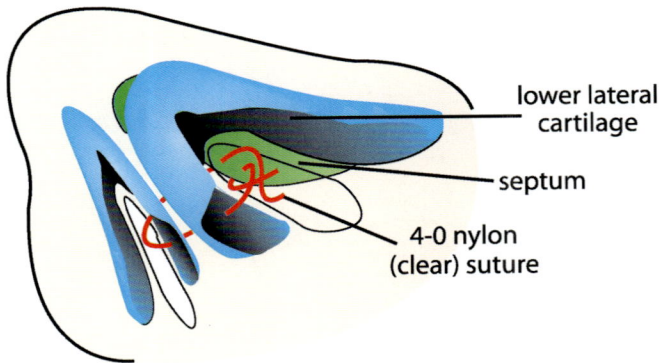

Figure 3–25 Placement of a "permanent" suture (4–0 clear nylon) between the caudal septum and medial crura (submucosal and subcutaneous placement) to combat tip ptosis occurring during the period of scar contracture.

Modification of the alae and columella, if necessary, is deferred until completion of the remainder of the rhinoplasty procedure (i.e., hump removal and osteotomies or dorsal augmentation with an implant). Alar-base surgery is often performed during the primary rhinoplasty procedure but can be delayed until resolution of perioperative edema. In many cases, alteration of the lobular configuration as described above will achieve satisfactory changes in alar size and shape, rendering external incisions unnecessary. If the patient desires additional alar refinement, this procedure is performed as a minor office operation and allows patient participation in the decision for a procedure that may leave external scars.

Reduction of the Cartilaginous and Bony Dorsum

The cartilaginous dorsum is reduced incrementally by shaving with a Bard-Parker no. 15 blade. As a guideline, sufficient lowering is performed so that the anterior

septal angle approximates the level of the apices of the nares (Fig. **3–26**). Both septal and upper lateral cartilages are reduced as a unit, the upper lateral cartilages being intentionally separated from the septum only if required for correction of a septal pathology.

The scrolls of the upper lateral cartilages are visualized and excised to reduce the width of the posterosuperior lobule as well as to obviate a possible contribution to postoperative supratip fullness.

If small, the bony hump is removed with a rasp. Larger humps are reduced using a chisel, followed by final adjustment with the rasp.

Following modification of the bony dorsum, lateral osteotomies are performed via a pyriform rim incision. These incisions are placed just above the level of the inferior turbinate, and a strut of bone is left in the pyriform rim to obviate airway narrowing in this area.

It is important to remove any accumulated bone dust or other fragments from the dorsum. Because the upper lateral cartilages may increase in height as they converge in the midline following infracture, final adjustment of the cartilaginous dorsal profile, using sharp dissection with a no. 15 blade, should be made prior to wound closure.

Postoperative Care

Postoperative care following reduction rhinoplasty in the Asian nose is identical to that following rhinoplasty in the Caucasian nose. Because of increased skin thickness, Asians are more likely to exhibit collagen proliferation in the supratip area. Triamcinolone injections should be considered at the first sign of supratip fullness; because of skin thickness, they are less likely to produce adverse sequelae, such as dermal atrophy, than in the Caucasian nose.

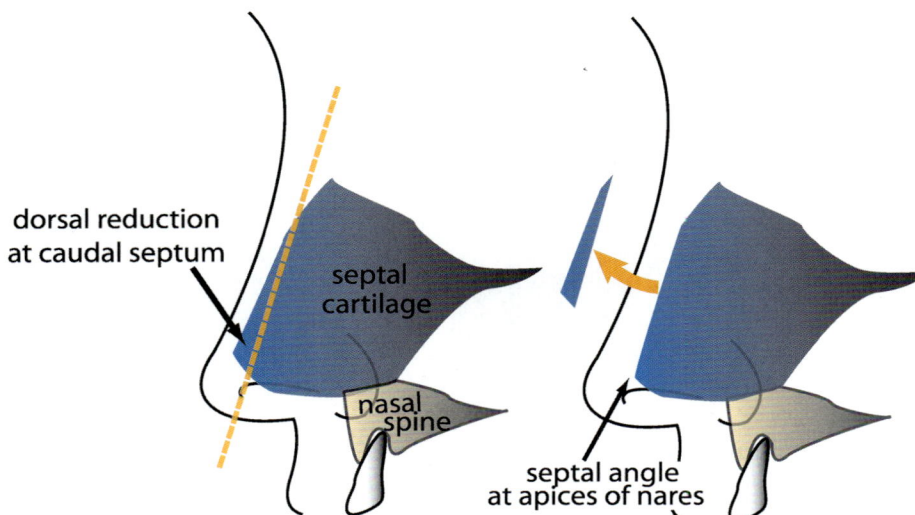

Figure 3–26 Reduction of the caudal dorsum so that the anterior septal angle approximates the level of the apices of the nares. Reduction is effected by an incremental shave excision with a no. 15 blade.

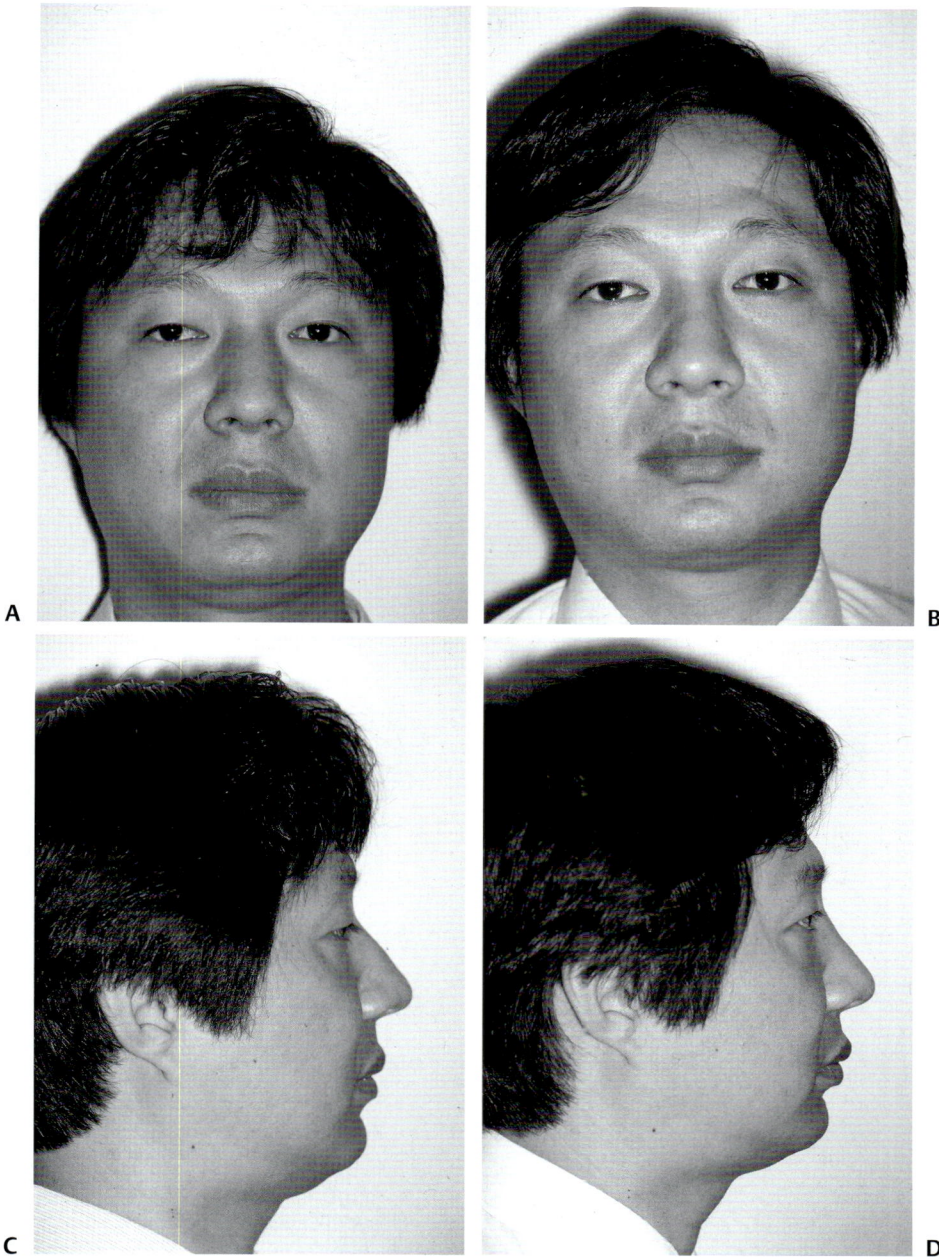

Figure 3–27 (A–D) Pre- and postoperative results of reduction rhinoplasty in the Asian nose.

Results of reduction rhinoplasty in the Asian nose are illustrated in Figs. **3–27** and **3–28**.

◆ Alar-Base Surgery

See DVD Disk Two, Alar-Base Reduction

Although surgery of the alar base is often beneficial in maximizing aesthetic implants in rhinoplasty, this procedure is used less frequently in the Asian nose than in other non-Caucasian populations. In my practice,

alar-base excision is performed in ~10% of augmentation rhinoplasties, the substantial majority of these procedures being undertaken in patients from the Philippines and Indochina, where Malay characteristics overlap with central and northern Asian traits.

As augmentation rhinoplasty does increase lobular projection, small degrees of alar flaring and flattening are often improved by the augmentation procedure itself. Patients in whom such improvement in alar configuration will likely be achieved by nasal augmentation alone are counseled to defer alar surgery until

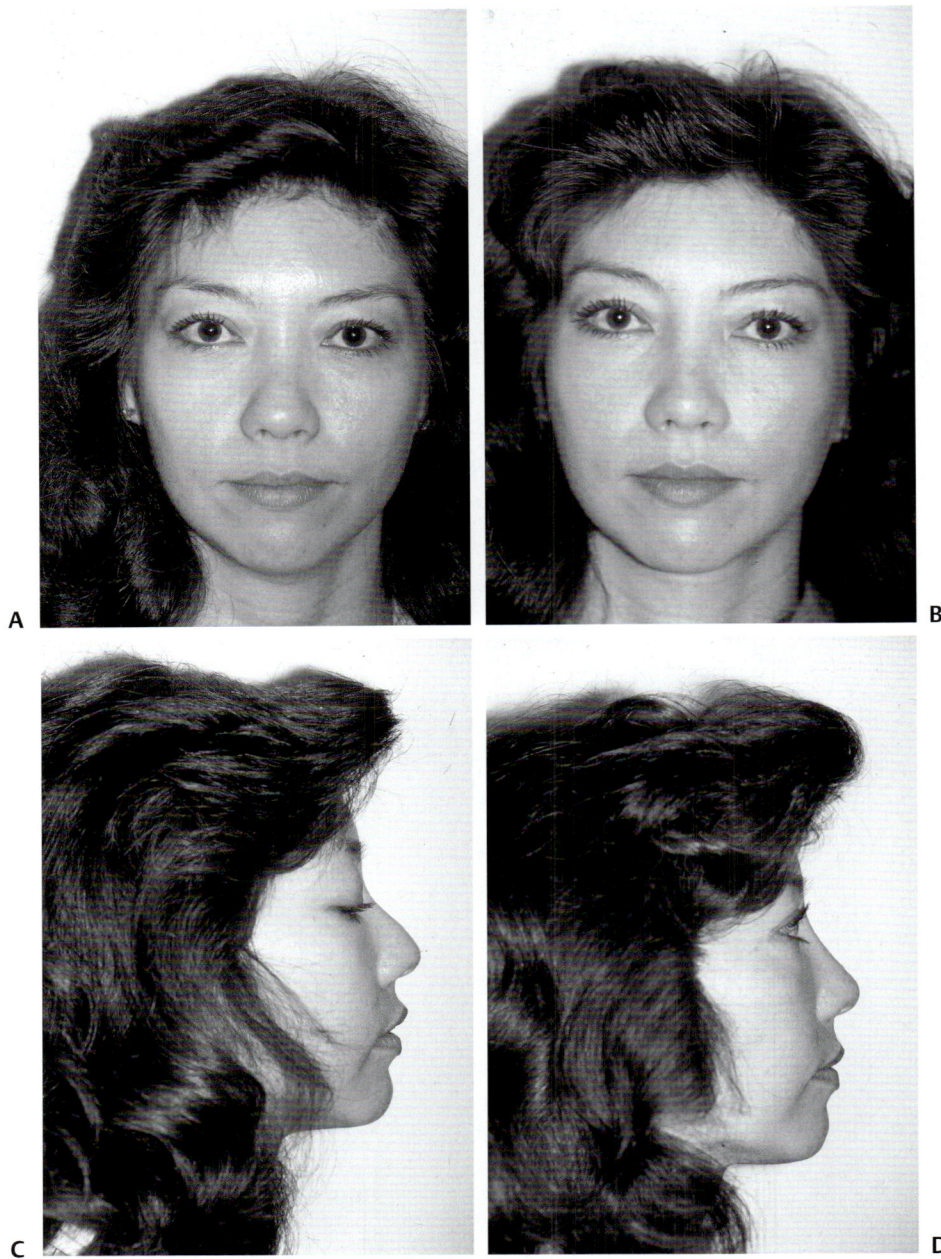

Figure 3–28   (A–D) Pre- and postoperative results of reduction rhinoplasty in the Asian nose.

they can personally assess the effect of the augmentation operation on the nasal base. If the patient feels that further reduction is desirable, alar-base excision can be performed in 3 to 6 weeks (or anytime thereafter), the operation perhaps being even more effective because planning of the excision takes into account the effects of prior augmentation.

If, however, the patient is satisfied following augmentation rhinoplasty, potential scarring resulting from an external incision is avoided. In this regard, surgeons should remember that, although a basically simple procedure, alar-base surgery is not without complications (scarring, alar notching, asymmetry) and is a procedure that even in the most experienced hands may contribute to the appearance of the "overoperated" nose. Thus, if possible, alar-base surgery is best avoided unless the aesthetic benefits clearly outweigh the possible disadvantages.

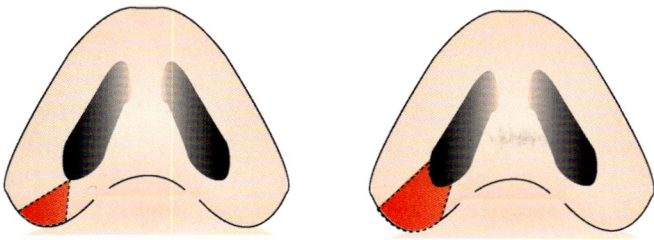

Figure 3–29 The relative contribution of nostril size and alar-skin excess dictates the type of incision used in alar-base reduction.

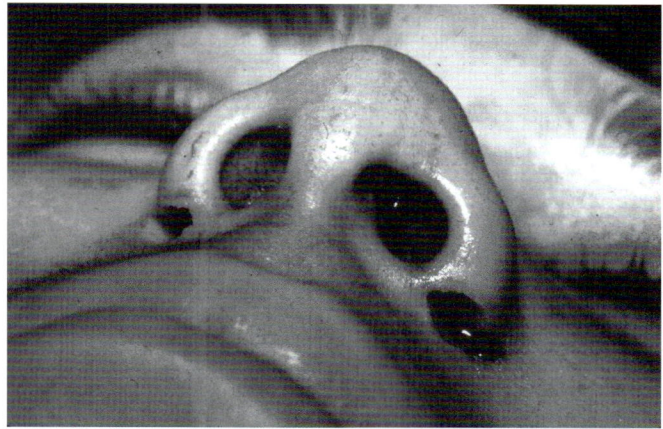

Figure 3–30 Alar reduction with skin excision avoids violation of the vestibular skin.

Planning Alar-Base Surgery

If alar-base surgery is to be undertaken, thorough analysis of this region is essential to formulation of a proper surgical approach. The relative contribution to the deformity of nostril size and alar skin excess must be ascertained (Fig. **3–29**). In some cases, lobular skin can be reduced without violation of the vestibular skin, a technique that avoids the possibility of an alar notch deformity (Fig. **3–30**). Extreme caution is indicated in noses exhibiting a wide lobule in association with a wide alar base. In such cases, alar reduction often results in a rectangular or square configuration of the lobule that is aesthetically less desirable than the original triangular lobular shape (Fig. **3–31**). Caution is also necessary in noses lacking a well-defined nostril sill, because scarring and notching are potentially more problematic (Fig. **3–32**).

When indicated, alar-base excisions are generally more substantial in the Asian nose than in Caucasian noses, especially with regard to the extent of excision of the lateral alar side wall and a corresponding length of excision posteriorly along the alar crease.

The markings for the medial aspect of the excision are placed in the alar crease (beginning the incision along the anterior aspect of this mark places the incision ~0.5 mm above the alar crease), and traversing one-third to one-half of the distance across the nostril sill. The incision is oriented perpendicular to the floor of the nostril sill at its terminus (Fig. **3–33A**). This creates a

modified medial flap that minimizes the tendency toward postoperative notching. The amount of alar side wall to be resected is determined by a gentle medial pressure on the alar side wall that results in visualization of a crease or natural demarcation point where the nostril "wants" to fold (Fig. **3–33B**). This point is marked and extended posteriorly to meet the previously marked line (Fig. **3–33C**). This procedure differs from other described techniques of alar-base surgery in that it does not involve direct measurement in planning the excision. In my opinion, given the high incidence of preexisting alar asymmetry, there is no valid reason to measure, ensuring that the amount of tissue excised on each side is identical. On the contrary, determining the point of natural demarcation by gentle medial pressure on the alar side wall has the best chance of creating postoperative asymmetry. It should be pointed out to the patient that in many cases of alar asymmetry, the cause of the asymmetry is not at the alar base but at the most anterior point (apices) of the nares. Obviously in such cases, alar-base excision will not completely correct the asymmetry.

The incisions are made with a Bard-Parker no. 11 blade, and wound closure is performed with 6–0 nylon

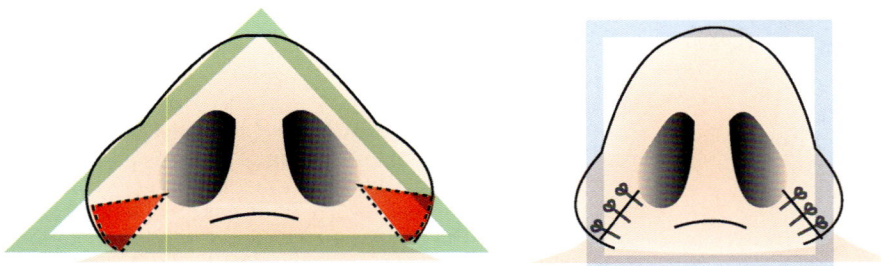

Figure 3–31 Alar reduction in a nose with a broad lobule may result in a rectangular or square lobular configuration that is less aesthetically desirable than the original triangular shape.

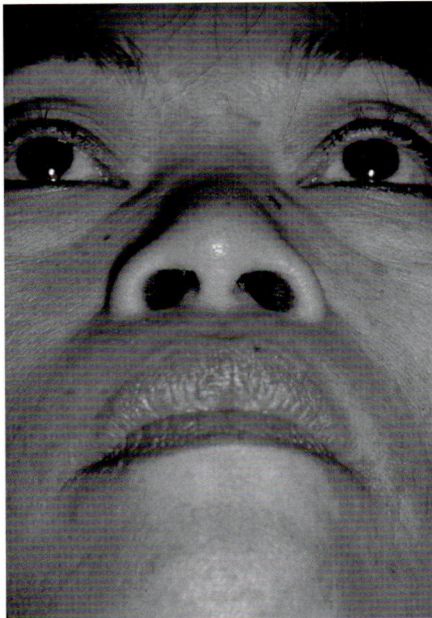

Figure 3–32 Deficiency of the nostril sill predisposes to visible scarring and notching following alar-base surgery.

without need for any additional subcutaneous closure. Sutures are removed 6 to 7 days postoperatively.

Variations in design of the alar-base excision as a function of alar and nostril configuration are demonstrated in Fig. **3–29**. Other procedures designed to thin the alar side walls and alter the size and shape of the nostrils have been described. I rarely consider these techniques because of the possibility for aesthetically unpleasing scars.

Fig. **3–34** illustrates the result of alar-base excision.

◆ Conclusion

Techniques of reduction rhinoplasty for the Asian nose are similar to those used in Caucasian rhinoplasty. Because of the thickness of lobular skin and the abundance of subcutaneous fibrofatty tissue, the response of the Asian lobule to these techniques is usually not as dramatic as Western surgeons expect, and if the tip requires additional projection, cartilage grafts (or

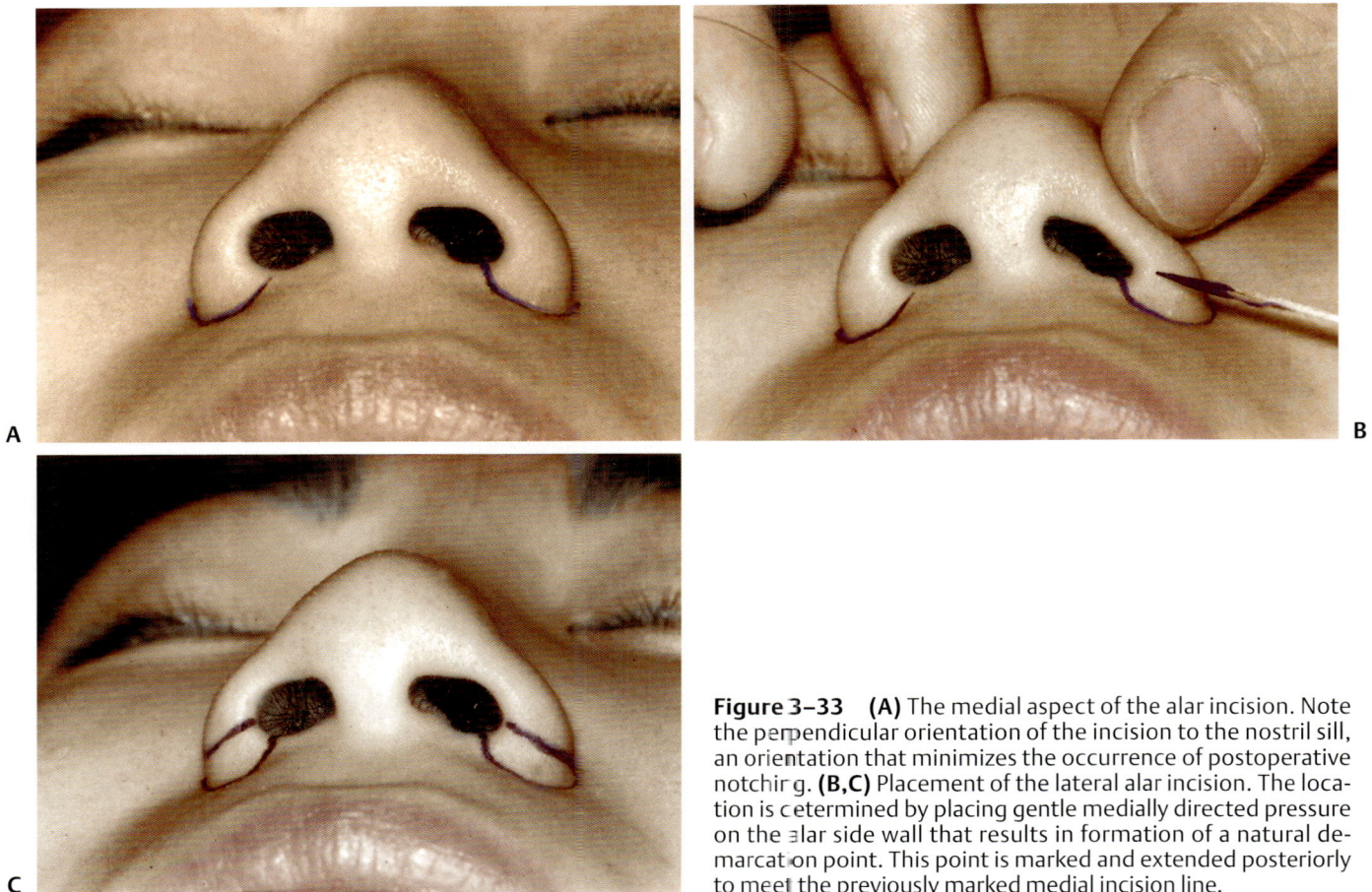

Figure 3–33 **(A)** The medial aspect of the alar incision. Note the perpendicular orientation of the incision to the nostril sill, an orientation that minimizes the occurrence of postoperative notching. **(B,C)** Placement of the lateral alar incision. The location is determined by placing gentle medially directed pressure on the alar side wall that results in formation of a natural demarcation point. This point is marked and extended posteriorly to meet the previously marked medial incision line.

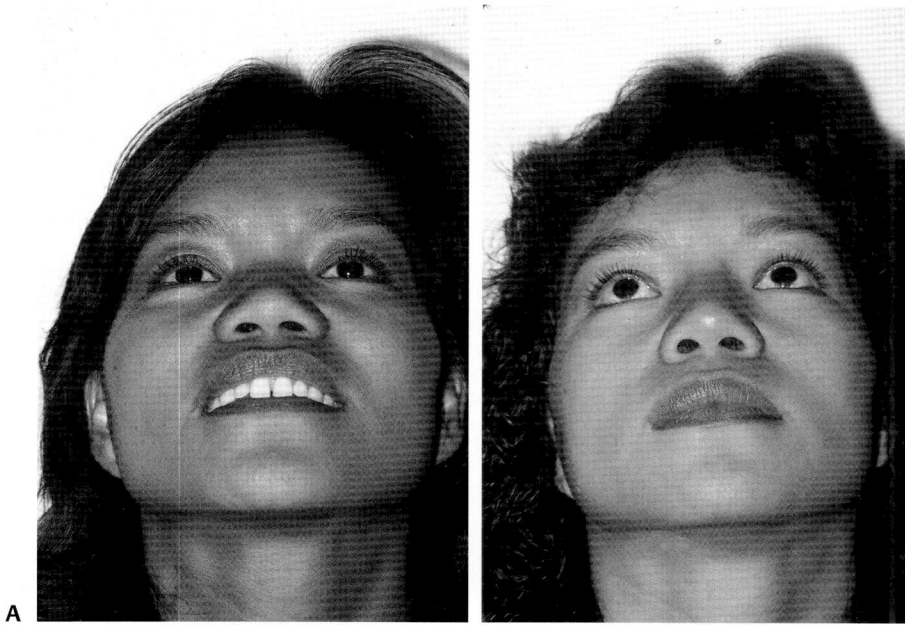

Figure 3–34   (A,B) Pre- and postoperative results of alar-base excision.

occasionally small alloplastic prostheses) are required to maximize aesthetic results.

Alar-base surgery may be a useful adjunct to both augmentation and reduction procedures, and a technique that stresses observation of natural points of demarcation rather than absolute measurement encourages natural and symmetrical results.

4

Cosmetic Surgery of the Asian Brow and Forehead

◆ Anatomic Considerations

The facial unit consisting of the eyebrows and forehead forms an important aesthetic component of the face and frequently benefits from surgical rejuvenation. In general, the distance between the brow and lashes of the upper eyelid is greater in Asians than in Caucasians. Furthermore, horizontal furrows tend to be less common perhaps due to increased dermal thickness as well as the presence of more abundant adipose tissue in the supragaleal plane, factors that reduce transmission of visible evidence of frontalis activity to the forehead skin. For these reasons, I find that indications for brow lift surgery are less common in Asians. My patients rarely request brow lifting procedures (unless they have actually seen one of my postoperative results); the majority are undertaken after I inform the patient that, in my aesthetic judgment, the appearance of the periorbital region would be enhanced by elevation of the brow. Indeed, many of my patients who request blepharoplasty have come to my office seeking a second opinion following recommendations by other surgeons for a coronal brow lift procedure. By far, the most common reason that I perform brow lift surgery in Asian patients is to rejuvenate a ptotic brow that has become aesthetically apparent years following upper blepharoplasty. Because of the relative lack of importance of forehead rhytidosis, by far the most common procedure I perform for brow lifting is the direct suprabrow approach. In spite of the general principle that lifting procedures are more accurate the closer the incision is placed to the structure requiring lifting, many surgeons have decried the suprabrow lift operation because of the possibility of visible scars. The enthusiasm, however, of Asian patients to undergo micropigmentation of the eyelids and brow provides a significant margin of safety regarding the issue of postoperative scars and has been proven to be extremely effective if necessary. (Chapter 13 covers the latest techniques for micropigmentation in detail.) For reasons to be discussed, there is no question that the accuracy and precision of eyebrow placement provided by direct suprabrow lifting exceeds that of coronal forehead lifting when performed by either open or endoscopic methods.

◆ Preoperative Considerations

As noted above, suprabrow and coronal forehead lifts are most commonly performed as a late sequel to upper-lid blepharoplasty, especially in cases in which creation of a large "double lid" with a deep palpebral sulcus (i.e., "westernization" of the eyelid; this situation does not occur following the more conservative "double lid" surgery) produces, most commonly in older patients, an apparent descent of the brow associated with deepening of glabellar frown lines, a combination that produces an angry look (Fig. **4–1**).

The decision whether to recommend a coronal forehead lift or a direct suprabrow lift depends on at least three factors:

1. The individual aesthetic situation, that is, the relative contribution of brow ptosis, horizontal forehead rhytids, and glabellar furrows to the aesthetic deformity

2. The desires of the patient with regard to correction of each of these contributing components

3. The experience, judgment, and preferences of the surgeon

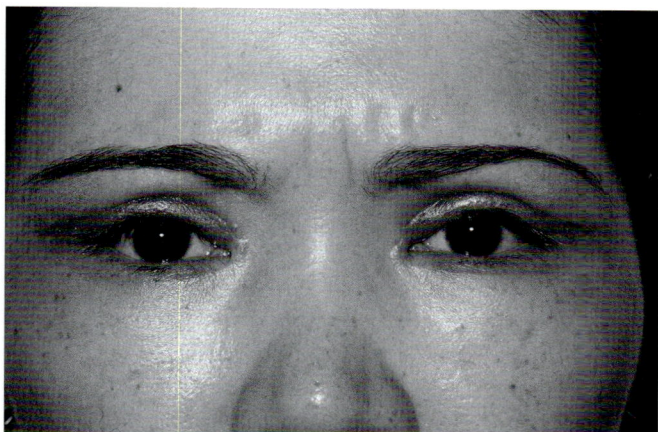

Figure 4–1   An angry look associated with an apparent brow descent and deepening of the glabellar frown lines following westernization of the upper eyelid.

Many patients, for example, are comfortable camouflaging forehead wrinkles with bangs, and are thus happy with the improvement in brow ptosis afforded by a direct suprabrow lift, a much simpler (and more accurate) procedure than a coronal forehead lift. The corrugator muscles responsible for glabellar furrows can be subtotally resected (although perhaps not as effectively as via the forehead lift exposure) during this procedure, if requested.

Patients who express concerns about deeper horizontal forehead wrinkles are obvious candidates for a coronal forehead lift as opposed to a direct brow lift.

As noted previously, Asian patients have enthusiastically embraced the technique of micropigmentation of the eyelids and brows, and use of this technique for camouflage of residual brow scars following suprabrow lifting has essentially obviated previous concerns about undesirable scars that occasionally follow this procedure.

◆ Direct Suprabrow Lift

Assuming that the general principle that the effectiveness of the "lift" of a facial component is directly related to the proximity of the surgical incision to that structure is valid, an accurate and long-lasting brow lift can be achieved with the suprabrow lift procedure.

Surgical Technique

1. With a patient in the sitting position, a line is marked in the suprabrow region corresponding to the location and shape of the brow that the surgeon wishes to create. In general, the maximum height of the brow is in the region of the lateral limbus, the

brow arching inferiorly from this point, terminating slightly higher at its lateral aspect than medially. The inferior skin incision is marked immediately adjacent to the most superior row of hair follicles, joining the superior incision medially and laterally (Fig. **4–2**).

2. The inferior skin incision is beveled in the direction of the hair follicles, and the superior skin incision is beveled at the same angle to encourage accurate skin approximation, ensuring formation of the thinnest possible scar.

Following skin excision, the frontalis muscle and underlying soft tissue within the wound are excised to the level of the periosteum. If indicated, the corrugator supercilii muscles are approached via the medial aspect of the wound. This is a semi-blind procedure, and accuracy relies on the surgeon's anatomic knowledge of corrugator anatomy. Although the excision can be initiated with small dissecting scissors, the majority of the technique is best achieved with an avulsion technique using tissue forceps, avulsion being less likely to injure the neurovascular bundle that courses through the corrugator musculature. In cases in which subtotal corrugator resection is undertaken, the glabellar skin is undermined to accommodate a thin sheet of expanded polytetrafluoroethylene (Gore-Tex) that is placed into the wound for two purposes:

1. The Gore-Tex serves as a volume replacement for the excised muscle tissue, thereby minimizing the incidence of localized depressions or irregularities.

2. The Gore-Tex acts as a barrier, decreasing the incidence of regenerating corrugator fibers attaching to the undersurface of the skin, which is a common cause of recurrent glabellar furrowing.

3. The tissue at the superior aspect of the excision is undermined several millimeters, creating a small flap that facilitates placement of fixation sutures and reduces tension during wound closure.

4. Fixation sutures (5–0 nylon) are placed between the orbicularis muscle just beneath the brow dermis and the frontal periosteum, "lifting" the brow into the desired position. The initial fixation suture is placed at the level of the lateral limbus (Fig. **4–3**), following which the lateral fixation suture is placed in the contralateral brow, and the resulting position carefully inspected for symmetry. The second fixation suture is then placed in like fashion at the mid-pupillary line (Fig. **4–4**), and a third fixation suture at an appropriate locus (determined by the surgeon in each individual case) is placed in the region between the medial limbus and medial brow terminus

Direct Browlift

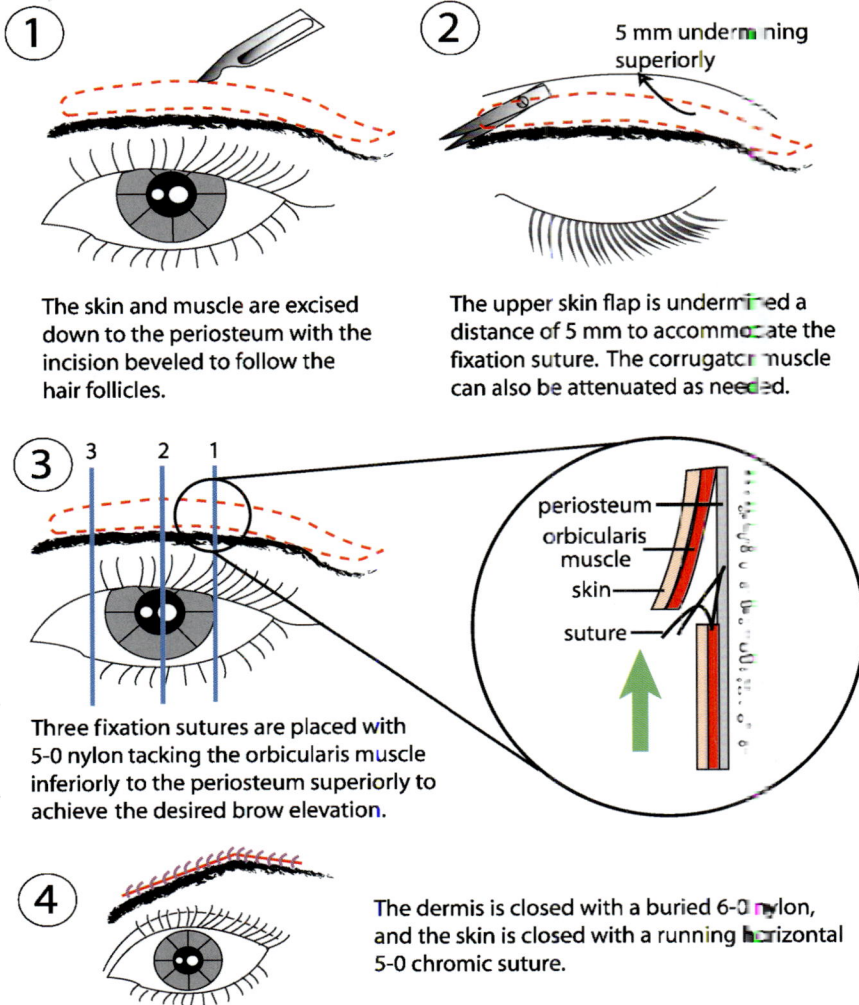

①

The skin and muscle are excised down to the periosteum with the incision beveled to follow the hair follicles.

②

5 mm undermining superiorly

The upper skin flap is undermined a distance of 5 mm to accommodate the fixation suture. The corrugator muscle can also be attenuated as needed.

③

3   2   1

periosteum
orbicularis muscle
skin
suture

Three fixation sutures are placed with 5-0 nylon tacking the orbicularis muscle inferiorly to the periosteum superiorly to achieve the desired brow elevation.

④

The dermis is closed with a buried 6-0 nylon, and the skin is closed with a running horizontal 5-0 chromic suture.

Figure 4–2   Incisions for the direct suprabrow lift.

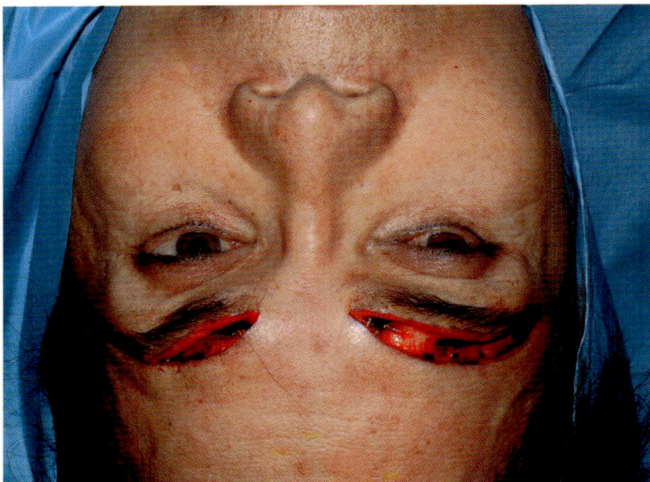

Figure 4–3   The lateral fixation suture has been placed in the left brow; note brow elevation as compared with the right side.

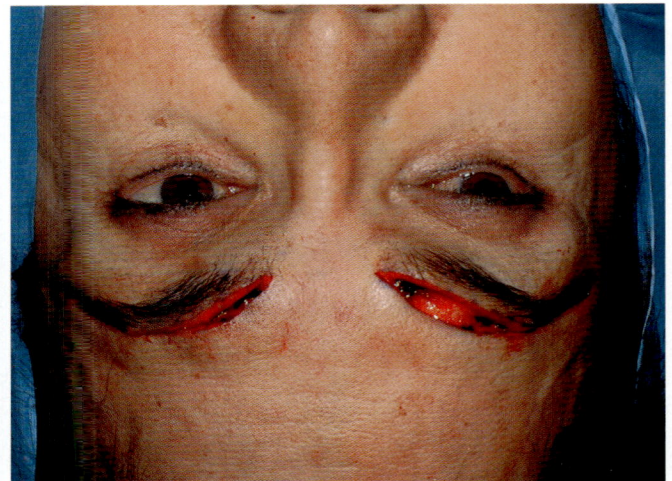

Figure 4–4   Lateral and middle fixation sutures have been placed in the left brow; a lateral fixation suture only has been placed in the right brow.

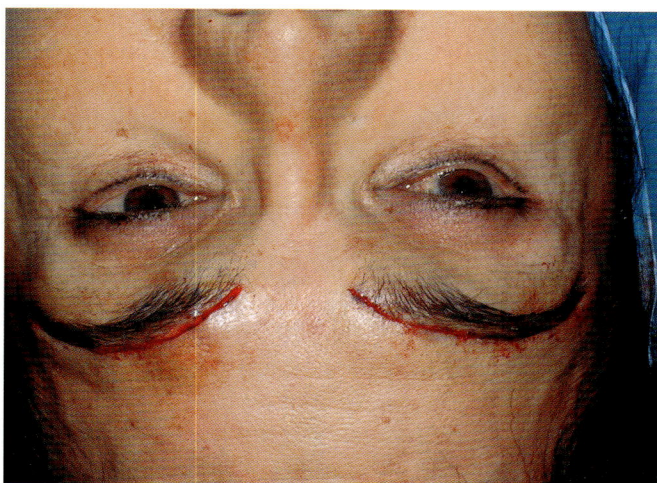

Figure 4–5 Three fixation sutures have been placed bilaterally. Note symmetrical "lift" with natural arch of brow.

(Fig. **4–5**). It is important that the needle enter the periosteum in a vertical direction to minimize the chance of strangulating nerve fibers in the suture, a situation that may produce excruciating postoperative pain of a tic-like nature. When properly placed, these fixation sutures result in close approximation of skin edges (encouraged in part by the previously described undermining of a superior flap), thus diverting considerable tension from the skin closure.

5. The dermis is approximated with buried sutures of 6–0 nylon, care being taken to minimize injury to the hair follicles, following which the epidermis is approximated with a running horizontal mattress suture of 5–0 plain gut, producing eversion of the skin edges (Fig. **4–6**). Use of absorbable suture avoids the requirement for suture removal, thus minimizing potential damage to delicate hair follicles.

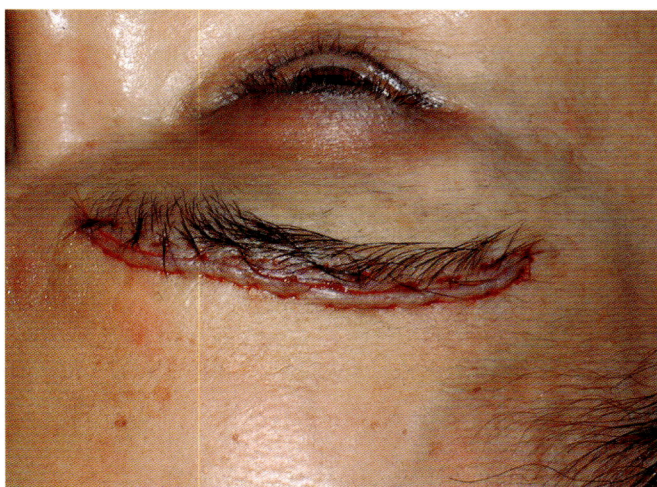

Figure 4–6 Closure with horizontal mattress suture of 5–0 plain catgut producing eversion of the skin edges.

Browlift Incisions

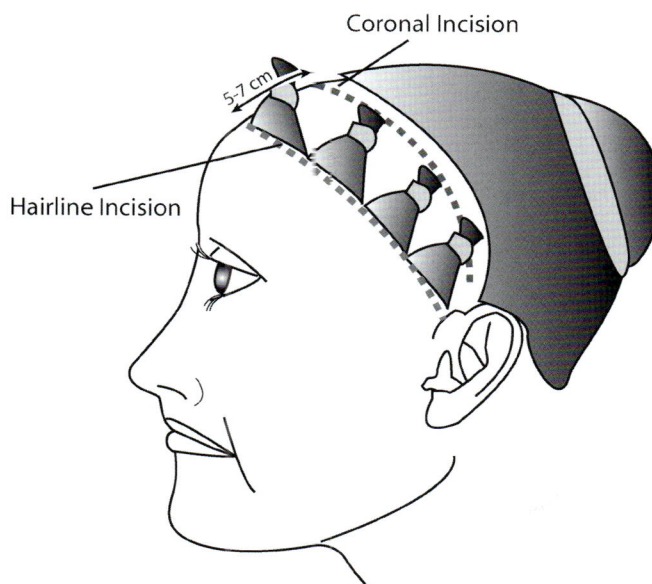

Figure 4–7 The coronal and hairline incisions for the forehead lift.

◆ Coronal Forehead Lift

In most individuals, the incision is placed 5 to 7 cm behind the hairline, but some patients are concerned about a "high forehead" and request placement of the incision directly at the frontal hairline (Fig. **4–7**). I try to discourage incision placement in this location, as the resulting scar is always somewhat visible, and the reduction of forehead dimension is minimal, considering the fact that the greatest amount of brow elevation, and therefore skin excision, occurs laterally rather than centrally.

When placed behind the hairline, the incision continues inferiorly into the temporal scalp to the level of the posterior helical border (~2 cm above the auricular attachment) and continues anteriorly 2 to 3 cm. An incision of this configuration facilitates inferior rotation of the flap during dissection. If placed in the hairline, however, the incision terminates in the temporal scalp just anterior to the auricular attachment.

1. The scalp incision is made using cutting cautery, and the flap is elevated in the supraperiosteal plane. Blunt dissection is generally effective until the suprabrow region is approached; care is taken to avoid segmental elevation of the periosteum by using sharp dissection to free adherent tissues.

2. Upon reaching the suprabrow region, a compilation of blunt and cautious sharp, "intrafibular" dissection mixed with a prying motion of the scissors best obviates injury to the neurovascular structures in this

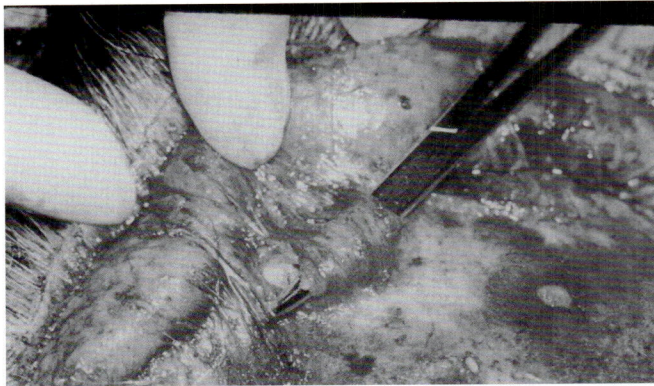

Figure 4–8 Isolation of a corrugator supercilii muscle in preparation for subtotal resection.

area. Upon identification of the superior orbital rim, subperiosteal dissection producing release of the arcus marginalis is undertaken. In the temporal region, flap elevation by blunt dissection proceeds to the level of the zygomatic arch in a plane deep to the facial nerve branches.

3. The corrugator supercilii muscles are defined and cautiously resected (subtotally), care being taken to avoid the small neurovascular bundles that course between the muscular fibers (Fig. **4–8**).

4. Using a cutting cautery, the frontalis muscle is crosshatched in both vertical and horizontal directions (Fig. **4–9**), creating a checkerboard interruption of this muscle. "Checkerboarding" greatly diminishes muscle function and allows avoidance of subtotal frontalis excision that is prone to produce localized forehead depressions or irregularities. This maneuver also partially releases the frontal aponeurosis, allowing more effective elevation of the brow.

5. Lifting is initiated in the lateral aspect of the flap, elevating each brow so that an aesthetically pleasing arch has maximal elevation at approximately the

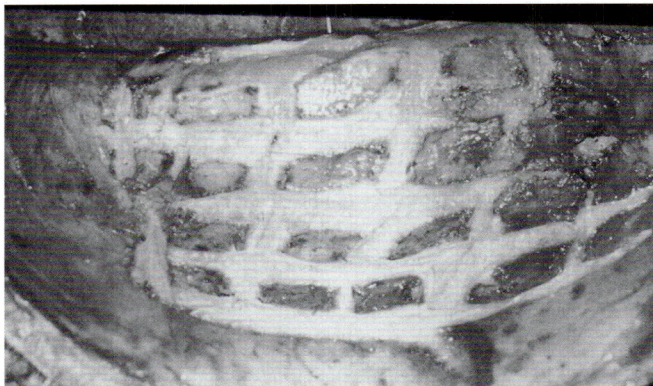

Figure 4–9 Reducing the function of the frontalis muscle by "crosshatching" or "checkerboarding" the muscle in both the horizontal and vertical directions.

level of the lateral limbus. Key sutures of 3–0 nylon are placed to accomplish this elevation; prior to proceeding, the brows are inspected for symmetry. The remainder of the flap is trimmed so that the skin edges approximate easily with little tension. The galea is approximated in three or four areas with 3–0 nylon, and the skin edges are closed with surgical staples.

Due to the coarseness and density of hair in most Asian patients, temporary hair loss following the coronal forehead lift is rarely of concern. However, segmental hypesthesia of the forehead may persist for 6 weeks to 6 months postoperatively but rarely constitutes a significant complaint. Occasionally, a patient experiences uncomfortable pruritus of similar duration that poses a treatment challenge: I use pramoxine with 1% hydrocortisone lotion (Pramosone cream 1%; Ferndale Laboratories Ferndale, MI) and add hydroxyzine if necessary.

Complications

Except for ticlike pain that may occur following the direct brow lift as a consequence of nerve strangulation with a fixation suture, and forehead hypoesthesia that may occur after the forehead lift (interbrow hypoesthesia may occur following direct suprabrow lift accompanied by subtotal corrugator resection), complications following this procedure similar to those that may follow other procedures for facial rejuvenation are discussed in Chapter 5.

Alternative Approaches to the Glabellar Frown Lines

As evidenced by the popularity of botulinum toxin, the glabellar frown lines are a matter of concern for a great number of individuals. Many patients inquire about surgical treatment of this area but feel that the most commonly recommended approaches (i.e., coronal or endoscopic forehead procedures) require a larger investment in time and expense than they are willing to undertake. I described a technique of subtotal corrugator resection via the direct brow lift approach, and I have had success in improving the glabellar frown lines by subtotal corrugator resection via an intrabrow incision that does not involve brow lifting.

1. An incision is made in the medial third of the brow, care being taken to bevel the incision in the direction of the brow hairs so as to minimize damage to the follicles.

2. Dissection is carried over the midline, connecting with a similar dissection on the contralateral side, resulting in elevation of skin beneath the entire extent of the vertical frown lines.

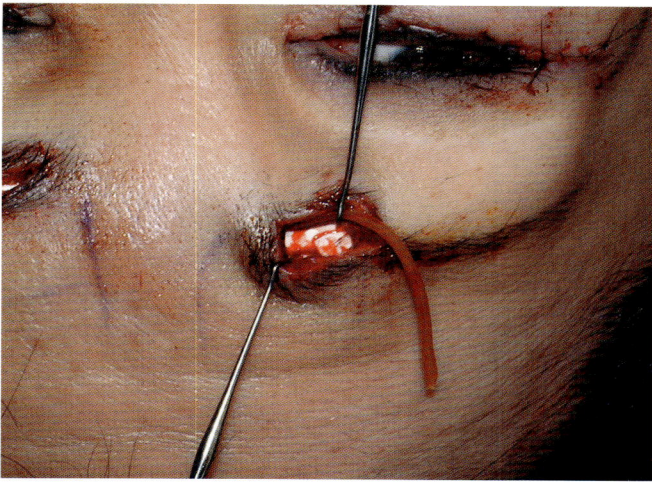

Figure 4–10   A tailored sheet of Gore-Tex placed beneath the glabellar frown lines.

3. Subtotal corrugator resection is undertaken by a combination of scissor dissection and avulsion with forceps so as to minimize damage to the neurovascular structures that course within the corrugator.

4. A sheet of Gore-Tex is tailored so that it fits the defect, and it is placed into the wound (Fig. **4–10**). I prefer to suture each lateral edge of the Gore-Tex with 6–0 nylon to minimize the chance of postoperative curling or bunching. The function of the Gore-Tex implant is twofold: to fill the small volume defect created by corrugator resection and to serve as a barrier to minimize reattachment of corrugator fibers to the dermis, a situation that leads to frown line recurrence.

5. A rubber-band drain is placed so that it exits through both brow incisions (Fig. **4–11**). The incisions are then approximated with interrupted sutures of 5–0 plain catgut.

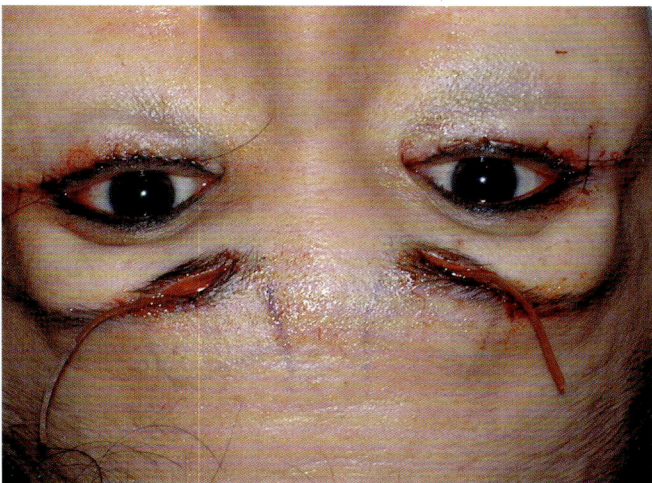

Figure 4–11   Rubber-band drains placed prior to wound closure.

A similar procedure can be performed via direct excision of one of the frown lines, preferably the deepest vertical rhytid. Most patients, however, prefer the intrabrow approach due to the absence of a visible postoperative scar. The key to success of this procedure is creation of a barrier to corrugator fiber reattachment using the Gore-Tex implant. Patients who undergo any of these procedures for effacement of the glabellar frown lines often benefit from postoperative treatment of residual depressions using various filler materials, as described in Chapter 13.

Forehead and Temple Augmentation

Occasionally, a patient requests augmentation of the central portion of the forehead for correction of a localized depression. Other patients request augmentation of depressions that may develop in the temporal fossa secondary to fat atrophy associated with the aging process. Correction of such defects with alloplastic implants is discussed in Chapter 11.

◆ Conclusion

Brow and forehead surgery, though rarely attracting the primary aesthetic concerns of Asian patients, are often a valuable adjunct to surgical enhancement of the eyelids and rejuvenation of the aging face. Many surgeons consider eyebrow position to be one of the most important factors in achieving rejuvenation of the aging upper face. In my practice, however, relatively few patients request either suprabrow or coronal forehead lifting as a primary procedure unless they have been impressed with postoperative results in one of their friends or acquaintances.

The results (and probably longevity) of coronal forehead lifting can be improved by careful attention to excision of subgaleal areolar tissue, enhancing fixation of the flap to the periosteum.

Considerable controversy exists regarding the best approach to browplasty. As a consequence of advances in endoscopic facial surgery during the 1990s, a considerable number of surgeons recommended an endoscopic approach for brow lifting, suggesting that, in addition to the procedure being less invasive, healing was more rapid and the incidence of complications substantially lower, further claiming that the coronal approach was obsolete and should be relegated to the dust bin of history. As is too often the case in contemporary cosmetic surgery, the experiences of most have not lived up to the hype surrounding the endoscopic approach (there are no definitive data indicating superiority in the efficacy or longevity of brow lifting, or any evidence

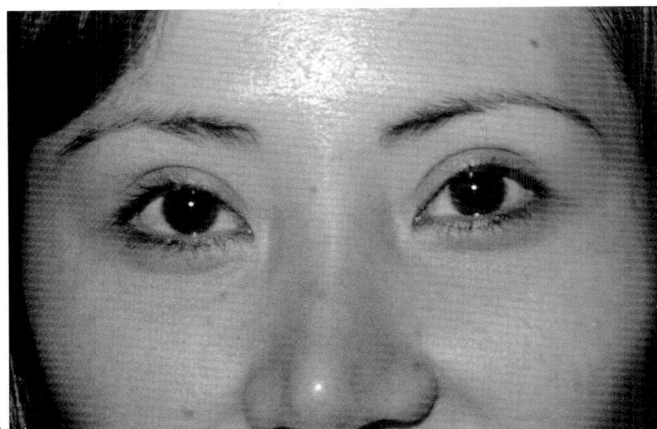

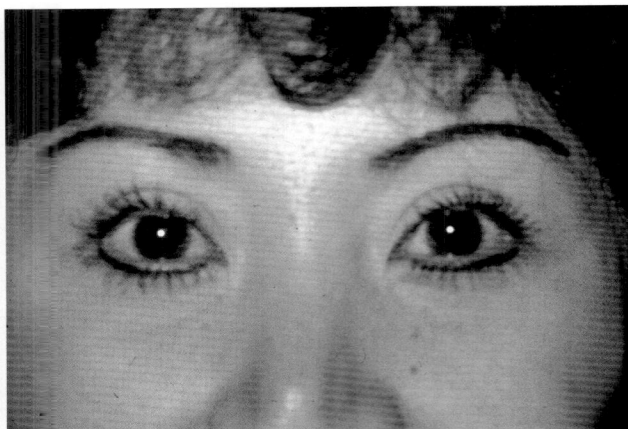

Figure 4–12   (A,B) Pre- and postoperative result following direct suprabrow lift.

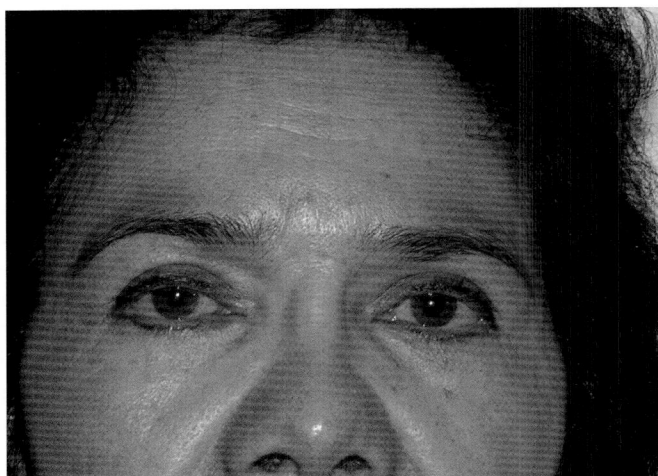

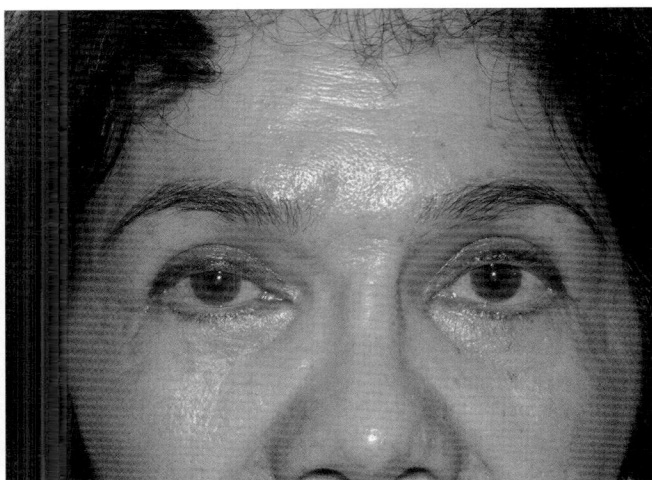

Figure 4–13   (A,B) Pre- and postoperative result following direct suprabrow lift.

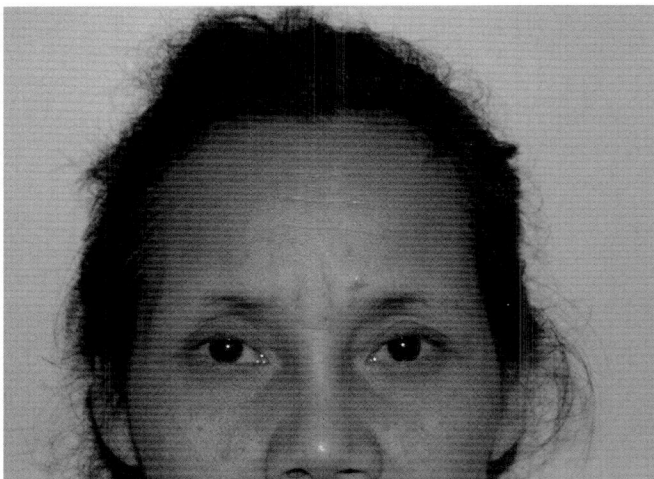

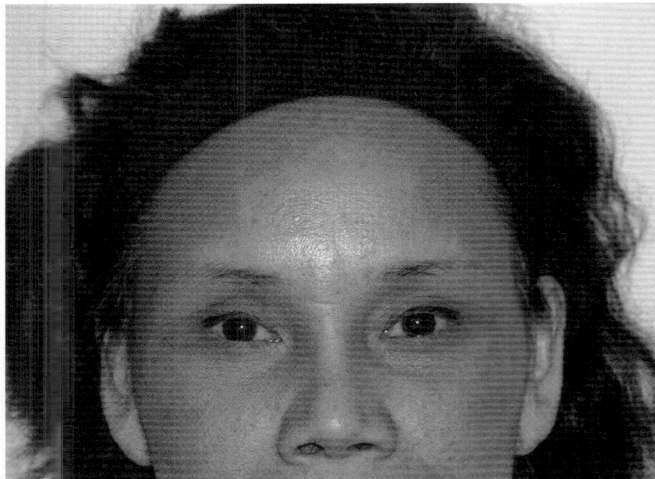

Figure 4–14   (A,B) Pre- and postoperative results following coronal forehead lift.

suggesting that the treatment of horizontal furrows and glabellar frown lines equals that of the coronal lift). Even the most enthusiastic endoscopic surgeons admit that many, if not most, of their colleagues are returning to the coronal lift as their method of choice.

I must disclose the fact that I have never personally performed endoscopic surgery for facial rejuvenation. A major reason is that, in my experience, most traditional Asian patients are somewhat suspicious about techniques that offer better results by minimizing surgical intervention, especially with regard to lesser degrees of skin removal. A patient dissatisfied with the results of this procedure would undoubtedly demonstrate considerable expressiveness (see Chapter 1) in demanding revision using a procedure that excised skin.

Lost in the battle over the endoscopic versus the coronal approach has been the efficacy of the direct suprabrow lift that I have described in detail. This procedure offers more precise reconstruction of optimal brow position and shape than either of its competitors (relying on direct visualization rather than a "formula" for the amount of skin excision per millimeter of desired brow elevation). Relatively speaking, the suprabrow lift is minimally invasive, and the only legitimate objection to this procedure—a visible scar—is largely obviated by the excellent results of scar camouflage using micropigmentation, if necessary.

Pre- and postoperative results of the direct suprabrow lift are illustrated in Figs. **4–12** and **4–13**. Fig. **4–14** demonstrates results of a coronal forehead lift.

5

Rejuvenation of the Aging Asian Face and Neck

Although the goals of rejuvenating the aging face and neck are the same in the Asian as in the Caucasian patient, certain anatomic differences, as well as biological manifestations of the aging process, are noteworthy, as they translate into variation in surgical approach to cervicofacial rhytidectomy.

◆ General and Anatomic Considerations

Differences between the Asian and Caucasian face and neck are manifested in skin thickness and texture, patterns of fat accumulation, and, perhaps most importantly, skeletal structure. When analyzing these anatomic differences, it is important to note that just as in the Caucasian population, considerable individual variations in anatomy exist among Asians, perhaps the most important variable being related to the geographic latitude of origin. In general, Asian skin tends to be thicker, and the face and neck tend to accumulate more fat during the aging process than the Caucasian. Prominent malar eminences accompanied by premaxillary retrusion and a relatively wide mandible combine to generate a more square, less angular configuration. A combination of heavier soft tissue and a flat facial skeleton translates into less resistance to gravitational forces with aging.

Skin

Although the classical Western description of Asian skin having a yellowish coloration is not without some biological justification, there is actually a wide variation in the color and texture of the skin. Generally, skin pigmentation is darker in Asians originating from southern latitudes, whereas individuals from northern areas tend to display light-colored, somewhat milky skin pigmentation. The yellowish tint of Asian skin is largely a consequence of the number and distribution of melanocytes rather than of variations in the skin lipoproteins.

As is the case with skin color, a wide variation in texture and thickness is apparent among Asians, the dermis tending to be more fibrous (or dense) in individuals with darker pigmentation. The skin of lightly pigmented Asians, however, is generally thicker and denser than of equivalently pigmented Caucasians. Greater collagen density is manifested in a tendency toward a more vigorous fibroplastic response toward wound healing, which may produce hypertrophic scarring and prolonged hyperemia during scar maturation, an incidence worthy of note even in lightly pigmented Asians (especially with regard to prolonged incisional hyperemia). Although I cannot recall ever having observed a true keloid in an Asian patient following cosmetic surgery, there is definitely an increased incidence of hypertrophic scar formation in the postauricular region, at the junction of the superior helical and temporal portions of rhytidectomy incisions, and in the medial canthal area. Curiously, hypertrophic scars are extremely rare in the alar crease.

Because of differences in dermal thickness, the Asian face undergoes photoaging differently than the Caucasian face, the Asian face tending to exhibit fewer fine wrinkles than a Caucasian of comparable age. The Asian face, however, shows a higher incidence of pigmented dermatoses (e.g., seborrheic keratoses, lentigines, and other melanocytic lesions) (Fig. **5–1**)

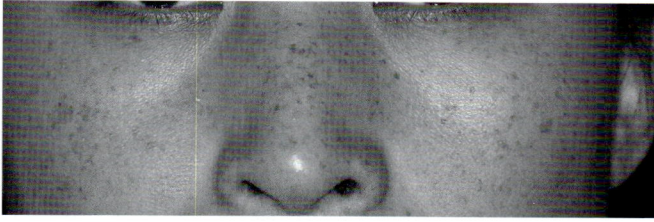

Figure 5–1   Lentigos in a 35-year-old Asian woman.

with aging, and fair-complexioned Asians often exhibit rhytidosis comparable to Caucasians of a similar age (Fig. **5–2**).

Skin flaps developed during cervicofacial rhytdectomy are more tolerant of tension; however, this is counterbalanced by an increased incidence of hypertrophic scar formation, as noted above. Some clinicians have described a more vertical orientation of subdermal vascularity in the Asian face and suggest that this anatomic pattern might reduce collateral circulation in skin flaps. I have noted no such differences in vascularity and conclude that such suggestions are of no clinical significance with regard to the tolerable extent of undermining.

Fat

During the aging process, the Asian face typically accumulates greater volumes of fat than its Caucasian counterpart. This fat accumulation tends to concentrate in the jowl, nasolabial mound, and buccal regions The

clinical significance of fat accumulated in these areas as accentuated by the skeletal structure of the Asian face has important implications for successful surgical management of facial aging.

Fat accumulation in the neck that contributes to the so-called double chin is less common in Asians younger than 40 years old than in comparably aged Caucasians; submental fat accumulation, however, occurs more frequently in the Asian than in the Caucasian neck after age 40.

Platysma Muscle

Although the platysma is generally thicker in the Asian neck, the incidence of diastasis is considerably less, occurring in ~30% of patients who undergo cervicofacial rhytidectomy (Fig. **5–3**), as compared with 60% of Caucasians undergoing this procedure.

Skeletal Structure

Perhaps the most significant anatomic differences between the Caucasian and Asian face are related to skeletal structure. As noted above, the Asian face is characterized by prominent malar eminences associated with relative deficiency of the premaxillary region that results in shallowness of the midfacial region. Wide, prominent mandibular angles are often present, contributing to a square, flattened face. Microgenia may be somewhat more common than in the Caucasian, but the

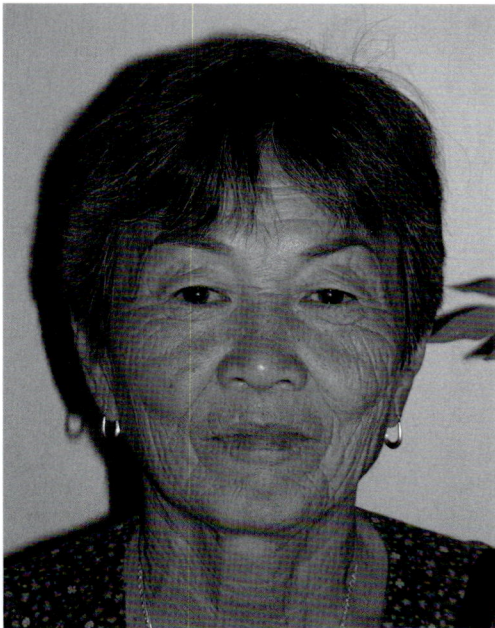

Figure 5–2   Extensive rhytidosis in 59-year-old Asian woman.

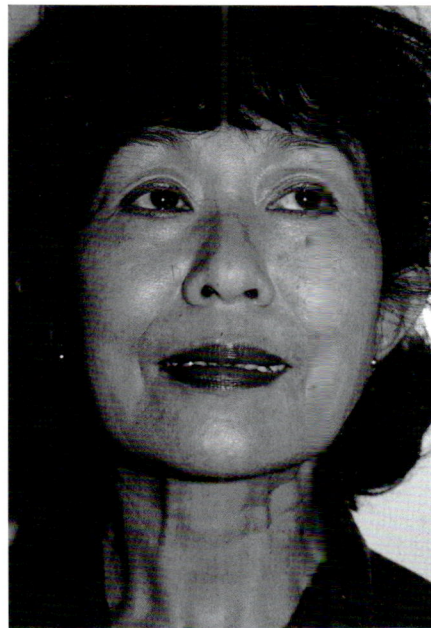

Figure 5–3   Diastasis of the anterior platysma.

cervical deformity attributed to a "low hyoid" bone is distinctly less common in the Asian neck.

◆ Formulating an Approach to Rejuvenation of the Aging Face and Neck

The basic subcutaneous face lift operation was described by Lexer in 1916, and, perhaps surprisingly, except for the extent of undermining, no substantial improvements or modifications in the basic procedure were introduced until the 1970s. Since that time there has been a vast proliferation of variations and modifications of the face lift operation; thus, not surprisingly, considerable controversy exists regarding the optimal surgical approach for facial rejuvenation. A brief historical survey of the evolution of face lift techniques is instructive and valuable in assisting the surgeon in formulating an approach to the aging face and neck.

The first such innovation was the Skoog technique introduced in 1973.[1] This procedure consisted of elevation of a platysmal flap in the neck and lower face without dissection of the overlying skin.

In 1976, Mitz and Peyronie[2] described the muscle and fascial complex of the lower face, which they termed the superficial musculoaponeurotic system (SMAS). Surgeons quickly became enamored with SMAS techniques, and numerous variations have been described (limited SMAS, lateral SMAS, conventional SMAS, extended SMAS, and anterior SMAS procedures); however, for the most part, the only actual modifications relate to the extent of flap elevation and/or the direction of flap suspension.

Experience has suggested that following any SMAS dissection, improvement is generally limited to the lower face (i.e., the jowl and mandibular regions). Incorporation of platysmal elevation and repositioning in conjunction with SMAS dissection extends improvement into the cervical region but does not improve the nasolabial folds, resulting in what some surgeons term "facial disharmony."

Of significance in assessing the role of SMAS dissection in cervicofacial rhytidectomy is the fact that the precise anatomy and clinical importance of this structure are currently matters of controversy, a situation that I term "SMAS confusion." Jost and Levet[3] claim that the anatomic interpretations of Mitz and Peyronie are erroneous, the SMAS layer that they described being merely a superficial fascial layer that lacks sufficient tensile strength to hold plication sutures. According to their anatomic studies Jost and Levet state that the true SMAS is actually a deeper structure contiguous with the parotid fascia that ne-

cessitates actual exposure of the lobular structures of this gland for proper dissection. Embryologic considerations, as well as histologic findings of muscle fibers in this tissue, support labeling the true SMAS as a vestige of the platysma aponeurosis.

Regardless of its precise anatomy, it is important to consider that the SMAS itself does not participate in facial ptosis, and thus any role that it may play in facial rejuvenation is limited to service as a vehicle to assist in repositioning of more anterolateral (or superficial) ptotic tissues, being of value by diverting tension from the skin flap.

Efforts to improve the nasolabial fold were largely unsuccessful until 1988, when Hamra[4] described the deep plane rhytidectomy. This procedure involved elevation of the malar fat pad following its dissection from the superficial surface of the zygomatic musculature. This dissection was accompanied by elevation of a SMAS flap in the lower face, and was the first technique that allowed true anatomic repositioning of cheek fat in an effort to efface the nasolabial folds.

Not completely satisfied with results of this procedure because, although the nasolabial fold did demonstrate improvement, stigmata of aging in the superior aspect of the malar region and the lower portion of the orbicularis muscle persisted, Hamra[5] enhanced the deep plane rhytidectomy by incorporating dissection of orbicularis oculi into the flap, producing a bipedicled musculocutaneous flap based on the platysma and orbicularis blood supply. This operation was termed composite rhytidectomy, and a key concept of this procedure involved the ability to suspend the flap under "extraordinary tension" to efface the nasolabial fold. Hamra maintained that the composite rhytidectomy was the only anatomically correct method for deep plane manipulation, and that, in contrast, SMAS dissection disrupted the normal relationships among the orbicularis, cheek fat, platysma, and skin.

Of major interest in this regard was a study published in 1996. Ivy, Lorenc, and Aston[6] compared various SMAS procedures and composite rhytidectomy, different procedures being performed on contralateral sides of the face in 21 patients. The surgeons reported that on the operating table, composite rhytidectomy produced more dramatic effacement of the nasolabial folds as compared with limited SMAS dissection, but that this difference disappeared within 24 hours postoperatively, and no difference was observed by a panel of three surgeons or the patients themselves on evaluation 6 and 12 months postoperatively.

Following long-term examination of his results, Hamra[7] stated that neither the deep plane nor early versions of the composite rhytidectomy resulted in substantial lasting effacement of the nasolabial fold (in contrast to the effect of SMAS dissection that yielded long-term improvement in the lower face), and that the only method of producing long-term improvement was direct excision (nasolabioplasty). He further suggested that an improved composite rhytidectomy incorporating superomedial repositioning of the orbicularis–zygomatic muscle reduced the incidence of postrhytidectomy facial disharmony that results from disparity between the longevity of SMAS dissection (lower face) and midfacial rejuvenation.

To summarize, SMAS dissection tends to improve results in the jowl and mandibular regions, but it is associated with relatively poor nasolabial effacement, a disparity that may produce "facial disharmony." One possible reason for this effect is the fact that SMAS may actually result in tethering of the zygomatic muscles, dissipating "lifting" forces applied intraoperatively by plication or suspension. Of importance is the fact that many surgeons feel that, in spite of the initial optimism surrounding the deep plane and composite face lifting techniques, there is little evidence of lasting benefit as compared with extended subcutaneous lifting.

Other surgeons approached the problem of midfacial ptosis utilizing subperiosteal dissection inspired by the techniques of Tessier, which were developed in his epic contributions to reconstruction of craniofacial deformities. In 1988, Psillakis and his associates[8] described a subperiosteal approach for which they claimed enhanced results but which was associated with a high incidence of facial nerve injury. Ramirez et al have been the most persistent disciples of the subperiosteal face lift, first describing this technique in 1991[9] and stating that their modifications reduce the incidence of facial nerve complications from 20 to ~2%.

The subperiosteal approach described by Ramirez et al begins with a coronal incision, thus allowing subperiosteal dissection to the level of the superior and lateral orbital rim. Laterally, the dissection continues deep to the temporoparietal fascia; at a point ~3 cm above the zygomatic arch, dissection is deepened through both layers of the temporalis fascia, continuing to the superior aspect of the zygomatic arch, at which point the deep temporal fascia and periosteum of the entire zygomatic arch are incised on its posterior surface with a scalpel. The subperiosteal dissection is connected with the superior and lateral orbital rim dissection plane, and dissection over the anterior surface of the zygomatic arch and body continues over the maxilla inferiorly to the pyriform aperture. Dissection is continued inferiorly over the masseter muscle, this freeing of the cheek tissues from the masseter being the key factor in allowing midfacial elevation.

Currently, there is much enthusiasm (although I sense that it is waning) for endoscopic,[10–12] transble-pharoplasty,[13,14] and transbrow[15] approaches to the midface. (Many such techniques depend on suture or "sling"(utilizing alloplastic or autogenous material) suspension of musculofascial tissues as a vehicle for skin–fat elevation.[16–18] Although I certainly applaud all attempts at innovation and technical improvement, I maintain a cautious attitude, given the surgical community's experience with enthusiastic embrace of previous techniques that all too often failed to yield the long-term benefits suggested by early results. At any rate, even the enthusiasts for such procedures suggest that they are most effective for younger patients who exhibit minimal redundant tissue. Given the tendency for the aging Asian face to accumulate large volumes of fat in the central cheek region, I feel that particular caution is warranted in application of such techniques to this population.

As might be expected, advocates of deep approaches to the midfacial tissues have been vigorously opposed by other surgeons concerned by the high incidence of prolonged edema, facial nerve injury, and associated complications. Several experienced surgeons have suggested that the pendulum has swung too far, recommending, in the interest of patient safety, as well as the lack of definitive evidence proving long-term efficacy, a return to more traditional techniques of facial rejuvenation.

In spite of this tangled web of controversy regarding the optimal surgical approach (that remains uncertain and in a state of continuing evolution and discovery), most surgeons do agree that regardless of the techniques employed, the goals of rejuvenation should be the same: a natural, long-lasting appearance associated with a relatively rapid healing period and a low incidence of complications.

Each individual surgeon has strong opinions regarding the relative importance of various facial components and the most efficacious method of achieving optimal results. Most, however, agree that achieving these goals requires repositioning of ptotic skin as well as some sort of manipulation (not necessarily dissection and/or elevation) of deeper structures. A major problem in face lift surgery relates to the fact that cosmetic surgery is not an exact science. Results are difficult to quantitate with scientific precision. Double-blind studies are impractical because of both ethical and logistical considerations, and reliable animal models are not available. A major reason for absence of proof of long-term efficacy is the fact that most satisfied patients do not return for extended follow-ups. Most individual surgeons are convinced, largely for anecdotal reasons, that their techniques produce the best results. Finally, the "herd instinct" seems to be particularly powerful in cosmetic surgery.

As a most interested observer and a participant in this continuing 30-year drama, my preferences have undergone significant metamorphoses as a function of time. I have chosen my current rhytidectomy techniques (which, of course, are subject to change as clinical evidence evolves) based on the following observations and convictions:

1. Skin and fat morphology are the key factors in determining whether the face and neck appear youthful or aged. Regardless of the amount of attention paid to deep tissues, successful rejuvenation requires that ptotic skin and fat be replaced in a more youthful position. The mindset of the surgeon when performing cheek lifting should be elevation of the midface; the mindset when rejuvenating the neck should be restoration of the submental and anterior cervical region, requiring platysma modification if anterior banding is present.

2. Most clinically significant ptosis occurs in the anteromedial aspect of the face and neck. Although the posterolateral portion of the face is traversed to gain access to these tissues, there is no evidence that elevation (repositioning) of the deeper tissues of this region (i.e., SMAS, periosteum, posterior platysma) serves any purpose other than acting as a vehicle for tension sharing in effective repositioning of the more medial tissues. Certainly mobilization and elevation of these posterolateral tissues (as a vehicle for tension sharing) have less effect on anteromedial ptosis per unit of elevation than the effect of direct elevation of the medial tissues enabled by wider skin undermining.

3. With regard to tension sharing, there appears to be an inverse relationship between the extent of skin undermining and tension placed on the skin flap. In other words, as the amount of skin undermining increases, the amount of flap tension required to reposition the skin decreases. Conversely, abbreviated skin undermining tempts the surgeon to apply more tension to effect repositioning of anteromedial tissues. To achieve optimal skin repositioning, undermining must be sufficient to release the osteofasciodermal ligaments (zygomatic, masseteric, parotid, mandibular). The barrier function of these ligaments must be appreciated (the structures act as barriers to ptosis of the aging skin and subcutaneous tissue resulting in characteristic and predictable sagging immediately inferior to their location). It is necessary to release these barriers (i.e., the cutaneous attachments of these ligaments) to maximize mobilization and subsequent lifting. This has been termed the "ironing" effect.

4. Repositioning of deeper structures is not necessarily a substitute for wide skin undermining, as optimal skin repositioning often requires wide release and mobilization, especially in the older patient. Deep tissue repositioning and skin undermining are often complementary procedures, but each must be evaluated and employed based on its individual merits. For instance, if repositioning of the malar fat pad is deemed to be of aesthetic benefit, mobilization and elevation via either a supra- or subperiosteal approach are appropriate, but such manipulation does not mean that additional aesthetic benefit cannot be achieved by extension of skin flap mobilization i.e., undermining) over the elevated malar fat.

5. Microliposuction, described in detail below, is often a valuable adjunct to management of certain problem areas, notably the nasolabial mound, the jowl, and the submental region. This technique offers a compromise between replacement of ptotic fat into a more youthful position and direct excision of fat (as in direct nasolabioplasty) and is accompanied by some degree of aesthetically beneficial skin contraction in the suctioned area. Microliposuction is of particular value in the Asian face because of its propensity for fat accumulation during the aging process.

Surgeons are understandably frustrated by the current state of affairs in cervicofacial rhytidectomy. To some extent, public relations agents have replaced peer review, "innovations" are hyped for their marketing value, and as a result many patients demand the latest techniques that lack proof of efficacy. Responsible surgeons recognize that rapid healing and restoration of social and occupational functioning as well as safety are important factors in patient satisfaction. In many respects, these factors exceed the importance of total eradication of all vestiges of facial aging, especially when more complex techniques involve prolonged healing and an increased incidence of complications.

The primary techniques that I employ for cervical facial rhytidectomy are described in the following sections.

◆ Rhytidectomy (Full Face Lift)

As noted above, since the description of SMAS in 1976, surgeons have attempted to devise an enhanced, longer lasting face lift based on dissection of the deep facial and cervical tissues. Although mobilization and modification of deep cervical structures (i.e., platysma muscle) have become accepted practice for most surgeons, many have been reluctant to incorporate the aggressive dissection of deeper facial structures into their surgical routines because of the seeming complexity of these procedures coupled with the increased risk of facial nerve injury (as well as prolonged facial edema). In addition, the initial enthusiasm for SMAS mobilization has waned somewhat, as it has become apparent that, although such techniques do enhance effacement of the jowl, little or no long-term improvement is noted in the midfacial (i.e., nasolabial mound and fold) regions following even the most extensive SMAS dissection.

New insights into the pathophysiology of midfacial ptosis have clarified understanding of the failure of SMAS dissection to rejuvenate this region. Because midfacial aging is largely a consequence of ptosis of the malar fat pad (not accompanied by ptosis or diminished tone of the mimetic musculature), in some cases associated with localized hypertrophy of cheek fat, rejuvenation of this area requires direct elevation (or other modification) of the ptotic malar fat pad and overlying skin.[19] Although this goal can be achieved via supra- or subperiosteal approaches, I initially felt that the subperiosteal approach provided a direct route associated with a lower incidence of complications than supra-periosteal dissection.

Since March 1994, I have used a direct, simplified approach to subperiosteal dissection of the midface[20] that obviates the need to initiate subperiosteal dissection via the coronal approach with time-consuming, tedious, and often frustrating attempts to release periosteum from the deep and superficial surfaces of the zygomatic arch to safely enter the midfacial region. This subperiosteal midfacial dissection is of special benefit in the Asian face, because the detrimental aesthetic effects of midfacial ptosis are accentuated in this population as a consequence of the skeletal characteristics noted previously.

At this juncture, I wish to emphasize that although the anatomic differences noted previously are important, the basic technique that I employ for the Asian patient is similar to that which I utilize for the Caucasian face, the major exception being the extra attention paid to modification of fat in the central face. This is consistent with the fact that the goals of facial rejuvenation are the same for all ethnic groups. In general, I do not subscribe to notions that occasionally originate from surgeons in Asian countries that the characteristic anatomy of the Asian face necessitates substantial modifications in surgical techniques (with the notable exception of skeletal surgery) for successful rejuvenation.

Surgical Technique: A Simplified Approach to Subperiosteal Dissection of the Midface

The basic operation of cervicofacial rhytidectomy is essentially the same in both Asian and Caucasian patients, with the exception of the requirement for increased attention to the midface in the Asian, as the combination of fat accumulation and skeletal deficiency allows malar fat pad ptosis to produce especially prominent nasolabial mounds

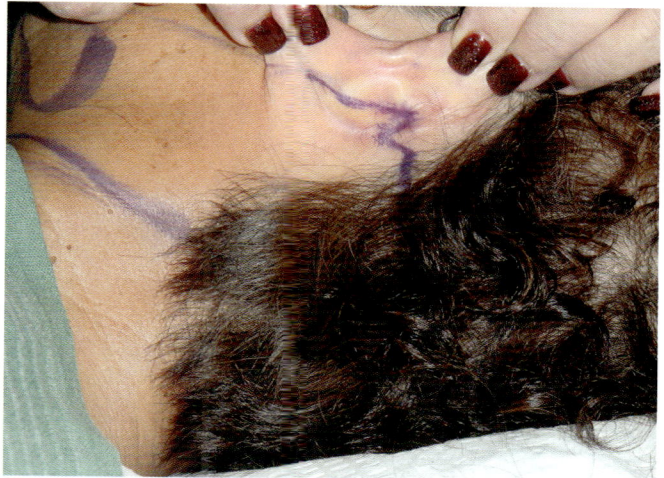

Figure 5–4   Half Z-plasty to minimize hypertrophic webbing of the postauricular incision.

and deep nasolabial folds. The skin incisions are the same in both populations, and any of the described incisional modifications in the temporal and cervical regions may be utilized. One particularly useful variation in the cervical region involves a dart or "half Z-plasty" just posterior to the postauricular crease that tends to minimize the incidence of postoperative webbing in this area (Fig. 5–4).

If subperiosteal dissection of the midface is to be performed, the temporal aspect of the incision is extended posterior to the hairline to a level superior to the lateral aspect of the brow. Undermining of the temporal scalp begins in the subdermal plane at a level sufficiently deep to preserve hair follicles. Dissection at this level (i.e., superficial to the superficial layer of temporal fascia rather than deep to this fascial layer) provides additional protection for the temporal branch of the facial nerve and provides a less vascular surgical plane. Undermining extends anteriorly to the lateral aspect of the brow, to the lateral periorbital rim, and to a point ~1 cm anterior to the anterior border of the masseter muscle (see preoperative facial markings, Fig. 5–5). The dissection extends over the mandibular margin to join the cervical flap if a full face/neck lift is to be performed.

Attention is then directed to the midfacial region. The anatomic foundation of this simplified approach to subperiosteal dissection of the malar fat pad/zygomatic muscle complex relates to the constant relationship between the temporal and zygomatic branches of the facial nerve in this region (Fig. 5–6). Initiation of the subperiosteal dissection just posterior to the junction of the zygomatic body and frontal process of the zygoma (i.e., essentially over the greatest prominence of the malar eminence) ensures that both branches are protected. I term this region the "window of opportunity." Following incision of soft tissue through the periosteum,

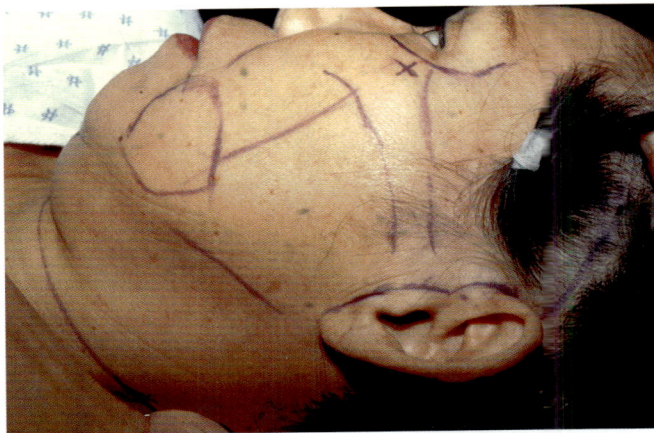

Figure 5–5   External preoperative markings for cervicofacial rhytidectomy with the subperiosteal malar flap. Note markings for jowl, anterior border of the masseter and lateral periorbital region, and zygomatic arch. The X marks the approximate locus for initiating dissection of the subperiosteal flap.

the subperiosteal dissection is initiated with a Freer elevator and proceeds inferiorly and medially into the canine fossa toward the pyriform aperture, beneath the nasolabial fold. As the dissection proceeds inferiorly and medially, the Freer elevator is exchanged for a blunt duckbill-type elevator, and the dissection is guided by a combination of the dissecting hand maintaining

elevator contact with bone and digital palpation of dissection progress through the skin surface with the other hand. The key to successful tissue mobilization and elevation is release of this composite flap (Fig. **5–7**) from its attachments to the tendinous (and thus avascular) anterior aspect of the masseter, easily and safely accomplished by blunt dissection. Should flap mobilization prove difficult, the tendency on the part of the inexperienced surgeon is to extend the dissection medially. Dissection in this direction, however, proves fruitless. Additional flap mobilization can only be obtained by dissecting more inferiorly along the tendinous portion of the masseter muscle and/or more posteriorly on the zygoma. Additional subperiosteal dissection over the body of the zygoma ensures that all fibers of the zygomatic ligament are released. Approximately 1 to 1.5 cm of posterosuperior composite flap advancement is then possible, resulting in improved effacement of the nasolabial fold and repositioning of the malar fat pad in a more youthful position (Figs. **5–8A,B**). Many surgeons advocate use of a buccal incision to assist subperiosteal elevation over the maxilla. I have found such an incision, however, to be unnecessary. Periosteum at the inferior and anterior aspects of this dissection is somewhat attenuated and is undoubtedly severed during the dissection, enhancing flap mobilization. The composite flap is not trimmed but is imbricated in a "pants over vest"

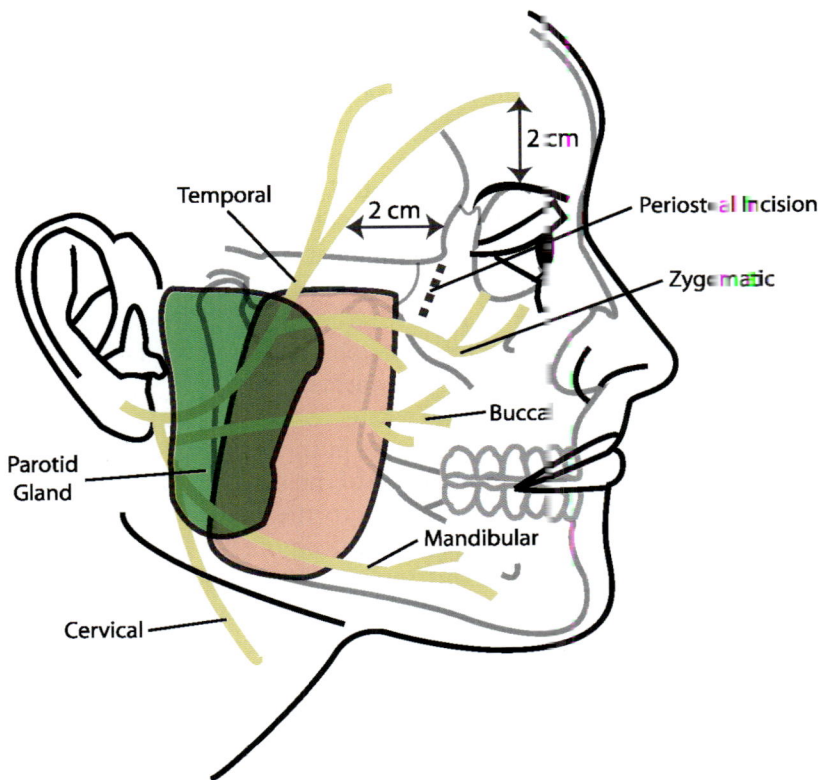

Figure 5–6   Anatomy of the facial nerve in the malar region.

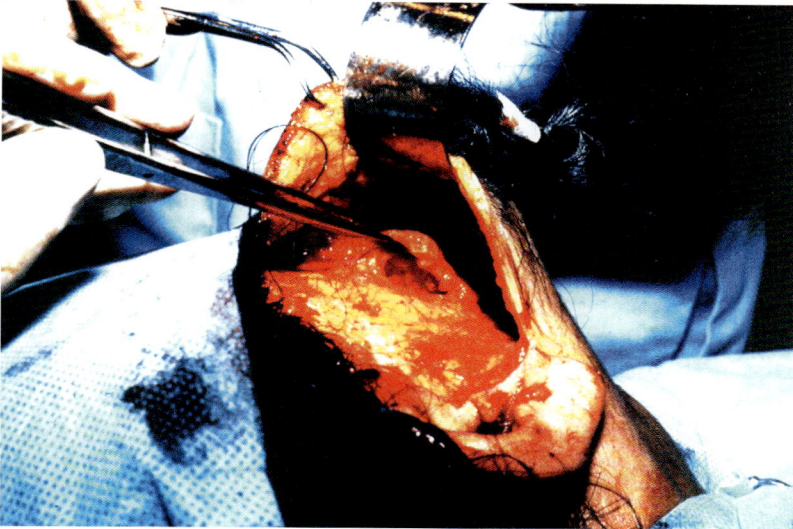

Figure 5–7 Intraoperative view of the subperiosteal malar flap.

fashion, being suspended to the superior aspect of the original flap incision (to avoid strangulation of more superiorly located facial nerve branches) with two or three sutures of 3–0 nylon to provide "permanent" fixation.

Because of the extensive mobilization and elevation of the midfacial region, the skin flap must be dissected to the level of the lateral orbital rim to avoid bunching. Such dissection allows exposure and modification of the orbicularis oculi muscle for treatment of lateral periorbital rhytids, if indicated. In some patients, the midfacial skin is dissected over the malar region and to the nasolabial fold to enhance draping of the skin flap. In spite of this increased skin undermining, reduced tension on the skin flap is enabled by advancement and suspension of the composite flap. Such management of the skin flap is in marked contrast to the "extraordinary tension" placed on the skin flap by advocates of the

deep plane or composite face lift operations who use the skin as a vehicle for advancement of the malar fat pad.

I must emphasize that, unlike the deep plane or composite face lift operations, the simplified subperiosteal malar flap dissection is not a substitute for reduced skin undermining. On the contrary, as noted above, utilization of the subperiosteal malar flap as described generally requires an increased extent of skin undermining. This is consistent with the fourth fundamental principle of surgical facial rejuvenation noted above, the necessity of sufficient skin undermining to allow "ironing" of the skin flap by adequate mobilization, suspension, and subsequent skin excision.

Because the nasolabial fold has been effaced by the composite malar flap, wide SMAS dissection toward the central face is unnecessary.

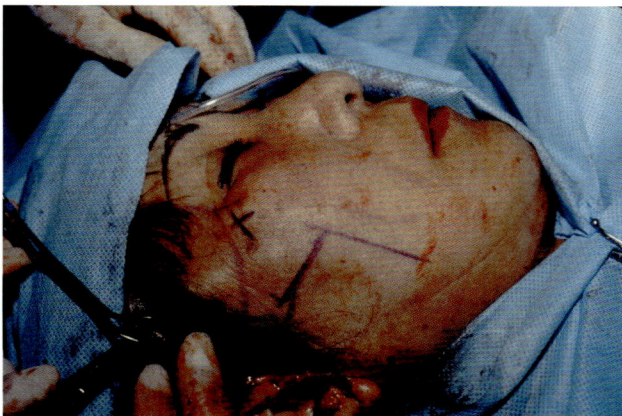

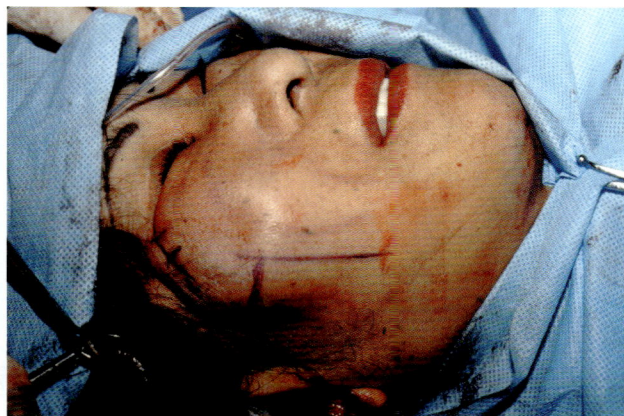

A   B

Figure 5–8 **(A)** View shows the subperiosteal malar flap before traction has been applied on it. **(B)** Effect of traction on the subperiosteal flap. Note the partial effacement of the nasolabial fold.

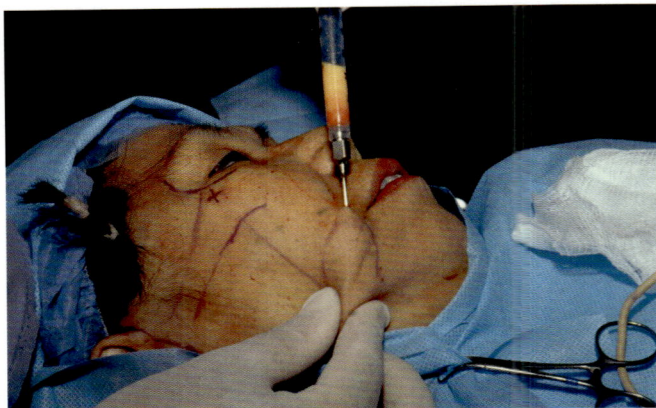

Figure 5–9 Microliposuction of the jowl.

Considerable improvement in the jowl region can be achieved by spot microliposuction of jowl fat via a stab wound in the labiomental fold with a 16-gauge needle cannula and syringe (Fig. **5–9**). Maximal effacement of the jowl may require skin flap elevation to the oral commissure to reduce the tethering effect of the mandibular ligaments. Occasionally, dissection of a small SMAS flap is initiated (dissection is initiated in a plane that exposes the lobular elements of the parotid gland as recommended by Jost and Levet) approximately 2 cm inferior to the zygomatic arch. The posterior border of this flap lies immediately lateral to the anterior border of the masseter (Fig. **5–10A,B**). Superiorly directed traction on the flap allows advancement of ptotic jowl tissue. Because the nasolabial fold has been effaced by suspension of the composite malar flap, wide

SMAS dissection toward the central face is unnecessary. In some cases, however, additional effacement of the nasolabial fold may be achieved by microliposuction debulking as described below.

Although the subperiosteal malar flap is suspended immediately following its dissection, skin flap rotation/elevation is deferred until the contralateral flaps have been dissected. Attention is then redirected toward the original side, which is carefully inspected for hematoma or bleeding prior to elevation, tailoring, and closure of the skin flap. This sequence offers a "second look" that reduces the incidence of postoperative hematoma. Pre- and postoperative photographs of the subperiosteal malar flap procedure are presented in Figs. **5–11** and **5–12**.

Anterior SMAS Plication: An Alternative to Dissection of a Subperiosteal Malar Flap

My initial enthusiasm for the simplified subperiosteal flap elevation has waned somewhat during the past several years as I became more sympathetic with the fact that patients undergoing this procedure did experience postoperative edema for a time substantially longer than those undergoing wide subcutaneous dissection. I also began to suspect that, although the initial results following this approach seemed to be superior to my skin flap procedures, the results after 12 to 18 months did not appear to show substantial improvement over my previous procedures. Consequently, I sought new methods, and the technique that I chose, anterior SMAS plication,[21] a procedure designed to effect effacement of the nasolabial folds, has yielded

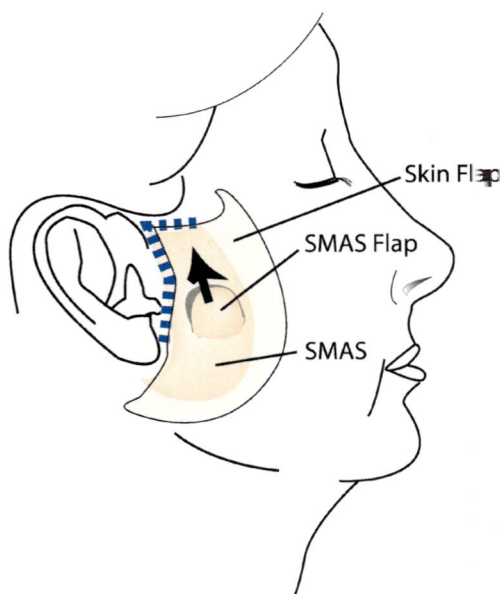

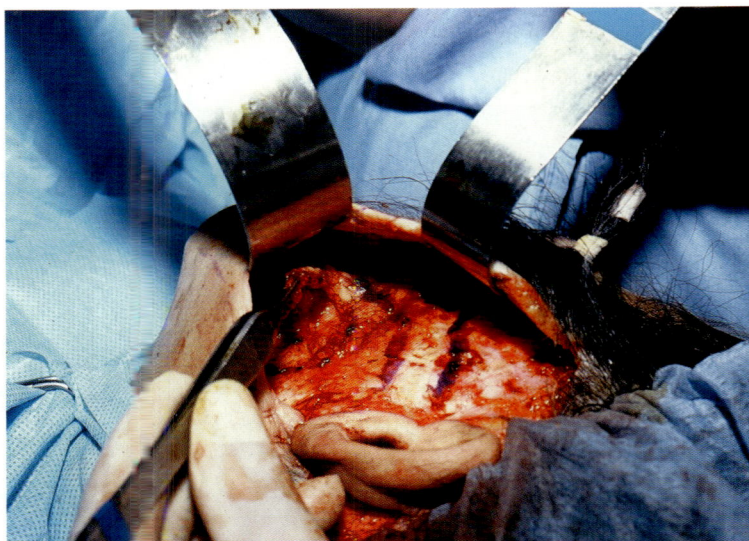

A

B

Figure 5–10 **(A,B)** Modified SMAS flap for effacement of the jowl.

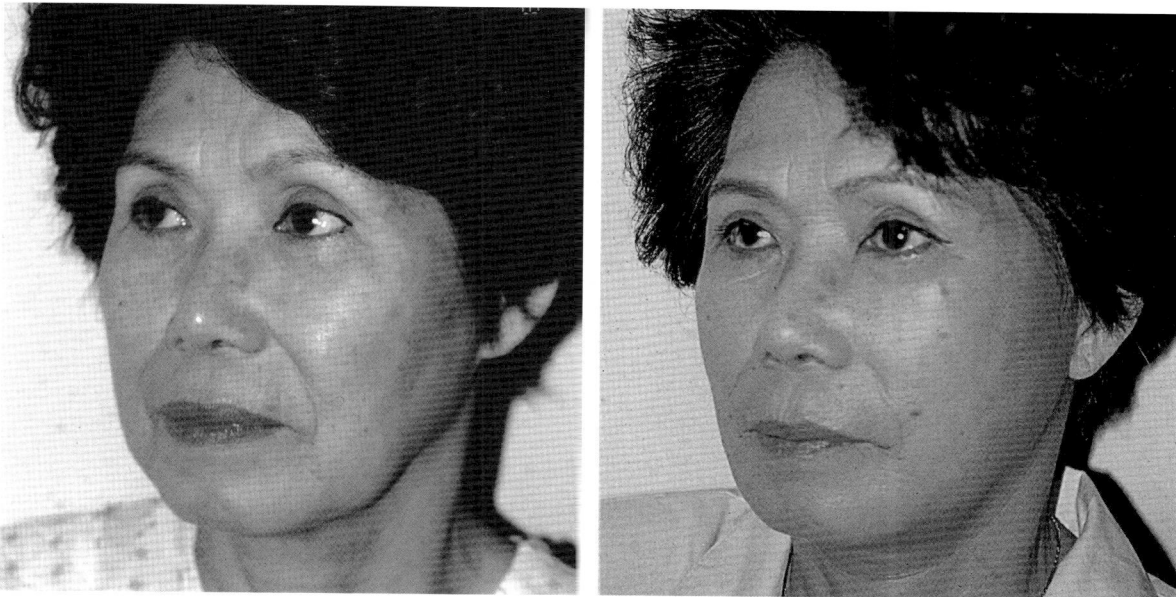

Figure 5–11   (A,B) Pre- and postoperative photographs of a cervicofacial rhytidectomy with a subperiosteal malar flap.

improved results with postoperative edema similar to that of subcutaneous procedures. My thinking in choosing this technique over alternative described procedures relates to my belief that the primary cause of facial aging is ptosis of the skin and subcutaneous fat in this region, and that the most direct and probably most effective technique of restoring this tissue to a more youthful position would, theoretically, involve direct mobilization and plication (or actual debulking of adipose tissue) rather than attempting to lift these tissues by traction on deeper structures located more posteriorly. This belief was reinforced by a study using MRI techniques that confirmed that the primary problem in nasolabial fold development is ptosis of the skin and subcutaneous tissue, rather than sagging of the musculofascial structures.[19]

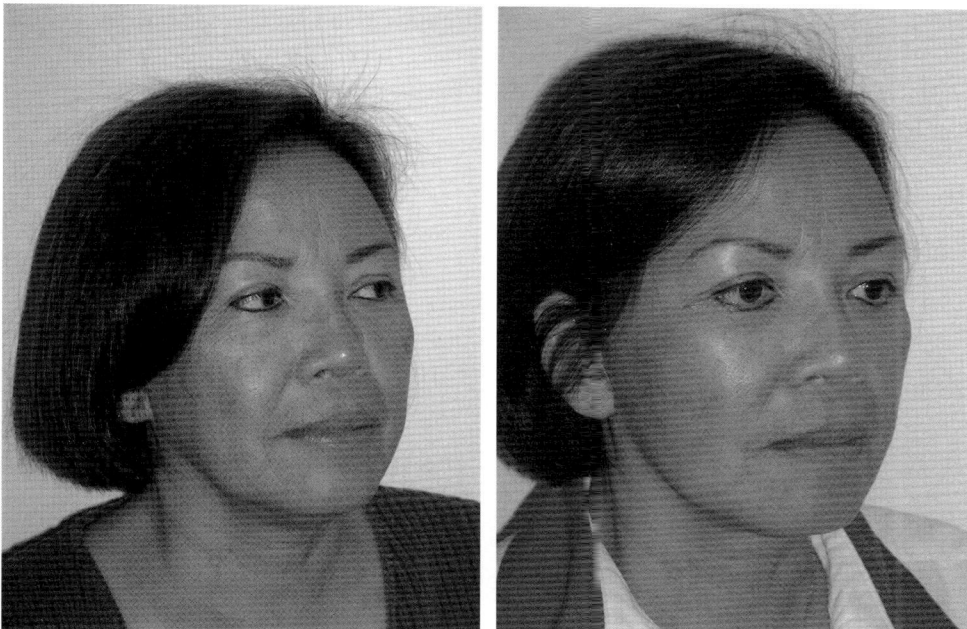

Figure 5–12   (A,B) Pre- and postoperative photographs of a cervicofacial rhytidectomy with a subperiosteal malar flap.

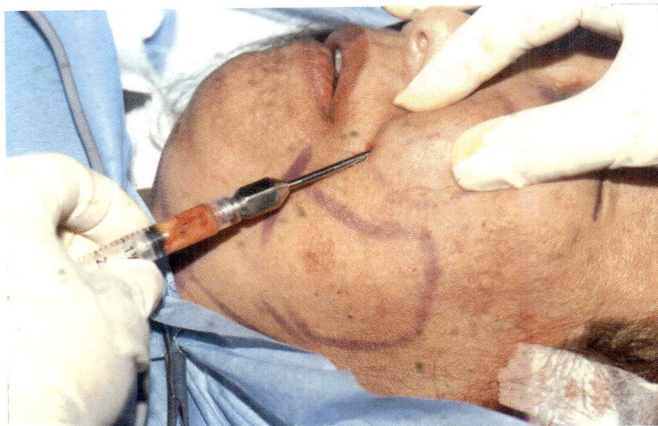

Figure 5–13   Microliposuction of the nasolabial mound.

Even if the surgeon chooses to elevate the malar fat pad into a more youthful position, aesthetic results in the midface are enhanced in many patients by debulking this region using syringe microliposuction (Fig. **5–13**) or a suitable alternative. Although surgeons whose primary patient population is Caucasian may dispute this contention, arguing that all ptotic facial fat should be elevated to replace it in a more youthful position, because removal of midfacial fat will result in postoperative hollowness, Asian patients seem to actually accumulate extra fat during the aging process, and it is this fat that benefits from removal using microliposuction techniques. An additional benefit of microliposuction is induction of some skin shrinkage over the treated area that follows this technique. Indeed, I find that I am employing this technique in an increasing number of patients in whom the malar fat pad is elevated using subperiosteal dissection or anterior SMAS plication.

It must be noted that the term *anterior SMAS plication* is actually a misnomer, as the tissue that is plicated is actually a condensation of fibroadipose tissue located just anterior to the actual SMAS, that is, the anterior border of the malar fat pad.

Surgical Technique: Anterior SMAS Plication

See DVD Disk Two, Cheek Lift

1. The incisions are the same as described for cervicofacial rhytidectomy using the subperiosteal malar flap (Fig. **5–14**). Cheek skin is undermined to a point ~50% of the distance between the anterior masseter border and nasolabial fold.

2. Just anterior to the masseter muscle, the anterior SMAS is easily identified as a condensation of fibrofatty tissue oriented in the direction of the nasolabial fold (Fig. **5–15**). Posterosuperior traction on this tissue with forceps results in elevation of the oral commissure and nasolabial mound (i.e., the malar fat pad).

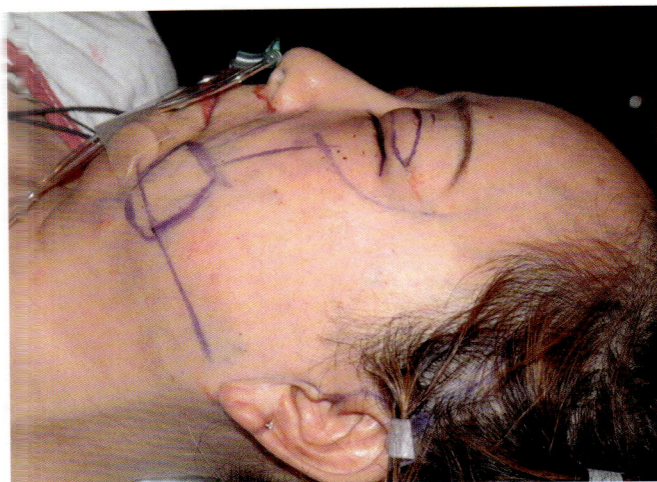

Figure 5–14   External markings for cervicofacial rhytidectomy with anterior SMAS plication.

3. Plication of the anterior SMAS is initiated with a 3–0 nylon suture placed at a point that produces the most effective elevation of the oral commissure. Additional plication sutures, generally numbering three or four, are placed superior and inferior to this initial suture to efface the nasolabial and labiomental folds.

4. Attention is then directed to the cheek skin. Inspection generally shows several dimples created by the fixation sutures. These dimples are released by additional skin undermining.

5. Hemostasis is secured, following which dissection is performed on the contralateral side of the face. The original flap is then rotated and tailored, following which the contralateral flap is closed in a similar fashion. Deferring closure of the original flap until completing dissection on the contralateral side offers a "second look" opportunity that diminishes the incidence of postoperative hematoma.

Although excellent elevation of the nasolabial mound is achieved by anterior SMAS plication, I find that, in many cases, additional benefit is achieved by debulking the nasolabial mound using syringe microliposuction. Judicious microliposuction often produces enhanced effacement of the jowl (Fig. **5–9**).

Pre- and postoperative photographs of cervicofacial rhytidectomy with anterior SMAS plication are presented in Figs. **5–16** and **5–17**.

Additional Considerations in the Management of the Nasolabial Fold

See DVD Disk Two, Gore-Tex Insertion and Liposuction of Nasolabial Folds

The nasolabial fold/mound complex is one of the most challenging areas in facial rejuvenation surgery, and classic methods of effacing this fold, including subperiosteal

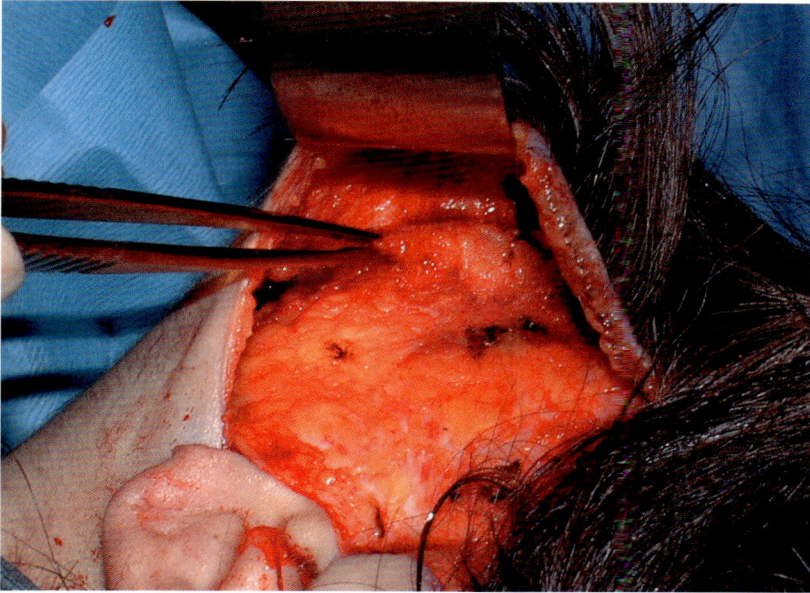

Figure 5–15 Intraoperative view of the anterior SMAS.

dissection and anterior SMAS plication, often yield suboptimal results. Microliposuction often improves the results of these techniques by adding controlled debulking of fat to the lifting procedure (Fig. **5–13**).

Microliposuction is performed via a stab wound in the inferior aspect of the nasolabial fold. A 16-gauge needle cannula is attached to a 3 cc syringe, allowing precise sculpturing of the nasolabial mound. Following debulking of this prominence, the cannula is employed as a dissector, extending beneath and medial to the nasolabial fold in an attempt to loosen its cutaneous attachments and thereby soften the fold.

Nasolabial liposuction is frequently performed as an isolated procedure for treatment of the nasolabial region in patients who do not wish or require cheek and/or face lift surgery.

The patient who undergoes nasolabial liposuction as an independent procedure or as an ancillary procedure in conjunction with cheek or face lifting must understand that the goal of this procedure is improvement, not perfection. If the patient is dissatisfied with the surgical result, several options are available. These include repeating the procedure and attempting further effacement of the fold using an injectable material.

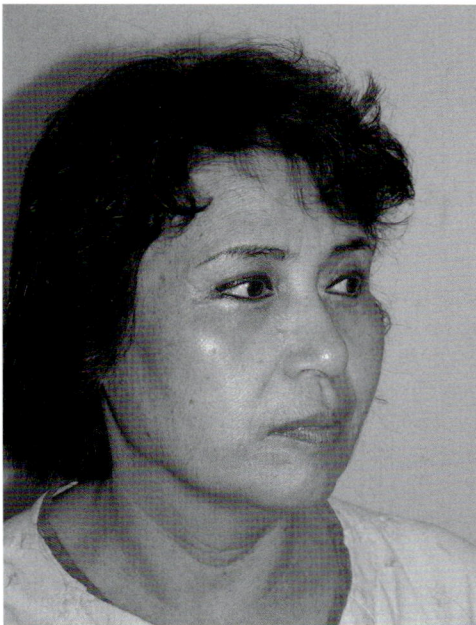

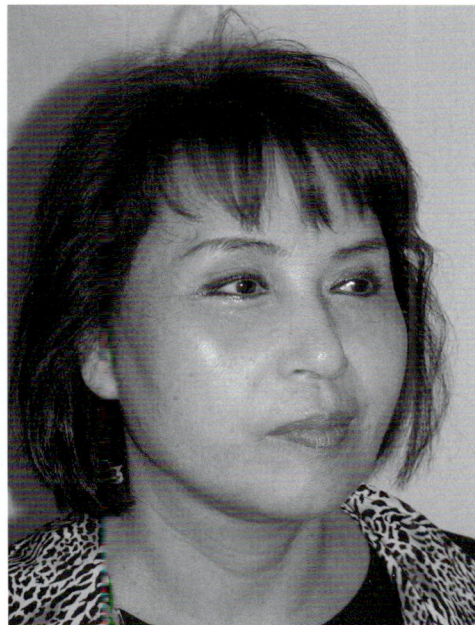

Figure 5–16 **(A,B)** Pre- and postoperative photographs of a cervicofacial rhytidectomy with anterior SMAS plication.

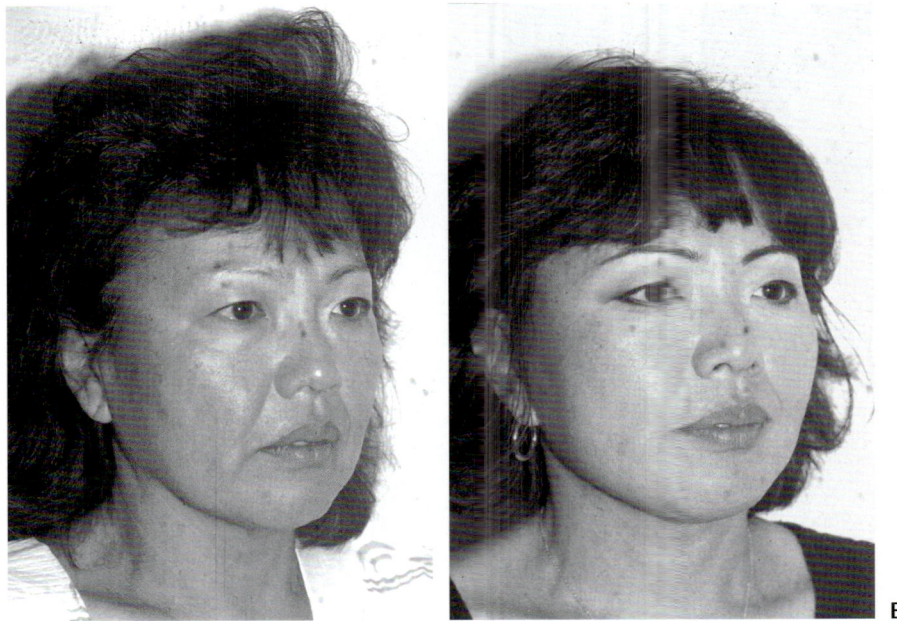

Figure 5–17 **(A,B)** Pre- and postoperative photographs of a cervicofacial rhytidectomy with anterior SMAS plication.

I inform patients that the nasolabial fold can be compared with a hill and valley, the hill being the nasolabial mound and the valley being the fold itself. Improvement, I explain, can be effected either by lowering the hill or by elevating the valley. Lowering of the hill, of course, is effected by microliposuction.

Raising the valley is achieved by augmentation of tissue beneath the fold either by implantation of fat or autogenous materials, ranging from Gore-Tex (Fig. **5–18**) to silicone premaxillary implants (see Chapter 11), or by injection of various substances postoperatively (see Chapter 13).

Perhaps the most predictably dramatic improvement of the nasolabial fold is achieved by direct excision of the mound via an incision placed precisely in the fold (Fig. **5–19A,B**). Unfortunately, most women refuse this procedure, and thus the only patients who benefit from this technique are the occasional men who agree, usually out of desperation, to undergo such surgery. The scar is generally difficult to distinguish from the natural nasolabial fold, and patients are invariably pleased with the outcome.

Liposuction of the Buccal Fat Pad

Many Asians exhibit fullness of the cheeks secondary to fat accumulation in the buccal space. Some surgeons feel that ptosis of the buccal fat during the aging process contributes to jowl formation, offering an explanation for early occurrence of jowling following standard cheek or face lifting procedures involving tightening of the skin and removal of subcutaneous fat only.

Because they are technically difficult and are prone to complications, classic procedures for buccal liposuction have seldom been used in association with surgical rejuvenation of the face. Use of liposuction techniques, however, enables safe and rapid removal of buccal fat via an intraoral approach. This liposuction-assisted fat removal under direct visualization is associated with a low incidence of complications that result from injury to neurovascular structures and the buccal space and often yields dramatic improvement in the cheek fold as well as in the jowl, reinforcing the concept that in some

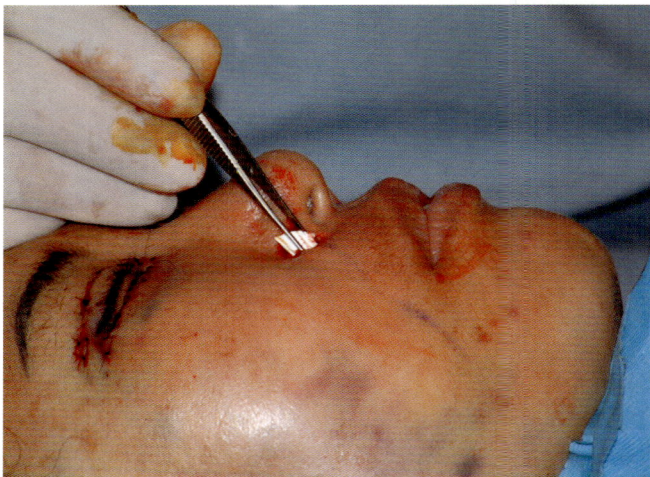

Figure 5–18 Placement of Gore-Tex in the nasolabial fold.

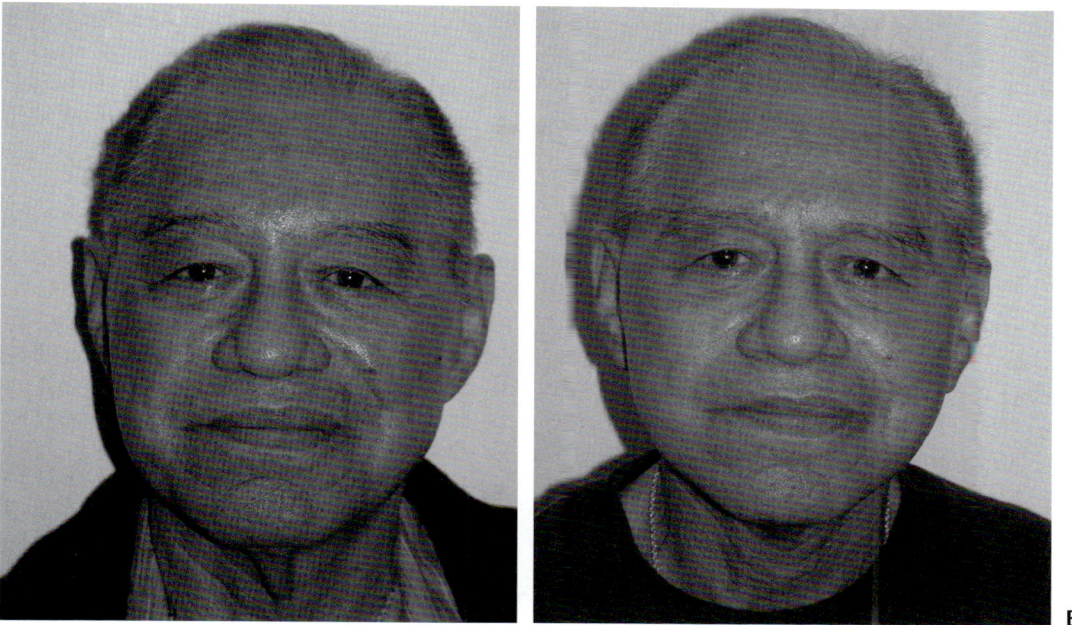

Figure 5–19   (A,B) Pre- and postoperative photographs of a direct nasolabioplasty.

individuals, ptosis of the buccal fat may indeed contribute to jowl formation.

Surgical Technique

1. Anesthesia of the anterolateral aspect of the gingivobuccal sulcus and buccal space is obtained by infiltration of local anesthetic (1% lidocaine with epinephrine 1:50,000).

2. A 1.5 cm incision is made so that the central portion of the incision is opposite the first maxillary molar.

3. Using blunt scissors, the buccal space is readily entered.

4. The anterior border of the masseter muscle is identified. This muscle forms the lateral boundary of the buccal space, and the fat to be removed therefore lies medial to this muscle.

5. The superficial fibrous septa surrounding the buccal fat are gently disrupted using scissors, following which a 6 mm buccal liposuction cannula (Fig. 5–20) is placed into the wound to facilitate fat dissection and removal.

6. Using the buccal suction cannula to maintain traction on the fat, the fat is teased from the buccal space using long forceps. Additional scissor

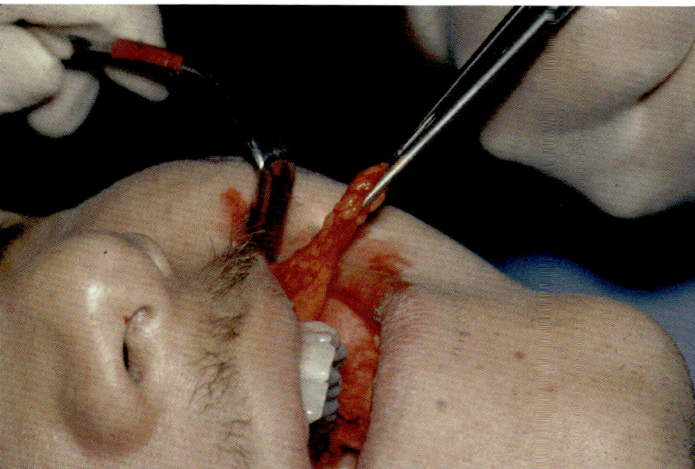

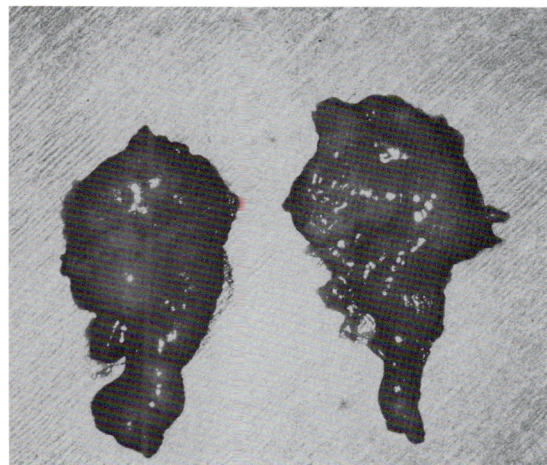

Figure 5–20   (A,B) Buccal liposuction.

dissection is only rarely required. Occasionally, vascular structures are visualized and may be cauterized if necessary.

7. Following extraction of buccal fat, digital palpation of the buccal space allows extension of a probing finger into the cheek and jowl region, further reinforcing the concept that there is an anatomic basis for descent of ptotic buccal fat into this area, accentuating jowl fullness.

8. The wound is approximated with a single suture of 4–0 chromic placed in the central aspect of the wound. This loose closure reduces postoperative swelling apparently by allowing drainage. Postoperative bleeding, however, is distinctly uncommon following liposuction-assisted extraction of buccal fat.

9. No external dressing is used except that which would normally be placed in conjunction with a face or cheek lift procedure.

In addition to its use as an ancillary procedure in conjunction with face and/or cheek lift surgery, liposuction of the buccal space is often performed as an isolated procedure in young individuals with cheek fullness (Fig. **5–21A–D**).

Suction-assisted buccal liposuction can also be performed via exposure achieved during face/cheek lift procedures (Fig. **5–22**).

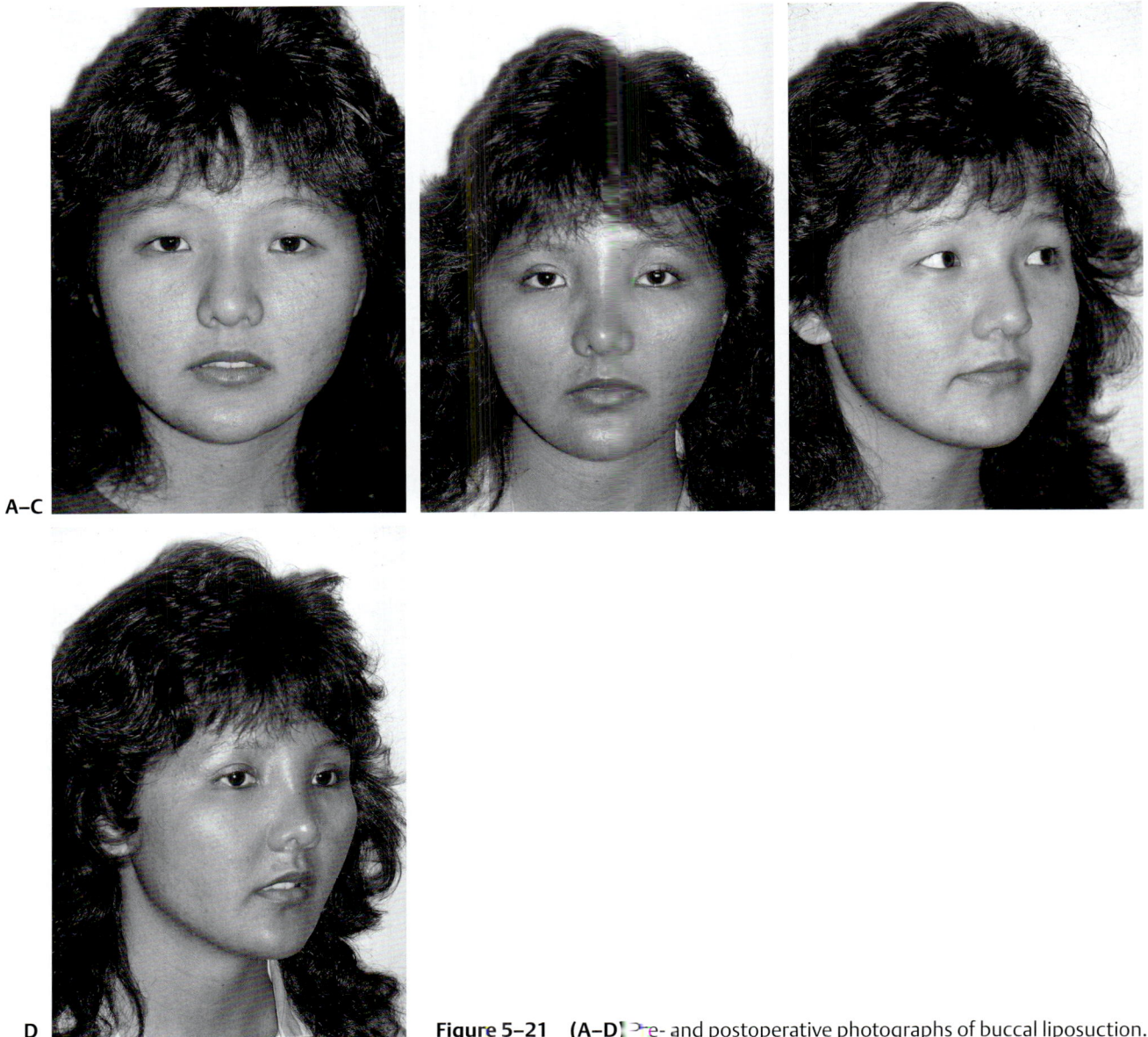

A–C

D

Figure 5–21   **(A–D)** Pre- and postoperative photographs of buccal liposuction.

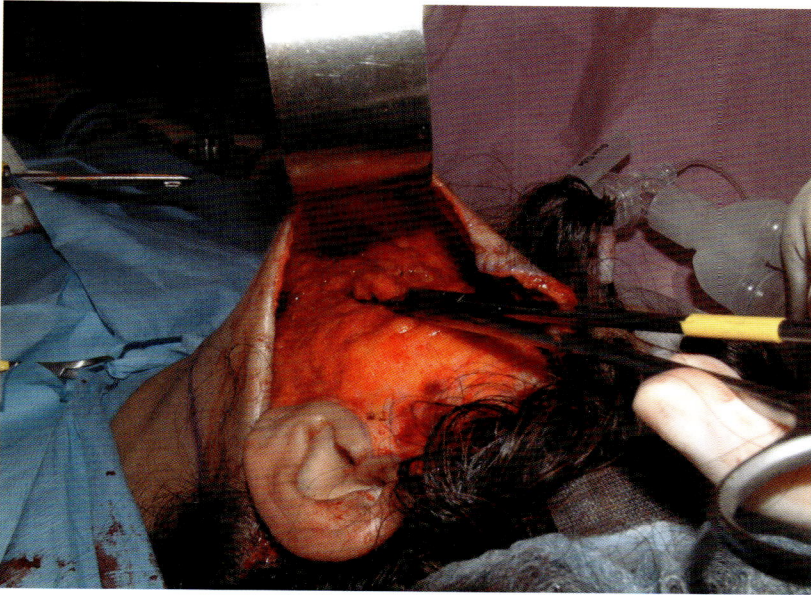

Figure 5–22 Buccal liposuction via a face lift exposure.

◆ Formulating an Approach to the Neck in Cervicofacial Rhytidectomy

The anatomic basis for deformities of the cervical region is well described. In addition to redundant skin, cervical aging is characterized by an accumulation of fat in the submental and submandibular regions producing distinct fullness. Midline diastasis of the platysma muscle produces objectionable bridle-like bands in the anterior aspect of the neck (Fig. **5–3**). Patients with a low hyoid bone demonstrate blunting of the cervicomental angle, which may appear as early as adolescence. Microgenia is often a contributing factor. Occasionally, fullness may be a consequence of ptosis of the submandibular glands.

Restoring a pleasing neck contour requires accurate preoperative analysis of the factors that contribute to the cervical deformity in each individual patient. Evaluation of each of these various components (skin, fat, platysma muscle, and facial skeleton) allows formulation of a systematic approach to surgical rejuvenation of this area. The classification proposed by Dedo (Fig. **5–23**) is a useful aid in preoperative analysis. Goals of neck rejuvenation include reconstruction of a cervicomental angle ranging between 105 and 120 degrees, highlighted by a visible depression in the subhyoid region as well as restoration of a well-defined mandibular line. Ideally, the anterior border of the sternocleidomastoid muscle should be visible.

Although surgical modification of the posterior aspect of the platysma muscle remains in vogue, long-term results of such surgery are often disappointing if fat accumulation and platysma diastasis contribute to the cervical "deformity." Wide undermining of the cervical skin is usually necessary in such cases to attack these problems. This presents little risk in the Asian patient, for the skin is generally thicker and well vascularized.

The surgical plan of attack on the cervical region is based on the presence or absence of fat as well as the presence of anterior platysmal banding. In the absence of significant submental and submandibular fat or platysmal banding, conservative skin undermining is performed (i.e., 3–4 cm anterior to the posterior border of the platysma muscle). At the present time, I rarely perform subplatysmal undermining in such cases, as I feel that direct undermining and elevation of the cervical skin yield a more effective "lift." Microliposuction of the submental and submandibular regions, even in the absence of substantial fat accumulation, encourages contraction of the overlying skin in this region, and this contraction, in my opinion, produces an effect superior to that following wide undermining of the cervical skin for patients in this category.

Patients who exhibit platysmal banding without fat deposition are managed by conservative skin undermining and midline approximation of the anterior aspect of the platysma muscles via a submental incision (subscribed subsequently in more detail in conjunction with the submental neck lift operation). In actuality, submental skin undermining necessitated by the need to release skin dimpling that follows anterior platysmal plication often connects the submental dissection with the lateral cervical flap.

Dedo's Neck Classification

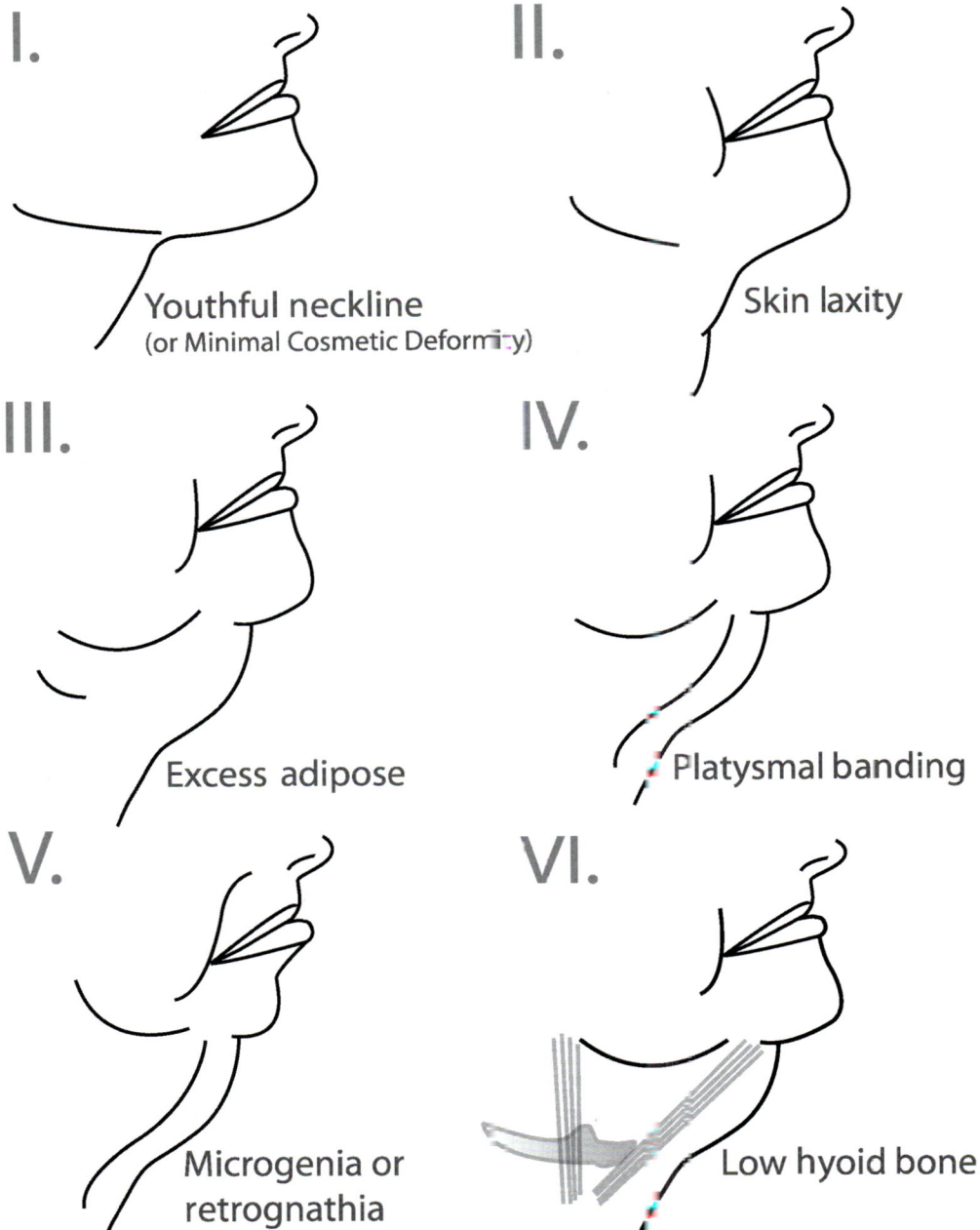

I.

Youthful neckline
(or Minimal Cosmetic Deformity)

II.

Skin laxity

III.

Excess adipose

IV.

Platysmal banding

V.

Microgenia or
retrognathia

VI.

Low hyoid bone

Figure 5–23   Dedo's classification of the aging neck. From Williams EF, Lam SM. Comprehensive Facial Rejuvenation: A Practical and Systematic Guide to Surgical Management of the Aging Face. Philadelphia: Lippincott, Williams & Wilkins; 2004. With permission.

Patients demonstrating cervical fat without platysmal diastasis are treated by wide skin undermining preceded by machine liposuction using a 3 or 4 mm cannula (Fig. **5–24A,B**). The platysma is not adjusted anteriorly and is not plicated posteriorly in these patients because the cervical skin has been completely separated from the platysmal surface, thus obviating any tension-sharing benefit provided by posterior platysmal plication. Removal of submandibular fat is also performed with liposuction, employing a flat 6 mm cannula introduced beneath the cervical skin flap—a procedure that has been called the "open" technique (Fig. **5–25**).

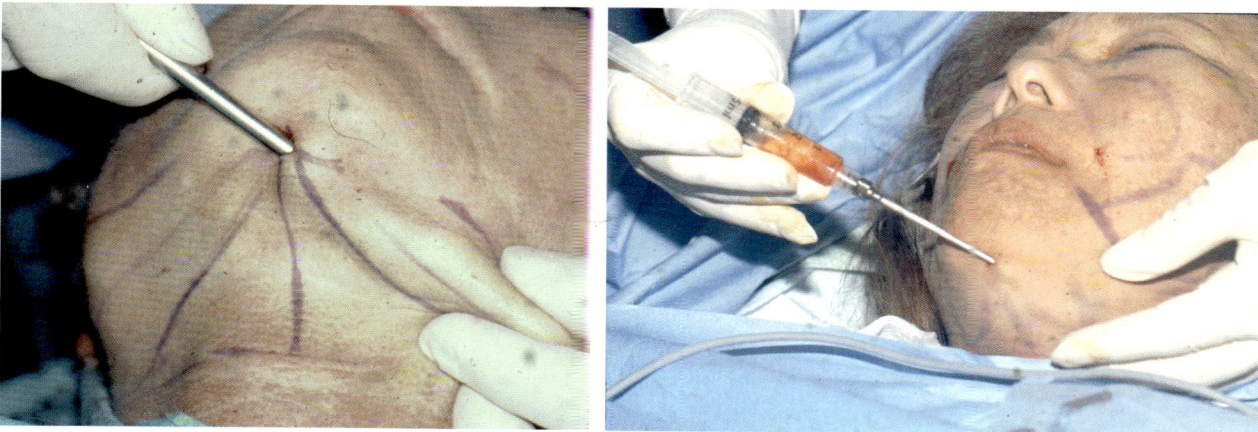

Figure 5–24   (A) Machine liposuction of the submental region. **(B)** Microliposuction of the submental region.

In patients with both cervical fat and anterior platysmal banding, machine liposuction is performed in the submental and submandibular regions, following which the cervical skin is undermined across the midline. The anterior borders of the platysma muscles are then identified (Fig. **5–26**) and approximated in the midline using interrupted sutures of 3–0 nylon. Some patients benefit from a 1 cm transection (Fig. **5–27**) of the anterior platysma just inferior to the level of the hyoid bone that may accentuate the cervicomental angle. Again, because cervical skin has been widely undermined, the platysma is not plicated posteriorly. Occasionally, a small amount of subplatysmal fat is removed using a combination of conventional dissection and liposuction. Conservative fat removal is necessary to avoid an objectionable postoperative submental depression.

Pre- and postoperative results of cervical rejuvenation (achieved with cervicofacial rhytidectomy) are presented in Figs. **5–28** and **5–29**.

Segmental Operations for Correction of Cheek and Temple Ptosis

Many Asian patients demonstrate manifestations of aging in the facial area without associated problems in the cervical region except for possible accumulation of submental fat. Such concerns are consistent with the observation that patterns of fat accumulation associated with the aging process tend to be initially accentuated in the facial region in Asian patients. Treatment of cheek ptosis and fat accumulation without associated neck fullness or redundancy can be managed successfully with the cheek lift operation, the incisions for which are illustrated in

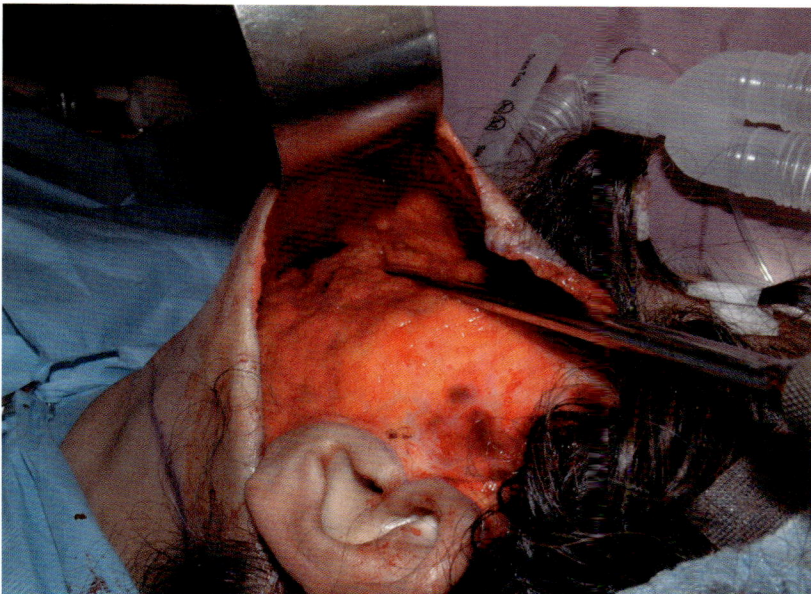

Figure 5–25   "Open" liposuction of the submandibular region.

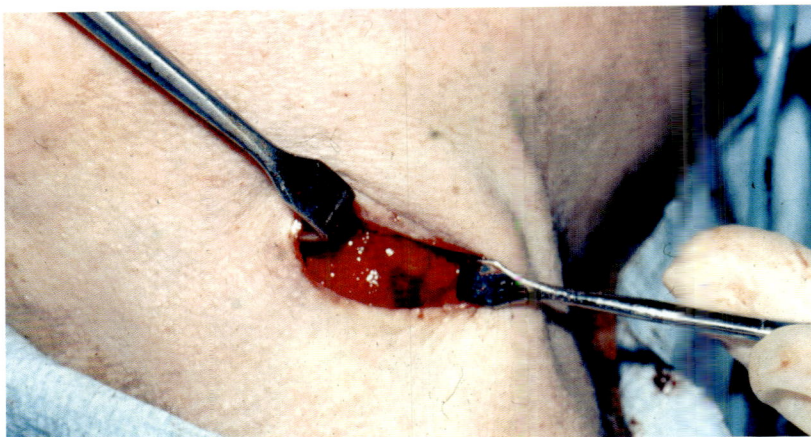

Figure 5–26 Identification of the anterior platysma prior to midline approximation.

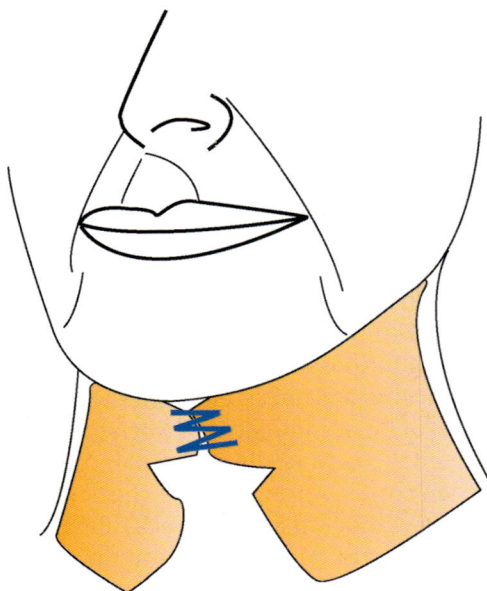

Figure 5–27 Anterior platysmal transection and plication.

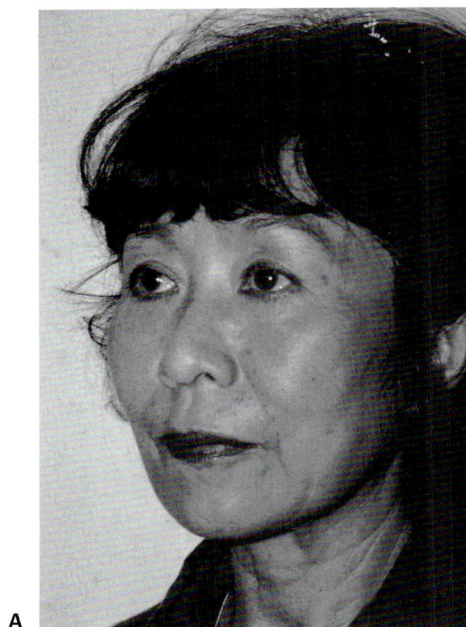

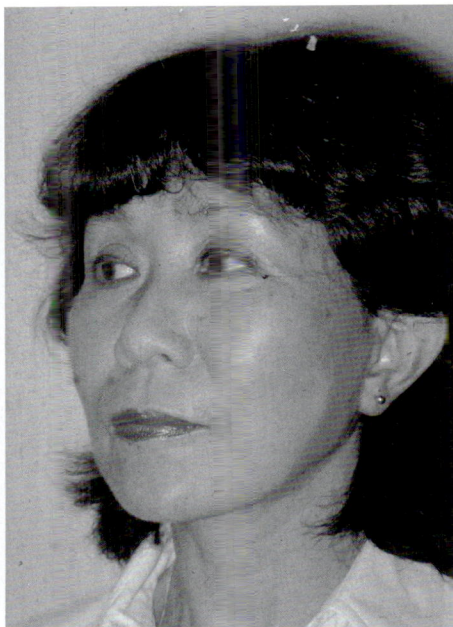

Figure 5–28 (A,B) Pre- and postoperative photographs following a cervicofacial rhytidectomy.

A

B

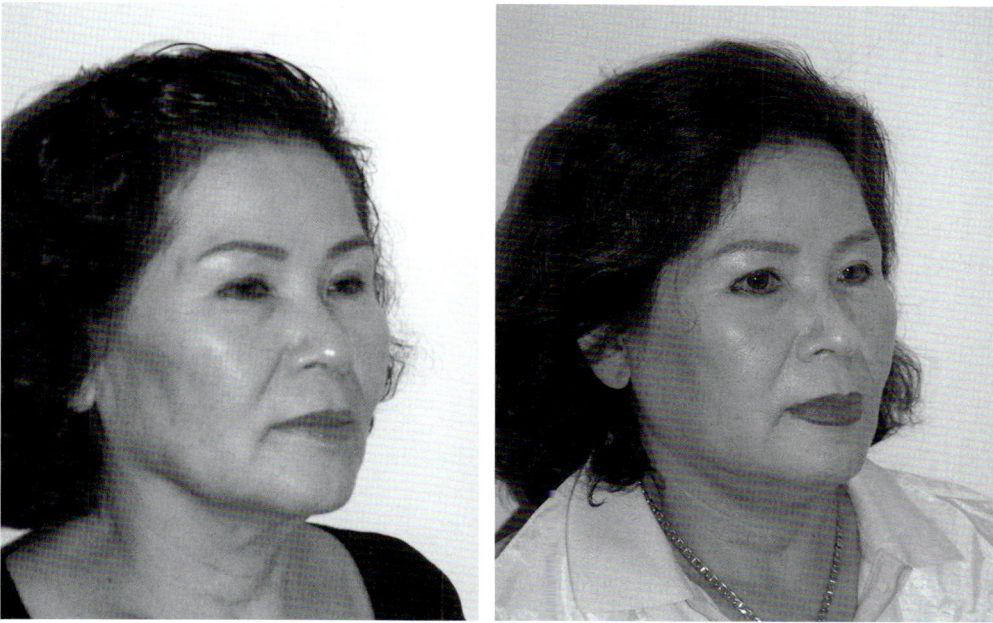

Figure 5–29   (A,B) Pre- and postoperative photographs following a cervicofacial rhytidectomy.

Fig. **5–30**. It must be stressed that this procedure is not a "mini-lift," as it involves wide skin flap undermining often accompanied by subperiosteal dissection of the midface or anterior SMAS plication. In actuality, the extent of temporal and facial dissection is virtually identical to that employed during a full cervicofacial rhytidectomy (Fig. **5–31**). The results of such procedures (Fig. **5–32A,B**) are often enhanced by spot microliposuction of the jowl and/or nasolabial mound using a syringe technique. If submental fat accumulation accompanies cheek ptosis, it can be addressed by either syringe microliposuction or machine liposuction, depending on its extent.

If indicated, the temporal aspect of the cheek lift incision can be extended superiorly (Fig. **5–30**), resulting in another segmental operation, the so-called cheek/temple lift.

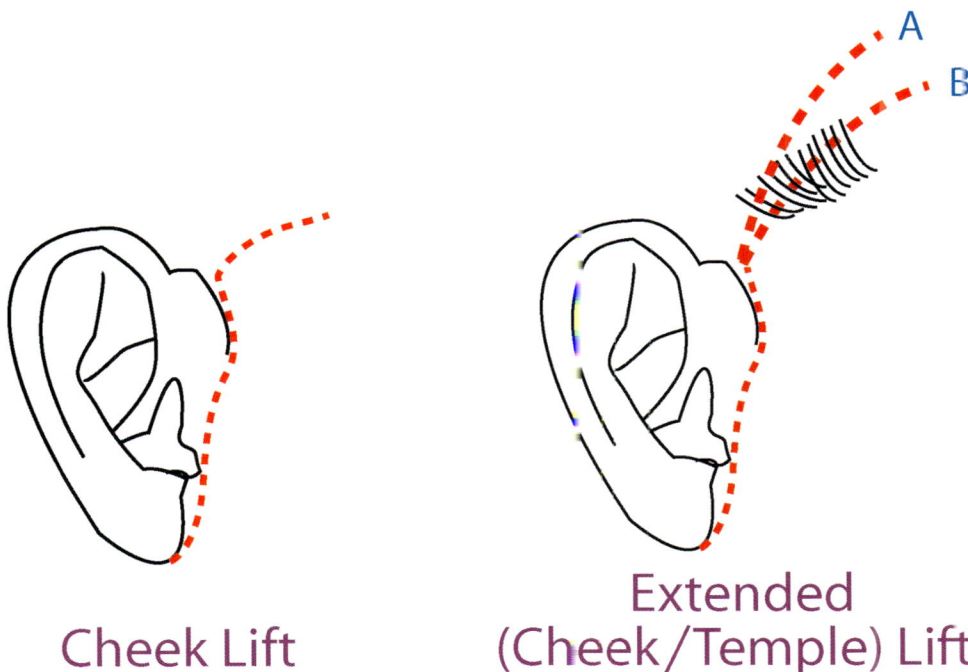

Cheek Lift

Extended
(Cheek/Temple) Lift

Figure 5–30 Incisions for a cheek lift and cheek/temple lift.

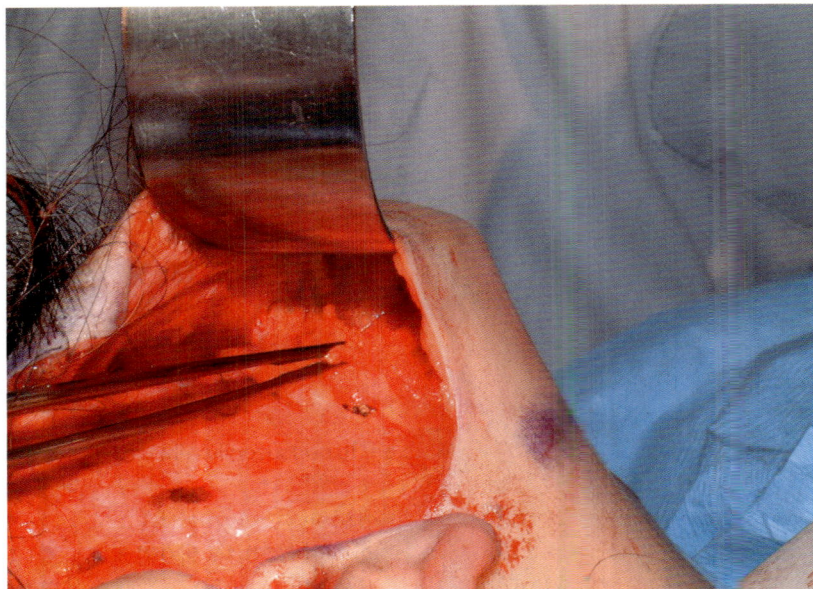

Figure 5–31   Extent of undermining for a cheek lift is essentially the same as for a cervicofacial rhytidectomy; a cheek lift is not a "mini-lift."

Occasionally, a patient with early cheek ptosis does not wish to undergo a lifting procedure. If early jowl and nasolabial mound fullness are the primary concerns, spot microliposuction of these areas using the syringe technique often yields satisfactory results (Figs. **5–9**, **5–33A,B**).

Segmental Procedures for Rejuvenation of the Neck

As is the case with cheek ptosis, a patient occasionally presents with deformities of the cervical region that are relatively isolated and do not require performance of a full cervicofacial rhytidectomy. I have conceptualized a series of three progressively more intensive segmental neck operations.

Cervical Liposuction

Patients in whom the neck deformity is limited to accumulation of submental or submandibular fat can be adequately managed by liposuction, either using microliposuction techniques with fine cannulas and

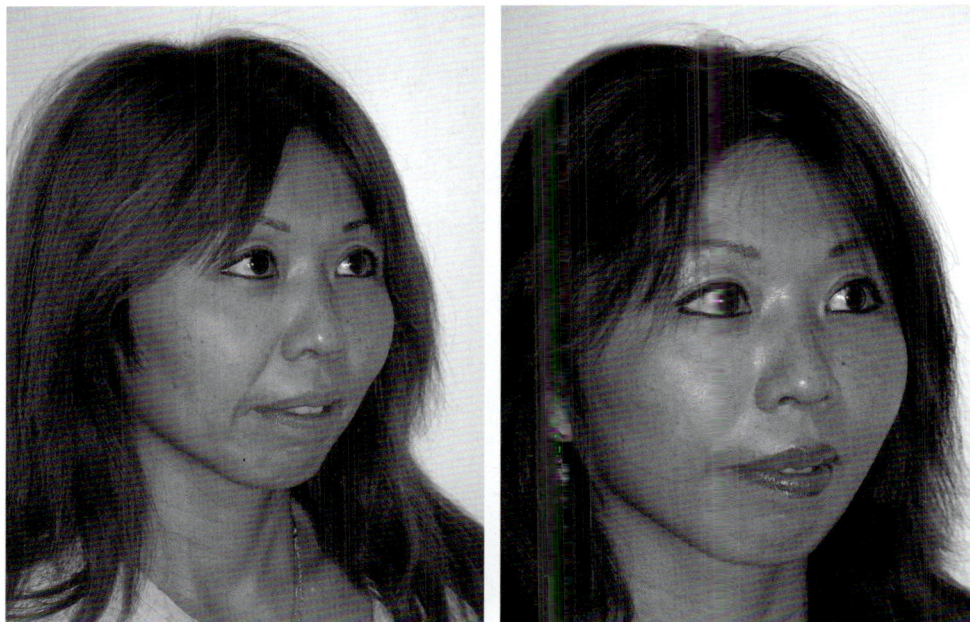

A   B

Figure 5–32   (A,B) Pre- and postoperative photographs following a cheek lift.

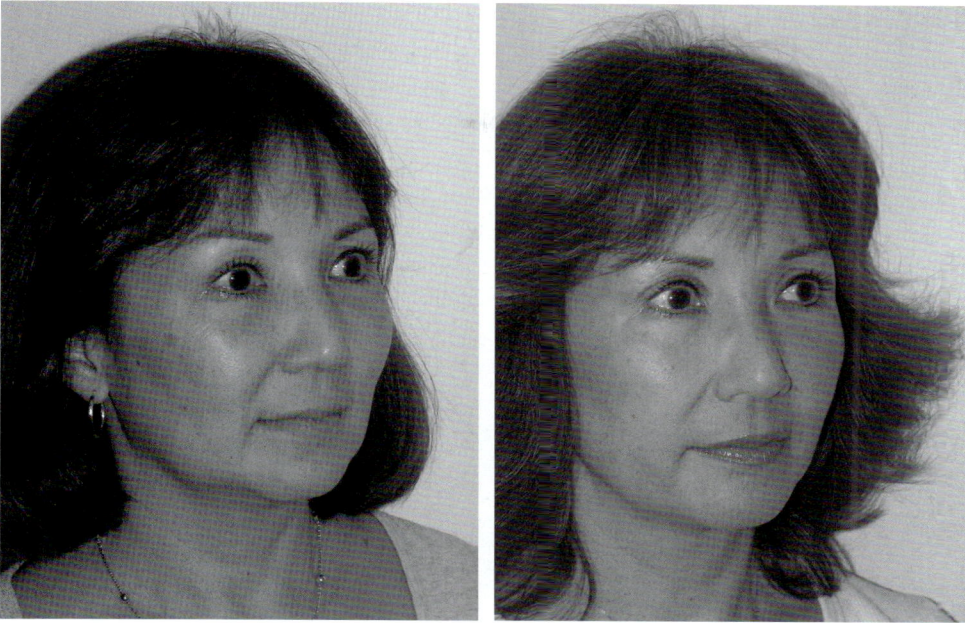

Figure 5–33   (A,B) Pre- and postoperative photographs of jowl liposuction.

syringe suction or 3 to 4 mm cannulas using machine suction. Liposuction of the neck has rendered the standard submental lipectomy virtually extinct (Fig. **5–34A,B**).

Submental Neck Lift

Patients who present with midline diastasis of the platysma muscle with or without cervical fat accumulation require anterior platysmaplasty in addition to fat removal as indicated, an operation I term the submental neck lift.

Cervical liposuction is performed using either syringe microliposuction techniques or machine liposuction with 3 or 4 mm cannulas. A 4 to 5 mm curvilinear incision is then placed in the submental crease, following which the submental and submandibular skin is widely undermined with scissors. Undermining is extended along the mandibular border laterally to a point corresponding to the anterior border of the sternocleidomastoid muscle. Inferiorly, undermining extends to the level of the cricoid cartilage. The platysma is identified (Fig. **5–26**), and each anterior border is undermined ~1 cm

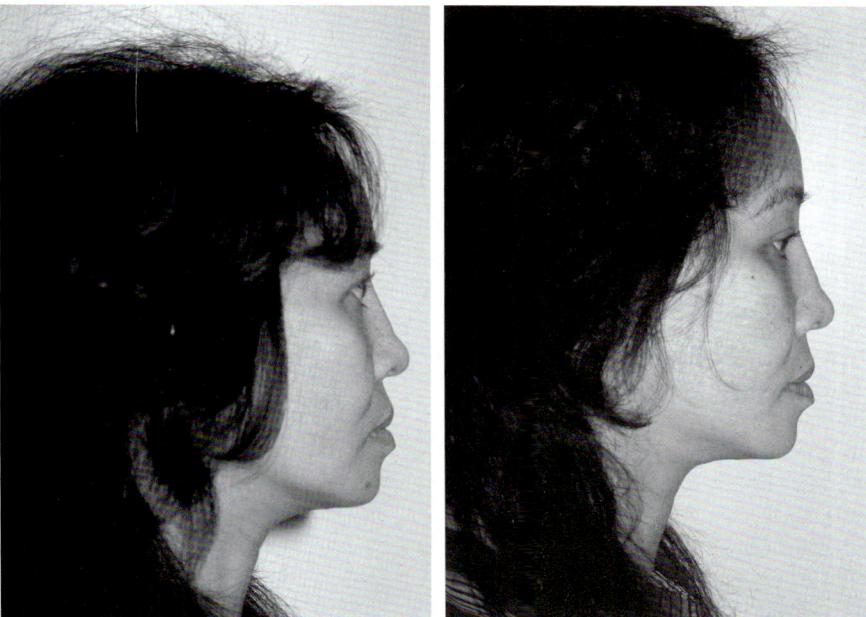

Figure 5–34 (A,B) Pre- and postoperative photographs of submental liposuction.

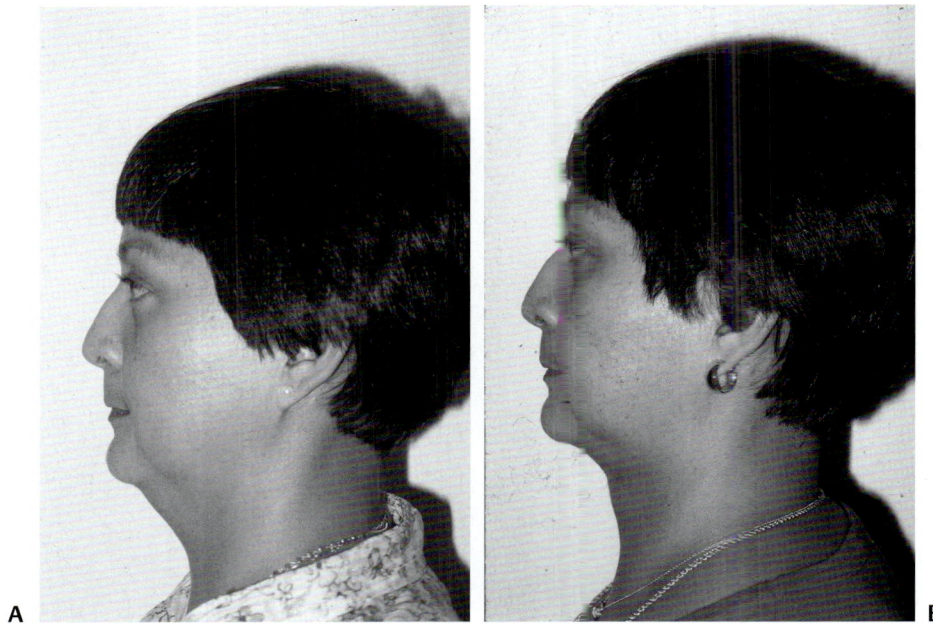

Figure 5–35 (A,B) Pre- and postoperative photographs of a submental neck lift.

along its posterior surface. If necessary, redundant muscle is excised (usually such excision is unnecessary), and a submental sling or corset is constructed by approximating the anterior borders of the muscles from the level of the hyoid bone to the mentum using sutures of 3–0 nylon (Fig. **5–27**). In earlier days, I had recommended transection of the platysma muscle at the level of the thyroid cartilage. Evidence, however, suggests that this maneuver is unnecessary (except occasionally, as noted above, in a patient in whom a 1 cm transection of the anterior border may assist in defining the cervicomental angle), and avoiding extensive muscle transection reduces the risk of dysfunction of the depressor anguli oris muscle.

The muscle must not be sutured under excessive tension as dehiscence is more likely. Sutures are placed at 1 cm intervals and tied so that the knots are buried. Following platysmal approximation, the lateral aspect of the neck is inspected for evidence of dimpling or skin bunching, indicating inadequate undermining. If dimpling is noted, skin undermining is extended into the affected areas. The wound is closed with 5–0 nylon around a small drain.

As more skin is required to fill the newly created cervical concavity, no cervical skin is excised in most cases. The skin flaps are secured with strips of paper tape similar to those applied following submental liposuction, and an occlusive dressing is applied for 24 hours. The drain is removed at this time, and a submental sling is worn constantly for 1 week and is recommended for continued use for an additional 3 weeks when the patient is alone. A typical result is illustrated in Fig. **5–35**.

Posterior Neck Lift

Patients with more advanced cervical redundancy who do not require correction of cheek ptosis can be managed with the posterior neck lift. Most candidates for this procedure also benefit from cervical liposuction or from the submental neck lift described previously. After completion of submental surgery, the posterior portion of a standard face lift incision is made (Fig. **5–36**). It is frequently necessary to extend this incision anteriorly around the ear lobule to facilitate distribution of cervical skin. If submandibular fat requires removal, skin

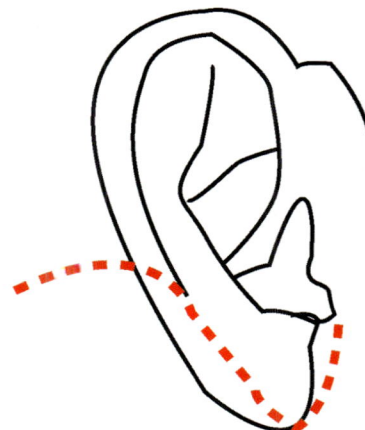

Posterior Neck Lift

Figure 5–36 Incisions for the posterior neck lift.

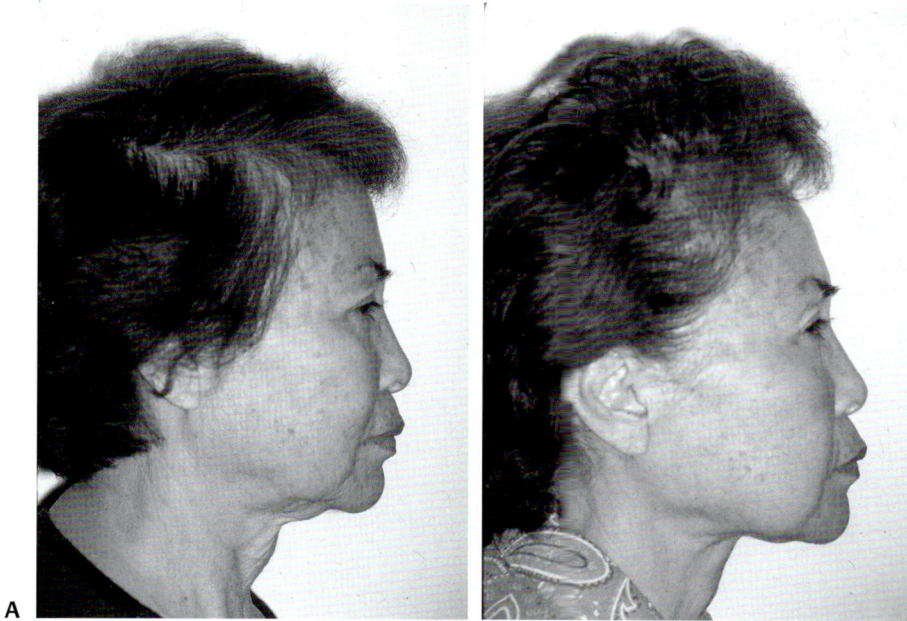

Figure 5–37   (A,B) Pre- and postoperative photographs following the posterior neck lift.

undermining extends across the midline, connecting with the submental dissection, and submandibular lipectomy is performed using a 6 cm flat liposuction cannula. The skin flap is rotated and advanced in an anterior and superior direction. The excess skin is removed and the incision closed, ensuring that no tension exists around the ear (Fig. **5–37A,B**).

Complications Following Face-, Cheek, and Neck Lifts

Complications following surgical rejuvenation of the Asian face are identical to those occurring following such surgery in the Caucasian (i.e., bleeding, hematoma, infection, scar formation, flap necrosis, hair loss, nerve injury, and asymmetry).

Older Asian patients have a higher incidence of hypertension than Caucasians of comparable age; thus, the surgeon should ensure that adequate control of blood pressure has been obtained preoperatively to reduce the risk of bleeding or hematoma formation. As is true in Caucasians, hematoma is more common following face lift procedures in males.

Flap necrosis is somewhat less common in Asians than in Caucasians because of the increased thickness of the skin. The incidence of hypertrophic scarring, however, is higher. Such scars occur most commonly in the postauricular region but occasionally manifest themselves in the preauricular and temporal regions. In most cases, satisfactory management of hypertrophic scarring is achieved with intralesional triamcinolone injections.

Although much less common when liposuction is performed in the neck, inadequate submandibular lipectomy may result in objectionable lateral bulges. Conversely, overly aggressive subplatysmal lipectomy may produce a central depression in the submental region. For this reason, the subplatysmal fat pad should be approached only if fullness persists following removal of subcutaneous fat in the submental region.

Induration of the platysma muscle may occur following anterior approximation and occasionally requires intralesional steroid injections. When undertaking midline approximation of the platysma, care must be taken to ensure that excessive tension on the suture line is avoided so that the incidence of postoperative dehiscence and recurrence of anterior banding is minimized.

Occasionally, transient asymmetry of the lower lip may occur as a result of temporary paralysis of the depressor anguli oris muscle. Spontaneous return of function, however, occurs in most if not all cases. Patients often complain of tightness in the neck for 6 to 8 weeks following anterior platysmal approximation. Some patients describe a choking sensation, but true dysphagia is not a problem.

◆ Conclusion

Successful rejuvenation of the aging face and neck demands a careful assessment of various factors that may contribute to the deformity as manifested by each individual patient. There are two keys to successful surgical rejuvenation: adequate management of midfacial ptosis (i.e., the nasolabial fold) and management of deformities related to the anatomic configuration of the platysma muscle, both of which constitute surgical challenges. Cervical lipectomy with liposuction and platysmal approximation, if indicated, enables dramatic and lasting rejuvenation of the neck. Understanding the mechanism of midfacial ptosis and the methods of its correction using either the simplified technique of subperiosteal midfacial

dissection or anterior SMAS plication accompanied by debulking of the nasolabial mound using microliposuction generally enables a successful attack on this problem.

Differences in the anatomy and manifestations of aging in the Asian face allow more frequent use of segmental procedures to correct localized ptosis of the cheek and cervical redundancy than is indicated in the Caucasian population.

References

1. Skoog T. Plastic Surgery: New Methods and Refinements. Stockholm: Almquistand Wiksell, 1974

2. Mitz V, Peyronie M. The superficial musculo-aponeurotic system (SMAS) in the parotid and cheek area. Plast Reconstr Surg 1976;58:80–88

3. Jost G, Levet Y. Parotid fascia and face lifting: a critical evaluation of the SMAS concept. Plast Reconstr Surg 1984;74:42–51

4. Hamra S. The deep-plane rhytidectomy. Plast Reconstr Surg 1990;86:53–61

5. Hamra S. Composite rhytidectomy. Plast Reconstr Surg 1992;90:1–13

6. Ivy EJ, Lorenc ZP, Aston SJ. Is there a difference? A prospective study comparing lateral and standard SMAS face lifts with extended SMAS and composite rhytidectomies. Plast Reconstr Surg 1996;98:1135–1143

7. Hamra S. A study of the long-term effect of malar fat repositioning in face lift surgery: short-term success but long-term failure. Plast Reconstr Surg 2002;110:940–951

8. Psillakis JM, Rumley TO, Camargos A. Subperiosteal approach as an improved concept for correction of the aging face. Plast Reconstr Surg 1988;82:383–394

9. Ramirez OM, Maillard GF, Musolas A. The extended subperiosteal face lift: a definitive soft-tissue remodeling for facial rejuvenation. Plast Reconstr Surg 1991;88:227–236

10. Ramirez OM. Endoscopic full facelift. Aesthetic Plast Surg 1994;18:363–371

11. Maloney BP, Schiebelhoffer J. Minimal-incision endoscopic face-lift. Arch Facial Plast Surg 2000;2:274–278

12. Freeman MS. Endoscopic techniques for rejuvenation of the midface. Facial Plast. Surg Clin North Am 2001;9:453–468

13. Hester TR Jr, Codner MA, McCord CD, et al. Evolution of technique of the direct transblepharoplasty approach for the correction of lower lid and midfacial aging: maximizing results and minimizing complications in a five-year experience. Plast Reconstr Surg 2000;105:393–408

14. Williams JV. Transblepharoplasty endoscopic subperiosteal midface lift. Plast Reconstr Surg 2002;110:1769–1777

15. Williams EF III, Vargas H, Dahiya R, et al. Midfacial rejuvenation via a minimal-incision brow-lift approach: critical evaluation of a 5-year experience. Arch Facial Plast Surg 2003;5:470–478

16. Sasaki GH, Cohen AT. Meloplication of the malar fat pads by percutaneous cable-suture technique for midface rejuvenation: outcome study (392 cases, 6 years' experience). Plast Reconstr Surg 2002;110:635–657

17. Yousif NJ, Matloub H, Summers AN. The midface sling: a new technique to rejuvenate the midface. Plast Reconstr Surg 2002;110:1541–1557

18. Keller GS, Namazie A, Blackwell K, et al. Elevation of the malar fat pad with a percutaneous technique. Arch Facial Plast Surg 2002;4:20–25

19. Gosain AK, Amarante MT, Hyde JS, Yousif NJ. A dynamic analysis of changes in the nasolabial fold using magnetic resonance imaging: implications for facial rejuvenation and facial animation surgery. Plast Reconstr Surg 1996;98:622–636

20. McCurdy J. A simplified approach to subperiosteal dissection of the midfacial region: preliminary observations. Am J Cosmetic Surg 1995;12:85

21. Robbins LB, Brothers DB, Marshall DM. Anterior SMAS plication for the treatment of prominent nasomandibular folds and restoration of normal cheek contour. Plast Reconstr Surg 1995;96:1279–1288

6

Otoplasty in the Asian Face

◆ General Considerations

In Western societies, prominent ears are regarded as an undesirable facial feature. Historically, protruding auricles have been associated with the lack of intelligence, insanity, and criminal tendencies. Although such feelings are not pervasive in the 21st century, young children with prominent ears are often subjected to teasing, derision, and ridicule, making surgical correction of this deformity at an early age commonplace.

Eastern cultures, in contrast, do not place negative connotations on prominent ears; thus, little social pressure for correction exists in Asia.

Consistent with the Asian preoccupation with physiognomy, however, the size and shape of the auricles are considered to be important markers of an individual's personality and potential for success. Because all facial features except for the ears undergo substantial metamorphosis during childhood and early adolescence, the ears are one of the few positive sources of predictive information during early life.

Large auricles are the most auspicious characteristic, although proportion relative to the face is important. Large ears on a small face suggest a shallow character, whereas large ears on a large face suggest honesty, power, and success. In my practice, I have seen several middle-aged Asian women who have undergone enlargement of the lobule by silicone injection to produce what they term "Buddha ears" (Fig. **6–1**) that are considered aesthetically desirable. Interestingly, I have never received a request to reduce lobular size in any of these individuals.

In Asia, the most desirable ears are flat, indicating good fortune, longevity, and stable family relationships. Prominent ears, however, are not an object of derision but suggest a need to draw on an inner reservoir of strength and ability to achieve success in life.

◆ Anatomic Considerations

Although the incidence of prominent ears appears to be somewhat greater in Asians than in Caucasians, native Asians rarely request otoplasty. Correction of prominent ears, however, is requested by Asians residing in Western countries. The surgical procedure is identical to that utilized for correction of protruding auricles in the Caucasian and is based on an analysis of the anatomic factors responsible for protrusion:

1. Conchal excess is corrected by reduction of conchal cartilage, achieved by shave excision of the posterior cartilaginous surface using a no. 10 Bard-Parker blade.
2. Deficiency of the antihelical fold is corrected by the Mustarde technique, employing mattress sutures of 4–0 nylon.
3. Prominence of the lobule is corrected by subtotal resection of the cauda helix. If lobular prominence does not respond to this maneuver, the "fishtail" skin excision described by Converse is employed (Fig. **6–2**).

Surgery is performed under local anesthesia in an outpatient surgical suite for adult patients, whereas general anesthesia is reserved for younger children.

◆ Surgical Technique

1. An ellipse of skin to be excised is marked on the posterior surface of the auricle, the medial aspect of

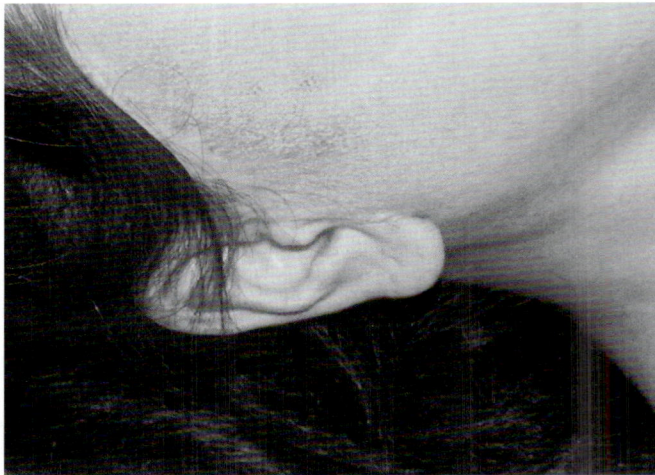

Figure 6–1 The so-called Buddha ear produced by the lobular injection of silicone.

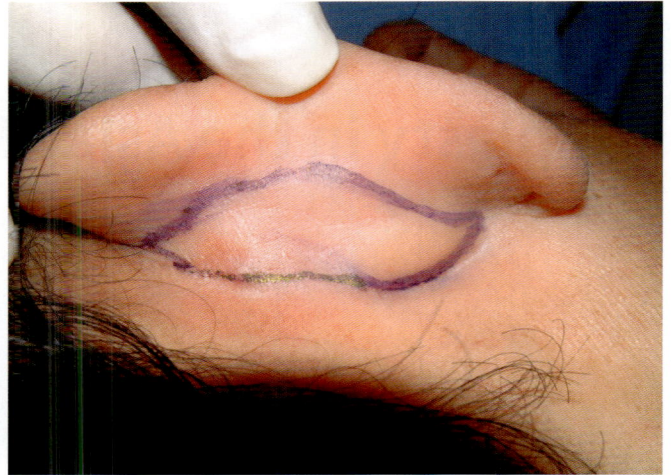

Figure 6–3 Postauricular elliptical skin excision for otoplasty.

the ellipse being placed in the postauricular crease so that the surgical scar will reside in the sulcus (Fig. **6–3**). If special anatomic considerations dictate (i.e., marked protrusion of the superior aspect of the auricle), the skin excision may be dumbbell shaped rather then elliptical.

2. Following excision of skin and underlying soft tissue, the conchal cartilage is separated from its mastoid attachments to the level of the posterior aspect of the external auditory meatus, care being taken not to violate the skin of the canal.

3. If deficiency of the antihelical fold will require placement of mattress sutures, the postauricular skin is undermined to the lateral border of the helix.

4. Auricular muscle and other soft tissue between the conchal cartilage and mastoid periosteum are excised, debulking this space so that the conchal cartilage can more closely approximate the mastoid, reducing its prominence (Fig. **6–4**).

5. Using a no. 10 blade, segments of cartilage are shave excised from the posterior surface, debulking the cartilage. Following each segmental shave excision, the surgeon manually approximates the concha to the mastoid, with shave excision being terminated when the conchal reduction allows the desired conchal "setback" (Fig. **6–5A,B**).

6. The new conchal position is maintained by two or three sutures of 4–0 nylon placed between the full thickness of conchal cartilage (and anterior perichondrium) and mastoid periosteum (Fig. **6–6**). If Mustarde sutures are to be used for deficiency of the antihelical fold, these conchomastoid sutures are not tied until the Mustarde sutures have been placed. It is often observed that prominence

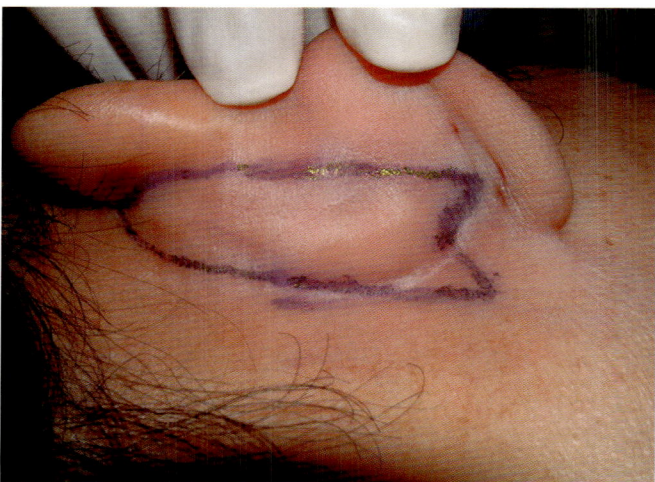

Figure 6–2 "Fishtail" skin excision for reduction of lobular prominence.

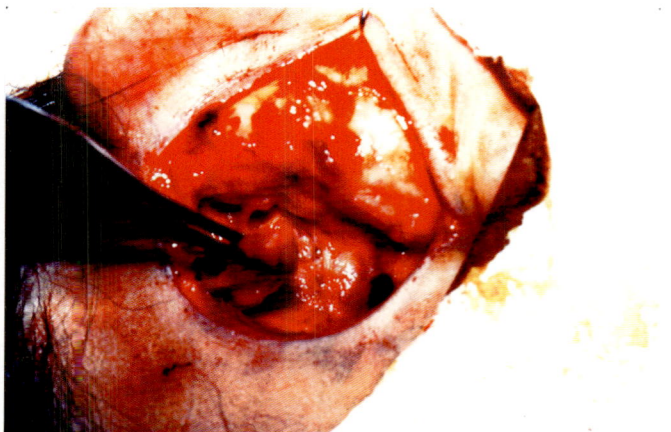

Figure 6–4 Excision of soft tissue over the mastoid.

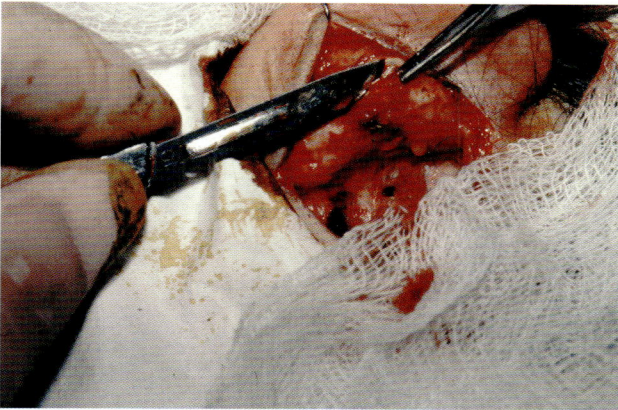

Figure 6–5 **(A)** Shave excision of the posterior conchal surface with a no. 10 Bard-Parker blade, resulting in reduced volume that allows the desired degree of conchal "setback." **(B)** Following shave excision (note the excised cartilage fragments in the foreground), the auricle is prepared for conchal "setback."

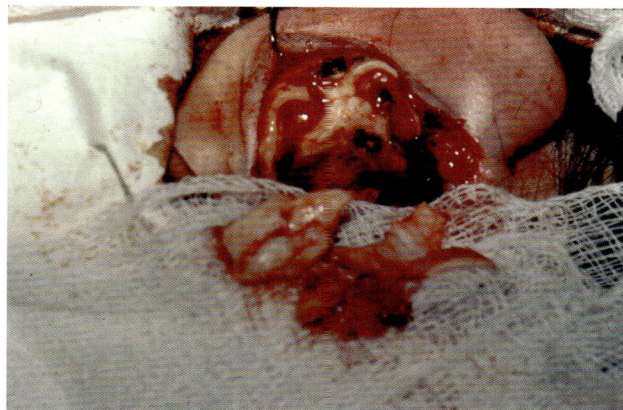

attributed to an antihelical fold deficiency is diminished following conchal setback, limiting (and sometimes altogether eliminating) the requirement for Mustarde sutures.

7. Two or three Mustarde-type mattress sutures are placed, incorporating the full thickness of the cartilage and anterior perichondrium. The sutures are tightened as necessary, forming the antihelical fold.

8. If required, lobular prominence is reduced by subtotal excision of the cauda helix. If not responsive to this maneuver, an L-shaped "fishtail" is drawn on the posterior lobular surface continuous with the existing skin wound. The corresponding one-half "fishtail" is "tattooed" onto the mastoid skin by pressing the lobule against the mastoid (Fig. **6–2**). Skin incorporated within these markings is excised and closed in continuity with the postauricular skin closure, resulting in reduced lobular prominence.

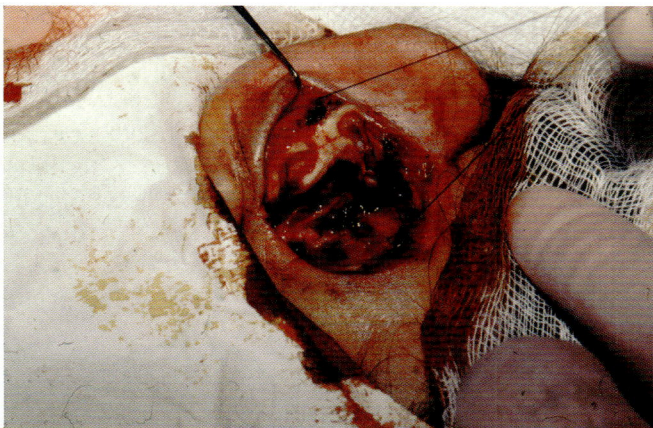

Figure 6–6 Conchal "setback" is achieved with two or three 4–0 nylon sutures.

9. Final hemostasis is secured, following which the postauricular wound is closed with a running suture of 4–0 chromic.

10. Several stab wounds are made into the anterior conchal skin to serve as "drain holes." This maneuver substantially reduces postoperative edema of the anterior conchal surface and obviates the use of a postauricular drain. The stab wounds heal with imperceptible scarring.

◆ Postoperative Care

A standard occlusive auricular dressing is placed and is usually removed on the first postoperative day. Subsequent compression is afforded by a terry cloth athletic headband. The patient is asked to wear this headband continuously for the first 48 hours postoperatively, and thereafter to wear it when sleeping, or actively exercising, for the next 30 days.

Antibiotic cream or ointment is applied three times daily to the postauricular wound and to the anterior auricular stab wounds for 7 days. Because chromic catgut is used for the postauricular closure, suture removal is unnecessary.

◆ Advantages of This Otoplasty Technique

Correction of auricular prominence by conchal setback is an easy, safe, and reliable technique that, in most cases, eliminates the need for more time-consuming and somewhat less reliable efforts to effect correction by enhancement of the antihelical fold alone. If antihelical fold definition is required, use of the Mustarde

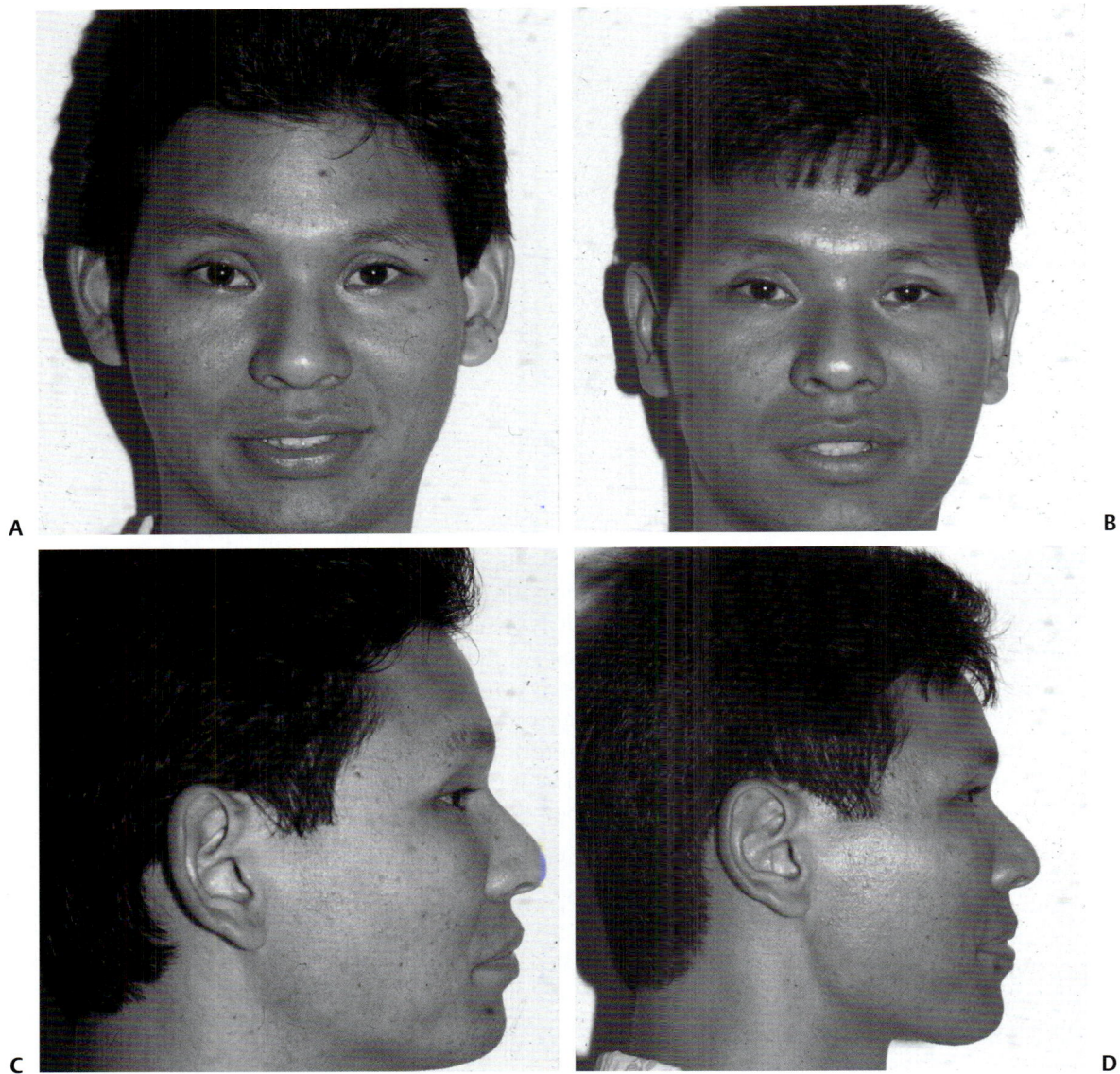

Figure 6–7   (A–D) Pre- and postoperative results of otoplasty.

technique eliminates the need for potential complication-producing incisions on the anterior surface of the conchal skin.

Conchal setback by incremental shave excision of the posterior surface of the conchal cartilage allows precise debulking (and reduction of cartilage "spring") while preserving the structural continuity and integrity of the concha. Following cartilage shave excision, conchomastoid sutures are under no tension, and thus recurrence of the conchal deformity is unlikely.

Although lobular prominence rarely requires a "fishtail" skin excision, this procedure, if necessary, allows precise positioning of the prominent lobule.

Postoperative results following otoplasty are illustrated in Fig. **6–7**.

◆ Complications

Hemorrhage or Hematoma

Because of the anterior auricular drain wounds, it is not uncommon for a moderate amount of blood to accumulate in the dressing during the first 24 hours. Frank hematoma, however, is uncommon, but if it occurs, drainage is necessary to minimize discomfort as well as to reduce incidence of subsequent wound infection and perichondritis (or suppurative chondritis).

Infection

Fortunately, infection is an unusual complication of otoplasty, and the incidence is further minimized if hematoma is recognized and promptly drained. The most devastating complication of otoplasty is chondritis and suppurative perichondritis. Although extremely rare, the incidence of this complication may be increased by inadvertent perforation of the posterior external auditory canal skin during conchal elevation. Irrigation of the wound with 5% povidone-iodine solution prior to closure may serve to diminish bacterial contamination and thus reduce the risk of postoperative infection.

Prophylactic antibiotics (oral cephalosporins) are begun on the night prior to surgery and continued postoperatively for 2 days.

Scar

Because skin excision is planned so that the scar is positioned in the postauricular sulcus, visible postoperative scarring is minimal. Although Asian skin characteristically exhibits an increased fibroplastic response during healing, hypertrophic scarring in the postauricular region following otoplasty is uncommon, even when lobular repositioning using the "fishtail" skin excision is utilized. If a hypertrophic scar develops, prompt treatment with triamcinolone injection is generally successful.

Residual Deformity

As conchal setback can be effected under little or no tension by employing the shave excision method, recurrent deformity in this area is uncommon. Occasional failure of the Mustarde mattress sutures occurs and is managed by suture replacement. Preoperatively, patients should be counseled about existing asymmetry of the auricles and informed that, because asymmetry is a natural phenomenon, precise postoperative symmetry is unlikely.

7
Radio-Frequency Resurfacing of the Asian Face

◆ **General Considerations**

Although skin resurfacing is recognized as a component of facial rejuvenation that equals or, in some cases, exceeds the importance of surgical lifting procedures, the search for an effective, precise, and relatively complication-free method of resurfacing continues.

The application of laser technology to cutaneous resurfacing ushered in a new age of operator-controlled skin peeling, an exciting development given the fact that chemical peeling, the previous gold standard of resurfacing, exerted its effects via a self-limiting chemical interaction with the skin that was not entirely under the control of the operator (even though its proponents argued that the self-limiting nature of the reaction provided an inherent margin of safety).

Indeed, the advent of the laser age did prove that, although operator controllability offered distinct advantages, it was, in actuality, a double-edged sword. In many cases, well-intentioned attempts to extend the therapeutic envelope with "one more pass" too often resulted in production of sufficient additional thermal damage to substantially prolong healing and, in some cases, to sabotage the clinical efficacy of the procedure as a result of complications, most notably pigmentary disorders and hypertrophic scarring.

These concerns have had particular influence in application of current technology to resurfacing of the Asian face. Although sporadic reports of successful skin resurfacing in this population using various types of lasers have appeared in the literature, most surgeons remain reluctant to employ these modalities in the Asian face.

An ideal skin-resurfacing method would be characterized by operator controllability coupled with an inherent margin of safety, resulting in an acceptable rate of healing and low incidence of complications. Radio-frequency resurfacing (Coblation, ArthroCare Corp., Sunnyvale, CA) exhibits a therapeutic profile that more closely approximates the characteristics of an ideal method than most other currently available modalities. Coblation provides, by virtue of its mechanism of action, a margin of safety that exceeds that of carbon dioxide (CO_2) laser systems. While early clinical reports suggested that the clinical efficacy of radio-frequency resurfacing fell between that of CO_2 and Erbium ER:YAG) lasers, more recent reports suggest that aggressive use of the radio-frequency unit (i.e., a greater number of passes) produces clinical improvement approximating that of the CO_2 laser while maintaining the healing profile of the Er:YAG laser.

I have found that radio-frequency resurfacing produces excellent results in the Asian face, although the time requirement for complete healing is somewhat longer than in the Caucasian face. Of special importance is my observation that the most debilitating pigmentary complication of resurfacing, hypopigmentation, has not occurred during my experience with this procedure.

◆ **Mechanism of Action**

A brief description of the mechanism of action of radio-frequency resurfacing will enhance appreciation of its clinical profile. An important concept is that the tissue interaction with radio-frequency energy is distinctly different and entirely unrelated to the mechanism of interaction with laser-generated energy. An electrically conductive solution (normal saline) is dripped over the target tissue via a port on the hand

A

B

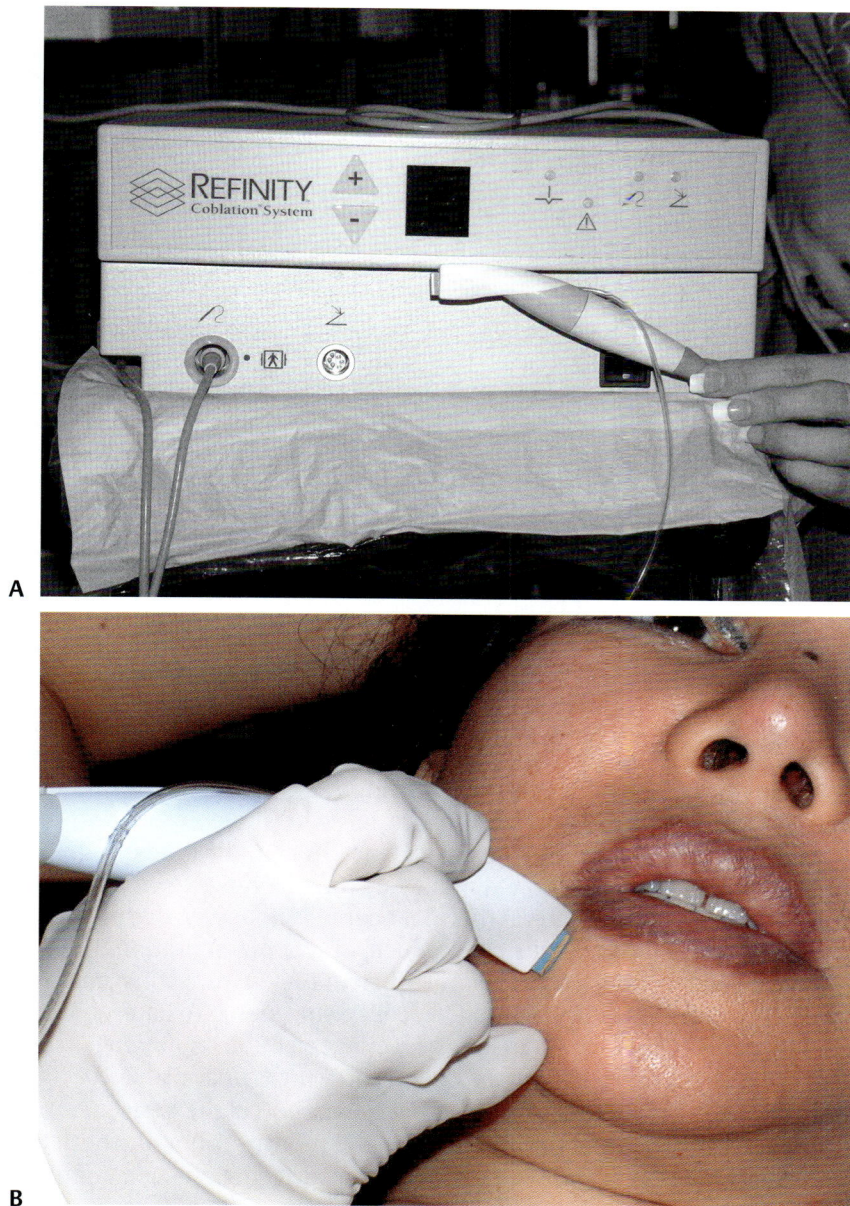

Figure 7–1   (A,B) Radio-frequency resurfacing device with wand used for skin contact.

piece (wand, Fig. **7–1A,B**) that maintains constant contact with the skin during operator activation. Three bipolar electrodes near the surface of the wand generate a variable, operator-controlled voltage gradient that converts the normal saline into a vapor, termed plasma, composed of energized ions that accelerate toward the epidermal surface (Fig. **7–2**). The kinetic energy of this activated ion plasma (rather than heat energy generated by laser systems) produces molecular dissociation of epithelial cells that ablates the epidermal layer. Because of the structural differences between the epidermis and dermis, the physical characteristics of the energized plasma are such that it is unable to produce dermal ablation even with multiple passes, although thermal damage sufficient to induce

collagenogenesis does occur in dermal tissue. Of significance is the observation that maximal heating of the dermis is in the range of 60 to 90°C, dramatically lower than temperatures of 200°C generated by the Er:YAG laser, and as high as 400°C during treatment with CO_2 laser systems. The lower operating temperatures of radio-frequency resurfacing account for the trade name of this procedure, Coblation, an acronym for cold ablation or controlled ablation.

Histologic studies of skin subjected to radio-frequency resurfacing show that the first pass results in ablation of the epidermis (20–40 millimicron zone of ablation) accompanied by a 10 millimicron zone of collateral thermal injury. A second pass increases the collateral injury zone (dermal) to ~50 millimicrons

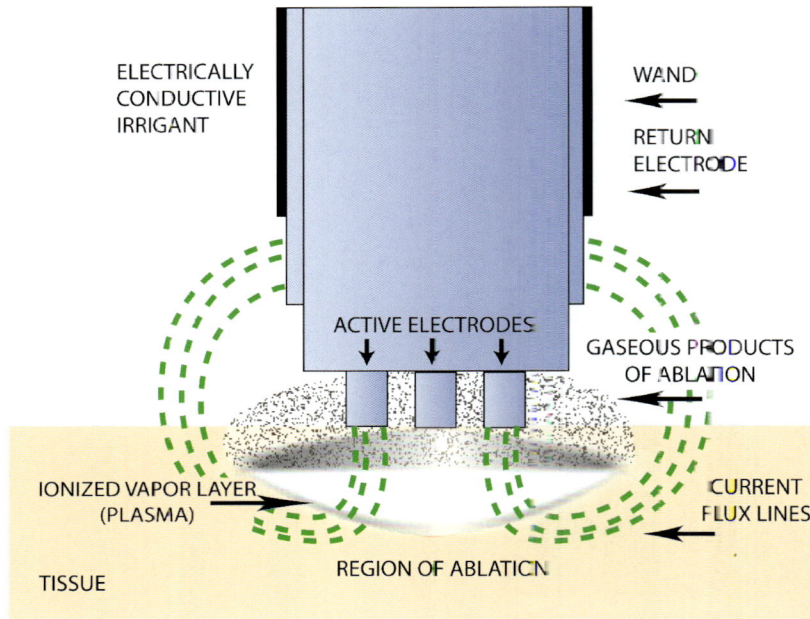

Figure 7–2 Mechanism of action of radio-frequency energy.

without actual ablation of the dermis, and a third pass increases the depth of thermal injury to ~80 microns. Subsequent passes result in minimal additive effect with regard to thermal injury of the dermis. These findings contrast with the effects of the CO_2 laser, which ablates tissue including dermis on each pass while extending the zone of thermal injury. Collateral damage following radio-frequency resurfacing is limited to the papillary dermis, and the reticular dermis is not affected. The zone of thermal injury is sufficient to result in denaturization of collagen, a finding that correlates with beneficial effects on neocollagenogenesis. Importantly, rapidity of healing after the injury and the incidence of adverse sequelae correlate directly with the extent of the zone of residual thermal injury of the dermis. A comparison of zones of ablation and collateral injury following radio-frequency, CO_2, and Er:YAG laser resurfacing is presented in Table **7–1**.

The major reason for limited collateral damage as compared with that produced by laser energy is the significantly reduced amount of heat to which dermal tissues are subjected during radio-frequency resurfacing. This reduced exposure has a positive correlation with healing time and incidence of complications. Temperatures generated in the target tissue range from 70 to 90°C, and collateral thermal energy is not extensive enough to produce side effects such as hypopigmentation. Thermal energy, however, is sufficient to denature collagen, causing shrinkage and neocollagenogenesis. To date, quantitative comparison of collagenization following radio-frequency versus laser resurfacing is unavailable.

Histologic studies have shown the presence of a band of dermal fibrosis at 3 months following both CO_2 laser and radio-frequency resurfacing, the band of fibrosis being more substantial following laser resurfacing, consistent with a greater degree of thermal injury.

Table 7–1 Comparison of Tissue Effects Following CO_2 and Er:YAG Laser and Radio-frequency Resurfacing

	CO_2	**Er:YAG**	**RF**
Temperature range	400°C	200°C	70–90°C
Tissue ablation (per pass)	20–30 mμ	2–3 mμ	70–80 mμ (first pass only)*
Collateral thermal injury	30–100 mμ	5–30	10 mμ (first pass)
			50 mμ (second pass)
			80 mμ (third pass)**

Er:YAG = TK; RF = radio frequency
*Epidermis only is ablated; dermal ablation does not occur with use at recommended parameters.
**Subsequent passes result in minimal additional thermal injury.

◆ Pretreatment Preparation

Because of the absence of evidence regarding efficacy of pretreatment with retinols and hydroquinone and the particularly high incidence of irritative dermatitis associated with these substances in the Asian face, no pretreatment other than sun avoidance is employed.

◆ Procedure

Regional treatment is performed using regional nerve blocks and or local infiltration anesthesia. All full-face procedures are performed under general anesthesia.

The periorbital region is treated with three passes at a power setting of 4 (125 V); all other areas of the face were routinely treated with three passes at a power setting of 5 (150 V). Deeper rhytids and acne scars are treated with four to six passes at a power setting of 5 in the affected areas only. Velocity of wand movement approximates 1 cm per second with application of sufficient pressure to maintain contact with the skin surface.

An important technical consideration in radio-frequency resurfacing is that the wand overlap the area treated on previous passes by one-third of its width to avoid uneven treatment, which might produce clinically evident "striping." The previously treated track is easy to ascertain after the first pass (Fig. **7–3**), as well as the second and all subsequent passes, because there is no readily visible change produced in dermal appearance and no discernible evidence of the treatment track; thus, determination of proper overlap is difficult. To obviate this problem, a deviation from the generally recommended technique is undertaken: following completion of the first pass, a second, third, and, if indicated, fourth and fifth pass is performed on the same treatment track, thus ensuring that each area is evenly treated. The degree of overlap is then easily determined for the next treatment track, which is treated with three sequential passes, this being repeated in the same fashion for each subsequent track until the entire target area is completed.

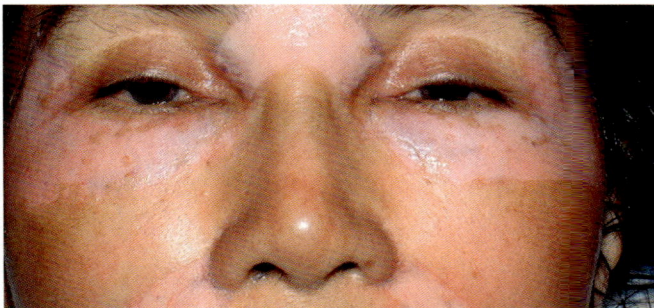

Figure 7–3 Well-defined treatment "track" following first pass with wand.

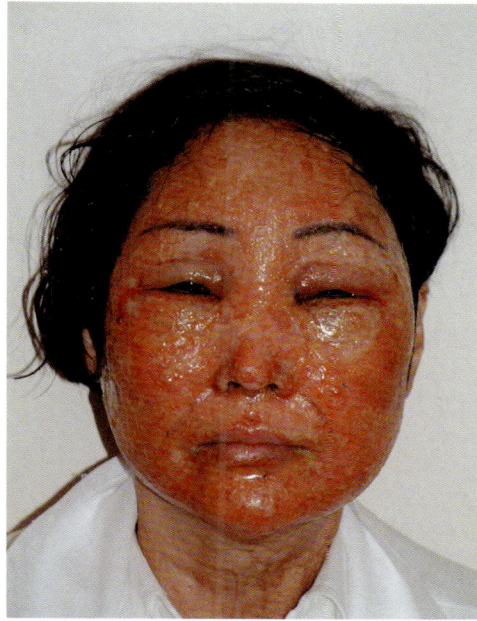

Figure 7–4 Appearance 48 hours posttreatment.

◆ Postoperative care

I prefer to manage patients with an open wound technique consisting of frequent application of petroleum ointment until epithelialization is completed in approximately 1 week. This is followed by use of a bland cream for 2 to 3 weeks. At this point, patients are allowed to resume their preoperative skin care regimen as tolerated.

Erythema is treated with 2.5% hydrocortisone cream. Patients who develop postinflammatory hyperpigmentation are treated with 4% hydroquinone (e.g., Glyquin or Lustra).

The early healing period is virtually identical to that observed following resurfacing with deep phenol peels or CO_2 laser treatment (Fig. **7–4**). After epithelialization is completed in approximately 1 week, the skin is intensely hyperemic but, once dry, can be camouflaged somewhat with cosmetics.

In Caucasian skin, erythema persists for an average of 2 to 3 months, whereas in Asian patients, hyperemia persists approximately 4 to 6 weeks longer.

Results of radio-frequency resurfacing are demonstrated in Figs. **7–5**, **7–6**, and **7–7**.

◆ Complications

Erythema sometimes evolves into postinflammatory hyperpigmentation, the incidence in my patients approximating 33% at 30 days and 20% at 90 days.

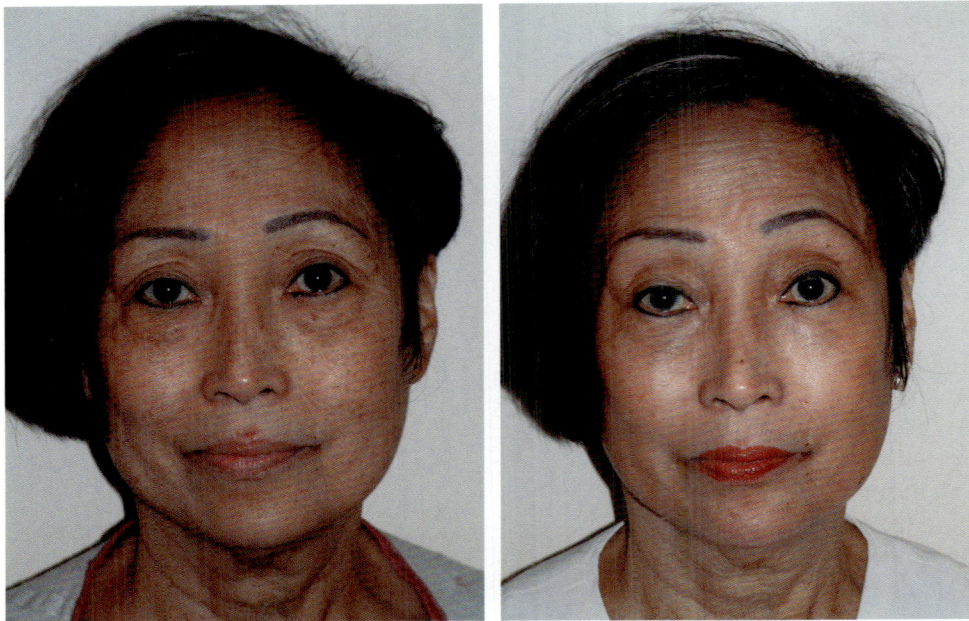

Figure 7–5   (A,B) Pre- and posttreatment results of radio-frequency resurfacing.

I have observed punctate hypertrophic scars on the lower-eyelid skin that have responded to topical corticosteroids. One of my patients developed herpetic dermatitis in the treated area that responded to therapy without residual scarring.

No patients have developed hypopigmentation.

◆ Discussion

All patients show improvement in skin texture and fine to moderate rhytidosis as determined by physician assessment and patient satisfaction. Most show continued incremental improvement for 6 months or longer. As would be expected, many Asian patients do express concern over the duration of erythema, but less concern is voiced regarding hyperpigmentation, as it is more easily camouflaged. After final healing, most patients feel that the improvement in skin appearance is "worth" the inconvenience of the postprocedure healing period.

Of interest is the fact that morbidity is somewhat greater in fair-skinned Asians as compared with those with darker skin. This suggests that the Fitzpatrick phototype that is useful in assessment of Caucasian skin may require modification for reliable application to Asian skin. Specifically, morbidity in fair-skinned Asians is characterized by prolonged erythema rather than by postinflammatory hyperpigmentation. With regard to the Fitzpatrick classification, most of these individuals indicated that in response to sun (ultraviolet [UV] light) exposure, the skin did not readily burn but developed relatively painless erythema that resolved rapidly, usually without frank sunburn. Such individuals are not described in the Fitzpatrick classification, and it should be noted that a substantial percentage of Asians exhibit skin of this type.

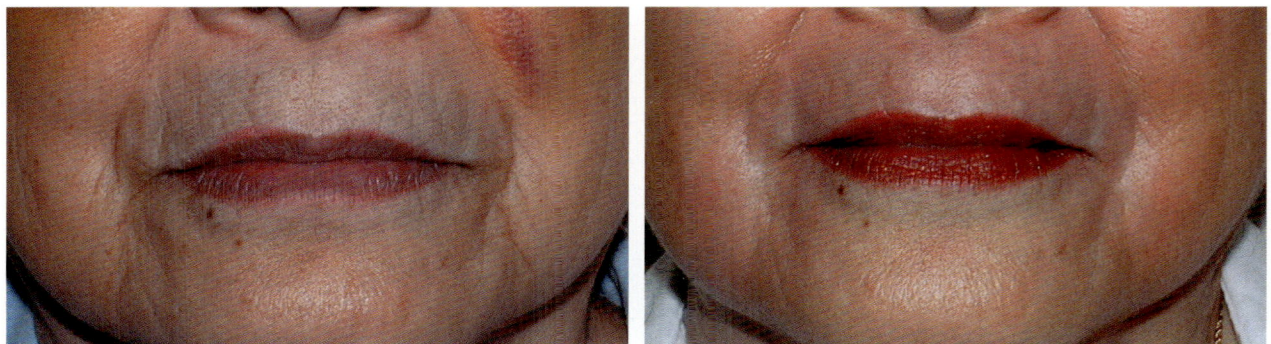

Figure 7–6   (A,B) Pre- and posttreatment results of radio-frequency resurfacing.

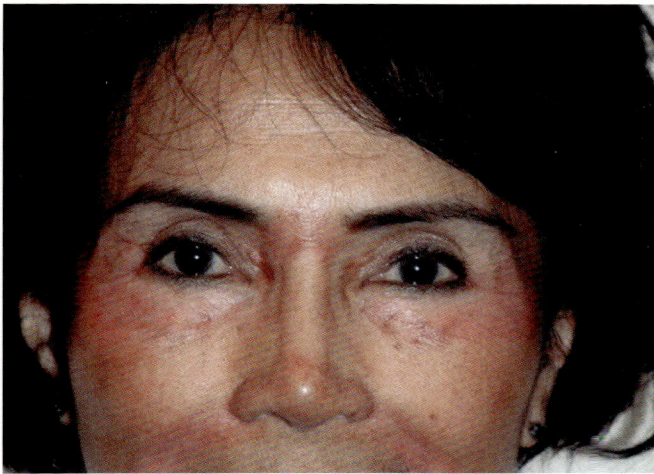

Figure 7–7 Punctate hypertrophic scars on lower-eyelid skin 30 days postresurfacing.

The prolonged erythema observed following radio-frequency resurfacing is consistent with erythema often observed after any insult to skin of this type, including surgical incisions made with "cold steel." The incidence of hypertrophic scarring, however, is not appreciably increased in these wounds, and the result of final maturation is generally a fine scar, as observed in other Asian skin types.

In some cases, erythema exhibits an uneven, mottled configuration rather than the uniform appearance generally associated with laser and chemical peeling. It has been speculated that this pattern may be a consequence of an even contact between skin and wand or nonuniform wand velocity, resulting in uneven dwell time over segments of target tissue. This pattern, however, does not appear to exert a discernible effect on the final result.

Erythema, being a measure of post-traumatic inflammation, is thought to be correlated with the extent of thermal injury, and informing a patient that it likely has a positive correlation with the final degree of

collagenization may be of benefit in acceptance of this sequela.

A major advantage of radio-frequency resurfacing is the absolute hemostasis associated with this procedure. The tactile feedback resulting from direct contact of the stylus at the skin surface is beneficial in the experience of most surgeons. In addition, because tissue vaporization does not occur, there is no smoke plume or particulate aerosolization. Eye protection is not required.

My experience suggests that radio-frequency resurfacing is a safe and effective modality for rejuvenation of Asian skin. Healing, however, is more prolonged than observed in Caucasians, and greater morbidity, in contrast with Caucasian skin, occurs in fair-complexioned individuals. Prolonged erythema is of greater patient concern than post-inflammatory hyperpigmentation, which resolves with time and treatment. The tendency of Asian patients to exhibit excessive concern about minor defects and the progress of healing tends to make the postoperative period challenging.

The mechanism of action of radio-frequency resurfacing provides an inherent margin of safety as a consequence of the limited extent of residual thermal damage accompanied by relatively precise volumetric tissue ablation. The practical result is that this technology allows clinically efficacious resurfacing with reduced healing time as compared with CO_2 laser resurfacing. A major advantage of radio-frequency resurfacing of pigmented skin relates to the fact that permanent change in pigmentation is rare. Therefore, treatment of isolated aesthetic units can be undertaken with confidence.

Although the above characteristics make radio-frequency resurfacing a relatively forgiving procedure with a large margin of safety, it is, like laser resurfacing, subject to operator variability, and a learning curve is involved. Experience is required to determine the most effective parameters when utilizing this technique to maximize clinical efficacy while minimizing erythema and pigmentary sequelae.

Suggested Readings

1. Mancini P. A new system for skin resurfacing: preliminary clinical and histologic reports. Aesth Surg J 1999;19:459–464
2. Grekin RC, Tope WD, Yarborough JM Jr, et al. Electrosurgical facial resurfacing: a prospective multicenter study of efficacy and safety. Arch Dermatol 2000;136:1309–1316
3. Acland KM, Calonje E, Seed PT, et al. A clinical and histologic comparison of electrosurgical and carbon dioxide laser peels. J Am Acad Dermatol 2001;44:492–496
4. Carruthers A. Radiofrequency resurfacing: technique and clinical review. Facial Plast Surg Clin North Am 2001;9:311–319
5. Alster TS. Electrosurgical ablation: a new mode of cutaneous resurfacing. Plast Reconstr Surg 2001;107:1890–1894
6. West TB, Alster TS. Effect of pretreatment on the incidence of hyperpigmentation following cutaneous CO2 laser resurfacing. Dermatol Surg 1999;25:15–17

Section II

Variations and Ancillary Techniques

Samuel M. Lam, M.D.

8

Asian Upper Blepharoplasty: The Partial-Incision and Suture Techniques

◆ General and Anatomic Considerations

Creation of a supratarsal crease for the Asian patient may be achieved through a variety of surgical strategies. In fact, the number of permutations of surgical technique that exists closely matches the number of surgeons who practice double-eyelid surgery, as every surgeon performs a slightly different modification to suit his or her own preference. Perhaps the simplest categorization that can offer the reader comprehension of the myriad techniques that exist for double-eyelid surgery is to divide the techniques into three major types: full-incision, partial-incision, and suture technique.[1] This simplified classification is not meant to imply that all techniques fall neatly into these groupings. For instance, some surgeons prefer to perform a near full incision but stop short laterally. Other practitioners advocate a suture technique via a limited, partial-incision approach.[2,3] Alternatively, a full incision can be undertaken, and only part of the levator length fixated to the dermis, as performed in the partial-incision method. All of these many techniques have been proven with considerable clinical experience and are viable in the right surgical hands.

The full-incision technique has already been thoroughly covered in Part I of this book and will not be reiterated herein.[4] This chapter is devoted to a detailed review of the two major alternative strategies for double-eyelid creation: the partial-incision and the suture technique. After reviewing numerous permutations of these two principal methods, the author has selected two techniques that celebrate simplicity and elegance and that are established upon a substantial clinical experience. The author relies principally on the partial-incision method to undertake most of his surgical endeavors and selects the full-incision technique only

when redundant skin must be removed, such as in the older individual seeking double-eyelid creation. The suture technique is reserved for patients who have relatively little adipose tissue (that would otherwise obstruct a favorable dermal-levator adhesion) and who express interest in this surgical modality.

◆ The Partial-Incision Technique

Method of Young Kyoon Kim
Preoperative Remarks

The partial-incision technique developed by Young Kyoon Kim offers an ideal balance between the full-incision and the suture methods.[5] The limited incision that spans only about one-third of the total eyelid length offers a rapid and reliable method for double-eyelid creation and limits postoperative edema and risk of scarring (Fig. 8–1). Unlike the aging eyelid, the medial fat compartment is rarely addressed in double-eyelid creation. Even if a full incision is undertaken, only the central fat compartment is resected, as removal of the medial fat may predispose toward scarring and is simply not necessary. Accordingly, the abbreviated incision involved with the partial incision affords easy access to the central fat compartment to reduce the "puffy" eyelid appearance characteristic of the Asian upper eyelid. Furthermore, an incision that extends toward the medial canthus increases the risk of cutaneous scarring and webbing, as the medial aspect of the Asian eyelid has a natural propensity for cicatricial formation. Therefore, the partial-incision technique permits removal of the only fat compartment that needs to be addressed and access to the levator aponeurosis for placement of

—1.5 cm—

8-10 mm

equidistant with contralateral side

incision commences along medial limbus

1 incision through skin & muscle

2 open orbital septum

3 preaponeurotic fat exposed

4 retain a 1 cm cuff of fat on each side

5
a. suture levator (partial-thickness)
b. suture dermis to include 0.1 mm of epidermis

6 skin closure

buried levator sutures

close skin between levator sutures

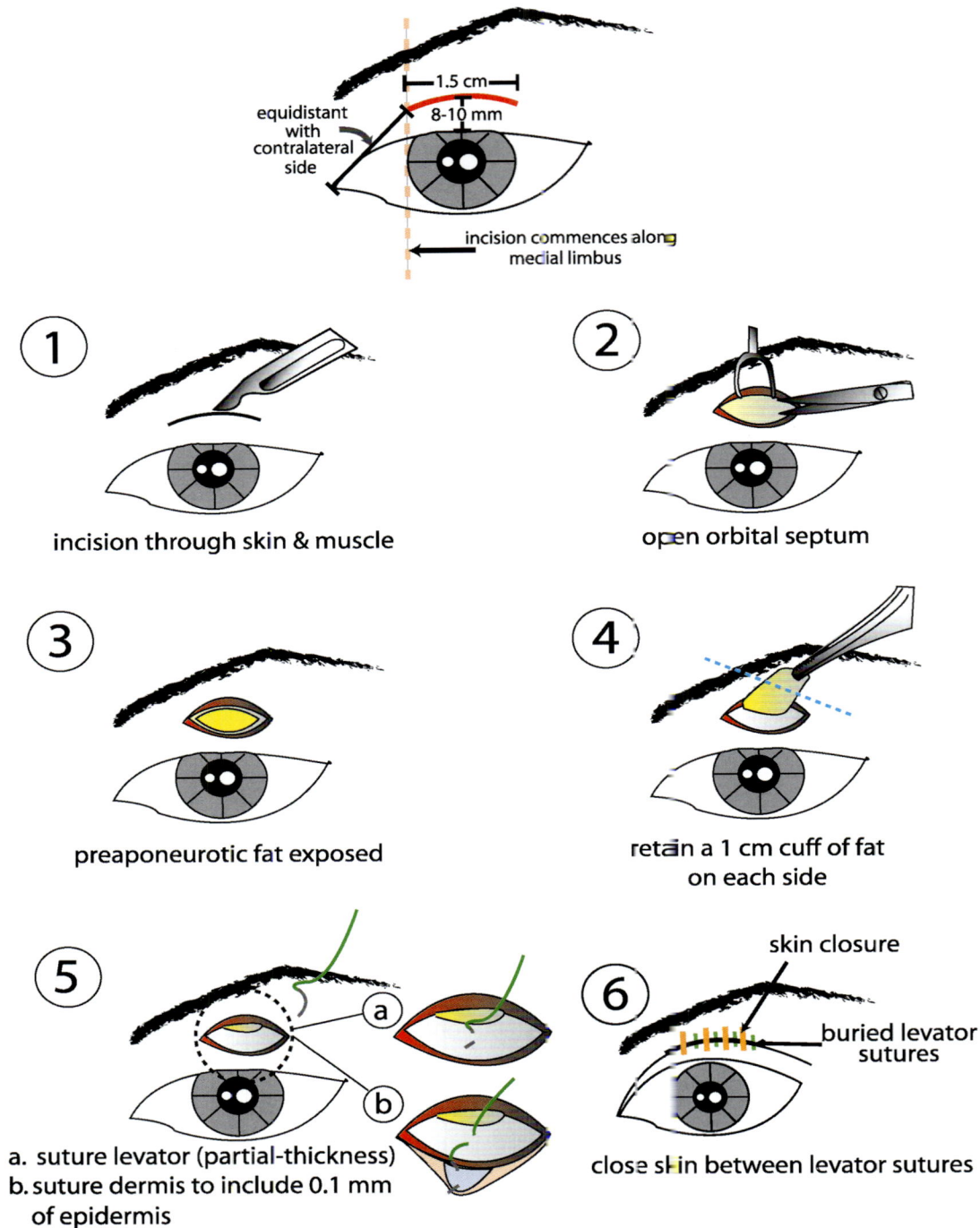

Figure 8–1   This schematic illustration demonstrates the step-wise approach to the partial-incision double-eyelid technique. The incision measures ~1.5 cm in diameter and begins medially at the medial limbus to span one-third of the eyelid distance. Symmetry should be well established with Castroviejo calipers before commencing surgery. Step 1: After a precise amount of local anesthesia is infiltrated into each incision (0.3 cc per side), the incision is made through the skin and muscle with a no.15 Bard-Parker blade. Hemostasis is achieved with bipolar cautery. Step 2: The orbital septum is incised and excised until the underlying postseptal adipose tissue is freely released. Step 3: With the preaponeurotic (postseptal) fat exposed, the contralateral eyelid should be approached in the same fashion until the fat is similarly encountered. Step 4: A 1-cm cuff of fat should be retained on each side to avoid a hollow-eye appearance. Step 5: The levator (**a**) to dermis (**b**) should be fixated passing the suture in a partial thickness fashion through the levator from superiorly to inferiorly then through the dermis up to include 0.1 to 0.2 mm of the epidermal edge from superiorly to inferiorly. The suture is tied down with one knot and the patient is asked to open his or her eyes to confirm adequate fixation and height of the eyelid crease as well as observation of slight eyelash eversion. The contralateral eyelid is undertaken in the same manner, and symmetry is confirmed. A total of seven levator-dermal fixation sutures are placed in each eyelid. Step 6: The skin is then closed with interrupted sutures between the buried levator sutures.

fixation sutures that will yield a fold that extends across the entire eyelid despite the relatively short length of suture fixation.

The partial-incision method offers the distinct advantage over the suture method in that the central fat compartment can be readily addressed and the longevity of crease fixation may be superior as well (although this point may be debated). As the length of fixation is shorter than with the full-incision technique, the chance of crease loss is potentially higher, but correction of this problem is simpler than with the full-incision technique. The full incision also permits modulation of the medial-canthal region by extending the incision toward the epicanthus if an epicanthoplasty is required. Nevertheless, an epicanthoplasty can still be undertaken concurrently with the partial-incision method using a separate, abbreviated incision along the epicanthus. The full-incision method also permits creation of a fold that follows a more precisely prescribed contour (e.g., an inside vs. outside fold). With the full-incision method, the outer shape of the eyelid can also be more effectively adjusted, for example, shaping an oval or round eyelid appearance.* In addition, excessive eyelid skin or muscle cannot be readily addressed with the partial-incision method. Accordingly, the partial-incision technique is ideally suited for younger patients who are in their teenage years and 20s. To compensate for the patient with excessive skin redundancy, the incision height may need to be adjusted superiorly to achieve the desired crease height. (The reader is referred to the following section on surgical technique for details.) Depending on the amount of skin redundancy and the height of the incision, an inside or outside fold will arise with the partial-incision method: greater skin redundancy and a lower crease height will predispose toward an inside-fold configuration, whereas less skin redundancy and a higher crease height will most likely yield an outside fold. If the patient does not express any significant desire to have one type of fold or the other, the partial-incision method may be undertaken for its technical ease, rapidity, and faster postoperative recovery. If the patient desires a precise shape and contour of the fold, then a full-incision method may be warranted. If revision surgery is required, the partial-incision method facilitates a faster, less labor-intensive undertaking compared with one that follows the full-incision method. As part of this spectrum, the suture technique is associated with the simplest and fastest revision surgery.

The patient should receive a detailed preoperative consultation that enumerates all of the potential advantages and disadvantages of each of the surgical methods so that an educated and informed judgment can be rendered as to the optimal technique for that individual.

Surgical Technique

1. The first step is to confirm with the patient the desired crease height in the following manner. Typically, the proposed incision should be measured ~8 mm above the ciliary margin for a low crease and at times slightly higher at 10 mm if the patient desires a larger crease. *The incision should be marked out when the patient is in a supine position with the eyes closed, and the skin is placed under tension until the eyelashes begin to evert to a perpendicular position* (Fig. 8–2). Use of Castroviejo calipers provides the most accurate method of measurement. Before formal marking of the entire incision length, a single point is marked with gentian violet at the desired crease height in the middle of the proposed incision on one eyelid using a toothpick dipped in gentian violet solution or a fine surgical marking pen. The patient is asked to return to a sitting position, and a curved wire is pressed into the marked point. When the patient returns to a sitting position, the lid height typically diminishes by half (e.g., a 10 mm marked lid height becomes 5 mm upon sitting). However, the greater amount of skin present and the larger proportion of fat removed may cause the

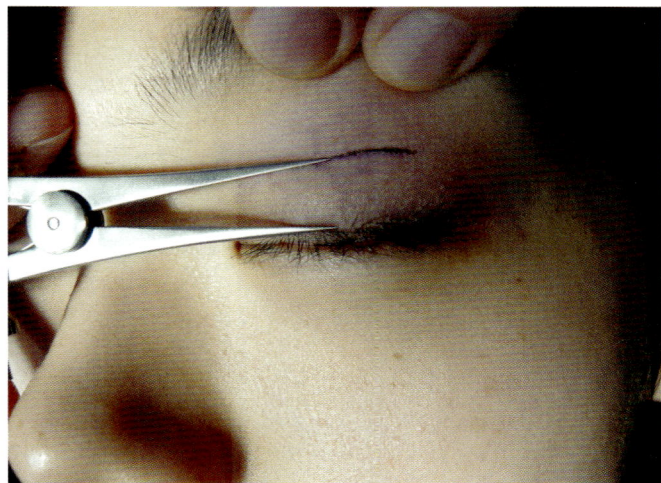

Figure 8–2 *The Partial-Incision Technique, Step 1:* The proposed incision for the supratarsal crease is measured between 8 and 10 mm above the ciliary margin: The incision should be marked out when the patient is in a supine position with the eyes closed, and the skin is placed under tension until the eyelashes begin to evert to a perpendicular position. A Castroviejo caliper is used for accurate measurement. (From Lam SM, Kim YK. Partial-incision technique for creation of the double eyelid. Aesthetic Surg J 2003;23:170–176; with permission.)

---

* The reader is referred to Chapter 2 for a detailed discussion of various strategies for epicanthal modulation, creation of an inside versus an outside fold, and construction of an oval versus a round eyelid.

crease ultimately to be lower than anticipated due to the draping of excessive skin over the incision line. While seated, the patient confirms that the crease height matches his or her aesthetic wishes, and the height is adjusted as necessary before continuing.

2. The technique, as for all double-eyelid surgeries, begins with careful, symmetrical marking of the proposed upper-eyelid folds. The desired lid crease is marked out with gentian violet, confirming the height with a pair of calipers in the manner described previously. The partial incision extends ~1.5 cm in length, with the medial extent of the incision situated at the medial border of the pupil, or medial limbus. The patient is asked to gaze directly forward in a neutral position to determine that the medial extent of the incision in fact aligns with the medial limbus. Because the patient's forward gaze may not be the most reliable indicator for precise symmetrical marking of the medial incision, the distance from the medial canthus to the medial extent of the incision is confirmed to be the same for both eyelids with Castroviejo calipers. In addition, the incision length and height are confirmed for symmetry with Castroviejo calipers before continuing.

3. Local anesthesia of 1 to 2% lidocaine with 1:100,000 epinephrine is infiltrated immediately below the incision line in the subcutaneous plane. Only 0.3 cc is used for each side. This limited amount of anesthetic contributes to less postoperative edema and permits accurate assessment of symmetry during the operation.[†] Injection should be placed in the central aspect of the incision and allowed to disperse naturally across the incision length rather than tunneling the needle across the proposed incision: this technique minimizes discomfort and ecchymosis. The anesthetic can be more evenly distributed by gently pinching the skin to disperse the anesthetic across the entire incision. Ten minutes are allowed to transpire for hemostatic and anesthetic effects to take effect.

4. Both incisions are then made with a no. 15 Bard-Parker blade through the skin and muscle to expose

the underlying orbital septum. The surgeon should make both incisions from the same side of the patient for simplicity and also to ensure that the angle of transection is the same. Bipolar cautery is used to achieve hemostasis along the transected muscle fibers and subdermal plexus before continuing on with the procedure. (The surgeon will consistently notice two parallel vessels that run transversely across the incision, which should be adequately cauterized before continuing.)

5. Attention is then paid to only one eyelid for dissection. The lateral portion of the orbital septum is gently lifted up with a pair of forceps, and a small wedge of orbital septum is removed with scissors along the superior border of the incision to expose the underlying preaponeurotic fat (Fig. **8–3**). Excision of a small portion of orbital septum must usually be repeated several times until the fat can be atraumatically teased out of its native position (Fig. **8–4**). (For patients with very little adipose tissue, the skin surrounding the incision can be depressed to encourage the fat to herniate through the incision to identify it more readily.)

6. With the central fat pad retracted out of the way, closed-tip scissors are passed under the orbital septum to ensure that an unrestricted plane exists between the overlying septum and the underlying levator. The remaining orbital septum can then be safely transected with the scissors along its entire length from a lateral to a medial direction (Fig. **8–5**). This maneuver is important to expose the entire levator complex for fixation.

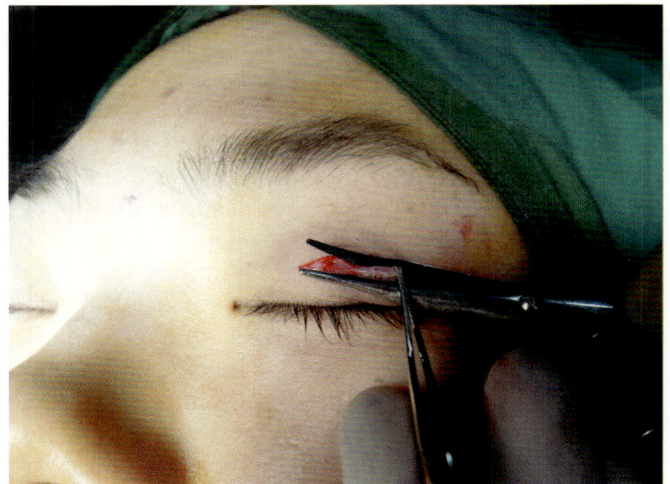

Figure 8–3 *The Partial-Incision Technique, Step 2:* After infiltration of local anesthesia and incision of the skin and muscle with a no. 15 Bard-Parker blade, the orbital septum (as well as any remaining orbicularis muscle) is incised centrally with a pair of fine scissors to expose the underlying preaponeurotic fat. (From Lam SM, Kim YK. Partial-incision technique for creation of the double eyelid. Aesthetic Surg J 2003;23:170–176; with permission.)

[†] The reader should note that additional anesthetic should not be placed when the levator is exposed for risk that the muscle might become anesthetized, leading to levator dysfunction that may last for several weeks postoperatively. In addition, when the patient cannot fully open his or her eyes, symmetry becomes an almost impossible task. If any anesthetic should fall directly on the levator muscle, a cotton-tipped applicator should be used to absorb the excess immediately and the patient's eye opening ability confirmed to be intact. If additional anesthetic is required during the case, the same amount should always be placed into both eyelids in the same distribution so that symmetry can still be evaluated. Furthermore, anesthetic placement along the skin edges to anesthetize the skin for skin closure should be avoided because of the added edema that ensues that may inhibit crease formation for 2 weeks, which magnifies the recovery period and may cause undue concern with the patient.

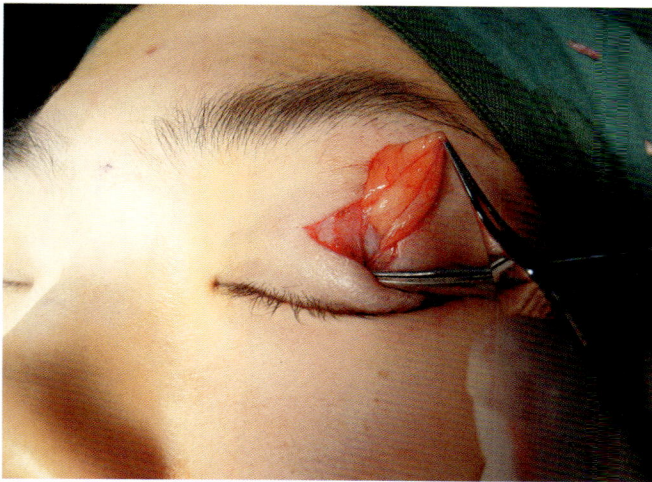

Figure 8–4 *The Partial-Incision Technique, Step 3:* The orbital septum is transected several times before the fat can be freely mobilized from its native position. The photograph shows the glistening white levator aponeurosis immediately below the postseptal, preaponeurotic adipose tissue. (From Lam SM, Kim YK. Partial-incision technique for creation of the double eyelid. Aesthetic Surg J 2003;23:170–176; with permission.)

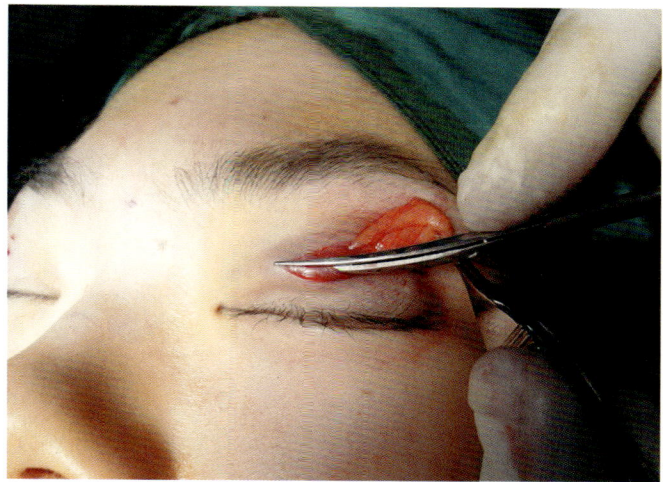

Figure 8–5 *The Partial-Incision Technique, Step 4:* With the central fat pad retracted out of the way, the remaining orbital septum is transected with the scissors along its entire length from a lateral to a medial direction. (From Lam SM, Kim YK. Partial-incision technique for creation of the double eyelid. Aesthetic Surg J 2003;23:170–176; with permission.)

7. A cotton-tipped applicator can then be used to sweep the fat pad away from the underlying levator complex, which should appear as a glistening white surface below the fat. (At times a false preaponeurotic plane is identified that may be confused with the levator. Fixation of the suture to this plane will contribute to early fold loss. If uncertain, the surgeon should grasp the tissue and ask the patient to open his or her eyes, with the inability to comply consistent with proper identification of the levator.)

8. Before the fat is removed, the exact same procedure is performed in the contralateral lid.

9. With both fat pads in view, a symmetrical amount of fat removal may be ensured. Both fat pads are first infiltrated with a small amount of 1% plain lidocaine: the reader is reminded never to infiltrate lidocaine with a vasoconstrictive agent (e.g., epinephrine) into the postseptal tissues to avoid the risk of vascular spasm and related blindness. Also, the same amount of anesthetic should be placed into each side so that a symmetrical amount of fat removal may be ensured.

10. *It is important that an excessive amount of fat not be excised*: exuberant removal of adipose tissue may eventually lead to an aged, hollow appearance to the upper lid (the "sunken eye" deformity). The intended fat pad to be excised is first clamped with a fine hemostat so that a 1 cm cuff of fat is retained under the clamp. The overlying fat is excised with scissors (Fig. **8–6**), and a small cuff of adipose should be retained above the clamp so that it can be cauterized with bipolar cautery before clamp removal.

The fat pad is then carefully inspected for hemostasis before venturing to the contralateral side.

11. The same technique of fat excision is applied to the other side, being mindful to retain the same 1 cm cuff of fat intact. Of note, an asymmetrical amount of fat may be removed, as patients often naturally have asymmetrical adipose deposits. Accordingly, a symmetrical amount of fat that is retained is more important than a symmetrical amount that is removed.

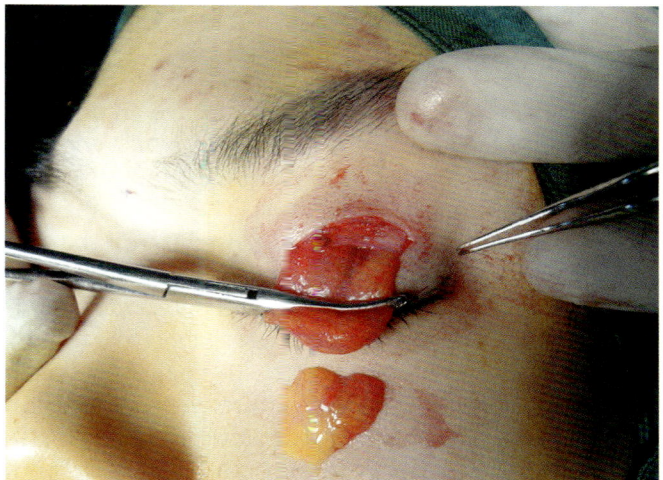

Figure 8–6 *The Partial-Incision Technique, Step 5:* Before the fat is removed, the exact same procedure is performed in the contralateral lid. With both fat pads exposed, a symmetrical amount should be retained, generally leaving a cuff of 1 cm of fat intact. The photograph shows a hemostat applied to remove a portion of the exposed fat pad with the already excised contralateral fat pad resting on the cheek. (From Lam SM, Kim YK. Partial-incision technique for creation of the double eyelid. Aesthetic Surg J 2003;23:170–176; with permission.)

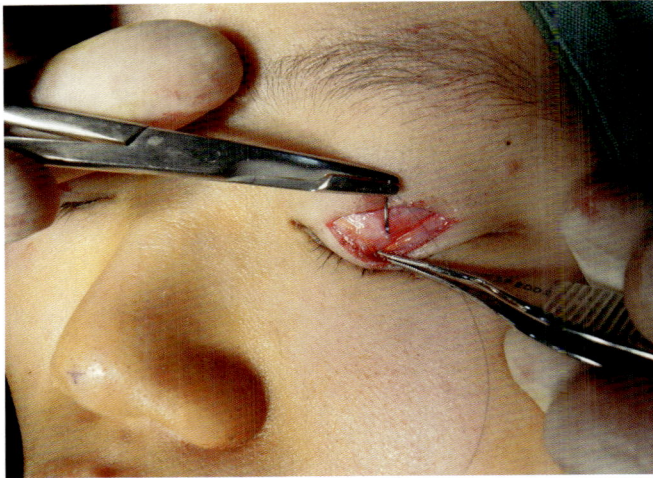

Figure 8–7 *The Partial-Incision Technique, Step 6:* To close, 7–0 nylon is used as the levator–skin fixation suture. With the levator in full view, the aponeurosis is pierced with the suture needle at the midheight and central aspect of the incision from a superior to inferior direction. Only a fraction of a millimeter of the levator (about the width of the needle) and only partial thickness need be purchased with the needle. (From Lam SM, Kim YK. Partial-incision technique for creation of the double eyelid. Aesthetic Surg J 2003;23:170–176; with permission.)

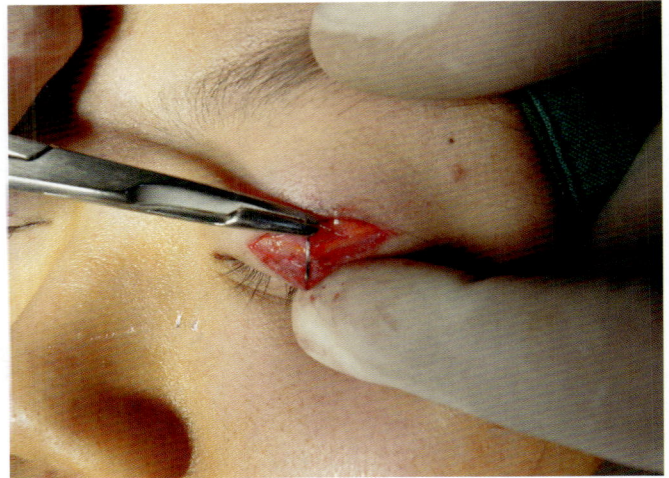

Figure 8–8 *The Partial-Incision Technique, Step 7:* The needle is driven through the inferior skin edge, purchasing the full thickness of the dermis to include 0.1 to 0.2 mm of epidermis. Inclusion of the cornified layer of epidermis may promote a foreign-body reaction and thereby more fully secure levator fixation. (From Lam SM, Kim YK. Partial-incision technique for creation of the double eyelid. Aesthetic Surg J 2003;23: 170–176; with permission.)

12. Next, 7–0 nylon or 8–0 polyglycolic acid (e.g., Dexon, US Surgical, Norwalk, CT)‡ is used as the levator–skin fixation suture. With the levator in full view, the aponeurosis is pierced with the suture needle at the midheight (the levator that lies immediately superior to the tarsal plate) and central aspect of the incision from a superior to inferior direction. Only a fraction of a millimeter of the levator (about the width of the needle) and only partial thickness need be purchased with the needle (Fig. **8–7**). Then, the needle is driven through the inferior skin edge, purchasing the full thickness of the dermis and ~0.1 to 0.2 mm of the epidermis (Fig. **8–8**). (The needle should pass into the cornified layer of the epithelium, which will promote better levator–skin adherence by virtue of a limited foreign-body reaction. The index finger of the nondominant hand can be used to roll the skin and apply countertraction while the needle is being passed through the skin edge to ensure a more complete purchase of the above described layers of skin. If the suture is placed correctly through a small portion of the epidermis, the suture will tent the skin edge in a gull-wing configuration (Fig. **8–9**) and also form a raised ridge of levator that spans from both

sides of the suture and that will serve to guide placement of the remaining fixation sutures.

13. After the suture is tied down with a single knot, the patient is asked to open his or her eyes to examine the adequacy of the crease position. (The reader is referred to Fig. **2–17B** for a profile view of the internal fixation suture that is used with this technique.) If the fold appears aesthetically pleasing *and the patient's eyelashes appear slightly everted*, then the remainder of the knots can be tied (typically a total of three square knots), and the suture tails can be

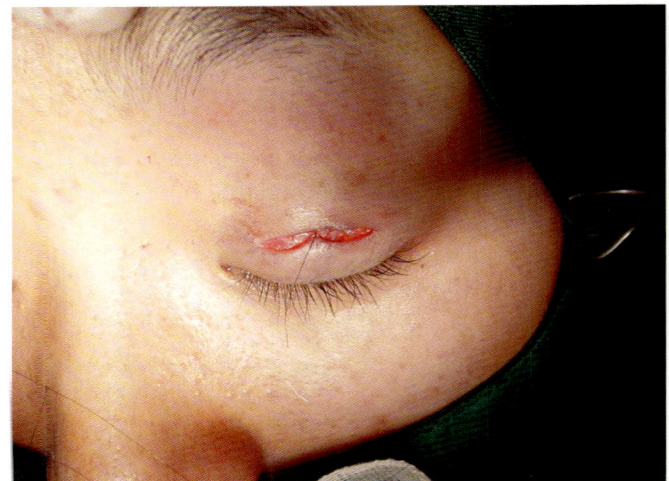

Figure 8–9 *The Partial-Incision Technique, Step 8:* After placement of one suture in the prescribed fashion, a gull-wing appearance of the skin edge should manifest. In addition, the fixation suture will engender a raised ridge of levator that facilitates placement of the remaining fixation sutures.

‡ If 8–0 polyglycolic acid is used, only three square suture throws are necessary. Tying down the suture should be done more gently than with nylon, as this suture material has a greater tendency to break with application of tension. The reader should note that 7–0 nylon has been used in the majority of operative cases (over 1500 cases), but polyglycolic acid has been used safely as well in over 40 cases. Use of an absorbable suture like polyglycolic acid will decrease the incidence of suture extrusion.

trimmed to the knot so that they will be buried as they are permanent sutures.

14. The surgeon should then pass to the contralateral lid to place the same suture through the central levator and lower-lid skin edge. A single knot is tied, and the patient is asked to open his or her eyes again to confirm that the crease height is symmetrical with the contralateral lid crease *and the patient's eyelashes are slightly everted.*

15. Once symmetry is confirmed with one fixation suture on each side, the remaining six sutures (per side) can be placed easily by following the raised ridge of levator aponeurosis that arises from the first fixation suture. The fixation suture is placed through the raised levator ridge to the skin in the same manner prescribed above for the first fixation suture. (Refer to step 12.)

16. To close, two or three interrupted sutures of 7–0 nylon are placed to approximate the skin, taking care to place the skin sutures between the fixation sutures to avoid inadvertent transection of the fixation suture. All of the skin-closure sutures are removed on the third postoperative day, and the buried, internal fixation sutures remain permanently.

17. If asymmetry is noted at the end of the procedure, the smaller fold can be elevated to match the contralateral side in the following manner: the levator is identified through a small opening in the skin (if it has been closed already), and an additional suture may be placed through the levator and the superior skin edge to raise the fold appropriately. Additional sutures may be placed as needed if further minor adjustments are needed. However any gross asymmetries will require a more formal undertaking of revision surgery by removing and replacing the previous fixation sutures.

Postoperative Remarks

Three notable complications that can occur after this surgery are asymmetry, loss of lid fold, and suture extrusion, all of which occur less than 1% of the time.

Asymmetry may arise despite the best surgical efforts, and proper surgical technique will limit the occurrence of this complication. Asymmetry that is evident in the early postoperative period (first two postoperative weeks) may be due to edema and should be carefully followed. Typically, the patient should return after 2 weeks to determine whether asymmetry is still present at that time. After 2 weeks, any asymmetry that remains should be addressed with surgical revision. After a 2-week period, revision surgery is rather straightforward, as the plane of the levator aponeurosis can be easily identified with gentle spreading of the scissors

after blade incision through the skin. Identification of the fixation sutures will also aid in confirmation that the correct surgical plane has been attained. The old sutures should then be removed, and any dermal-levator adhesion should be broken. Care must always be taken not to transect the levator muscle, which can be a disastrous maneuver. Placement of fixation sutures should follow the same alternating fashion as prescribed in the preceding section. Albeit tempting, *the surgeon should never revise a single eyelid to correct asymmetry, as success of this endeavor is almost always elusive.* If asymmetry is corrected several months after surgery, then identification of the levator aponeurosis may be more difficult. The surgeon is advised to progress methodically and deliberately to ensure that the muscle is not damaged. Progressing laterally to medially as superiorly as possible will help prevent damage to the muscle. Furthermore, identification of any remaining adipose tissue will help guide dissection, as the levator should lie immediately below this plane. If the surgeon is uncertain whether the levator is in view, he or she can grasp the tissue with forceps and ask the patient to open his or her eyes. If the patient cannot open the eyelid that is held by the forceps, then the surgeon has successfully grasped the levator. Conversely, if the patient can still open his or her eyes, then the surgeon most likely has not arrived at the plane of the levator. As mentioned, finding the old fixation sutures should also provide a helpful guidepost. Gentle tissue spreading with scissors rather than forceful sharp knife dissection will also help limit the risk of levator injury.§ After the plane of the levator aponeurosis is fully exposed, placement of fixation sutures progresses as prescribed before.

Because the technique that is elaborated herein relies on internal fixation sutures (Fig. **2–17B**) that remain permanently, suture extrusion may occur. No more than four knots should be placed per suture to minimize the likelihood of this complication. Suture exposure typically manifests after the first postoperative month. If this should arise, then the surgeon should wait until after the third postoperative month to remove the suture, as it is at this time that permanent lid adhesion has been established. The patient should be explained this fact and be asked to wait patiently. Fortunately, the suture oftentimes is not visible on casual inspection because the skin folds over the incision line to cover the exposed suture, and the suture typically only becomes visible when the eye is fully closed. Albeit infrequent, loss of the lid fold may also occur, which may be due to early removal of any extruded sutures. Revision surgery should follow the sequence mentioned above for cases of asymmetry.

---

§ The reader is advised to review the accompanying DVD video (Disk One) on lowering the eyelid crease, which shows a stepwise dissection to find the levator muscle in a previously dissected surgical bed.

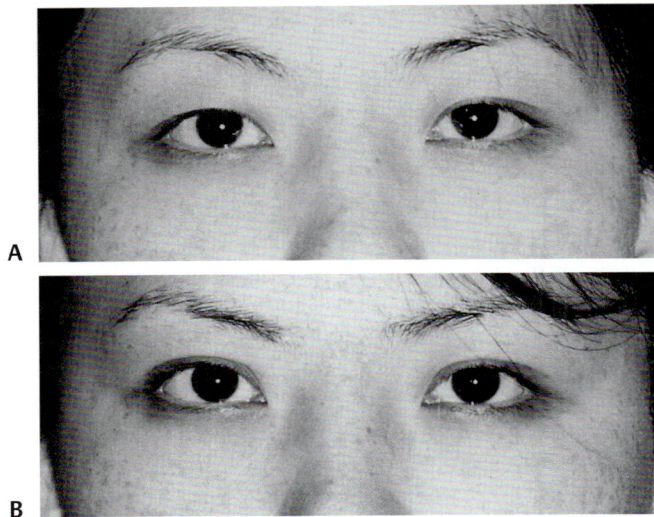

Figure 8–10 **(A)** Preoperative view of a 28-year-old woman with minimal upper-lid fat and a relatively wide palpebral fissure. **(B)** Postoperative view 1 year after double-eyelid surgery, involving the partial-incision technique, in which minimal fat was removed and a lid crease of 10 mm was marked in the supine position. (From Lam SM, Kim YK. Partial-incision technique for creation of the double eyelid. Aesthetic Surg J 2003;23:170–176; with permission.)

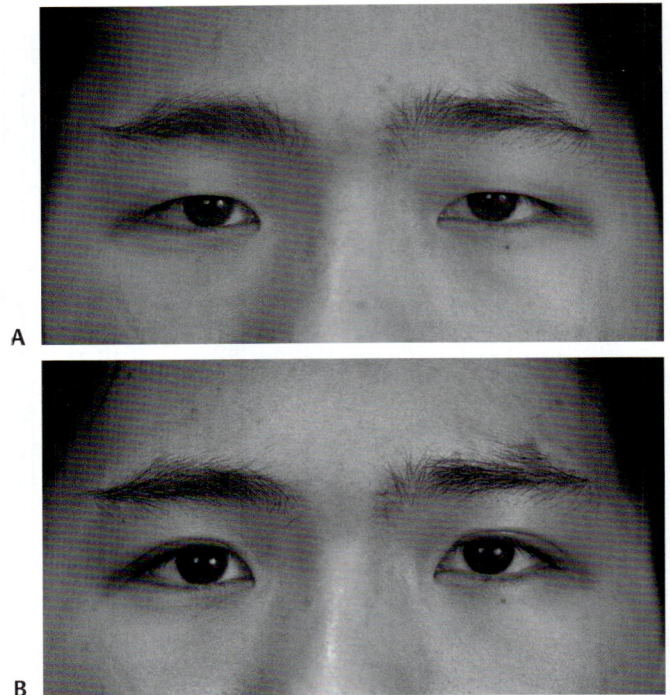

Figure 8–11 This 16-year-old Chinese male is shown preoperatively **(A)** with a narrower palpebral fissure and immediately postoperatively **(B)** following a partial-incision technique for double-eyelid creation with a measured incision 8 mm above the ciliary margin and modest fat removal.

Despite potential complications, the partial-incision technique has proven to be a safe, simple, and reliable method for double-eyelid creation, and it offers an ideal balance between the suture and the full-incision methods (Figs. **8–10A,B, 8–11A,B**).

◆ The Suture Technique

Method of Tetsuo Shu Preoperative Remarks

The suture technique developed by Tetsuo Shu represents the oldest method for double-eyelid creation,[6] but it remains a viable alternative to and offers several advantages over incision-based techniques. Placement of a suture through the upper eyelid does not require any formal knowledge of upper-lid anatomy, as the surgeon simply places the suture through the full thickness of the eyelid from the skin to the conjunctiva and back through again (Fig. **8–12**). Accordingly, no surgical dissection is required, and identification of anatomic landmarks (orbicularis oculi, postseptal fat, and the levator aponeurosis) is obviated, which makes this technique relatively ideal for the novice surgeon. Furthermore, the rapidity with which this technique can be accomplished is favorable for the surgeon and patient alike, as the surgeon may complete the task quickly without considerable technical labor, and the patient can be afforded the fastest recovery compared with incision-based surgery. Typically, patients experience very little postoperative edema, with return to a natural appearance within

several hours to days after surgery. The partial incision may require several weeks of time compared with several months for the full-incision method. As would be expected, the suture technique also offers the distinct advantage that no external scar is present. Incisions in Asian skin may require a longer recovery period to heal because of the chance of scarring, hyperpigmentation, hypopigmentation, and prolonged erythema. However, the surgeon should not be overly concerned about scarring if proper surgical technique is followed. After surgery, the lid crease can be lowered within the first postoperative month if the patient is unsatisfied with the height of the crease, whereas it can be raised for an indefinite period after surgery, as the higher level of fixation replaces the former lower point of adherence. Because no surgical dissection need be undertaken in revision cases (as the levator may be more difficult to identify safely with incision-based methods), the ease with which a revision operation may be accomplished stands as another advantage over incision-based surgery.

Several disadvantages of the suture technique have been cited in the literature and should be brought to the attention of the patient. The most criticized drawback that is associated with this technique concerns the potential temporary nature of the crease fixation. A 2000 report, however, contradicts this assertion.[7] Scarification between the levator and the dermis that ensures

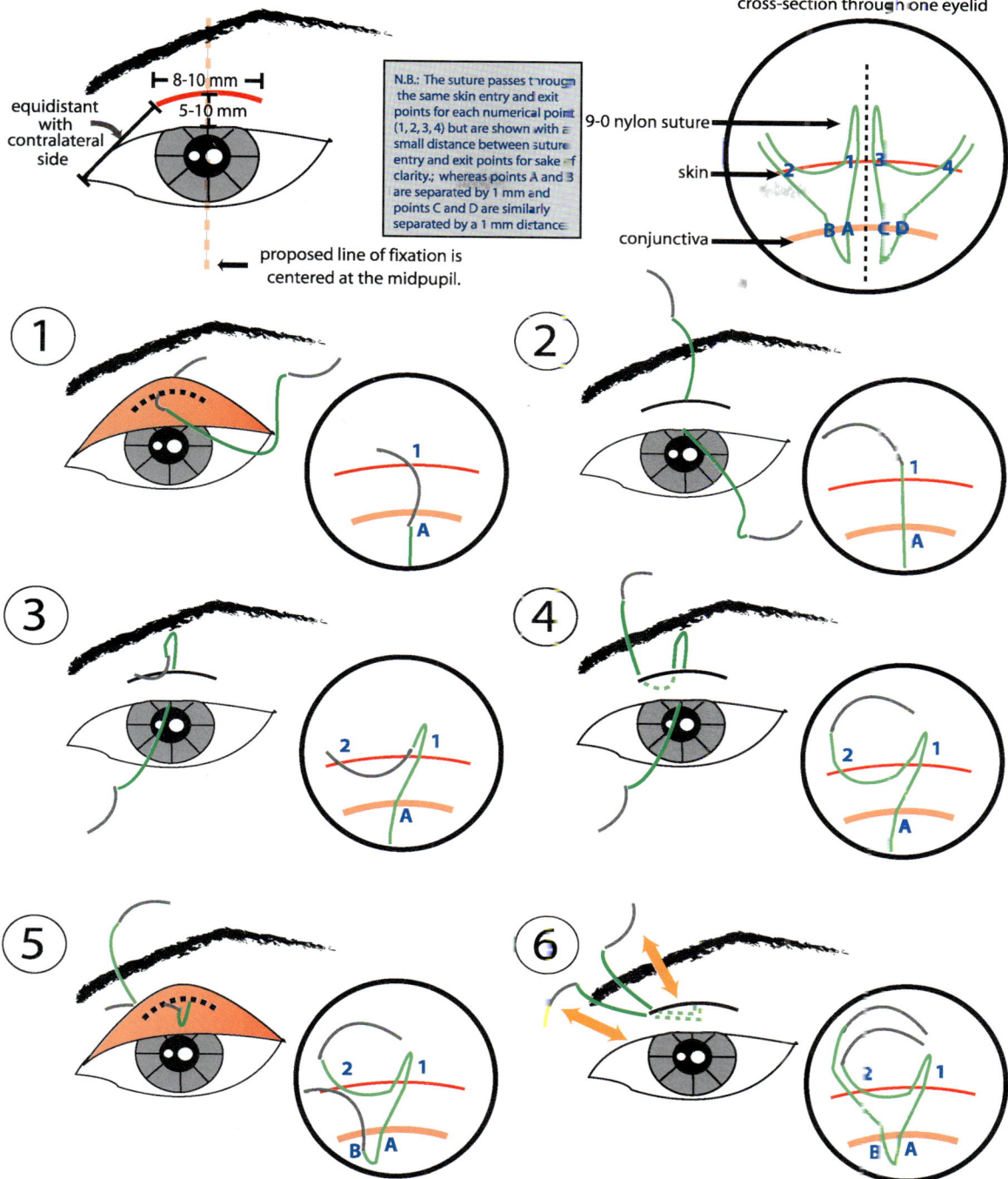

Figure 8–12 This schematic illustration demonstrates the stepwise approach to the suture-based double-eyelid technique. The proposed line of suture fixation measures ~1 cm in diameter and is centered at the midpupil. Symmetry should be well established with Castroviejo calipers before commencing surgery. The following steps demonstrate how to perform half of an eyelid crease, and the remaining half of the same eyelid crease is completed in a mirror fashion. *Step 1:* After local anesthesia has been administered (topical tetracaine to the globe and conjunctiva and 1% lidocaine with 1:100,000 epinephrine to the skin and the conjunctiva), a double-armed 9–0 nylon suture is passed through the midsection of the proposed fixation line (just lateral to the midsection of the fixation line) from the conjunctiva to the skin. A round retractor is used to expose the conjunctiva adequately. *Step 2:* The illustration shows the full passage of the needle from the conjunctiva through the skin discussed in step 1. *Step 3:* The same needle is passed back through the exact same skin exit point to tunnel under the skin toward the lateral end of the fixation line. *Step 4:* The illustration shows the full passage of the needle discussed in step 3. *Step 5:* The other needle of the double-armed suture is then passed through a point in the conjunctiva close to the first needle's entry (about a 1 mm distance away) and passed through to the skin to exit the skin laterally through the same exit point mentioned in step 4 for the first needle (i.e., at the lateral terminus of fixation line). *Step 6:* The two ends of the suture are then gently seesawed back and forth to bury the exposed suture on the conjunctival side and thereby minimize the risk of corneal abrasion. The suture is then tied down with a minimum of five square knots, and the tails are left in place until the remaining half of the fixation line is completed in a mirror fashion. (See cross section of suture passage at the upper right corner of the illustration.) The contralateral eyelid is completed in the same prescribed manner, and symmetry is confirmed before the suture tails are trimmed. The suture tails are then buried with a toothed forceps under the skin.

longevity of the surgical result may be compromised in the suture method. Intervening adipose tissue that remains compressed between the levator and dermis may prevent formation of a permanent adhesion between the muscle and the skin. Patients with excessive adipose tissue may also be unsuitable candidates for another reason: their adipose tissue cannot be removed via the suture method, and therefore their lid fullness may not be adequately addressed. Some surgeons also advocate partial resection of the orbicularis oculi muscle to reduce lid fullness, which clearly cannot be accomplished with the suture method. Furthermore, if a medial epicanthoplasty is required, the suture method fails to address this anatomic feature, and a full-incision method should be elected (as the partial-incision technique also cannot improve this condition.) In contradistinction, a lateral canthoplasty that can aesthetically widen the palpebral aperture further may be undertaken simultaneously, as the incision for this ancillary procedure is completely separate from any double-eyelid procedure (whether incision-based or not).

Despite these shortcomings, the originator of this technique, Tetsuo Shu, has reliably undertaken this procedure with great success. He notes that his crease retention rate exceeds 98% and that most of his patients do not require an incision-based procedure, which he undertakes only as deemed necessary. Curiously, he has also received the request from a few patients to create a small lid crease height first with a subsequent procedure to raise the height so that their friends and colleagues will not notice the abrupt transition to a full double lid—a procedure that is really only feasible with the suture technique. The technique described herein represents many years of modifications before arriving at its current incarnation.

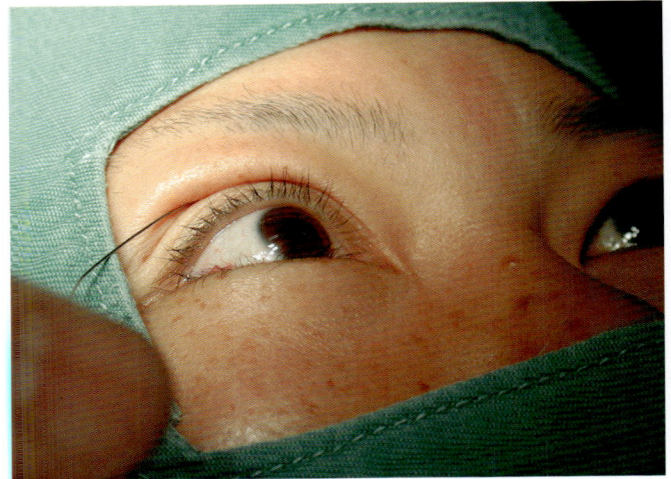

Figure 8–13 *The Suture Technique, Step 1:* The patient has a curved wire pressed into the upper eyelid to simulate the desired crease height. (Courtesy of Tetsuo Shu, M.D.)

Surgical Technique

1. The lid-crease position is marked either low (at 4–5 mm above the ciliary margin) or high (8–10 mm above) depending on patient preference, which is demonstrated to the patient with a curved wire that creates an impression in the upper lid at the desired level to simulate an upper-lid crease (Fig. **8–13**). (Of note, the crease marking is performed without tension on the upper eyelid described for the partial- and full-incision methods, as per Dr. Shu's technique.)

2. The upper lid is then marked at the preferred height at the midpupil, at another point 4 to 5 mm medial, and at yet another point 4 to 5 mm lateral to the midline (Fig. **8–14A,B**). The points are then connected as a line that should extend approximately one-third of the total distance of the upper lid, or ~8 to 10 mm

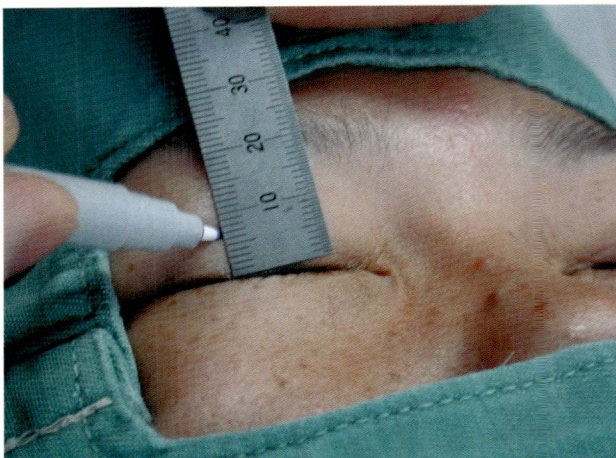
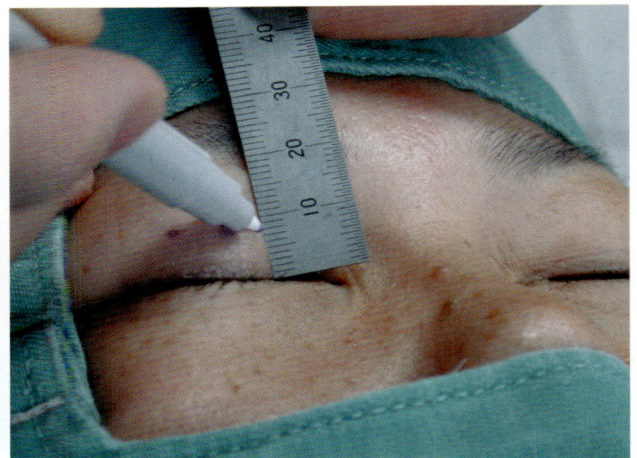

Figure 8–14 **(A, B)** *The Suture Technique, Step 2:* The upper lid is then marked at the preferred height at the midpupil, at another point 4 to 5 mm medial, and at yet another point 4 to

5 mm lateral to the midline. The points are then connected to form the proposed line for suture fixation. (Courtesy of Tetsuo Shu, M.D.)

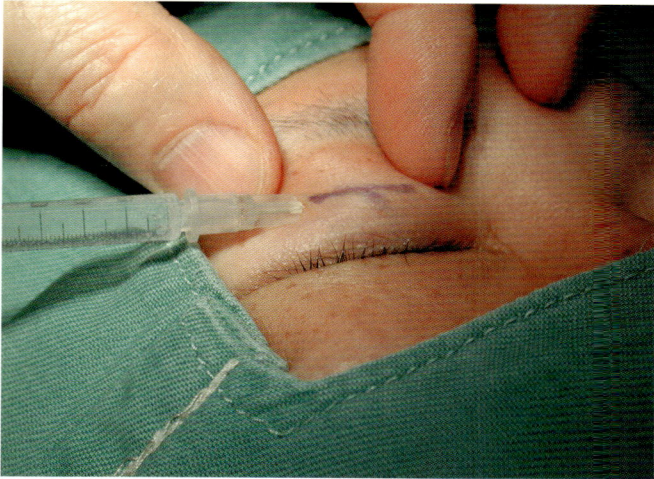

Figure 8–15 *The Suture Technique, Step 3:* After tetracaine is instilled onto the globe and conjunctiva, 1% lidocaine with 1:100,000 epinephrine is infiltrated into the subcutaneous tissue below the line of fixation. (Courtesy of Tetsuo Shu, M.D.)

total in length. Only one-third of the upper lid needs to be fixated to create a permanent double lid.

3. Tetracaine is instilled topically onto the globe and the conjunctiva. Next, 1% lidocaine with 1:100,000 epinephrine is infiltrated into the subcutaneous tissue along the marked-out line (Fig. **8–15**), as well as into the conjunctiva, using round forceps to evert the conjunctiva (Fig. **8–16**).

4. Two double-armed 9–0 nylon sutures are employed to create the double lid. Using the round retractor to evert the conjunctiva, the first needle is passed from the everted conjunctival side (at point A)#

These references to alphanumeric points correspond to those indicated in the schematic illustration, Fig. **8–12**.

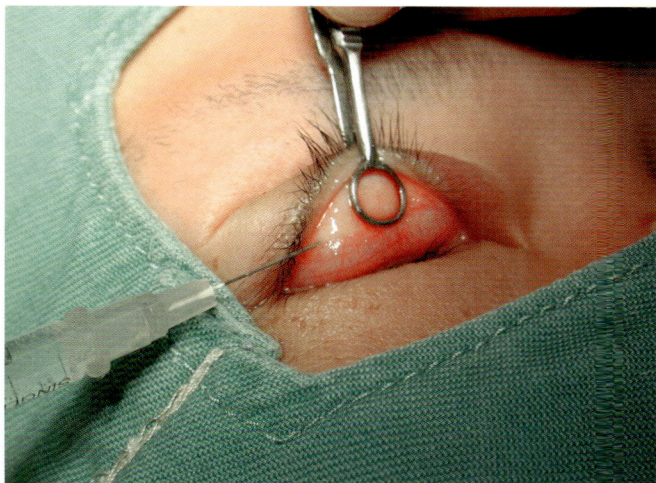

Figure 8–17 *The Suture Technique, Step 5:* One needle of the double-armed 9–0 nylon suture is passed through the conjunctiva (at point A) just lateral to the midpoint of the marked line. (Note: The references to alphanumeric points in Figs. **8–17** through 8–24 correspond to those indicated in the schematic illustration, Fig. **8–12**.) (Courtesy of Tetsuo Shu, M.D.)

(Fig. **8–17**) through the skin just lateral to the midpoint of the marked line (at point 1) (Fig. **8–18**).

5. That same needle is then passed back through the skin (at point 1) and tunneled under the skin to exit at the lateral margin of the marked line (at point 2) (Fig. **8–19**); the needle is then removed from the suture.

6. The other needle on the double-armed suture is passed from the conjunctiva (at point B, which is situated 1 mm adjacent to point A) through the skin (at point 2) to exit at the same position that the first suture did (Fig. **8–20**); the needle is removed from the suture.

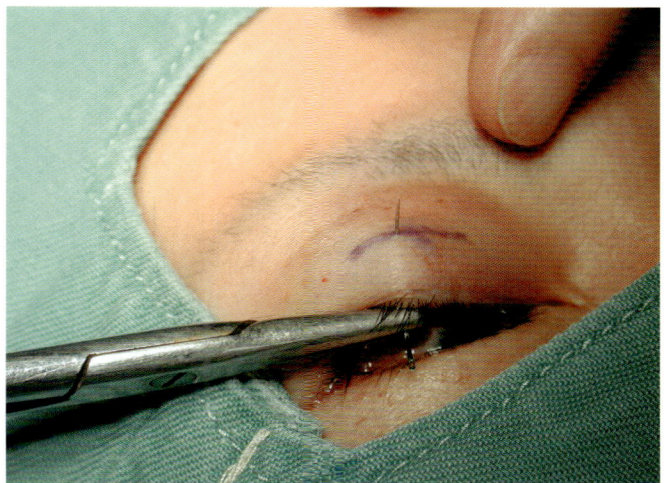

Figure 8–16 *The Suture Technique, Step 4:* The conjunctiva is everted with round forceps, and additional local anesthetic is injected directly into the conjunctiva. (Courtesy of Tetsuo Shu, M.D.)

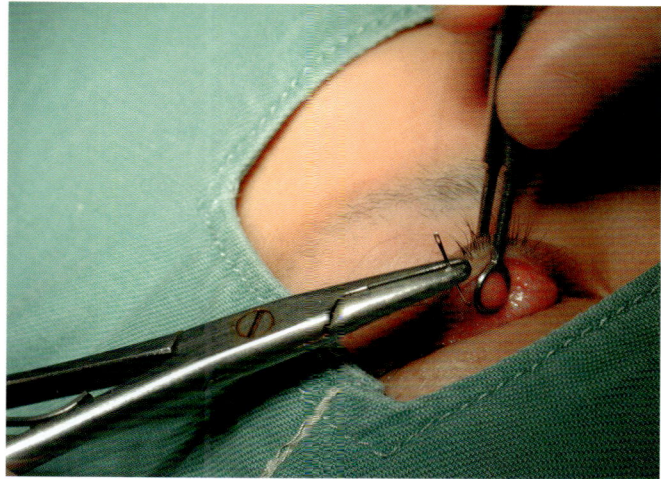

Figure 8–18 *The Suture Technique, Step 6:* The photograph shows the same needle after having passed through the skin just lateral to the midpoint of the marked line (at point 1). (Courtesy of Tetsuo Shu, M.D.)

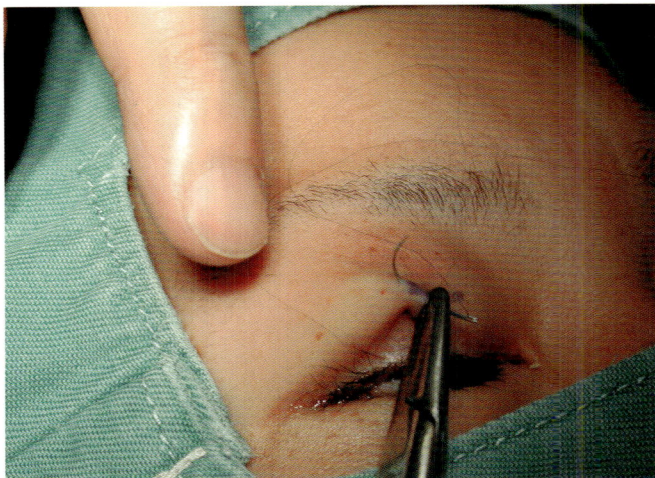

Figure 8–19   *The Suture Technique, Step 7:* The same needle is then passed back through the exact same skin exit point (at point 1) and tunneled subcutaneously to exit at the lateral margin of the marked line (at point 2). (Courtesy of Tetsuo Shu, M.D.)

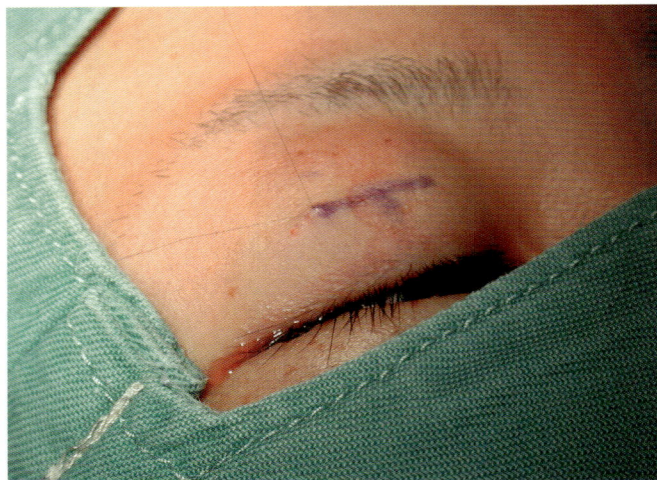

Figure 8–21   *The Suture Technique, Step 9:* The two ends of the suture are then slid gently back and forth in a sawing motion so that the exposed conjunctival suture will bury itself into the conjunctiva and not abrade the cornea. (Courtesy of Tetsuo Shu, M.D.)

7. The two ends of the suture are then gently slid back and forth in a sawing motion so that the exposed conjunctival suture will bury itself into the conjunctiva and not abrade the cornea (Fig. **8–21**). The suture ends are then tied with a minimum of five square knots, and the suture tails are left uncut until the patient is asked to ascertain whether the height of the lid crease is acceptable at the end of the case.

8. The other half of the crease is created as an exact mirror to the first half. The first needle passes from point C to point 3 (Fig. **8–22**) back through point 3 under the skin to exit at point 4 (Fig. **8–23**). The second needle passes from point D (Fig. **8–24**) to exit at point 4 (Fig. **8–25**), and the two ends of the suture are again gently slid back and forth to bury the conjunctival side of the suture (Fig. **8–26**). Similarly, the knot is secured with a minimum of five square knots, and the suture tails are not trimmed until the completion of the procedure (Fig. **8–27**). The crease of the other eyelid is then undertaken in the same manner as described above. If the appearance is acceptable, then all four sutures are cut with almost no suture tail above the knot.

9. A fine-toothed forceps is used to bury the four exposed sutures under the skin (Fig. **8–28**).

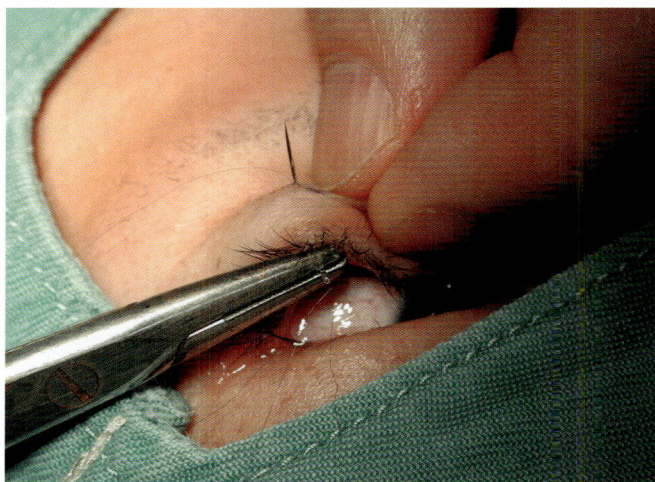

Figure 8–20   *The Suture Technique, Step 8:* The other needle on the double-armed suture is passed from the conjunctiva (at point B, which is situated 1 mm adjacent to point A) through the skin (at point 2) to exit at the same position that the first suture did, and the needle is removed from the suture. (Courtesy of Tetsuo Shu, M.D.)

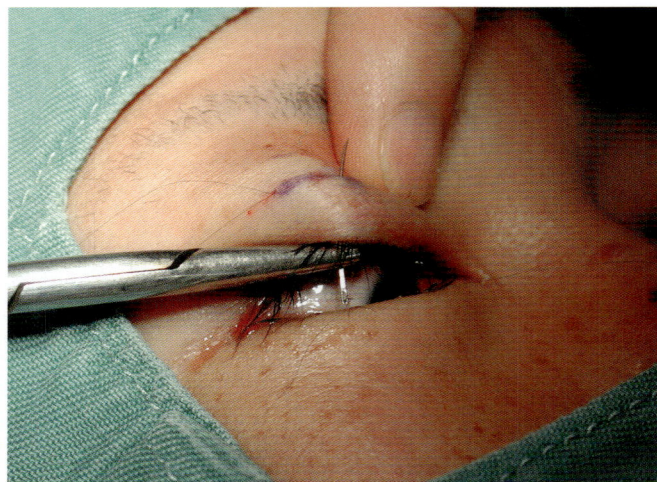

Figure 8–22   *The Suture Technique, Step 10:* The other half of the crease is created as an exact mirror to the first half. The first needle passes from point C (just medial to the midpoint of the fixation line on the conjunctival side) to point 3 (just medial to the midpoint of the fixation line on the skin side). (Courtesy of Tetsuo Shu, M.D.)

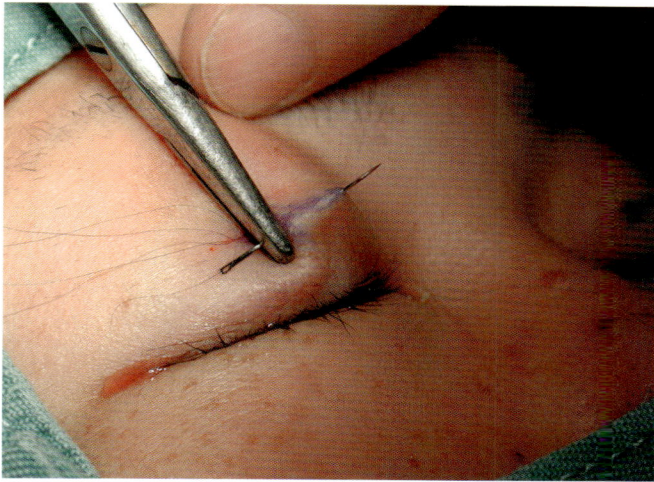

Figure 8–23 *The Suture Technique, Step 11:* The same needle is then driven back through point 3 under the skin to exit at point 4, at the medial limit of the fixation line. (Courtesy of Tetsuo Shu, M.D.)

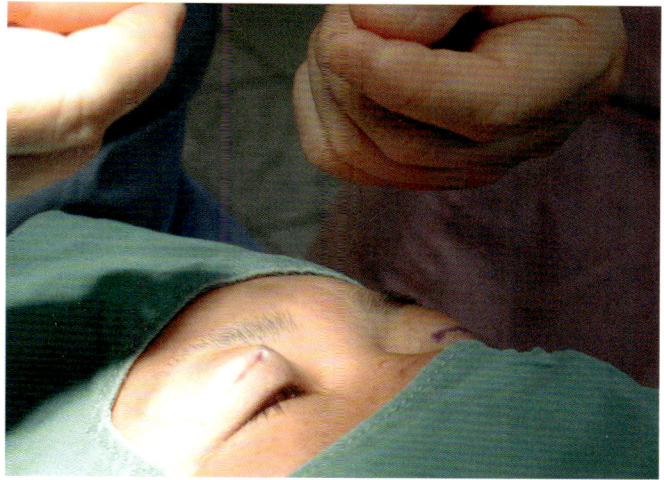

Figure 8–26 *The Suture Technique, Step 14:* The two ends of the suture are again gently slid back and forth to bury the conjunctival suture. (Courtesy of Tetsuo Shu, M.D.)

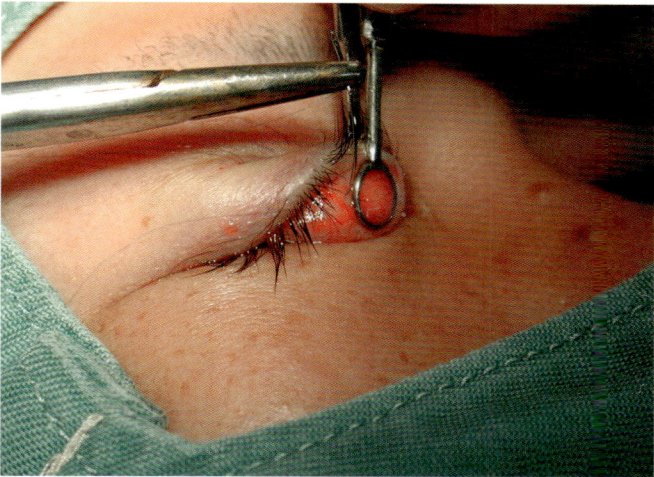

Figure 8–24 *The Suture Technique, Step 12:* The second needle passes from point D (located 1 mm medial to point C on the conjunctival side). (Courtesy of Tetsuo Shu, M.D.)

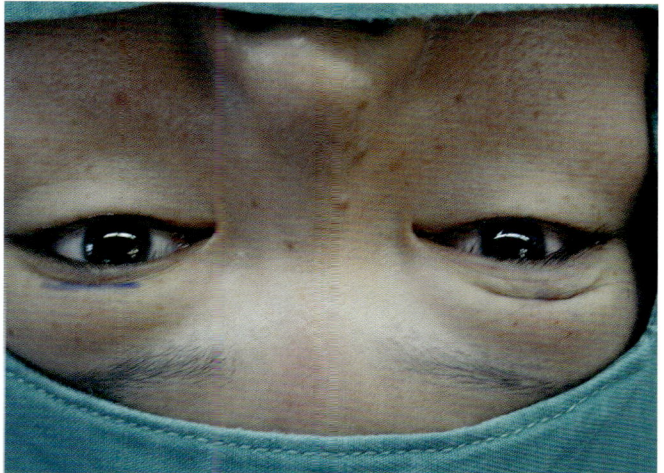

Figure 8–27 *The Suture Technique, Step 15:* The patient is shown at the completion of the right crease fixation, with the suture tails left untrimmed until the completion of the contralateral eyelid. (Courtesy of Tetsuo Shu, M.D.)

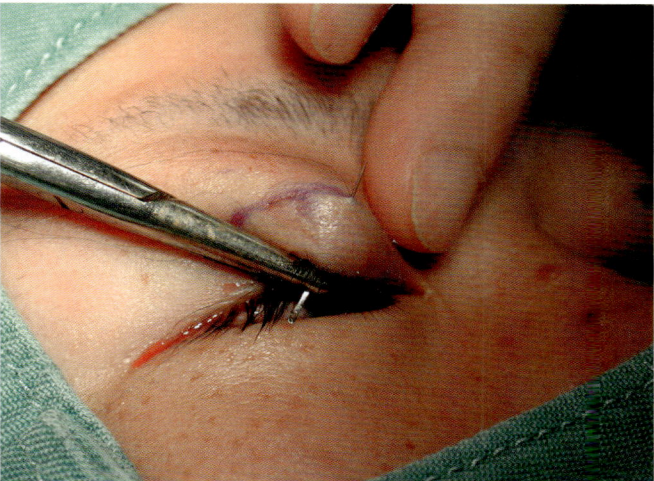

Figure 8–25 *The Suture Technique, Step 13:* This needle exits at point 4, the same exit point for the first needle described in Figure 8–23. (Courtesy of Tetsuo Shu, M.D.)

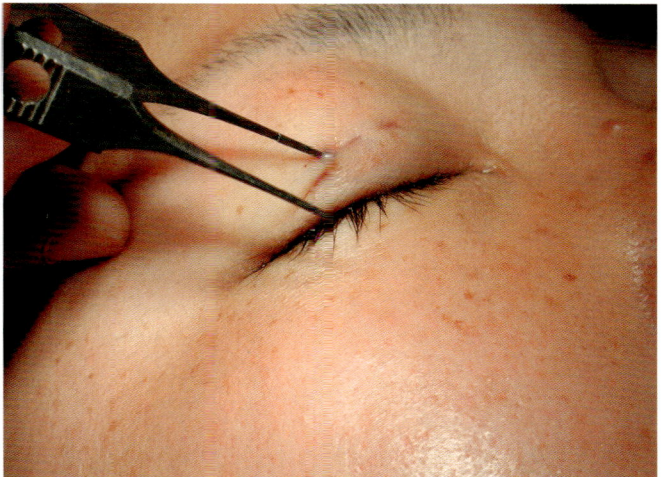

Figure 8–28 *The Suture Technique, Step 16:* After both eyelids have been completed and symmetry and height are deemed to be satisfactory, the suture tails are trimmed close to the knot and buried with a toothed forceps under the skin. (Courtesy of Tetsuo Shu, M.D.)

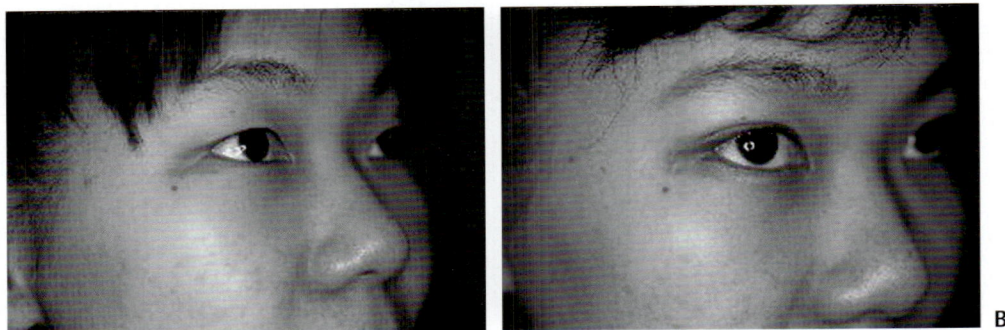

Figure 8–29   **(A,B)** This patient underwent the suture technique for double-eyelid creation and is shown with notable aesthetic improvement. (Courtesy of Tetsuo Shu, M.D.)

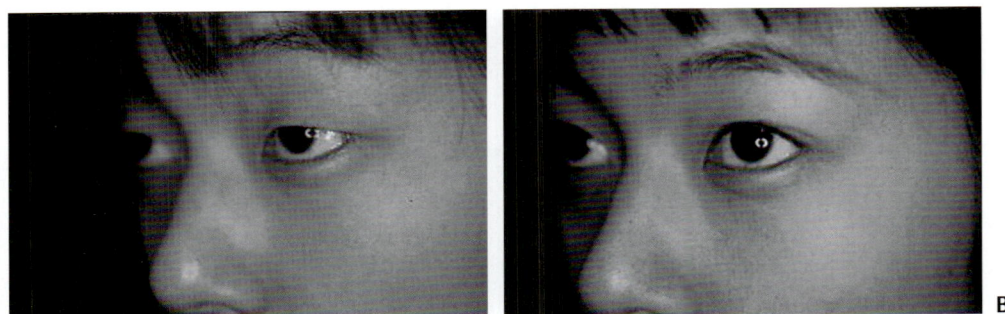

Figure 8–30   **(A,B)** This patient underwent the suture technique for double-eyelid creation and is shown with notable aesthetic improvement. (Courtesy of Tetsuo Shu, M.D.)

Postoperative Remarks

No sutures need to be removed during the postoperative visit, and the patient is followed up at 1 week for evaluation. The patient is informed that if the lid crease remains after 3 months, the likelihood that it will be permanent is almost guaranteed. However, if any sutures should fail within a 6-month period, Dr. Shu offers his patients additional surgery at no added expense. The suture technique has proven to be a reliable and expedient method for double-eyelid creation (Figs. **8–29**, **8–30**).

References

1. Choi AK. Oriental blepharoplasty: nonincisional suture technique versus conventional incisional technique. Facial Plast Surg 1994;10:67–83
2. Lee CS. Asian blepharoplasty. Available at: www.emedicine.com
3. Yang SY. Oriental double eyelid: a limited-incision technique. Ann Plast Surg 2001;46:364–368
4. McCurdy JA Jr. Upper lid blepharoplasty in the Oriental eye. Facial Plast Surg 1994;10:53–66
5. Lam SM, Kim YK. Partial-incision technique for creation of the double eyelid. Aesthetic Surg J 2003;23:170–176
6. Lam SM. Mikamo's double-eyelid blepharoplasty and the westernization of Japan. Arch Facial Plast Surg 2002;4:201–202
7. Homma K, Mutou H, Ezoe K, Fujita T. Intradermal stitch blepharoplasty for Orientals: does it disappear? Aesthetic Plast Surg 2000;24:289–291

9

Special Topics in Asian Rhinoplasty

◆ General and Anatomic Considerations

The Asian nose differs from that of the Caucasian in fundamental respects: the cartilage tends to be weaker and in short supply for grafting, the skin envelope is much thicker, and the nose is typically underprojected and the tip, amorphous. Given these dissimilarities, an entirely different strategy than traditional Western rhinoplasty must be envisioned for the Asian nose to achieve the intended aesthetic objectives.[1,2] The primary method for augmentation rhinoplasty of the Asian nose is silicone implantation, which has remained a steadfast and safe material for rhinoplasty in Asia. Because Chapter 3 has already outlined a systematic approach to rhinoplasty using this method, this chapter will focus instead on specialized topics concerning this subject in greater detail.

Besides augmentation of the tip and dorsum with a silicone implant, other ancillary procedures may benefit the Asian nose as well. The premaxillary component tends to be underdeveloped in the Asian nose, leading to an acute nasolabial angle that imparts an unaesthetic simian-like appearance to the nose–lip complex. The author does not favor use of an extended silicone implant that spans the entire columellar distance to address this deficiency: this type of implant risks extrusion and may contribute to pressure necrosis of the nasal tip. Instead of pushing the nose forward with this unfavorable "tent pole" type of implant, a separate premaxillary implant should be fashioned that can improve the nasolabial angle. Premaxillary augmentation is covered in detail in Chapter 11 on facial implants.

Another aspect of the Asian nose that imparts an overly ethnic appearance, which cannot be addressed with a silicone implant alone, is a wide alar base. Flared nostrils are particularly prevalent in the darker complected Polynesian races but is found to some extent in almost all Southeast Asian ethnicities. Alar-base reduction may effect a more favorable tip configuration in select Asian patients. Oftentimes, the alar base appears to be overly wide only because the nasal tip is relatively underdeveloped. Tip enhancement alone with a silicone implant may be sufficient to achieve the desired balance of the nasal tip vis-à-vis the side alae. This chapter will discuss both the aesthetic criteria that should be followed to determine the candidacy of a prospective patient for alar-base reduction and the technical details on proper surgical technique.

Although augmentation of the nasal tip and dorsum serves as the primary directive in Asian rhinoplasty, not all Asian noses follow this precise model. In particular, the Japanese nose stands in contradistinction to other Asian ethnicities in its shape and contour that mandates an alternative surgical strategy. The nasal dorsum appears to be at times overly projected and even may exhibit a dorsal convexity similar to the Caucasian nose, whereas the tip may remain retruded and ill-defined like the typical Asian nose. A combination of Western and Asian techniques should be exercised to address this nasal configuration. A systematic approach will be outlined for noses that tend to exhibit a mixture of leptorrhine and mesorrhine features. It should be emphasized that not all Japanese noses exhibit these characteristics, which may also be commonly found in other Asian ethnicities as well. Considering the increasing rise of interracial unions, a judicious selection of Western and Asian techniques may need to be employed for noses of a mixed heritage.

Although augmentation rhinoplasty of the Asian nose with silicone is a very safe and reliable method, complications may arise that are unique to this type of rhinoplasty. Like breast augmentation with silicone implants, the nasal tip may undergo contraction over time, usually due to repeated insertions or bouts of infection. Contraction of the nose may also occur idiopathically. Nevertheless, this complication may be a relatively difficult entity to treat and may require unique surgical strategies, which will be set forth in this chapter. Depending on the degree of contraction, the nose may be addressed in a relatively straightforward manner or may require more elaborate techniques to rectify the problem.

◆ Alar-Base Reduction

Preoperative Remarks

The decision to undertake an alar-base reduction is contingent upon several factors: a careful analysis of the patient's nasal and facial features, an investigation of the patient's aesthetic motivations, and a review of the postoperative course. Although many patients may seem like suitable candidates for this type of surgery, only a select few will meet all of the criteria to justify alar-base reduction (Fig. **9–1A–H**).

The lower third of the patient's nose should be studied assiduously to determine the patient's eligibility for alar-base reduction. Oftentimes, the nasal width appears to be overly wide simply because the nasal tip is retruded and amorphous. Augmentation rhinoplasty with a silicone implant can restore the balance between the nasal tip and the alae, so that alar-base reduction may be unnecessary. Furthermore, if the alae appear to be approximately the same width as the nasal tip preoperatively, alar-base reduction may regrettably serve to accentuate the width of the nasal tip vis-à-vis the narrowed alae rather than improve tip refinement. The patient can be shown this unfavorable outcome by manually pinching the alae together and demonstrating the illusion that the nasal tip increases in width. Accordingly, alar-base reduction should be reserved only for patients who exhibit a greater ala-to-lobule ratio (Figs. **9–2, 9–3**).

The nose should also be evaluated in the context of the patient's other facial features. The rule of horizontal fifths may be recalled as a starting point for aesthetic analysis: the nasal width should be roughly equivalent to the width of the patient's eye (Fig. **9–4**). Although this rule is indeed not infallible, it should be thought of as a general guideline. If the surgeon is uncertain how a narrowed nasal base will look for the patient, he or she can

again pinch the nasal base until the desired look is achieved. Alternatively, digital morphing can render an easily viewable image for the patient and physician to analyze, with the declared recognition that technology should not be equated with a guaranteed surgical outcome. If a patient has a very wide face, narrowing the nose significantly may create an unbalanced look (Fig. **9–5A–H**). As with any rhinoplasty endeavor, the patient's specific facial features must be thoughtfully assessed when deciding on the proper course of action.

Besides being an unaesthetic attribute, wide nostrils that are visible *en face* may be deemed a sign of bad fortune. Asian patients who subscribe to this cultural folklore believe that very wide nostrils represent a portal through which monetary wealth is drained out. In contradistinction, a high nasal bridge and prominent nose signify wealth and wisdom. These cultural biases that inform patient motivation must be carefully elucidated before surgery should be undertaken. Clearly, an operation that is intended simply to dispel bad omens should be undertaken with caution. An overly rotated nose can expose the nostril aperture excessively, but derotation of the nasal tip with a nasal implant will not decrease nostril show significantly. Even alar-base reduction may not satisfy the patient, as the nostrils will remain visible despite some reduction in overall width. As suggested, visible nostrils may not indicate the presence of a wide alar base but instead that of an overly rotated nose. Accordingly, alar-base reduction would only exacerbate the nasal tip appearance in this condition, as stated before.

Finally, if the patient's motivation is appropriate, and the aesthetic objective is favorable, the patient must still be instructed thoroughly about the postoperative course. Typically, augmentation rhinoplasty with silicone offers a relatively abbreviated recovery period, lasting only several weeks in length. However, alar-base reduction requires an external incision that may remain conspicuous for many months, a fact that should be clearly articulated to the patient. Given the predilection for Asian skin to respond unfavorably to injury, the patient should be fully cognizant of the potential for a longer recovery. The author contends that any external incision on the central aspect of the Asian face risks being visible for a prolonged period of time. Unlike a face lift or brow lift incision that is hidden away near the hairline, an external nasal incision may draw an observer's attention more readily. Even a blepharoplasty (if hidden entirely within the supratarsal crease) will fade

Figure 9–1 **(A–H)** This 38-year-old Vietnamese man exhibits a wide, flat nasal configuration in which the alar width exceeds the nasal lobule, or tip, width. For this reason, he is a suitable candidate for alar-base reduction surgery. He also exhibits an overrotated and underprojected nasal tip and dorsum, which contribute to a feminized appearance to his nose. To attain a balanced look to his nose, he underwent concurrent alar-base reduction and augmentation rhinoplasty with a silicone implant.

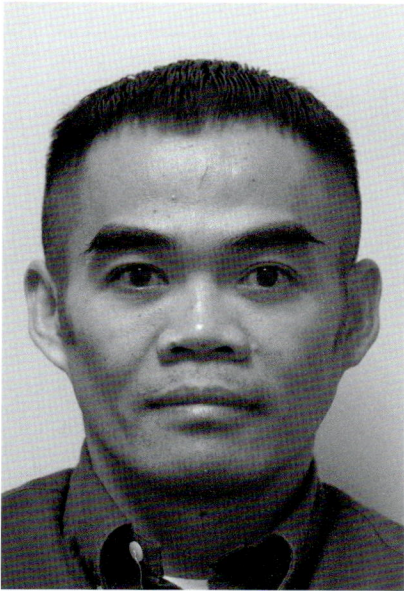 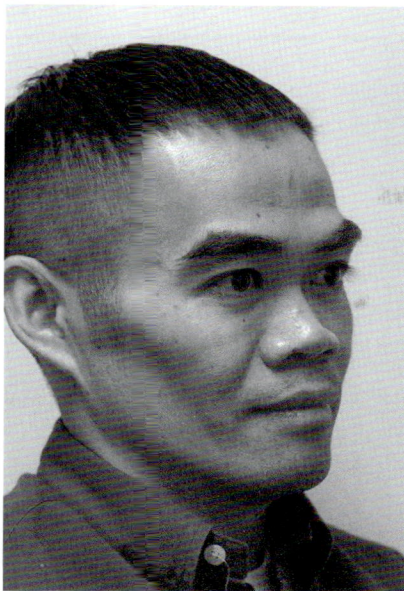 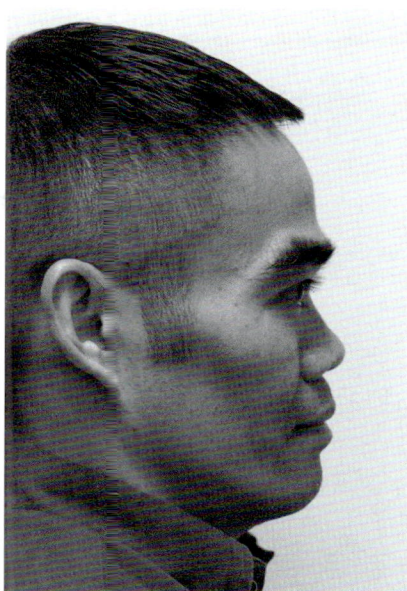

A–C

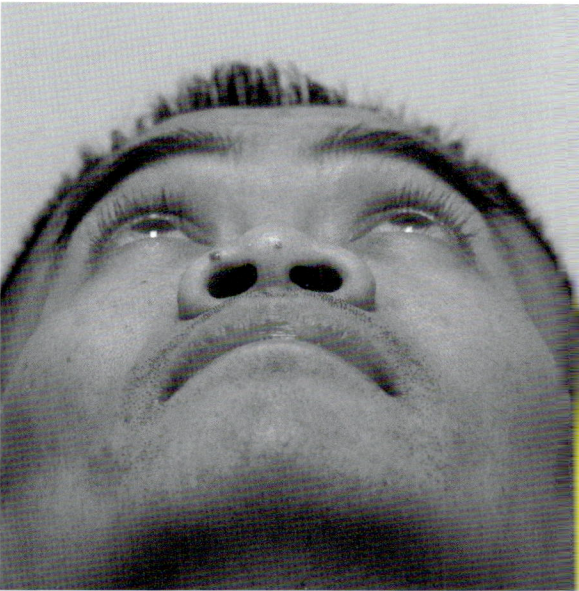 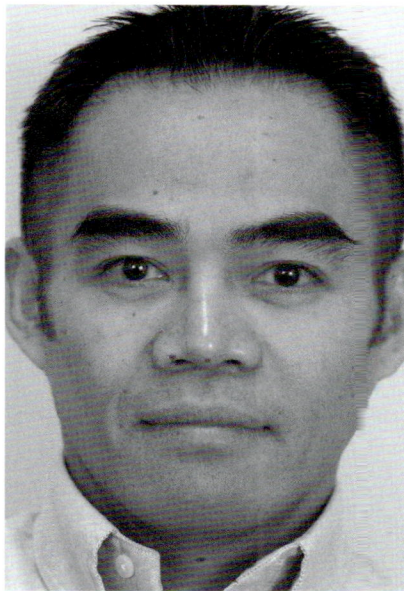

D–E

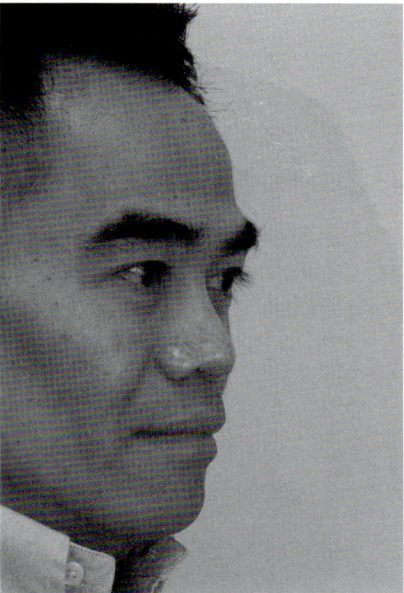 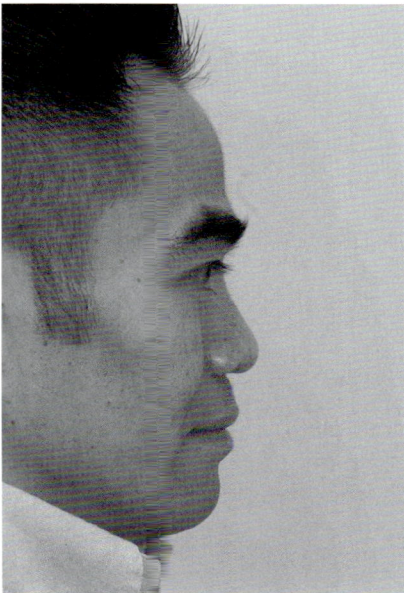 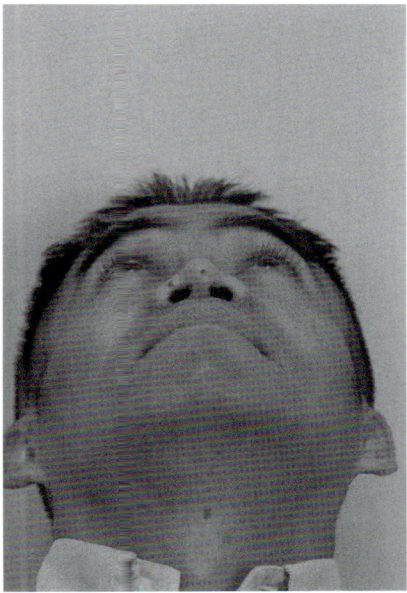

F–H

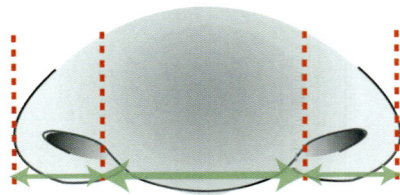

Unbalanced Tip-Ala Relationship

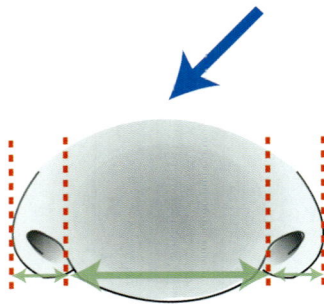

**Relationship Worsened
After Alar-Base Reduction**

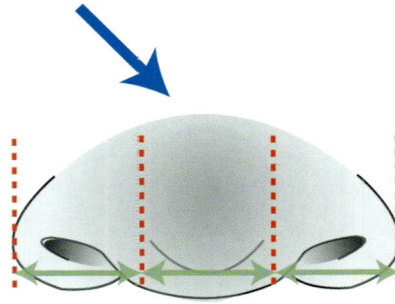

**Relationship Improved
After Nasal Implant**

Figure 9–2 A nasal base that appears overly wide must be carefully evaluated to determine whether the nasal lobule or the nasal alae are responsible for this appearance. Alar reduction for a patient with a wide nasal lobule and narrow alae will only make the lobule appear even wider. Augmentation rhinoplasty of a wide nasal lobule with a silicone implant will impart the illusion that the nose appears narrower.

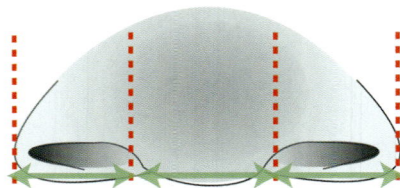

Flared Alae Make Nose Look Too Wide

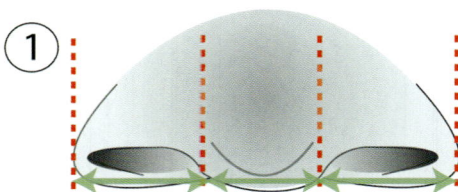

① **Nose Appears Narrower
After Insertion of Nasal Implant**

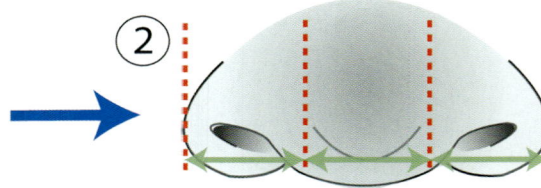

② **Nose Further Narrowed
After Alar-Base Reduction
(And Tip-Ala Relationship Restored)**

Figure 9–3 A patient who exhibits flared nasal alae will benefit from alar-base reduction, and the nose can be made to appear even narrower with augmentation rhinoplasty of the nasal lobule using a silicone implant.

away more quickly than an alar incision. Proper preoperative counseling will reduce potential postoperative headaches. The reader is reminded again that only a minority of patients (< 5%) qualify for all the criteria that justify alar-reduction surgery.

Surgical Technique

Many types of alar-base excisions have been advocated in the literature[3–5] (Fig. **9–6**). The extent of soft-tissue excision and the shape of the wedge to be excised are

Ideal Facial Aesthetics

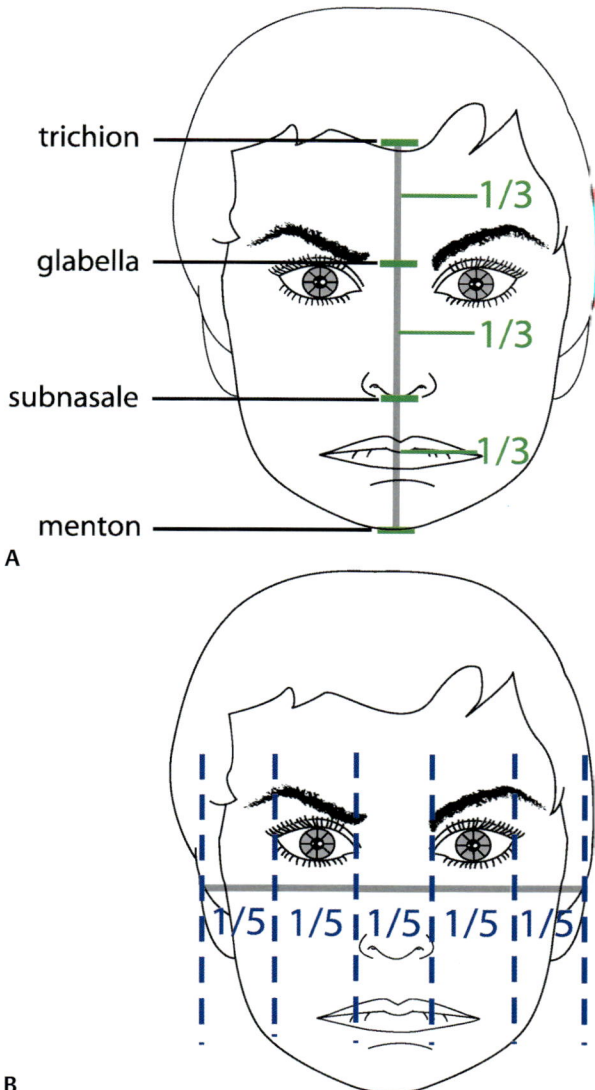

A

B

Figure 9–4 Nasal width should always be viewed in the context of other facial features. A very wide face may not tolerate the appearance of a narrow nose. **(A)** The nasal length (from glabella to nasal tip, or subnasale) should occupy approximately one-third of the total vertical height of the face. The upper one-third of the face should extend from the hairline (trichion) to the glabella, and the lower one-third should cover the distance from the bottom of the nose to the lower aspect of the chin, or menton. **(B)**: Horizontally, the nasal width should equal that of the eye, forming one-fifth of the total distance across the face. The distance from the lateral canthus to the lateral aspect of the ear should occupy the remaining fifth of the face. (From Williams EF, Lam SM. Comprehensive Facial Rejuvenation: A Practical and Systematic Guide to Surgical Management of the Aging Face. Philadelphia: Lippincott, Williams & Wilkins; 2004; with permission.)

dependent upon the amount of reduction that is desired. Furthermore, narrowing is partly accomplished by a cinching suture, as will be elaborated. When designing the wedge excision, the surgeon should consider the

thickness of the ala and the risk of unnatural notching along the nasal sill. Accordingly, crossing the nasal sill should be undertaken with caution, experience, and judgment. The reader is referred to Sheen and Sheen's textbook for a lucid discussion of this matter.[6]

1. Prior to infiltration of anesthesia, the area intended for alar resection is outlined with a surgical marking pen. The incision line should fall slightly less than 1 mm medial (on the nasal side) of the alar-facial groove rather than directly within the alar-facial junction. An incision that resides within the alar-facial junction does not heal as well as one that is placed entirely on the nasal skin, and skin closure is less precise with the former technique. Furthermore, an incision on the nasal skin will eventually migrate toward the alar-facial junction with continued wound contracture. When marking out the proposed incisions for soft-tissue resection, the surgeon should err on the conservative side for two reasons. First, a greater amount of soft tissue can always be removed if deemed necessary after placement of the cinching suture. Second, the cinching suture will provide further narrowing of the nose than soft-tissue wedge excision alone will do.

2. If augmentation rhinoplasty with a silicone implant will be undertaken concurrently, it should be completed prior to alar-base reduction for several reasons:

   a. Only after the nasal tip has been augmented can the surgeon more reliably determine how much alar reduction is still required.

   b. It is easier to insert the implant when the nostrils are still broadly configured.

   c. In addition, insertion of the implant after alar-base reduction can disturb both the delicate sutures placed along the alar margin and the cinching suture.

3. Local anesthesia (1% lidocaine with 1:100,000 epinephrine) should be infiltrated both directly into the proposed incisions for alar resection and along the entire base of the nose through which the cinching suture will be passed.

4. A no. 15 blade is used to resect the proposed alar soft tissue in a full-thickness wedge that tapers toward the nostril.

5. Hemostasis is achieved with judicious bipolar electrocautery when needed, as a tributary of the labial artery may be transected during wedge resection.

6. A 3–0 nylon suture is then passed through the pedicled ala to run in a circular fashion across the nasal base to the other ala and back again through the nasal base to the side of the original ala (Fig. **9–7**). Of note,

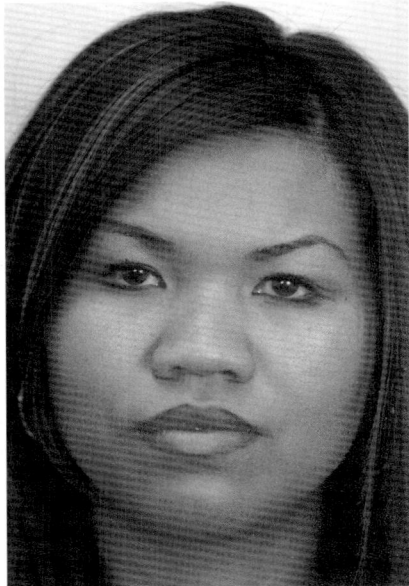
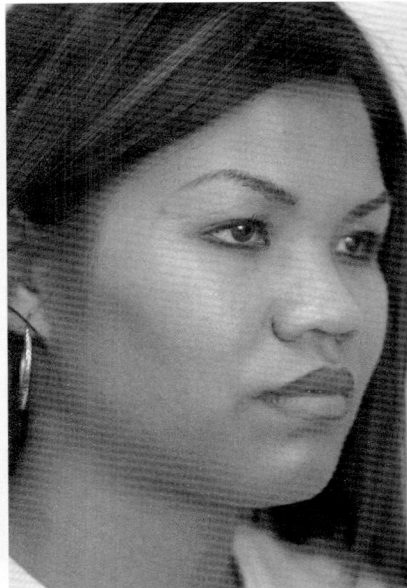
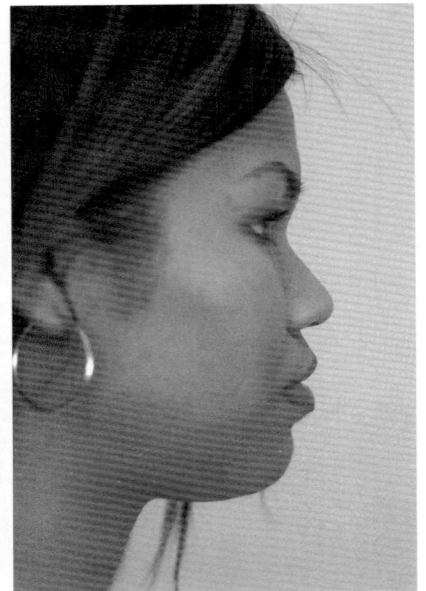

A–C

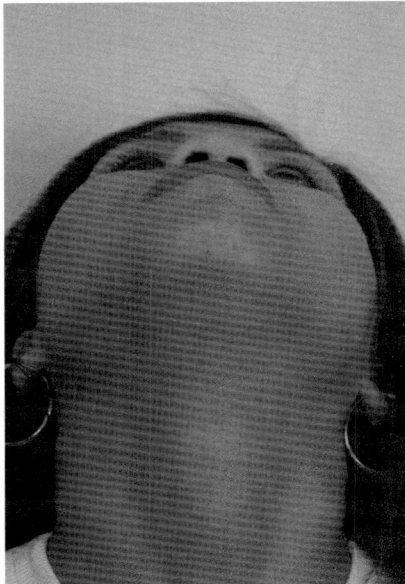
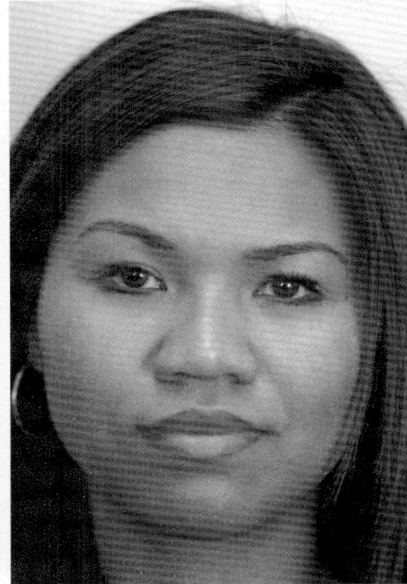
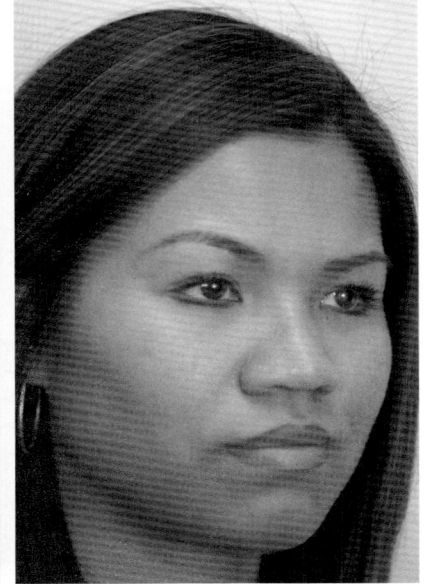

D–F

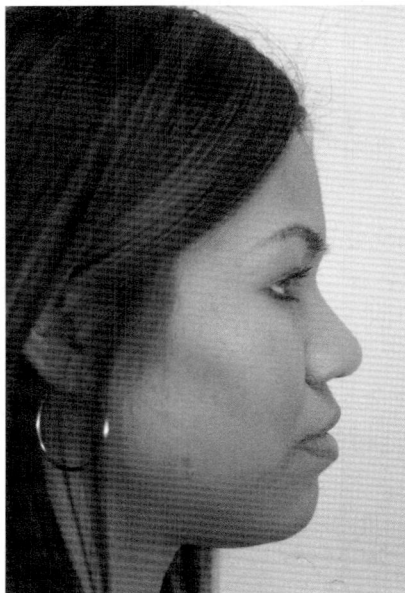
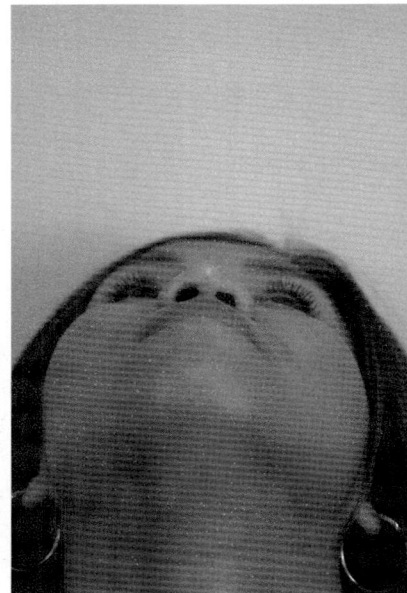

G–H

Figure 9–5 This 22-year-old Cambodian woman shows a very flat nasal appearance and relatively wide alae. However, given her broad face, overly narrowing her nose with alar reduction may have yielded an unbalanced appearance. Also, her dark complexion predisposes her to a potentially longer recovery period after alar-base reduction, including the risk of hyperpigmentation, hypopigmentation, and scarring. On profile view, the patient exhibits a retruded premaxillary component and would have benefited from an implant in this region, but she declined this ancillary surgical procedure. She underwent augmentation rhinoplasty with a silicone implant, with notable aesthetic improvement in her nasal appearance. She was informed that if she were unsatisfied after augmentation rhinoplasty alone, she could defer alar-base reduction for a separate session, but she was pleased with the results and did not desire any further surgical intervention.

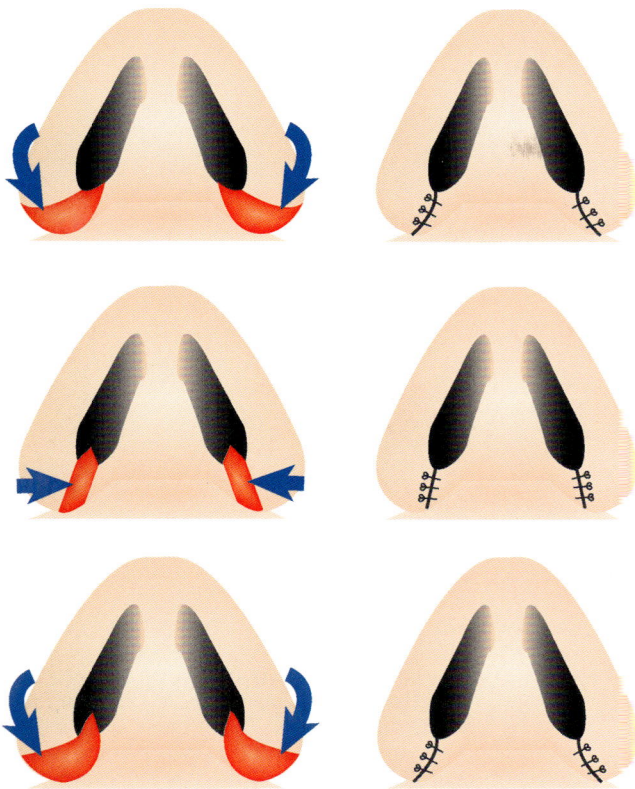

Figure 9–6 Many types of alar-base reduction excisions have been advocated in the literature. However, the author uses a simple wedge excision along the alar margin to accomplish most of his reduction surgeries, modifying the extent of soft-tissue resection based on what the patient should require aesthetically.

the needle should be a sufficiently large caliber to pass easily through the entire expanse of the nasal base.

7. The suture is then tied in a surgeon's knot and cinched until the degree of alar reduction is achieved. As the knot is cinched progressively tighter, the surgeon should observe that the desired aesthetic end point is achieved but also ensure that the nostrils do not begin to buckle unnaturally inward. If the nostrils appear to buckle inward before the surgeon arrives at the desired amount of reduction, then the suture can be removed and a greater amount of alar soft tissue, can be resected depending on the amount of observed buckling.

8. The remaining suture throws are placed to secure the 3–0 nylon in place before the suture tails are trimmed.

9. The alar incisions are then approximated with running, locking 6–0 polypropylene suture.

Postoperative Remarks

The postoperative care after alar-base reduction is rather straightforward. The patient should be advised to clean the incision with hydrogen peroxide two or three times per day during the first week and to dress the in-

cision with a topical antibiotic ointment immediately after cleaning, as per regular wound-care routine. The sutures can be removed on the seventh postoperative day and may be deferred later if the incision appears not to be healed completely. Three or four days after suture removal, the patient can begin application of vitamin E oil twice daily to minimize scar formation, and the patient should return 3 weeks postoperatively to monitor for any early signs of scarring. If the incision appears hypertrophic, triamcinolone acetonide (Kenalog 10 mg/cc) may be infiltrated directly into the incision, and the patient should be followed every 3 weeks until complete resolution. Subsequent mechanical dermabrasion may also be required in select patients who have persistent contour irregularity of their incision.

◆ Surgical Approach to the Japanese Nose: Combined Augmentation and Reduction Strategies

Method of Yukio Shirakabe The Asian nose has been thought of as requiring augmentation in almost all circumstances. Conversely, the Caucasian nose principally benefits from reduction rhinoplasty. Some Japanese noses share mesorrhine (Asian) and leptorrhine (Caucasian) features that at times mandate a unique surgical strategy, combining techniques of augmentation and reduction.[7] Unlike the majority of noses throughout Asia, the Japanese nasal dorsum occasionally exhibits an adequate dorsal height and at times even mild convexity that may require reduction surgery. However, the nasal tip is often amorphous, with a retruded columella that would profit from augmentation. Four clinical scenarios are proposed with which a surgeon can approach the Japanese nose: (1) dorsal augmentation with or without tip augmentation (Fig. **9–8A,B**), (2) tip augmentation and dorsal reduction (Fig. **9–9A,B**), (3) tip augmentation alone (Fig. **9–10A,B**), and (4) dorsal reduction alone (Fig. **9–11A,B**). After discussion of these four types of clinical presentations, a more detailed description of cartilaginous tip augmentation (used for scenario 3 and at times for scenario 2) and dorsal reduction (used for scenario 4 but not scenario 2) will be presented. The method described here was developed by Dr. Yukio Shirakabe.

The first clinical scenario, that is, dorsal augmentation with or without tip augmentation, represents the classic Asian augmentation rhinoplasty (Fig. **9–8A,B**). In the past, patients were principally interested in dorsal augmentation without modification in the tip, as they desired a more conservative alteration of their appearance. In this case, an I-shaped silicone implant is favored for dorsal augmentation alone. However, for combined dorsal and tip augmentation that is more common

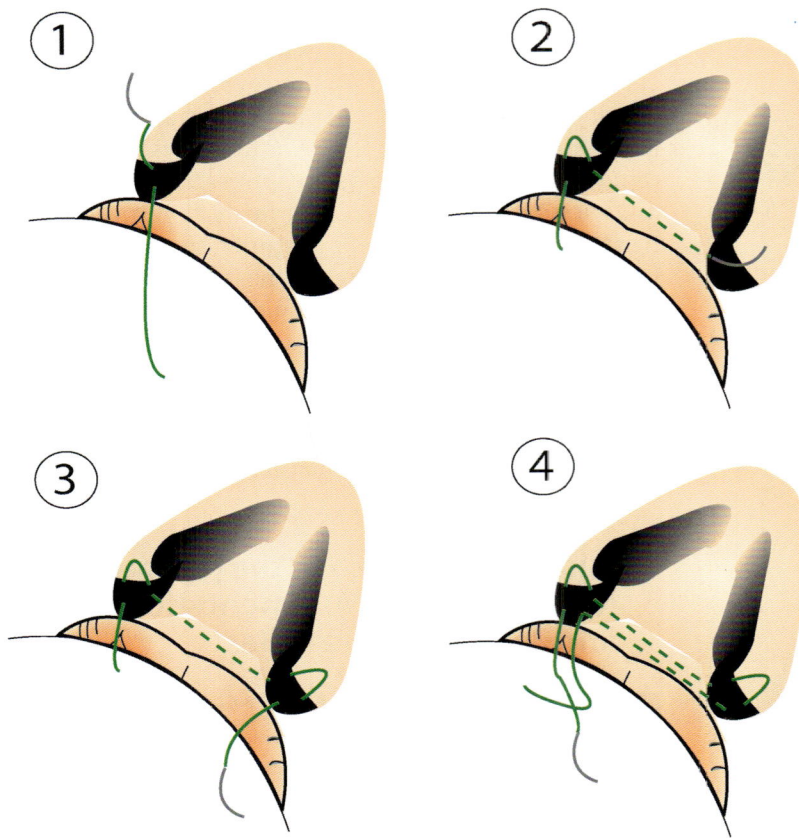

Figure 9–7 A 3–0 nylon suture is passed through the pedicled ala to run in a circular fashion across the nasal base to the other ala and back again through the nasal base to the side of the original ala. The suture is then tied in a surgeon's knot and cinched until the degree of alar reduction is achieved.

today, an L-shaped silicone implant that is tailored (i.e., carved) to fit each particular nose is employed.[8]

In the second clinical scenario, the dorsum is reduced and the tip, augmented (Fig. **9–9A,B**). It is unlikely that a Japanese nose will be significantly overprojected, but a mild dorsal convexity may be pre-

sent. In this case, the dorsal hump can be removed, and the consequent open-roof deformity can be camouflaged with an L-shaped silicone implant that augments both the dorsum and the tip. If the surgeon does not wish to overaugment the nasal dorsum with a nasal implant, then the dorsum can be reduced in the manner

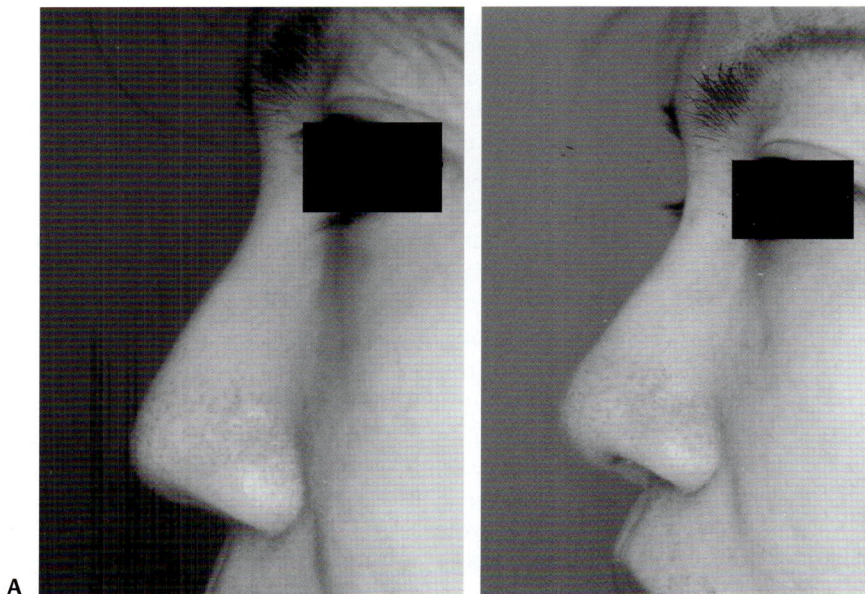

Figure 9–8 (A,B) This 23-year-old Japanese woman underwent augmentation rhinoplasty with an L-shaped silicone implant to attain both dorsal and tip enhancement. (Courtesy of Yukio Shirakabe, M.D.)

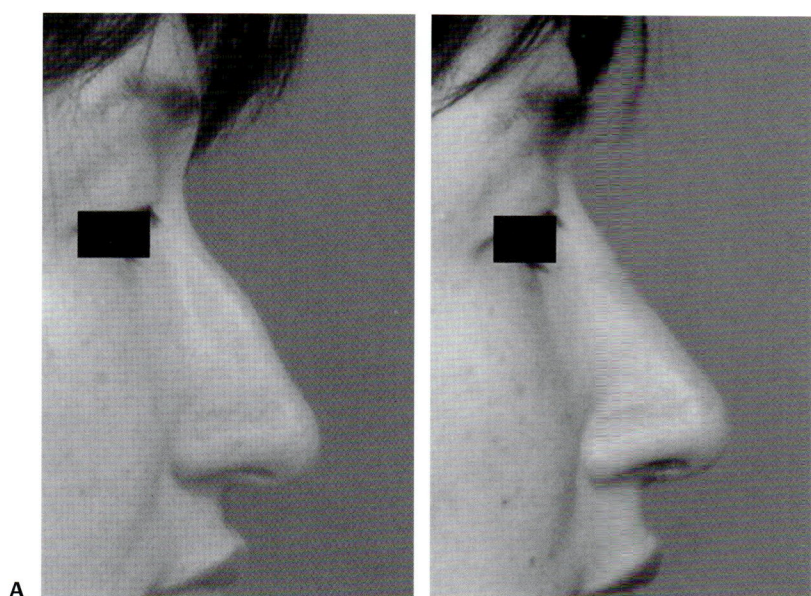

Figure 9–9   (A,B) This 37-year-old Japanese woman underwent reduction of her dorsal convexity followed by augmentation rhinoplasty with an L-shaped silicone implant. (Courtesy of Yukio Shirakabe, M.D.)

to be described for clinical scenario 4, and a cartilaginous tip graft can be fashioned by the method to be described for clinical scenario 3. Although a dorsal silicone implant can remain secure without a proximal tip component, a free-standing tip alloplast is unstable and is not advocated. Therefore, cartilaginous tip augmentation is preferred in this situation.

In the third clinical scenario, dorsal projection is adequate, but the tip requires augmentation (Fig. 9–10A,B). As mentioned above, this circumstance mandates autogenous cartilage grafting for tip augmentation. Another case that would require cartilaginous tip augmentation is observed in the patient who has a very scarred tip from prior surgery or trauma in whom a silicone implant may extrude due to the inelastic tissue.

Similarly, a patient who desires significant nasal augmentation may benefit from an autogenous graft so as to minimize the likelihood for extrusion, to which an alloplast may be predisposed. Also, a patient who has a foreshortened columella and a longer lobular segment may benefit from a carefully constructed autogenous graft that can reverse the ratio by lengthening the columella relative to the lobule.

In the aforementioned clinical cases, autogenous tip augmentation is warranted. The nasal septum tends to provide limited and flimsy grafting material in the Asian patient, and auricular cartilage is preferred. The cartilage for tip augmentation is harvested from one entire concha and divided into four portions: a columellar strut, a V-shaped onlay graft, a diamond-shaped onlay

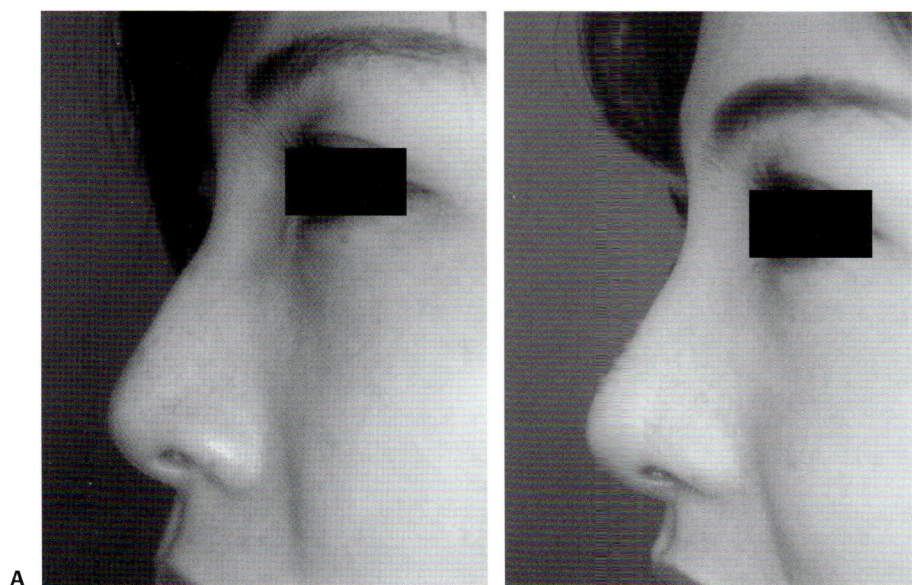

Figure 9–10   (A,B) This 31-year-old Japanese woman exhibits adequate dorsal height but a retruded nasal tip and underwent conchal-cartilage enhancement of her nasal tip. (Courtesy of Yukio Shirakabe, M.D.)

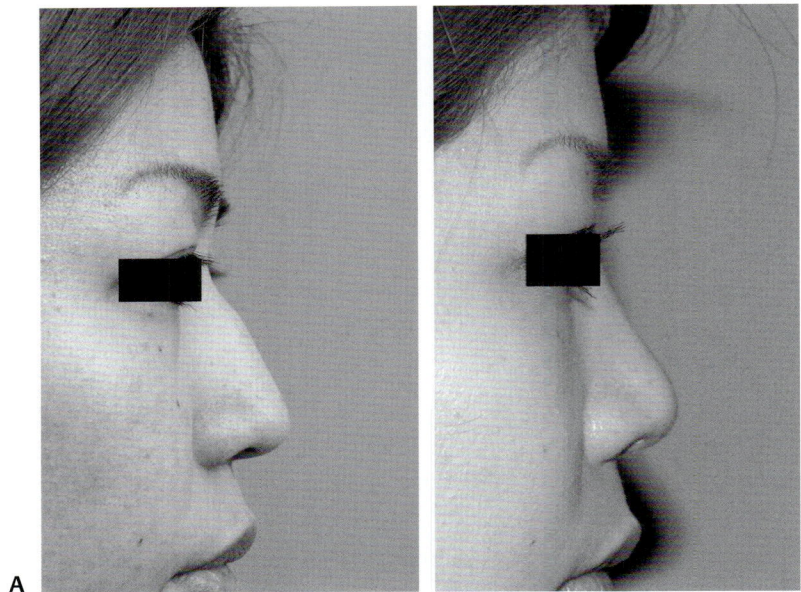

Figure 9–11   **(A,B)** This 27-year-old Japanese woman exhibits a dorsal convexity but adequate nasal tip projection. She underwent a modified Skoog technique for dorsal hump reduction. (Courtesy of Yukio Shirakabe, M.D.)

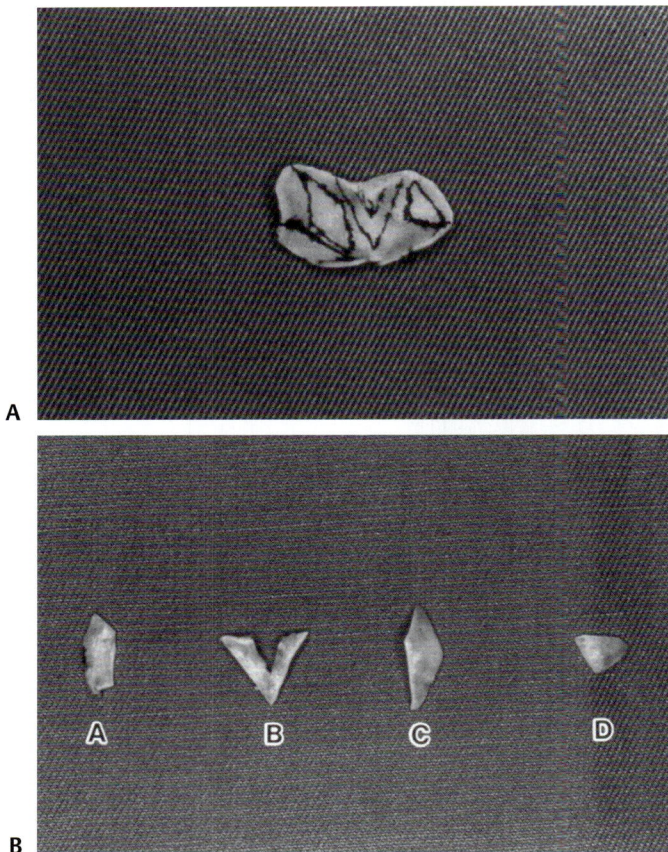

Figure 9–12   The left conchal cartilage with the derivation of the four cartilaginous onlay, tip, and strut grafts. (From Shirakabe Y, Suzuki Y, Lam SM. A systematic approach to rhinoplasty of the Japanese nose: a thirty-year experience. Aesthetic Plast Surg 2003;27:221–231; with permission.)

graft, and a triangular-shaped tip graft (Fig. **9–12**). The columellar strut is removed from the posteroinferior aspect of the cavum concha. The V-shaped onlay graft is taken from the junction of the cavum and cymba concha anteriorly. The diamond-shaped onlay graft is harvested from the anterior cavum concha, situated between the V-shaped graft and the columellar strut. Finally, a triangular tip graft is taken from the superior aspect of the cymba concha.

Unlike the endonasal approach favored for alloplastic augmentation, an external rhinoplasty incision is preferred to expose and manipulate the nasal tip. An inverted-W transcolumellar incision is performed (Fig. **9–13**), and the sub–superficial musculoaponeurotic system (SMAS) elevation is performed until the alar cartilages are fully exposed. A pocket is tunneled with fine scissors between the medial crura down to the nasal spine to accommodate the columellar strut, which is

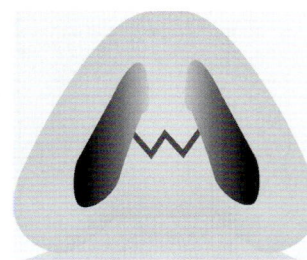

Figure 9–13   The transcolumellar inverted-W incision used for external rhinoplasty.

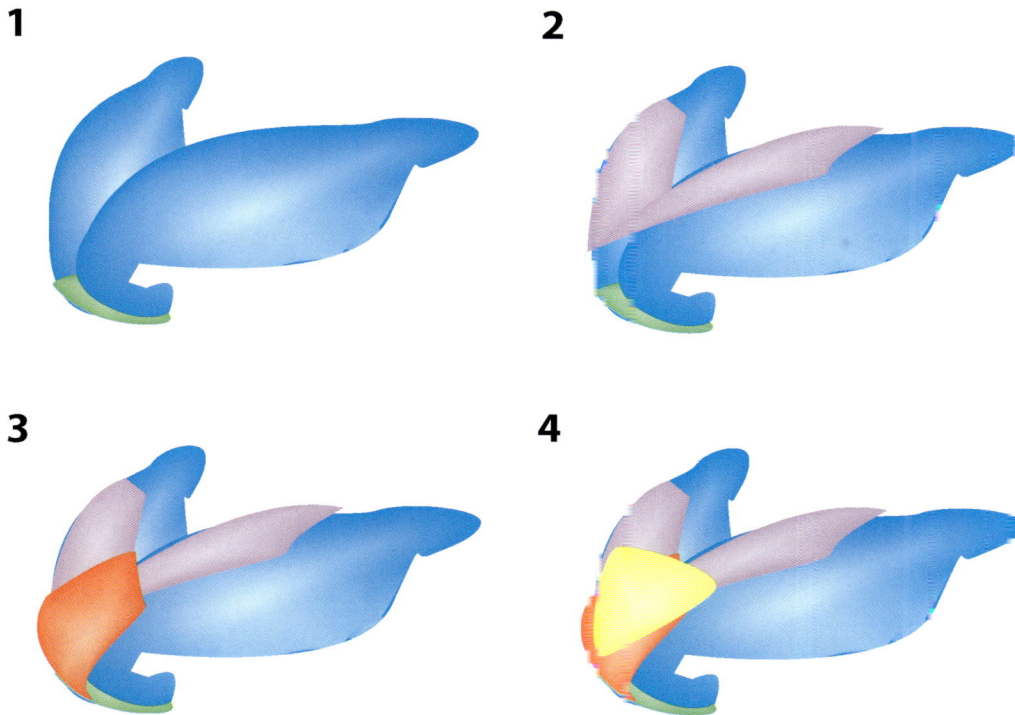

Figure 9–14   Three-dimensional illustration showing the cartilaginous grafts for tip augmentation.

secured into place with two horizontal mattress sutures of 6–0 nylon (Fig. **9–14**). The V-shaped cartilage is turned over so that the posterior convex surface assumes a superficial orientation to match the curvature of the ala, and the cartilage is sutured to the tip of the lower lateral cartilages with three simple 6–0 nylon sutures—one suture through each ala and one in the midline. The diamond-shaped cartilage graft is then affixed on top of the columella in an onlay fashion to increase columellar show. Finally, the remaining triangular-shaped cartilage is grafted on top of the V-shaped piece to yield additional projection and definition. If further augmentation is required, then any remaining cartilaginous piece may be layered on top to provide additional projection. Fibrin adhesive is applied intranasally prior to closure. The transcolumellar incision is then approximated in two layers. First, a single buried 5–0 polydioxanone suture is placed to reduce wound tension. Then, simple interrupted sutures of 5–0 nylon are used to close the external skin incision and the lateral intranasal incisions. All the lateral intranasal sutures and half of the external columellar sutures are removed after 3 days, and the remaining columellar sutures are removed at 5 days postoperatively.

In the fourth clinical scenario, dorsal reduction is all that is needed (Fig. **9–11A,B**). Unlike the technique described in clinical scenario 2, a modified Skoog method is used.[9] The nasal dorsum is accessed via an open, transcolumellar incision. The excess upper lateral cartilage is first trimmed with a no. 11 Bard-Parker blade up

to the bony-cartilaginous junction, and the remainder of the bony excess is removed as one piece with the cartilage segment using a sharpened and guarded Ruben osteotome. Of note, approximately one-third of the prominent hump consists of cartilage and two-thirds of bone; this condition is contrary to that of the Caucasian, in which the reverse is true: that is, two-thirds of dorsal convexity is usually due to cartilage and one-third, or less, to bone. After the dorsal hump has been transected, it is removed as one piece and inspected. The underlying septal component and at times a portion of the central upper lateral cartilage are shaved off to create a flat segment, which in turn is reinserted into its original position to camouflage the open-roof deformity. At times, the segment may need to be positioned slightly more cephalad to create the desired profile. The returned segment is held in position with fibrin adhesive. This type of dorsal reduction can be undertaken without the need for lateral osteotomies to close the open-roof deformity. However, Skoog originally described this method with the use of lateral osteotomies. Avoidance of lateral osteotomies is important because the nasal bones in Asian patients should not be overly narrowed, as the Asian face is quite wide in comparison. Further narrowing of the nasal bones would make the Asian face appear even wider.

Because the Japanese nose has unique features that differentiate it from other Asian noses as well as Caucasian noses, a unique strategy has been proposed that will offer the optimal aesthetic outcome. Certainly, these techniques can be successfully employed in all Asian noses that exhibit these characteristics.

◆ Management of the Contracted Nose

Method of Dong-Hak Jung

Although alloplastic implantation has a long legacy of safety in the Orient,[10] complications can arise,[11] the most devastating of which is a contracted nasal tip[12]

(Figs. **9–15, 9–16, 9–17**). The foreshortened nasal tip arises typically after repeated alloplastic implantation, related infection, or foreign-body reaction that causes capsular contraction. Management of this entity is a difficult surgical enterprise that requires a systematic thought process and careful analysis of the severity and nature of the problem.[13–15]

The two principal constituent anatomic structures that must be assessed are the lower lateral cartilages and the overlying skin envelope. The lower lateral

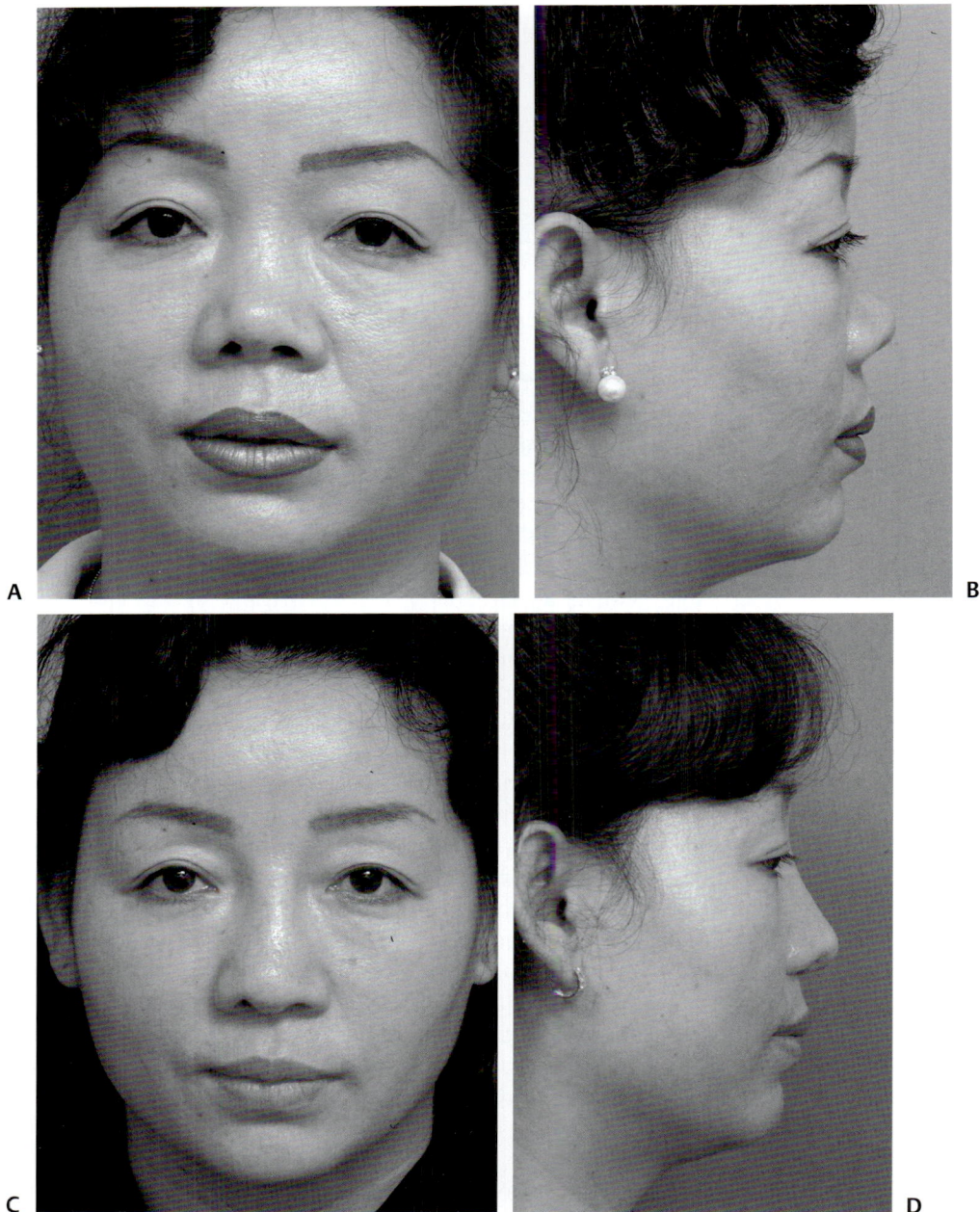

Figure 9–15 (A–D) This patient underwent three rhinoplasties with silicone with a notable contraction of her nasal tip. She is shown 2 years after revision surgery in which she had rib cartilage used as an extended spreader graft bilaterally and as a single onlay shield graft. (Courtesy of Dong-Hak Jung, M.D.)

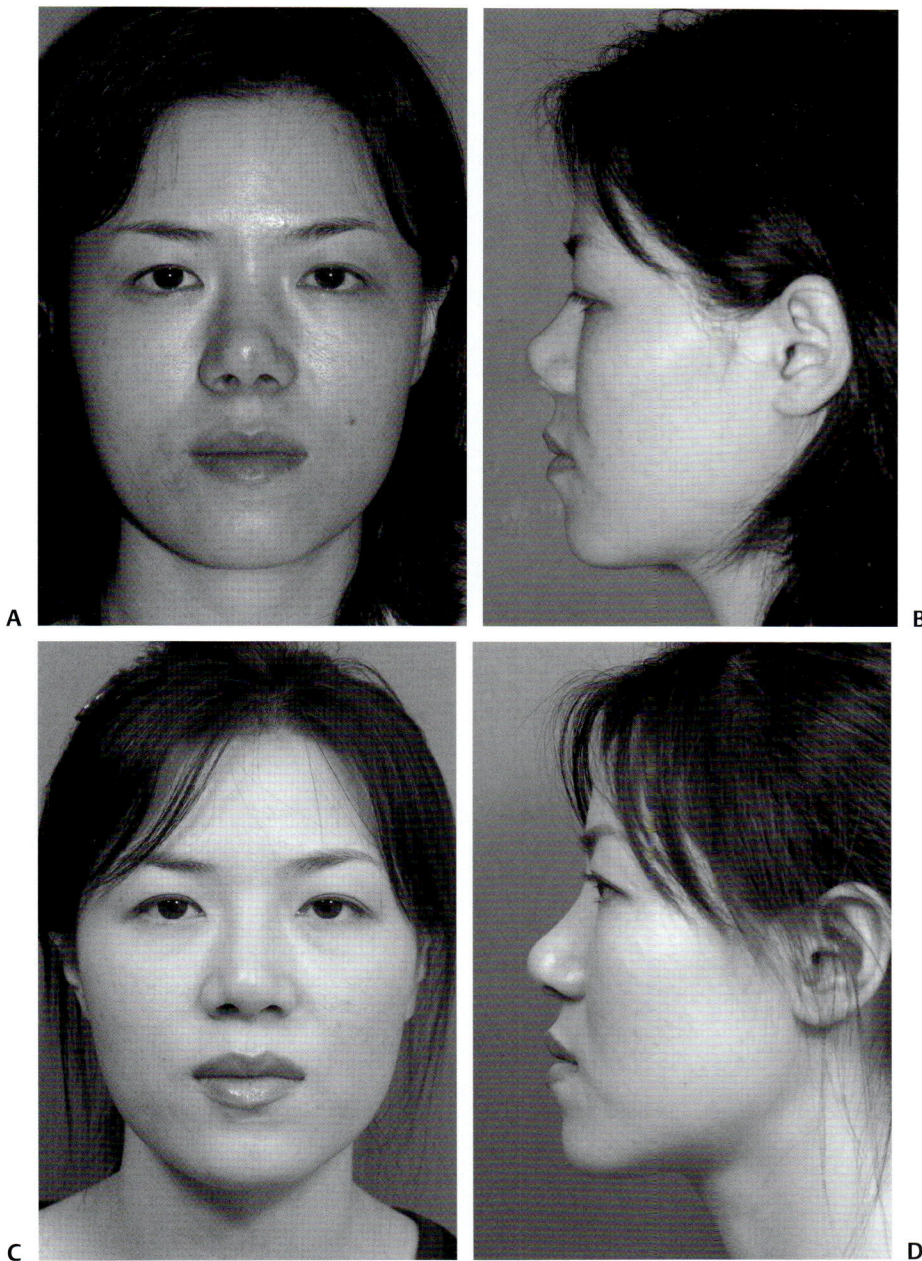

Figure 9–16   (A–D) This patient underwent several rhinoplasties with silicone and is shown 6 months after surgery in which she had septal and auricular cartilage used as extended spreader grafts and had two additional onlay shield grafts. (Courtesy of Dong-Hak Jung, M.D.)

cartilages are usually entirely intact but are oriented in a recessed, cephalic position. Given the difficult dissection in revision rhinoplasty, the need for better visualization, and the more extensive reconstruction, an external rhinoplasty approach is advocated. Unlike in standard primary and secondary rhinoplasties, the transcolumellar incision is made at the columellar-labial junction in a widely configured V shape to permit columellar lengthening if so needed (Fig. **9–18**).

The lower lateral cartilages are carefully dissected free from the surrounding scarred tissue, and their integrity is verified. To provide adequate length and to maintain that length in the postoperative period, an extended spreader graft is placed that continues past the caudal border of the septum and to which the reoriented alar cartilages may be affixed (Figs. **9–19, 9–20, 9–21, 9–22**). Septal and/or alar cartilages are usable graft material for construction of the extended

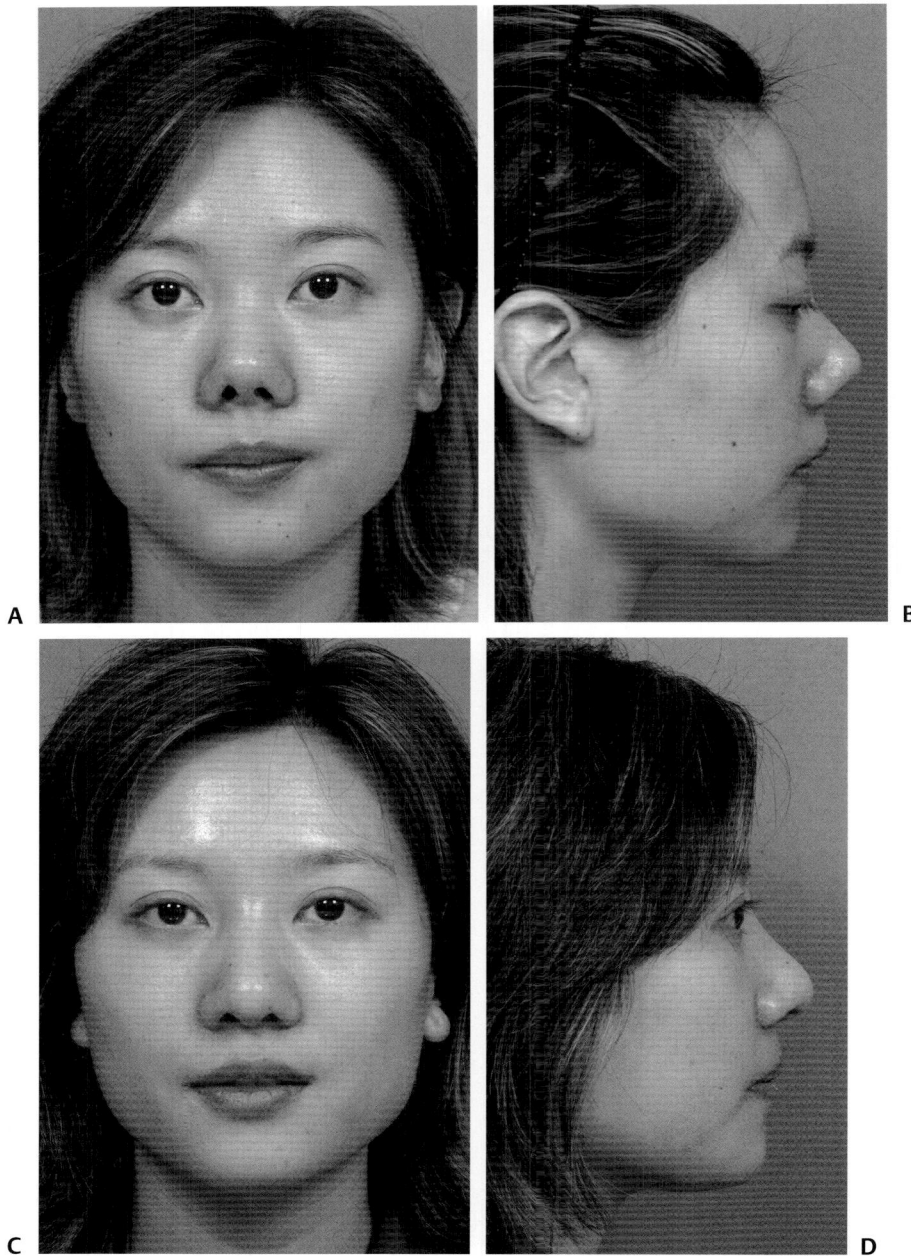

Figure 9–17 (A–D) This patient underwent two prior rhinoplasties and is shown after revision rhinoplasty in which she had an extended spreader graft placed using septal cartilage and two additional onlay shield grafts with auricular cartilage. (Courtesy of Dong-Hak Jung, M.D.)

spreader graft. However, if these sources of grafting have been depleted, costal cartilage may serve as a viable alternative. Generally, bilateral extended spreader grafts are preferred for symmetry and greater stability, but a unilateral graft may suffice in the face of an insufficient reserve of grafting material. Rib cartilage graft may provide greater tensile strength than septal or auricular cartilage and can be placed unilaterally as a spreader graft. Nevertheless, bilateral placement will enhance postoperative symmetry. If the integrity of the alar cartilages is violated, then onlay auricular cartilage grafts taken from bilateral cymba concha can restore the natural contour of the alae. Furthermore, if tip projection is still deemed inadequate after placement of an extended spreader graft, then onlay shield and tip grafts, single or multiple, may be used to obtain additional projection (Figs. **9–23, 9–24**). All grafts are sutured in place with 5–0 polydioxanone suture.

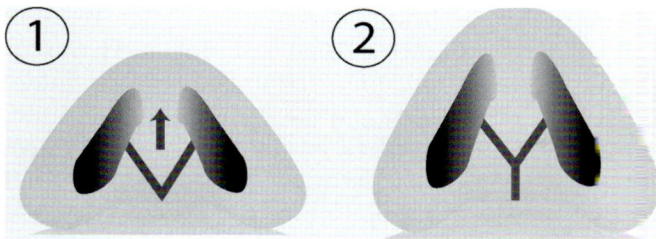

Figure 9–18   The illustration shows the extended transcolumellar V-shaped incision that approaches the nasolabial junction that is used for columellar advancement in a V-to-Y fashion. Oftentimes, the columella must be undermined down to the upper lip to permit tissue advancement, and the upper lip would then need to be taped upward toward the nose for a week to minimize tension on the incision.

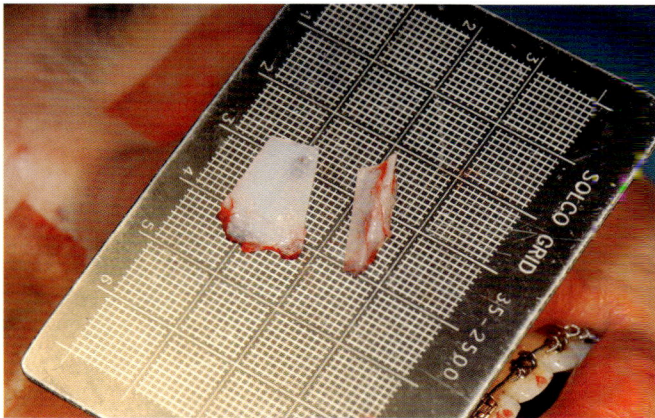

Figure 9–19   *Correction of the Contracted Nose, Step 1:* The first step in revision rhinoplasty for the contracted nose is to harvest all available grafting material. The septum is the first choice for ease of harvesting and for its straight, rigid profile. The photograph shows the harvested septal cartilage to be used as an extended spreader graft. (Courtesy of Dong-Hak Jung, M.D.)[EQ3]

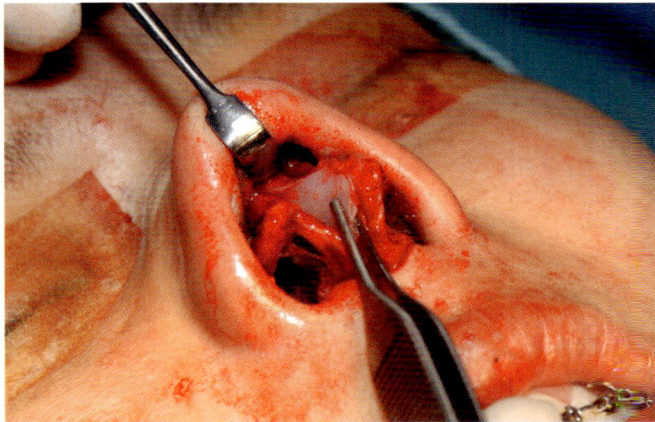

Figure 9–20   *Correction of the Contracted Nose, Step 2:* The nasal tip is approached via the external rhinoplasty method using the extended-V incision described in Fig. 9–18. The lower lateral cartilages are carefully identified, and the upper lateral cartilages are separated from the septum to accommodate the extended spreader graft. The photograph shows placement of the septal cartilage as an extended spreader graft to be ensconced between the lower lateral cartilages. (Courtesy of Dong-Hak Jung, M.D.)

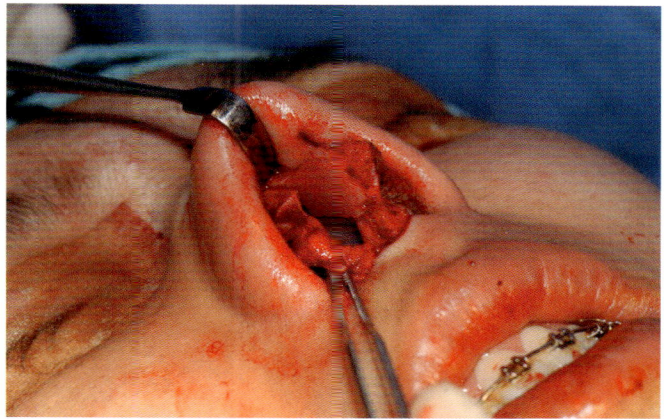

Figure 9–21   *Correction of the Contracted Nose, Step 3:* The extended spreader graft is affixed to the upper lateral cartilage with 5–0 polydioxanone suture. (Courtesy of Dong-Hak Jung, M.D.)

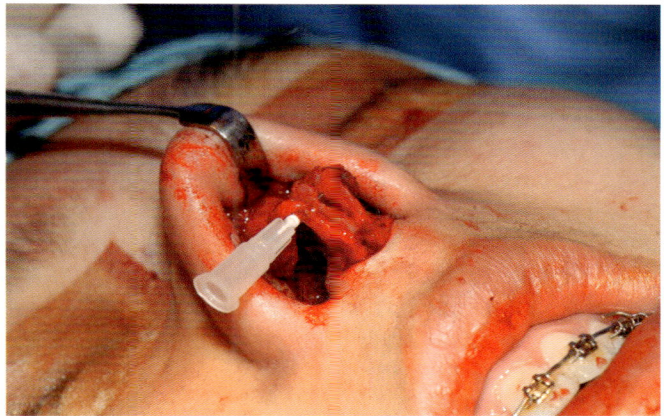

Figure 9–22   *Correction of the Contracted Nose, Step 4:* The lower lateral cartilages are then brought down to the septal spreader graft and held temporarily in place with a 5–0 polydioxanone suture. The lower lateral cartilages are then sutured to the spreader graft also with 5–0 polydioxanone. (Courtesy of Dong-Hak Jung, M.D.)

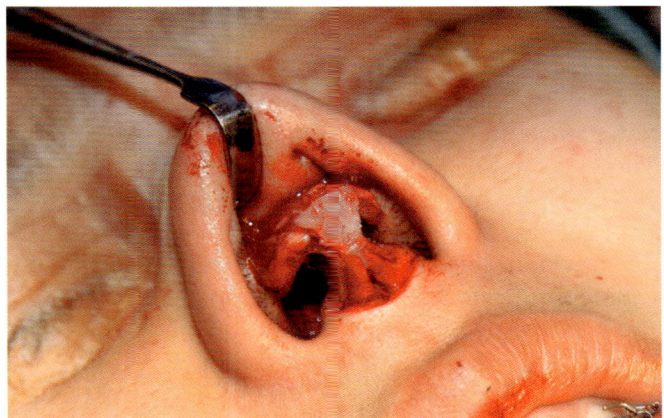

Figure 9–23   *Correction of the Contracted Nose, Step 5:* An onlay tip graft is used to provide additional projection and derotation of the nasal tip and is affixed into position with 5–0 polydioxanone suture. (Courtesy of Dong-Hak Jung, M.D.)

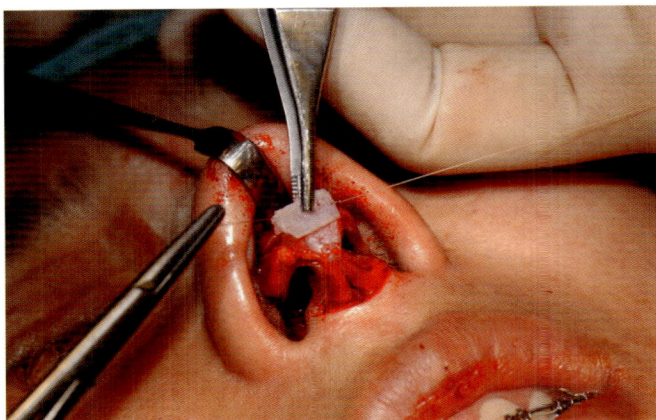

Figure 9–24 *Correction of the Contracted Nose, Step 6:* An additional onlay tip graft is placed to achieve greater projection and derotation. Multiple onlay grafts can be used to arrive at the desired nasal-tip configuration. (Courtesy of Dong-Hak Jung, M.D.)

The second important anatomic structure that must be addressed is the overlying skin envelope. In mildly contracted cases, the contracted skin is sufficient to drape over the new framework with relatively little tension. However, in moderate cases, the upper-lip skin must be undermined and taped upward for 1 week to relieve tension on the closure. For severe cases, the skin may lack both quantity and quality, and the radical solution of a paramedian forehead flap may serve as the most viable option at this point. The inner mucosal layer is generally deficient in these cases as well and also requires reconstruction. The existing dorsal skin may be turned over and pedicled downward at the nasal tip to reline the internal columella. The contracted alar skin can also be turned over and inward in a bipedicled, bucket-handle manner to reline the interior of the new alae. After appropriate cartilaginous reconstruction of the nasal framework, the forehead flap may be dissected, elevated, and inset. The pedicle should be transected after 4 weeks at a minimum, if not longer, due to the attenuated vascularity of the postoperative tissue bed. In cases in which the skin is sufficient but the mucosa is deficient, the septum can be rotated as a local flap to cover the internal columella and/or the soft triangle. When bilateral flaps are raised, the septal cartilage should not be harvested to minimize the risk of a septal perforation. However, patients who have a severe aesthetic deformity are often willing to tolerate a limited septal perforation.

Several complications can occur after revision surgery of the contracted Asian nose. The poorly vascularized tissue is prone to infection and necrosis. Infection can be devastating and is a frequent complication. All patients are placed on an intensive postoperative prophylactic regimen that includes broad-spectrum oral antibiotics. However, if an infection should arise, the inevitable outcome is a frank abscess and cellulitis. Therefore, early hospitalization with institution of broad-spectrum parenteral antibiotics may seem like an aggressive solution but has proven to be a necessary treatment strategy in these difficult cases. A minimum course of 5 to 7 days or until resolution of the infection is warranted to manage the infection. Skin necrosis can also occur along the columellar incision, predisposing to cartilage exposure and potential infection. Use of prostaglandin emollients has served to hasten wound healing and prevent infection in many cases.

Although the columella is lengthened in revision surgery, the surgeon should not attempt to address the alar deficiency in the same operative setting. Conchal composite grafts may be needed to reduce the alar-columellar disparity, but a full 6 months should transpire before electing to do so. This grafting is usually required only ~10% of the time. Most often, the restored nasal length provides patients with considerable satisfaction, and the alar retraction is not perceived as a noticeable deformity. Furthermore, composite free grafts at the time of surgery usually do not survive due to the already compromised vascularity of the dissected surgical bed and the contracted state of the nose. The alar-columellar relationship is difficult to gauge in the immediate postoperative period; but the final disposition of the ala and columella will be apparent after 6 months when mild retraction has already taken place. Oftentimes, the extended spreader graft can be trimmed slightly through a marginal incision at this time to reduce the alar-columellar disparity. This surgical sleight of hand is an expedient method of correcting this problem.

The contracted nose is a more prevalent problem after Asian rhinoplasty compared with Caucasian rhinoplasty. Fortunately, this complication remains relatively rare. However, if this problem should arise, the above algorithm and treatment protocol has served as a reliable method for revision surgery in over 40 cases in the past 10 years of practice.

References

1. Lam SM, Kim YK. Augmentation rhinoplasty of the Asian nose with the "Bird" silicone implant. Ann Plast Surg 2003;51:249–256
2. McCurdy JA Jr. The Asian nose: augmentation rhinoplasty with L-shaped silicone implants. Facial Plast Surg 2002;18:245–252
3. Ellis DA, Dindzans L. The geometry of alar base resection. J Otolaryngol 1987;16:46–48
4. Guyuron B, Behmand RA. Alar base abnormalities: classification and correction. Clin Plast Surg 1996;23:263–270

5. Watanabe K. New ideas to improve the shape of the ala of the Oriental nose. Aesthetic Plast Surg 1994;18:337–344

6. Sheen JH, Sheen AP. Aesthetic Rhinoplasty (2nd ed.). St. Louis, MO: Quality Medical Publishing; 1997

7. Shirakabe Y, Suzuki Y, Lam SM. A systematic approach to rhinoplasty of the Japanese nose: a thirty-year experience. Aesthetic Plast Surg 2003;27:221–231

8. Shirakabe Y, Shirakabe T, Takayanagi S. A new type of prosthesis for augmentation rhinoplasty: our experience in 1600 cases. Br J Plast Surg 1981;34:353–357

9. Skoog T. Plastic Surgery: New Methods and Refinements. Stockholm: Almquist & Wiksell International; 1974

10. Deva AK, Merten S, Chang L. Silicone in nasal augmentation rhinoplasty: a decade of clinical experience. Plast Reconstr Surg 1998;102:1230–1237

11. Ham KS, Chung SC, Lee SH. Complications of oriental augmentation rhinoplasty. Ann Acad Med Singapore 1983;12(2 Suppl):460–462

12. Jung DH, Moon HJ, Choi SH, Lam SM. Secondary rhinoplasty of the Asian nose: correction of the contracted nose. Aesthetic Plast Surg 2004;28(1):1–7

13. Naficy S, Baker SR. Lengthening the short nose. Arch Otolaryngol Head Neck Surg 1998;124:809–813

14. Gruber RE. Surgical correction of the short nose. Aesthetic Plast Surg 2002;26(1 Suppl):5

15. Tabbal N. Lengthening of the postoperative short nose: combined use of a gull-wing concha composite graft and a rib costo-chondral dorsal onlay graft. Plast Reconstr Surg 2000;105:2200–2201

10

Management of the Aging Face: Alternative Approaches

◆ General and Anatomic Considerations

Although the Asian face typically does not experience as much aging as that of the lighter-skinned Caucasian, facial rejuvenative surgery is warranted in the majority of Asian patients to varying degrees.[1] The darker Asian complexion renders the face more impervious to the ravaging effects of the sun and thereby aids in the preservation of a youthful countenance. Despite relatively fewer fine to coarse rhytids that manifest in the Asian skin, ptosis of facial tissues remains a prevalent condition, especially in the brow/upper-eyelid complex vis-à-vis the lower face and neck. Accordingly, brow lift procedures are a mainstay of intervention for the mature Asian face. Similarly, ablative skin resurfacing is less often necessary and is also less tolerated in the Asian skin (refer to Chapter 14).

Because the Asian skin often responds poorly to ablative skin therapy, surgical incisions may also remain conspicuous for an unacceptably protracted period of time. Any incisions in the central aspect of the face should be thoughtfully reviewed with the patient, and every effort should be made to avoid these types of incisions. This chapter will outline a surgical treatment strategy that relies on incisions that are created for maximal camouflage.[2] For instance, brow incisions are abbreviated in length and placed behind the hairline. Upper-eyelid incisions for upper-lid blepharoplasty do not extend past the lateral canthus in an area that may be more visually noticeable. Lower-eyelid surgery is performed via a transconjunctival approach so that no external incision will be observed. Face lift incisions are performed in a curvilinear and post-tragal fashion and are hidden high in the postauricular sulcus and hairline. The surgical philosophy and techniques outlined in this

chapter are also well suited for other races, as the author relies on the same methodology for all of his patients irrespective of race. The author contends that the brow lift, face lift, and blepharoplasty techniques described herein offer the benefits of a natural rejuvenation and a rapid recovery.

◆ Rejuvenation of the Brow: The Minimal-Incision Brow Lift

Preoperative Remarks

Over the past decade, the upper face/brow complex has assumed an increasing role in facial rejuvenation for two principal reasons. First, the advent of the minimally invasive, endoscopic brow technique has revolutionized brow surgery. The patient wary of the larger transverse incision involved with the coronal lift may be more readily accepting of the shorter scars in the hairline that accompany this type of brow lift. However, champions of the coronal or pretrichial lift advocate the more precise brow positioning and better exposure with the these traditional techniques. The direct brow lift, which has fallen into some disrepute in the Western world, may still remain a minimally invasive viable alternative to many Asians in that micropigmentation (eyebrow tattooing or permanent makeup) is much more prevalent in Asians and may effectively camouflage any suboptimal, more visible scarring associated with this technique. However, if micropigmentation is undesirable to the patient, a direct brow lift may yield a very obvious scar in the Asian skin. In the West, the midbrow lift has been used as a mainstay of brow lifting by certain staunch proponents of this technique, who even propose the suitability of midbrow elevation in the younger rhytid-free female population.[3] However, the darker complected Asian patient may manifest a fine white incision line, or worse yet a hypertrophic cicatrix, in the very conspicuous midforehead that would otherwise go unnoticed in the more alabaster Caucasian or lighter toned Asian patient. The surgeon now has an unprecedented, wider selection of options for upper facial rejuvenation than ever before: all of these modalities offer unique benefits and drawbacks. Despite the many varied techniques that exist, the author contends that the minimal-incision brow lift offers the best solution for the majority of Asian patients, as this technique avoids obvious incisions on the face (which can be particularly problematic for the Asian patient), does not require any excision of hair and facilitates a rapid recovery.

The second reason that brow rejuvenation has risen in prominence over the past 10 years is the increased comprehension that the scientific community has gained about the importance of the brow in facial aging. In the past, the face lift represented the central method by which the face was restored to a more youthful expression. However, today the brow has caught up and perhaps even exceeded the rejuvenative potential of a rhytidectomy in certain respects. Empirical observation has revealed that the brow may begin to age 10 years before the lower face does in many patients. However, patients may remain oblivious to brow descent and simply complain of looking more tired and aged than they feel. They may come to the facial aesthetic surgeon seeking to recapture their youthful appearance by demanding a blepharoplasty be performed but ignorant that a brow lift may be a more suitable undertaking. This fault may be accorded in part to the mass media, which have erroneously indoctrinated the public into equating tired eyes with eyelid surgery. The author has

also noted that Asian patients suffer more frequently from brow descent than lower facial aging, compared with the Caucasian patient, in whom the lower face ages at an equal rate as the upper face.

At this point, a simplified algorithm should be introduced that may facilitate easy analysis (but should be used with discretion and judgment). An imaginary vertical line can be drawn through the midpupil. Any tissue ptosis medial to this line may be thought of as upper eyelid in origin and may be corrected with an upper-lid blepharoplasty. Conversely, any ptosis that presents lateral to this invented line may be assumed to be principally due to brow ptosis rather than excessive upper-lid skin (or dermatochalasis) (Fig. **10–1**). The fallacy that bedevils many junior surgeons is the same unsophisticated thinking that encumbers patients, namely, that all upper-lid tissue ptosis is a by-product of redundant eyelid skin rather than brow ptosis. Quite the contrary is true: the brow tends to descend chronologically earlier than the onset of upper-eyelid skin redundancy. Anatomic studies have also highlighted the weaker development of the lateral-brow musculature that may serve as the principal cause for more significant lateral-brow ptosis.[4-6] If an upper-lid blepharoplasty is performed in lieu of a recommended browplasty, the brow may actually be further depressed; and if excessive upper-lid skin is removed, a brow lift may be precluded in the future due to risk of lagophthalmos (Fig. **10–2A,B**). Also, an aggressive upper-lid blepharoplasty alone, especially if the adjacent, thicker brow skin is removed together with the thinner upper-lid skin, may result in an unnatural appearance.

The aesthetic position of the brow should always be recalled when considering a brow lift. In the ideal female eyebrow, the eyebrow configuration assumes a tapered contour with a thicker, medial club of the eyebrow narrowing laterally to a fine point. The medial

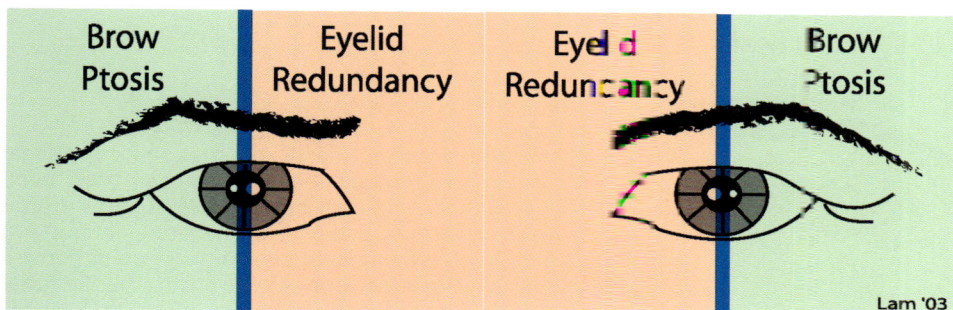

Figure 10–1 An imaginary vertical line can be drawn through the midpupil. Any tissue ptosis medial to this line may be thought of as upper eyelid in origin and may be corrected with an upper-lid blepharoplasty. Conversely, any ptosis that presents lateral to this invented line may be assumed to be principally

due to brow ptosis rather than excessive upper-lid skin (or dermatochalasis). (From Lam SM, Chang EW, Rhee JS, Williams EF. Rejuvenation of the periocular region: the unified brow, midface, and eyelid complex. Ophthal Plast Reconstr Surg 2004;20:[1-6]; with permission.)

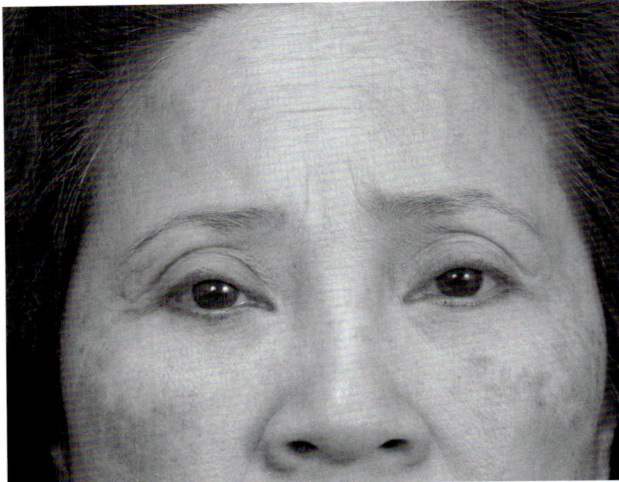

A

B

Figure 10–2   (**A**) This 55-year-old Vietnamese woman underwent upper-eyelid blepharoplasty in Vietnam several years before and is shown with noticeable asymmetry, in which the right upper eyelid is positioned farther down than the left. Manual elevation of her right eyelid showed that the patient could not close her eyelid, whereas she could on the left side; therefore, physical examination confirmed that overzealous upper-eyelid blepharoplasty resulted in notable brow ptosis, right greater than left. Any further upper-eyelid skin removal would exacerbate her tired, worried expression, as the brow would be brought farther down and would also risk lagophthalmos. Brow lift was undertaken with caution to avoid risk of lagophthalmos. (**B**) The patient underwent a minimal-incision brow lift with removal of right upper-eyelid fat from the medial pocket through a small incision. No upper-eyelid skin was removed. She is shown 3 months after brow lift with some improvement in symmetry and in her tired, worried expression without any lagophthalmos.

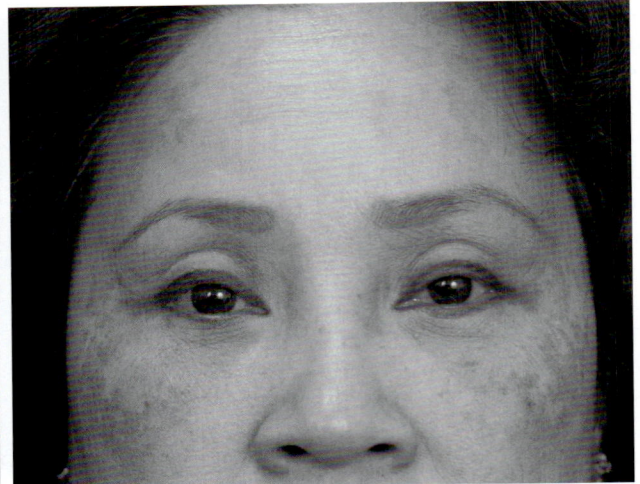

brow should rest at or slightly below the orbital rim, with the peak of the eyebrow situated either at the lateral limbus (classic description, Fig. **10–3**) or at the lateral canthus (revised description, Fig. **10–4**) lying above the orbital rim. Laterally the eyebrow descends somewhat to end at a point drawn through the imaginary line that joins the alar-facial groove through the lateral limbus or lateral canthus. The descended brow often assumes a more flattened appearance that resembles the ideal male eyebrow, that is, a straight line that runs along the orbital rim (Fig. **10–5**). Because the ideal female brow is arched laterally and because the brow descends disproportionately laterally, all efforts to raise the brow position should be concentrated laterally. As will be discussed, all fixation sutures are laterally based, and no medial suspension is undertaken. This surgical

Ideal Female Eyebrow
Classic Definition

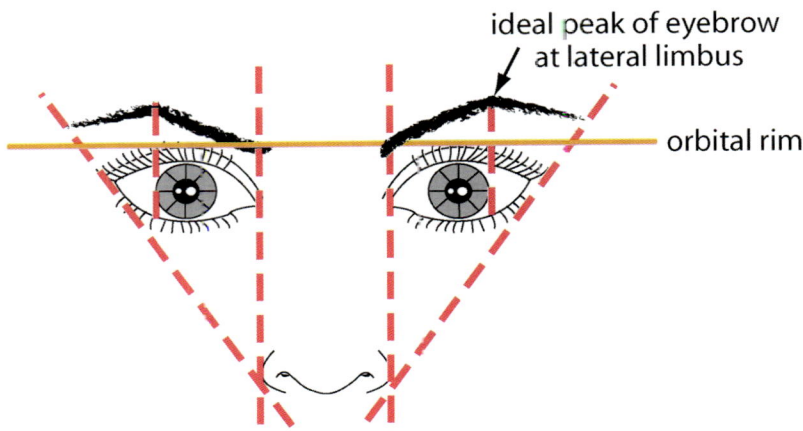

ideal peak of eyebrow at lateral limbus

orbital rim

Figure 10–3   Classic description of the ideal female brow position. The medial brow head starts at or slightly below the level of the orbital rim, arching to a peak at the lateral limbus and tapering laterally to an imaginary point derived from the intersection of two points: the alar-facial groove and the lateral canthus. (From Williams EF, Lam SM. Comprehensive Facial Rejuvenation: A Practical and Systematic Guide to Surgical Management of the Aging Face. Philadelphia: Lippincott, Williams & Wilkins; 2004; with permission.)

Ideal Female Eyebrow

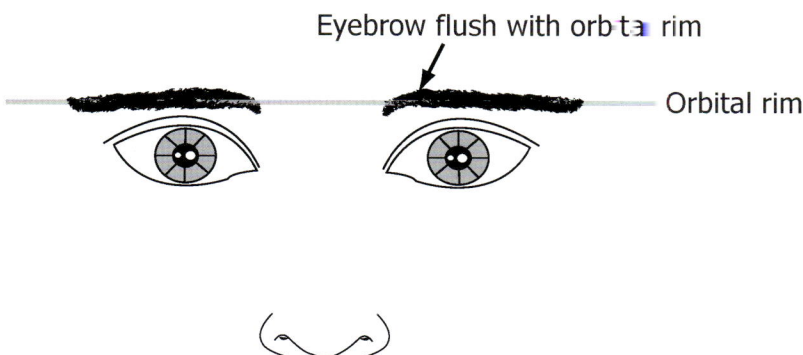

Revised Definition

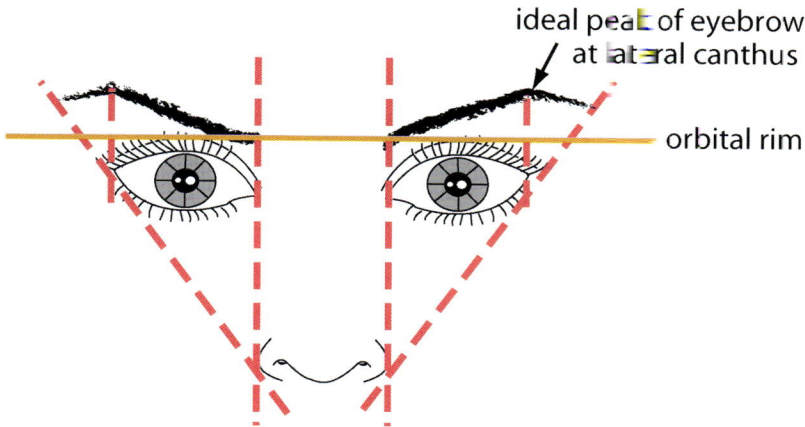

ideal peak of eyebrow
at lateral canthus

orbital rim

Figure 10–4 Revised description of the ideal female brow position. The description of the revised brow configuration matches that of the classic description, except the height (or peak) of the brow should lie above the lateral canthus rather than the lateral limbus. Both descriptions are acceptable alternatives, although some feel that the latter is more ideal given the less "startled" look that this shape imparts. Fashion and style change, so there are no absolutes to these guidelines. (From Williams EF, Lam SM. Comprehensive Facial Rejuvenation: A Practical and Systematic Guide to Surgical Management of the Aging Face. Philadelphia: Lippincott, Williams & Wilkins; 2004; with permission.)

technique properly restores the ptotic brow without unnaturally producing a startled or frightened appearance that is a stigma of an improper brow lift (Fig. **10–6A–D**)

Another fallacy that has ensnared the neophyte surgeon is the thought that the eyebrow (the hairy portion of the brow) is the exclusive aspect of the brow that requires rejuvenation. Instead, the entire lateral brow complex should be viewed as a unit, which includes both the hair-bearing eyebrow and the adjoining soft tissue. As part of the physical assessment, the surgeon should place his or her thumb along the ptotic lateral brow and lift the tissue upwards, carefully observing the improved position of the descended soft tissue and hair-bearing eyebrow. The patient should also be educated about this aesthetic deficit and confronted with the rejuvenated appearance using a mirror while the sur-

geon gently lifts the ptotic brow. Digital imaging should be used only with patients who have marked brow ptosis, as subtle aging may escape the visual capacity of this technology. Any excessive eyelid skin that remains after appropriate brow elevation may be pinched with forceps or between the surgeon's fingers to illustrate how a concomitant blepharoplasty would further enhance the intended objective. If the patient, however, desires only an upper-lid blepharoplasty, despite a thoughtful education, the surgeon should plan for a conservative upper-lid skin excision that would not compromise a prospective future brow lift or exacerbate the brow ptosis.

A relatively unique problem that may be encountered in the Asian patient is improper micropigmentation: the mature patient who undergoes late

Ideal Male Eyebrow

Eyebrow flush with orbital rim

Orbital rim

Figure 10–5 The ideal male brow is heavier than the female counterpart, in terms of the soft-tissue component, the hairy eyebrow itself, and the bony orbital rim. Classically, it should rest along the orbital rim in a flatter, straighter configuration as opposed to the arched shape of the ideal female eyebrow that extends superior to the bony rim. (From Williams EF, Lam SM. Comprehensive Facial Rejuvenation: A Practical and Systematic Guide to Surgical Management of the Aging Face. Philadelphia: Lippincott, Williams & Wilkins; 2004; with permission.)

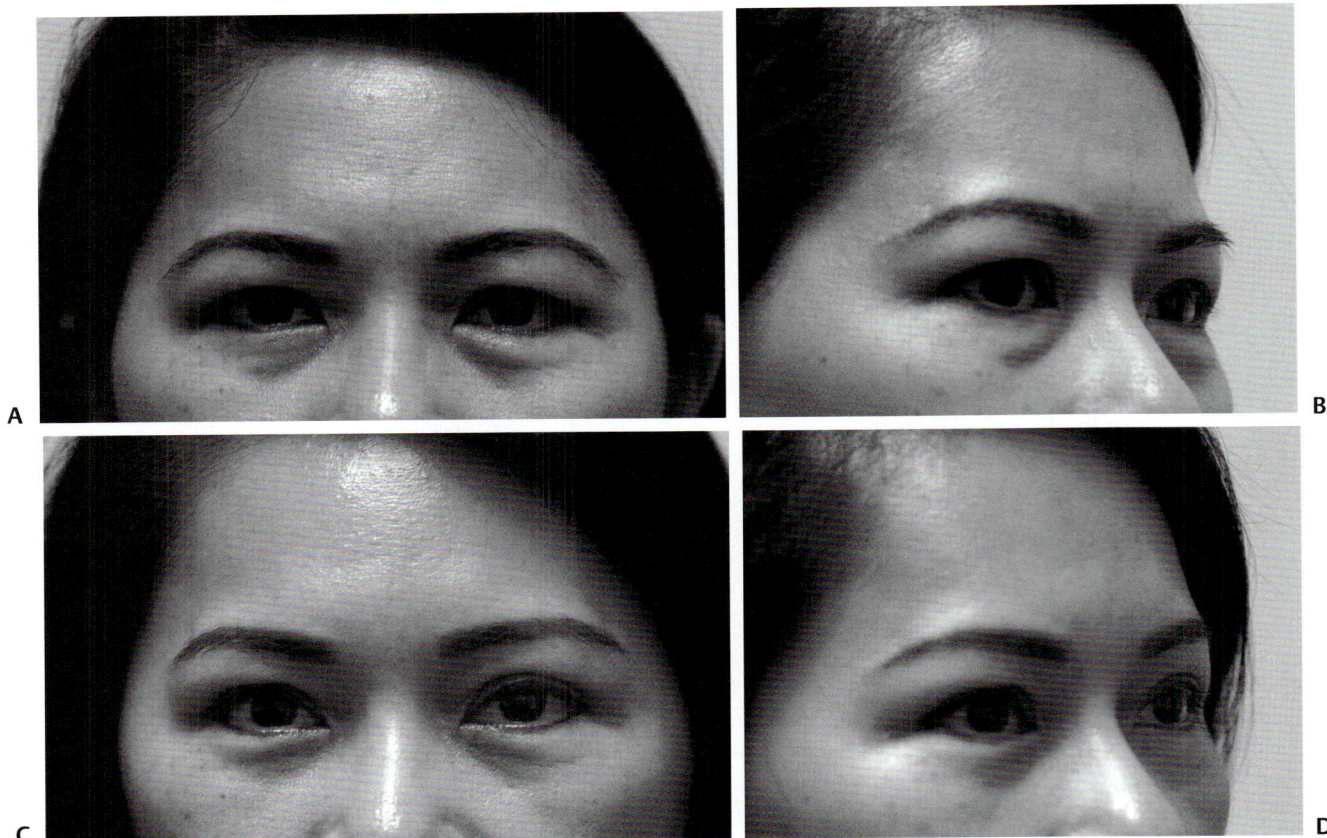

Figure 10–6   (**A,B**) This 44-year-old Chinese woman appears tired and worried principally due to her descended brow. The extent of brow hooding is evident by the shadow cast over the upper portion of her eye. Her lower-eyelid pseudoherniation of fat is more readily observed in the close-up oblique view and involves only the medial two fat pockets. (**C,D**) The patient underwent a minimal-incision brow lift, upper-eyelid blepharoplasty, and transconjunctival lower-eyelid blepharoplasty (of only her medial two lower-eyelid fat pockets with no skin removal). She is shown 3 months postoperatively, and her countenance appears less tired. The brow is elevated only laterally to avoid a startled expression. Also, the amount of brow elevation is minimal to effect a dramatic change in her appearance, as the goal of brow elevation is typically only several millimeters of lift and less often measured in centimeters of elevation. The removal of lower-eyelid fat reveals a more pronounced orbicularis oculi roll near the eyelid margin, which the patient should be aware of as a possible outcome postoperatively. The author feels that the appearance of a prominent orbicularis oculi is evident in all patients regardless of age and does not impart an aged appearance. Accordingly, the orbicularis oculi is almost never excised, as the author relies on a transconjunctival approach for the majority of his operative cases.

micropigmentation may try to compensate for a descended brow by tattooing a higher, peaked eyebrow. After the eyebrow has been tattooed in this fashion, surgical elevation of the descended soft tissue may render this drawn line unnaturally high following a brow lift. Accordingly, judicious eyelid surgery may be required instead, or laser removal of the tattoo should be undertaken before a brow lift is entertained.

Surgical Technique

The advent of the endoscopic brow technique has offered patients brow rejuvenation without any discernible, visible forehead incisions and without the large transverse scalp incision involved with the coronal-type lift. The recovery period is shorter than the coronal brow lift, and the scalp anesthesia is less global and of shorter duration than experienced with the coronal lift. Many surgeons have now evolved the technique such that endoscopic equipment has altogether been abandoned, and instead a so-called smart hand technique is used based on tactile feedback and gentle lifting rather than shearing movements, especially near neurovascular structures.[7] A more accurate term that reflects the technique is *minimal-incision brow lift* rather than *endoscopic brow lift*, as endoscopes have been eliminated in the technique described herein. Only three types of elevators are used for dissection: a small flat elevator, a large flat elevator, and a round elevator (Fig. **10–7**). The author uses this style of brow lift for the vast majority of his operative endeavors. Patients have been receptive to the advantages that this technique offers, and its popularity will certainly continue to gain.

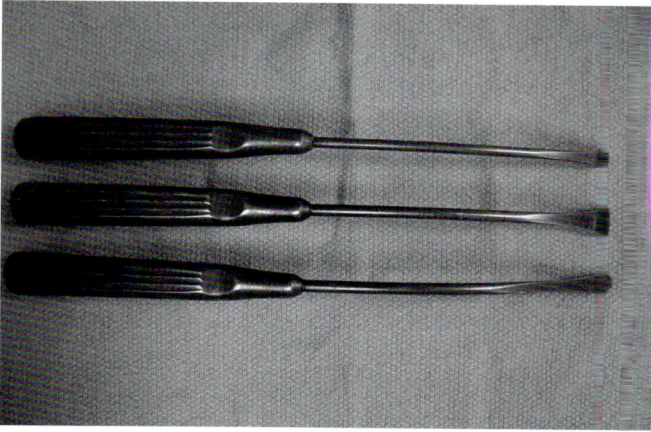

Figure 10–7 Three types of elevators are used for dissection: a small flat elevator, a large flat elevator, and a round elevator. The small flat elevator is used to initiate subperiosteal dissection and to complete periosteal release along the arcus marginalis. The large flat elevator is designed to elevate the broad area of periosteum between the incision and the arcus marginalis both quickly and uniformly. The round elevator is used to dissect the lateral, temporal pocket atraumatically to minimize risk of temporal nerve injury. However, the small flat elevator is still used to initiate the dissection in the lateral, temporal pocket a short distance behind the hairline and to achieve final release along the arcus marginalis and the conjoined tendon. All of the elevators have an ebonized finish to minimize reflection off their surface. (From Williams EF, Lam SM. Comprehensive Facial Rejuvenation: A Practical and Systematic Guide to Surgical Management of the Aging Face. Philadelphia: Lippincott, Williams & Wilkins; 2004; with permission.)

1. After the patient's hair is secured with $^{1}/_{2}$ inch paper tape (Micropore) to expose the planned surgical incision sites, five, standard "endoscopic" brow lift incisions are marked out with a surgical marking pen, with one situated in the midline; two located lateral to the midline in the paramedian position (approximately at the lateral canthus) just posterior to the hairline; and two additional, longer incisions located more temporally, also camouflaged by the hairline and extending over a 4 cm distance above the helical crus and over the temporalis muscle and fascia (Figs. **10–8A,B, 10–9**). In addition, the supraorbital notch is palpated, and marks are placed above each notch to guide dissection near the neurovascular structures.

2. One percent lidocaine with 1:100,000 epinephrine is infiltrated along the orbital rim and along each incision site but is not necessary over the intervening expanse of forehead. The usual 10 minutes should be allowed to transpire before the start of the surgical procedure to permit adequate time for anesthesia and hemostasis.

3. First, the midline incision is performed to access the medial brow complex. The incision is made with a no. 15 Bard-Parker blade down to the periosteum

(Fig. **10–10**). The periosteum is fully incised with a monopolar cautery, which also may be used to arrest any observed bleeding (Fig. **10–11**). The principal objective is release of the periosteum at the arcus to achieve unrestricted brow elevation; aggressive dissection of the musculature is abandoned in favor of possible chemical ablation with botulinum toxin A at a later date (or before surgery). The small sharp, flat periosteal elevator is used to dissect subperiosteally for a distance of a few centimeters circumferentially around the incision site. Little additional dissection is performed posterior to the incision site beyond the initial few centimeters, as extensive dissection toward the occiput provides limited benefit in transposition of the brow upward. The large flat periosteal elevator is then used to dissect down toward the arcus marginalis. As the orbital rim is approached, the small, flat elevator is then used to complete periosteal release along the arcus marginalis. Care is taken to remain medial to the marked-out neurovascular bundles.

4. This midline brow incision is then closed with surgical staples (Fig. **10–12**).

5. Next, the right paramedian incision (vertically situated in the hairline approximately above the lateral canthus) is dissected in the same fashion prescribed above for the midline incision. Care is taken to release the periosteum near the neurovascular bundle in a gentle lifting motion rather than a forward shearing motion to avoid injury to the supraorbital/supratrochlear nerves. The small flat elevator can be used to lift and release the periosteal attachment on either side of the marked-out neurovascular notch to ensure that the periosteum is sufficiently released (Fig. **10–13**). The nondominant, "smart" hand can be used to guide periosteal release. Furthermore, dissection from the paramedian incision always remains medial to the conjoined tendon.

6. A bone tunnel is then created in the posterior aspect of the paramedian incision through which the frontalis muscle will be anchored toward the conclusion of the operative case. A bone-tunnel guidance device (Browlift Bone Bridge System, Medtronic Xomed, Jacksonville, FL) may be used to create the bone tunnel (Fig. **10–14A,B**). After the bone tunnel has been created, the device designed to pull the suture through the bone tunnel may also be used to test whether a communicating tunnel has been established (Fig. **10–15**).

7. The left paramedian incision is then made, and the same method of bone-tunnel creation and periosteal release is performed as previously described for the contralateral paramedian incision.

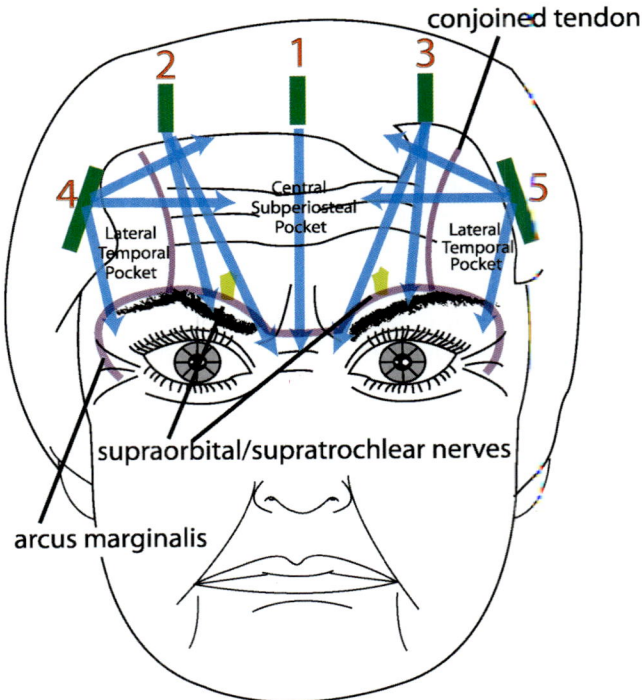

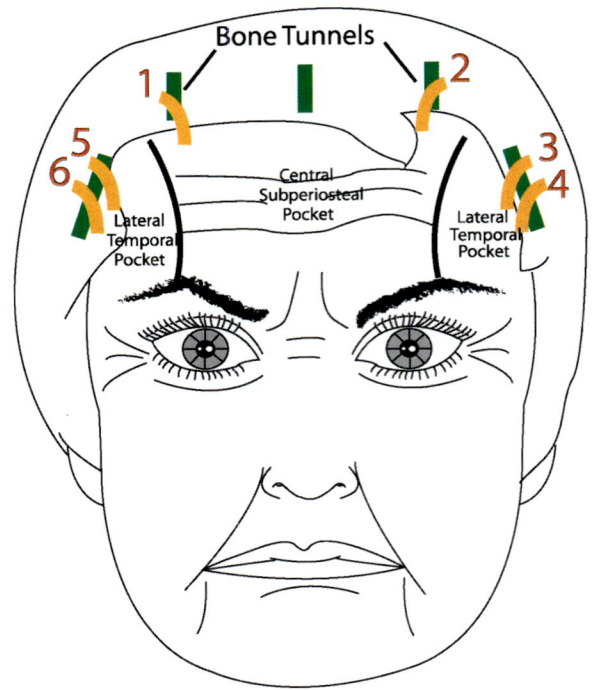

Figure 10–8 **(A)** Five standard brow lift incisions are used, with one situated in the midline; two located lateral to the midline in the paramedian position (approximately at the lateral canthus) just posterior to the hairline; and two additional, longer incisions located more temporally, also camouflaged by the hairline and extending over a 4 cm distance above the helical crus and over the temporalis muscle and fascia. Dissection occurs in the subperiosteal plane in the central pocket and below the temporoparietal fascia in the lateral pockets, with careful regard to avoid the supraorbital/supratrochlear neurovascular areas using the "smart hand" technique described in the text. Complete release along the arcus marginalis across the orbital rim and along the conjoined tendon (between the lateral and central pockets) is necessary before suspension can be undertaken. **(B)** All suspension sutures are placed laterally so as to avoid any unnatural elevation of the medial brow complex. The surgical order of suspension follows the numbers in the diagram. The first two sutures suspend the frontalis to the bone tunnels; then the temporoparietal fascia immediately inferior to the incision is suspended to the temporalis fascia immediately superior to the incision, with two sutures placed on each side.

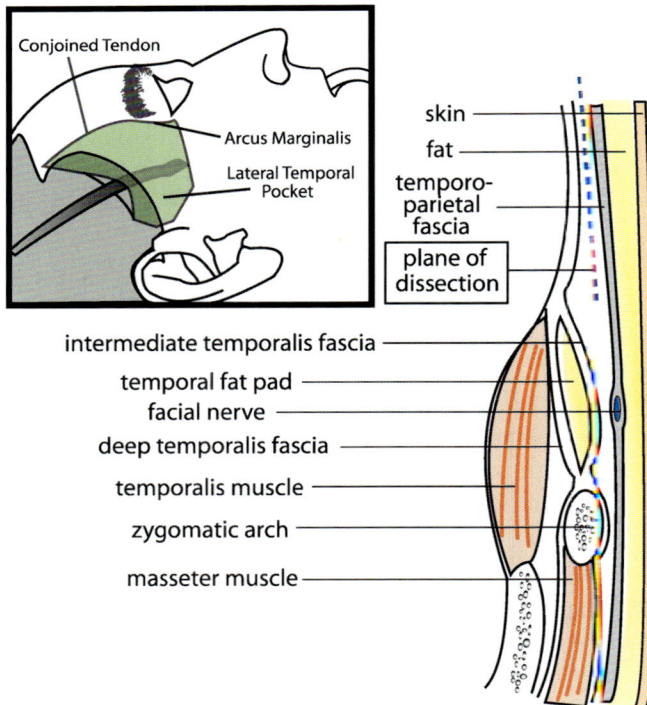

Figure 10–9 Dissection in the lateral temporal pocket is undertaken between the temporalis fascia (deep) and the temporoparietal fascia (superficial) to avoid injury to the temporal branch of the facial nerve, which resides above in the substance of the temporoparietal fascia.

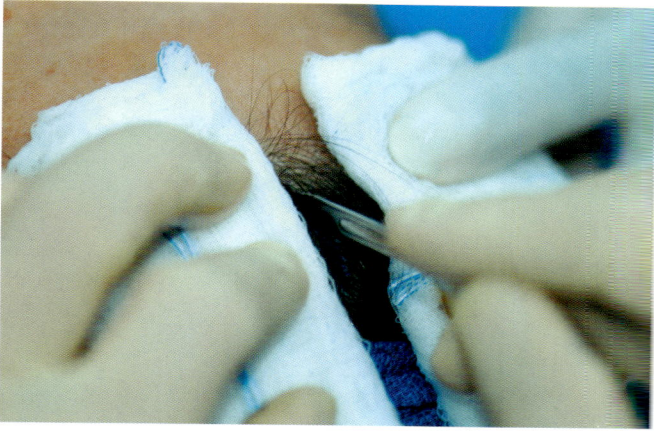

Figure 10–10 *Minimal-Incision Brow Lift, Step 1:* The midline incision is performed first with a no. 15 Bard-Parker blade. Two folded, moistened 4 × 4 gauze pads assist in lateral retraction and also to absorb any bleeding that may ensue.

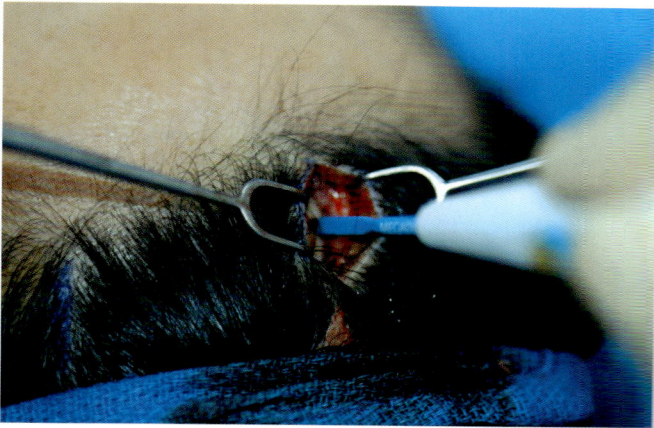

Figure 10–11 *Minimal-Incision Brow Lift, Step 2:* The wound is retracted with wide double-pronged hooks, and a monopolar cautery is used to dissect down through the periosteum to facilitate subperiosteal dissection. Any excessive bleeding can also be managed with cautery before continuing. The small sharp periosteal elevator is used to elevate the periosteum down to arcus marginaus centrally (not shown).

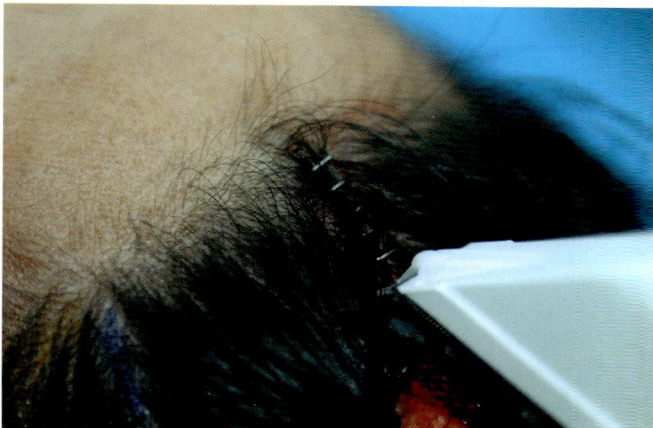

Figure 10–12 *Minimal-Incision Brow Lift, Step 3:* The midline incision is closed with surgical staples before continuing with the remaining incisions. Of note, only this incision is closed immediately after dissection, as no suspension sutures need to be placed at this site.

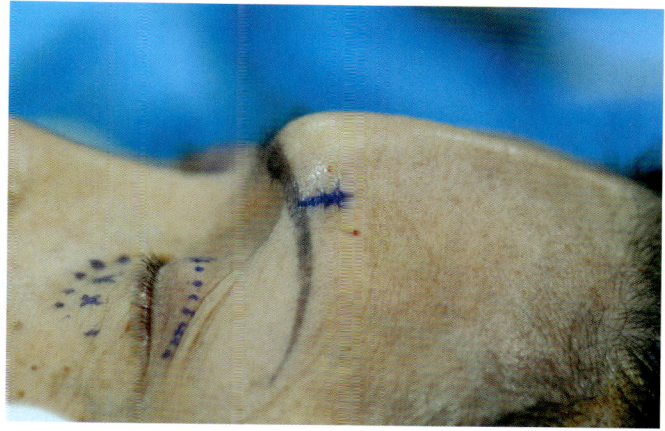

Figure 10–13 *Minimal-Incision Brow Lift, Step 4:* After completion of dissection in the midline, subperiosteal pocket, the right paramedian port is approached in the same fashion. As the arcus marginalis is approached near the supraorbital notch, the surgeon should take care to release the periosteum in only a lifting motion so as to avoid neurovascular damage. The photograph shows the elevator tenting up the skin along the arcus marginalis adjacent to the supraorbital notch marked out in gentian violet.

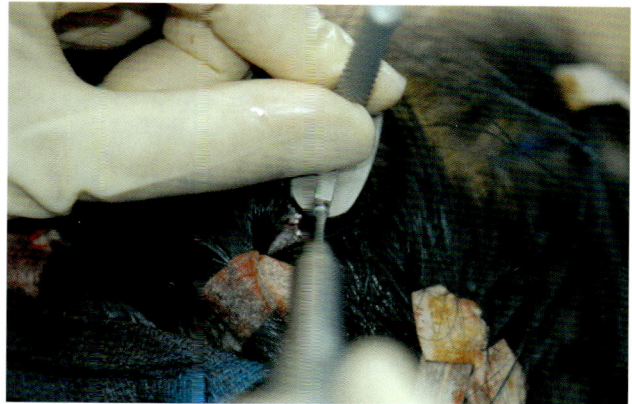

A

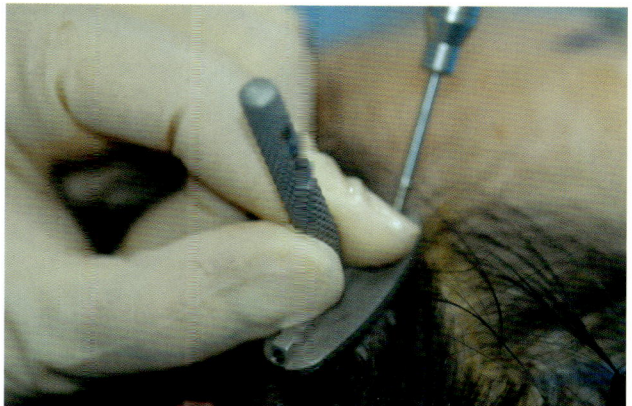

B

Figure 10–14 *Minimal-Incision Brow Lift, Step 5:* The bone-tunnel guidance device is used to guide the drill to create a safe, communicating bone tunnel, which will be used later to suspend the frontalis muscle.

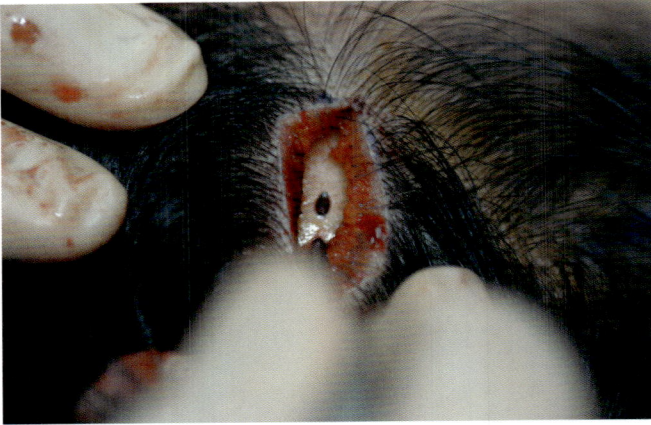

Figure 10–15 *Minimal-Incision Brow Lift, Step 6:* After the bone tunnel has been created, the device that comes with the kit is used to confirm that a communicating bone tunnel has been established. The same device may be used to pull the suture through the bone tunnel. The contralateral, paramedian incision is performed in the same fashion as described for the right side in Figs. **10–13** to **10–15**.

8. After the surgical maneuvers have been completed in the central pocket (medial to the conjoined tendons of the temporalis muscle), the longer lateral temporoparietal incision is then addressed on the right side. The incision should be situated ~1 cm behind the hairline to lie over the temporalis muscle and not more posteriorly to avoid transection of the superficial temporal artery (Fig. **10–16**). Dissection is carried down through the temporoparietal fascia (TPF) so that a proper tissue plane may be achieved between the TPF and the true temporalis fascia to avoid injury to the frontal branch of the facial nerve. The surgeon should be absolutely certain that he or she is in the correct surgical plane of dissection. Use of fine scissors to dissect through the filmy TPF can aid in establishing the correct tissue plane

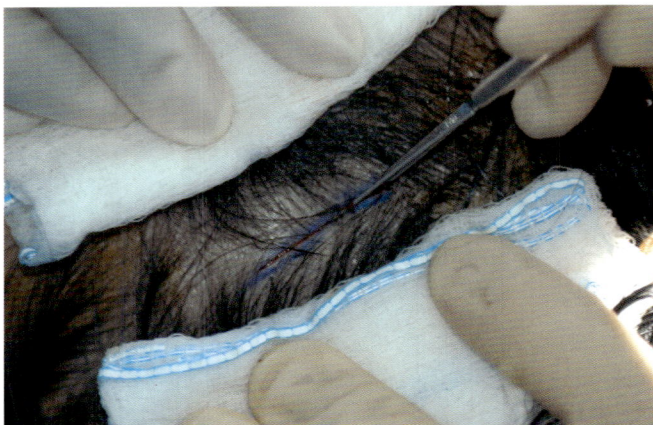

A

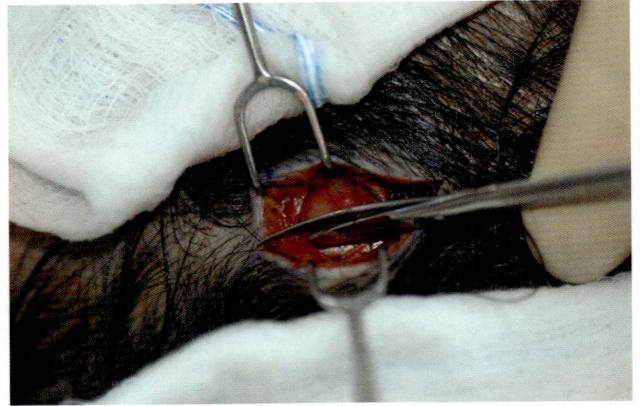

B

Figure 10–17 *Minimal-Incision Brow Lift, Step 8:* **(A)** Dissection is carried down through the temporoparietal fascia using fine scissors to ensure that all of the temporoparietal fascia fibers have been incised. **(B)** A thin remaining film of temporoparietal fascia fibers is left to transect before arriving at the glistening white surface of the true temporalis fascia.

(Fig. **10–17A,B**). Then, vigorously abrading the temporalis fascia with a 4 × 4 gauze pad can help guarantee that all of the filmy TPF has been stripped away. Finally, a small incision can be made in the glistening temporalis fascia to expose the underlying muscle for ultimate assurance that the surgeon has entered the correct surgical plane.

9. Initial dissection is performed with a small flat periosteal elevator over the true temporalis fascia toward the hairline (Fig. **10–18**). The round elevator is then used to continue the dissection toward the conjoined tendon and the arcus marginalis. Upon approaching either the conjoined tendon or the arcus marginalis, the small flat elevator is used again to break through each of these structures precisely and definitively.

10. The paramedian suture (located at the lateral canthus) is fixated first. The CV-3 Gore-Tex, or equivalent, suture is used to secure the overlying frontalis muscle through the bone tunnel in the paramedian incision (Fig. **10–19**). The needle is passed first through the bone tunnel: bending the tip of the

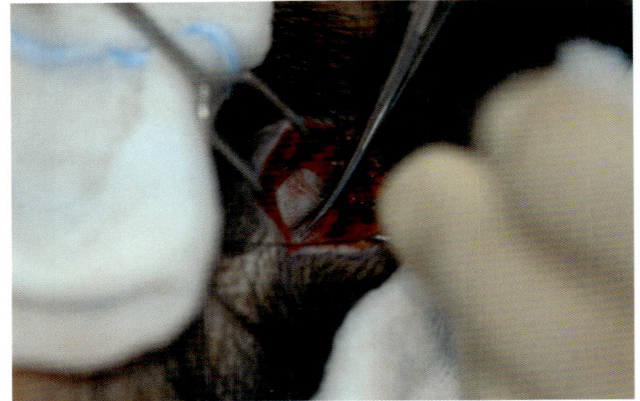

Figure 10–16 *Minimal-Incision Brow Lift, Step 7:* The lateral temporal incision is then made with a no. 15 Bard-Parker blade ~1 cm behind the hairline.

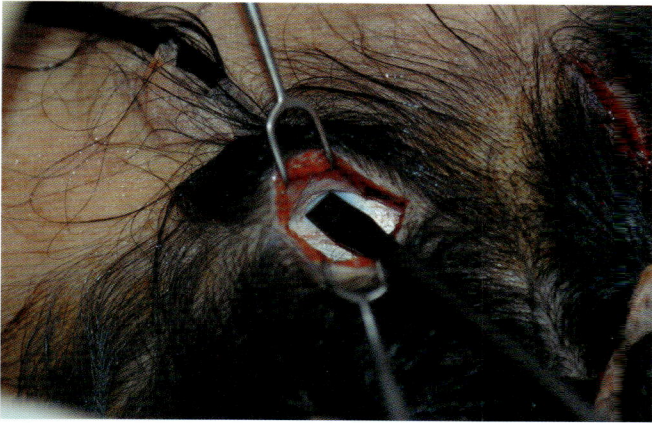

Figure 10–18 *Minimal-Incision Brow Lift, Step 9:* The photograph shows the initial dissection with a small flat periosteal elevator over the true temporalis fascia toward the hairline. The round elevator is then used to continue the dissection toward the conjoined tendon and the arcus marginalis. Upon approaching either the conjoined tendon or the arcus marginalis, the small flat elevator is used again to break through each of these structures precisely and definitively.

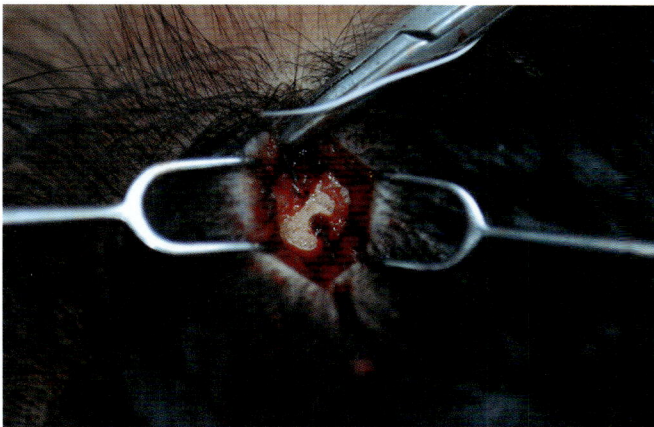

Figure 10–20 *Minimal-Incision Brow Lift, Step 11:* A generous bite of frontalis muscle needs to be grasped with the suture needle to achieve a secure and adequate suspension. This suture is then tied down securely. The same suspension is performed in the contralateral, paramedian incision.

needle slightly facilitates passage of the suture through the tunnel. (If the needle caliber is too thick to pass through the bone tunnel, then the back end of the suture can be passed using the aforesaid suture-passing device instead.) Then, a generous bite of frontalis muscle needs to be grasped with the suture needle to achieve a secure and adequate suspension (Fig. **10–20**). To ensure that sufficient frontalis muscle has been grasped, the surgeon can tug firmly on the suture to determine whether it will pull through the purchased muscle. CV-3 Gore-Tex is first tied as a square knot in midair and cinched down to position. Seven or eight suture throws are necessary to avoid slippage of the knot. The wound is then closed with surgical staples.

11. The same suspension is performed in the contralateral paramedian incision.

12. Next, the temporoparietal fascia just anterior to the temporal incision (but behind the hairline) is sutured to the temporalis fascia more superiorly with the CV-3 Gore-Tex suture to pull the overlying brow and soft tissue superolaterally (Figs. **10–21, 10–22**). This suture placement is undertaken twice. It is easier to place both sutures first before tying down each one (Fig. **10–23**). These sutures cannot be overly pulled, as some degree of brow ptosis will return over time. All incisions are then closed with surgical staples (Fig. **10–24**).

13. The same technique is used to dissect the contralateral, left temporal pocket.

14. Bacitracin ointment is applied to the external incisions, and a pressure dressing is fashioned into place.

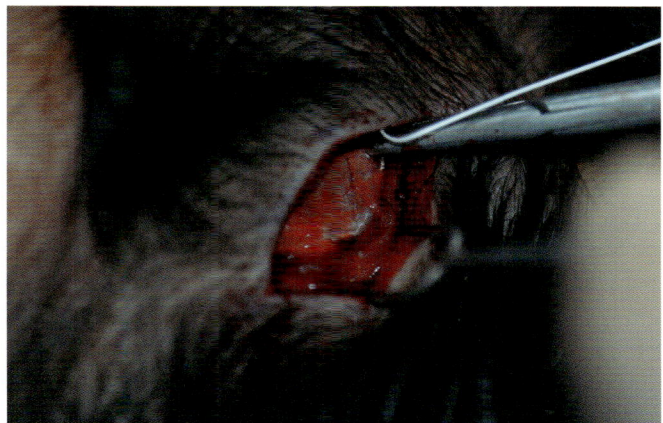

Figure 10–19 *Minimal-Incision Brow Lift, Step 10:* The CV-3 Gore-Tex suture is placed through the created bone tunnel first. Bending the tip of the needle slightly will facilitate passage of the suture through the tunnel.

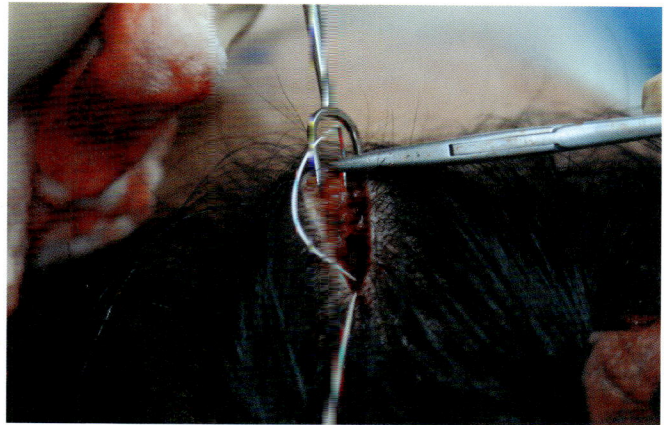

Figure 10–21 *Minimal-Incision Brow Lift, Step 12:* The lateral brow suspension is performed by first placing a suture through the temporalis fascia.

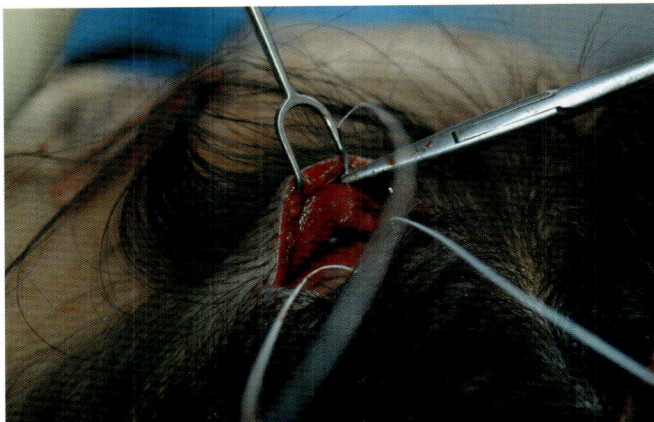

Figure 10–22 *Minimal-Incision Brow Lift, Step 13:* The same suture is then passed through the overlying temporoparietal fascia immediately anterior to the incision (but posterior to the hairline).

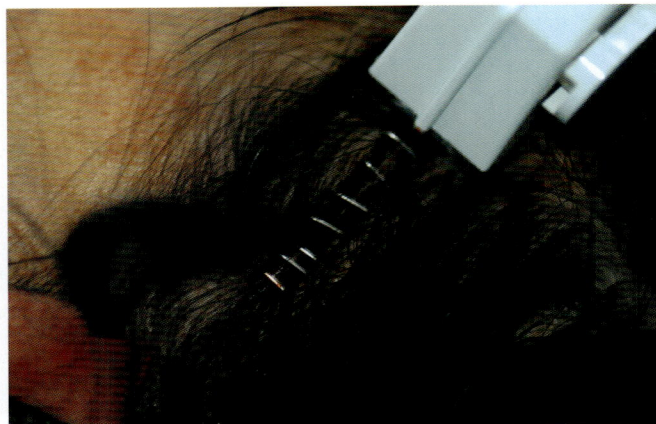

Figure 10–24 *Minimal-Incision Brow Lift, Step 15:* The incision is then closed with surgical staples. The contralateral, temporal incision is suspended in the same fashion.

Postoperative Remarks

The patient is seen on the first postoperative day for dressing change and for clinical evaluation. The heavy circumferential bandage applied at the time of surgery is removed; the wounds are inspected and cleaned, and kacitracin is reapplied. The patient should be evaluated for facial nerve movement. Oftentimes, despite proper surgical dissection, the facial nerve may be immobile for 1 to 3 weeks after surgery due to neuropraxia engendered from dissection and edema. The patient should be reassured of this eventuality. Small fluid collection under the raised flap is normal and should not raise alarm. As a reminder, no drains are needed in this type of brow lift. On the sixth or seventh postoperative day, the patient has all of the surgical staples removed. The patient may complain of tightness in the brow region on jaw opening, which will resolve in several weeks' time.

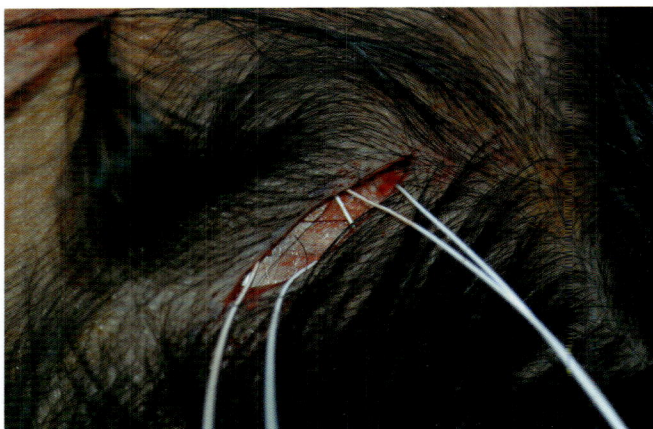

Figure 10–23 *Minimal-Incision Brow Lift, Step 14:* Before the suture is tied down, the same suture is placed adjacent to the first suture, as shown in the photograph. Then, both sutures can be easily tied down.

◆ Rejuvenation of the Upper Eyelid: Upper Blepharoplasty

Preoperative Remarks

What may appear to be excessive upper-eyelid skin in the aging face at first glance may be largely attributed to brow descent, as carefully explained in the preceding section (Fig. **10–2**). During the aging process, redundant skin does not mysteriously materialize: Instead, most of the extra tissue arises from ptosis of brow tissue. Accordingly, the author rarely performs an exclusive upper-eyelid surgery without a concomitant brow lift. If the surgeon should elect to undertake an aggressive removal of eyelid skin without a concurrent brow lift, then several potential problems may arise. First, an incision must extend quite far laterally past the lateral canthus to encompass all of the extra tissue, which truly represents descended brow tissue. When this incision is closed, the thicker brow tissue that is approximated to the thinner eyelid skin oftentimes leads to a conspicuous scar, especially in the Asian skin. Although this extended incision may be acceptable in fairer-skinned Caucasians, it may be more noticeable in Asians, who have a tendency to manifest scarring, prolonged erythema, hyperpigmentation, and hypopigmentation. Instead, the author prefers to terminate an upper-blepharoplasty incision within the supratarsal crease for maximal incision camouflage. Furthermore, excision of excessive eyelid tissue may exacerbate brow descent, as removal of intervening tissue may act to draw the brow farther downward, rendering the patient even older in appearance (Fig. **10–2**). Finally, aggressive upper-eyelid blepharoplasty may render a subsequent brow lift untenable due to the risk of lagophthalmos. For all of these reasons, upper-eyelid blepharoplasty is rarely undertaken without a brow lift.

A few exceptions to this general rule should be elaborated to guide the reader. Many men do not want to entertain a brow lift and may staunchly refuse to undergo this type of surgery. Accordingly, an upper-lid blepharoplasty may be performed in lieu of a brow lift but with the understanding that the rejuvenative potential will be suboptimal. Alternatively, patients who have undergone a brow lift in the past may require a modest skin pinch to remove some of the excess skin that remains. Patients who have a very high lid crease from older "westernization" double-eyelid procedures in the past may benefit from skin removal below the surgically created crease to achieve a more natural fold. Oftentimes, simple skin removal is insufficient to lower the crease height, as the high crease may already be tenaciously fixed in the superior location. The reader is referred to Chapter 2 and the enclosed DVD (Disk One) video for revision, double-eyelid surgery.

Because the height of the supratarsal crease is an important aesthetic attribute for many Asians, the new position of this anatomic landmark after brow lift, blepharoplasty should be a point of consultation with the patient. Over the past decade, the trend has been toward a more natural-appearing crease height (3–5 mm). However, after a brow lift and upper blepharoplasty, the height of the crease may be considerably higher than before surgery only because the patient has grown unconsciously acclimated to the lower crease after years of brow and upper-eyelid descent. The author has encountered patients who claim that their lid crease appears "unnatural" after brow lift and upper blepharoplasty, even though the lid crease height had been restored to its former position. If the mature patient is entertaining a double-eyelid procedure along with a brow lift, the double-eyelid surgery should be deferred for a minimum of 6 weeks until all brow edema has resolved. Furthermore, double-eyelid surgery should be undertaken under local anesthesia to gauge crease symmetry and height by virtue of patient cooperation. Clearly, no skin removal should be undertaken at the time of the brow lift if a double-eyelid surgery is planned at a later date so that an untrammeled surgical field can be encountered when eyelid surgery is undertaken.

If the patient has only a single eyelid crease configuration and desires upper blepharoplasty, then the surgeon can either counsel the patient about a delayed double-eyelid procedure or a concurrent upper blepharoplasty in which the incision is made at a predetermined height. The patient should understand that the incision would most likely not lead to a well-defined supratarsal crease. However, for the sake of symmetry a consensual supratarsal crease height should be chosen and marked out immediately before the procedure (see below).

Surgical Technique

1. If a concurrent brow lift is planned, the upper blepharoplasty should always be performed only after the brow lift portion of the procedure is completed. The remaining redundant eyelid skin can then be accurately assessed for removal. If the patient has had prior upper blepharoplasty, care should be taken to err on the conservative side for eyelid skin removal to avoid the potential for lagophthalmos. If a concurrent brow lift will be undertaken in an individual who has undergone previous upper blepharoplasty, it may be wiser to abstain from skin removal for 6 weeks to 3 months to ensure that too much skin is not removed.

2. Prior to entry into the operative theater, the supratarsal crease should be marked out with gentian violet, and symmetry can be confirmed with visual inspection and with a Castroviejo caliper measurement. If the patient has a poorly defined or not visible crease, the surgeon can gently roll the eyelid skin downward with the patient in the supine position to attempt to accentuate the natural crease. If this maneuver fails, then the surgeon and patient should elect to determine an arbitrary height for the supratarsal crease. To ensure that precise symmetry is maintained, the height of the crease should be measured with the lid under tension (until incipient eyelash eversion is noted), with the patient in the supine position. If the patient would like to have the supratarsal crease lowered, the extra skin can be removed below the existing crease line rather than above it, as would normally be undertaken. The crease can be lowered only depending on how much extra skin exists and only to match the side with less skin present to ensure symmetry.

3. With the patient in the supine position and the eyes in the closed position, an Allis clamp is used to pinch the redundant skin, with the inferior tine placed at the supratarsal crease (Fig. **10–25**). The amount of redundant skin to be removed is determined by the resulting eyelash position after clamping the skin: when the eyelashes begin to evert to a perpendicular position, the proper amount of skin has been grasped. The skin should be clamped down firmly at this point so that the narrow island of crimped skin will be observed.

4. The contralateral side is crimped in the same fashion, and symmetry of the proposed incision length and incision height is confirmed before skin excision is undertaken. A pair of fine scissors is used to trim the crimped skin island (Fig. **10–26**). As the skin is being removed, the surgeon should carefully inspect to ensure that he or she does not take more

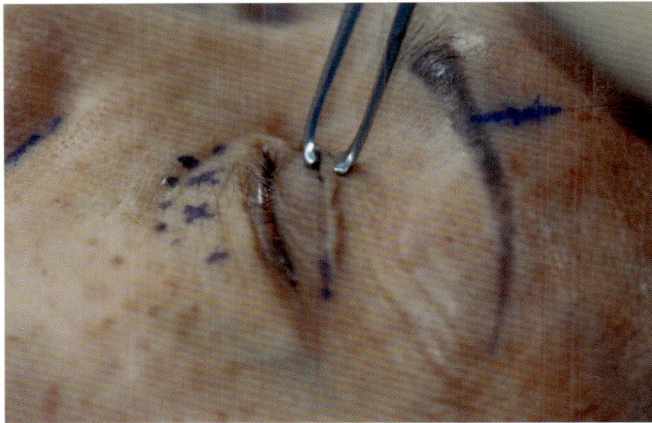

Figure 10–25 *Upper-Eyelid Blepharoplasty, Step 1:* An Allis clamp is used to crimp the redundant eyelid skin with the inferior tine placed along the marked-out supratarsal crease. The amount of skin that should be crimped is attained when the eyelash position achieves a perpendicular orientation. The contralateral side should be undertaken in the same manner, and the surgeon should ensure that symmetrical length and height of crimped skin are observed bilaterally before excising any skin.

skin than has been crimped. Typically, only skin is removed, and the underlying orbicularis muscle is left intact. This technique permits more rapid healing and less ecchymosis that would result from transection of the muscle. Of note, the skin edges may appear to be uneven after skin removal, but the surgeon must resist the temptation to trim these edges further, as this maneuver is unnecessary and may risk the potential of lagophthalmos.

5. Hemostasis is achieved with selective bipolar cautery.

6. The contralateral crimped skin island is then excised.

7. If any prolapsed medial fat was noted preoperatively, then removal of this fat should follow next. A hot-tip, handheld cautery device is used to fenestrate the orbicularis muscle and orbital septum medially over the medial fat pad. Tiny double-hook retractors are used to retract the divided muscle–septum on opposing sides. The globe is gently balloted until the fat begins to herniate through the defect. If the fat appears still to be retained behind the orbital septum, the fenestration can be widened and more deeply transected until the fat easily escapes through the defect.

8. The fat is then clamped in a hemostat and the excess amount trimmed away with a pair of fine scissors. A small cuff of adipose should remain above the clamp so that bipolar cautery can be applied along the entire length.

9. Before the hemostat is released, fine-toothed forceps are used to grasp the adipose tissue below the hemostat to ensure that there is no bleeding that could retract upon release of the hemostat tines. (The author has also made a small incision medially to remove fat only when a full incision is not required for skin removal. Generally, selective fat removal has been performed without skin removal only in the patient who has already undergone an upper blepharoplasty in the past and may risk persistent postoperative lagophthalmos.)

10. The contralateral adipose pocket is addressed in the same manner.

11. The skin is then closed with a running, nonlocking 7–0 nylon suture, carefully purchasing only a very small amount of skin on both sides of the incision to avoid lagophthalmos (Fig. **10–27**). After skin closure, it is typical to observe 1 to 2 mm of lagophthalmos that should resolve in 1 to 2 days.

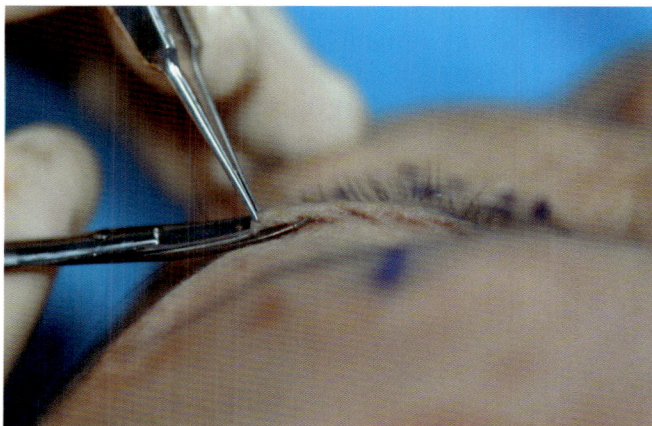

Figure 10–26 *Upper-Eyelid Blepharoplasty, Step 2:* The crimped skin island is then removed with fine scissors, ensuring that no more than the crimped skin is excised. The contralateral side is performed in the same manner.

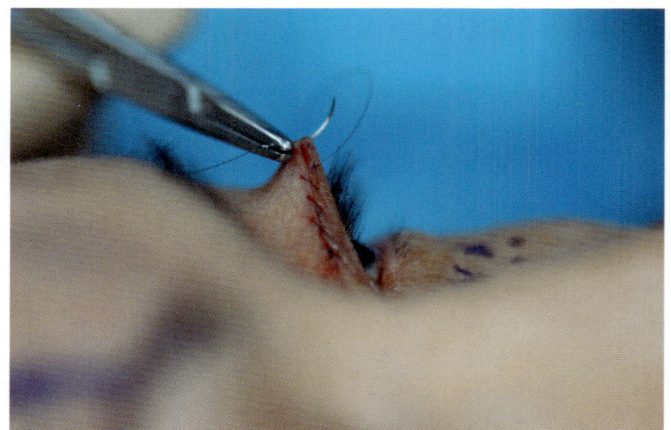

Figure 10–27 *Upper-Eyelid Blepharoplasty, Step 3:* The skin is then approximated with 7–0 nylon suture in a running, nonlocking fashion. Only the skin edges should be approximated rather than an overly generous bite of skin on each side that would otherwise predispose toward excessive lagophthalmos. The contralateral side is approached in the same manner.

12. The contralateral skin incision is then closed in the same manner.

13. Finally, 0.1 cc of triamcinolone acetonide (Kenalog) 10 mg/cc is prophylactically infiltrated into the medial aspect of the incision to minimize the risk of scarring, as the Asian skin tends to form a scar principally near the medial canthus.

Postoperative Remarks

If the patient demonstrates any evidence of lagophthalmos immediately after the procedure, the surgeon can provide the individual with a lubricating ointment (e.g., Lacrilube or an ophthalmic antibiotic solution) to be used at night until the condition resolves. Like general wound care, the incision should be cleaned two or three times per day with hydrogen peroxide so that no blood lingers over the incision site, then dressed with an antibiotic ointment (e.g., bacitracin, Neosporin, etc.) The sutures should be removed on the seventh postoperative day. The patient can then begin to apply vitamin E oil to the incision lines ~3 days after suture removal to limit scar formation. Earlier application of vitamin E may cause local irritation. Cosmetic makeup should be deferred for ~10 to 14 days, depending on patient tolerance. If the patient wears contact lenses, he or she should refrain from using them for 14 days after surgery to avoid disruption of the incision line. Unlike lower-eyelid blepharoplasty, topical ophthalmic drops are generally unnecessary except for immediate postoperative lubrication mentioned above. Milia may arise several weeks after suture removal due to trapped epithelial remnants under the approximated skin edges. Typically, these inclusion cysts will resolve spontaneously but their resolution may be expedited by unroofing them with a no. 11 blade (or 18-gauge needle) followed by gentle pressure with opposing cotton-tipped applicators to express the cyst contents. If they recur or persist, topical tretinoin (Retin-A) can also be helpful so long as the patient is counseled to be cautious about inadvertent entry of this noxious agent onto the globe.

◆ Rejuvenation of the Lower Eyelid: Transconjunctival Lower Blepharoplasty

Preoperative Remarks

Transconjunctival blepharoplasty may offer distinct advantages for rejuvenation of the Asian lower eyelid over the conventional skin–muscle technique. As an external incision in the Asian may prove to be a conspicuous entity in the postoperative setting, the transconjunctival approach offers a method of addressing the pseudoherniation of fat without risk of scar formation (Fig. 10–28A,B). Besides hypertrophic scarring, the external incision may remain obvious due to prolonged erythema or eventually become noticeable as a hypopigmented incision line contrasted against the darker surrounding skin. Furthermore, the transconjunctival approach may be associated with a lower incidence of postoperative lower-lid malposition (e.g., scleral show or frank ectropion). However, in experienced hands, these complications should remain low with either technique.

Unlike the Caucasian, the Asian eyelid exhibits the principal pathology of fat herniation rather than combined skin redundancy and fat herniation. Accordingly, the transconjunctival approach allows easy removal of fat without the need for an external incision. In the rare circumstance, a pinch of skin can be performed to remove the excess skin. By maintaining the orbicularis

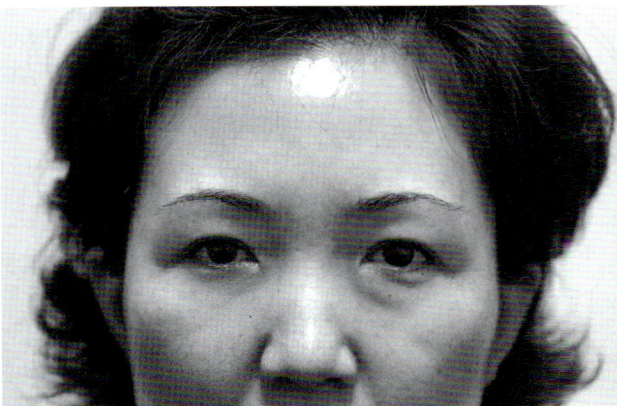

Figure 10–28   (A) This 44-year-old Korean woman underwent a skin–muscle lower-eyelid blepharoplasty 2 years before in Korea and now has return of fat herniation on the left side along with notable scars along both lower eyelids. She also exhibits some fold left sided lower-lid rounding malposition. If another skin–muscle flap would be undertaken, the hypertrophic scar and eyelid position could be further exacerbated. **(B)** Instead, the patient underwent a left-sided only transconjunctival blepharoplasty with removal of her medial and middle fat pockets. She is shown 1 week after surgery with minimal swelling and bruising and good aesthetic improvement.

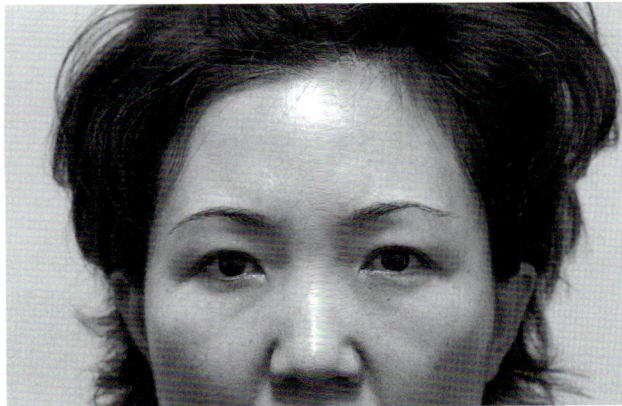

oculi sling with the transconjunctival approach, the lower-lid position is favorably maintained even when a conservative skin pinch is undertaken. To reiterate, removal of excess skin is typically not required in most Asian lower eyelids and can be deferred for 6 weeks or more after the initial operation to ensure that this additional procedure is in fact necessary.

Another benefit of a transconjunctival blepharoplasty with skin pinch over a skin–muscle flap is the relatively shorter skin incision that is possible with the former strategy. If a skin pinch is necessary, the incision ends at or just medial to the lateral canthus. When a skin–muscle flap is raised, the incision typically originates lateral to the lateral canthus. This extension of the incision past the lateral canthus with the skin–muscle flap may exhibit a greater tendency toward obvious scar formation for several reasons. The incision line falls in an area that is not camouflaged by the ciliary margin, and the thicker cheek skin does not align well with the thinner eyelid skin when approximated.

Fine rhytidosis in the lower-eyelid region is also less frequent in the Asian patient than in the Caucasian counterpart. Nevertheless, creeping and wrinkling of the skin may occur, but they are not as easily addressed. Ideally, a chemical peel offers the benefit of effacing fine wrinkles and contributes favorably to overall skin contracture, with less risk of vertical lid shortening (compared with direct skin removal). However, in darker complected Asian patients, the risk of hypo- to depigmentation is ever present, especially with higher concentrations of peeling agent. A line of demarcation may also arise between the peeled and unpeeled areas that can be aesthetically unpleasing. Accordingly, if the patient would benefit from a lower-lid peel and is fully cognizant of the attendant risks of pigmentary changes, then a chemical peel can be combined with a lower-lid transconjunctival blepharoplasty. Clearly, a lower-lid chemical peel is contraindicated with a skin–muscle flap due to the risk of flap compromise, which serves as another reason that the transconjunctival approach may be justly entertained. Furthermore, if a chemical peel is performed, a skin pinch should be deferred for several weeks to avoid the chance of vertical lid shortening. To minimize the development of any obvious line of demarcation between peeled and unpeeled skin, the chemical peel solution can be feathered by adjusting the concentration (e.g., using 35% trichloroacetic acid [TCA] in the immediate lower-eyelid region and 20% TCA more inferiorly) or by applying fewer passes of the same concentration of chemical peel as one approaches the cheek. (For more details about chemical peeling and related techniques, please consult Chapter 14.) If the patient's wrinkles are only or principally evident during animation, then botulinum toxin is the only acceptable modality to address this aesthetic problem. The patient should be fully informed of this limitation in the preoperative setting, so as to minimize confusion about the perceived benefits of lower-eyelid surgery.

Surgical Technique

1. After careful preoperative evaluation of the patient's aesthetic concerns and anatomic constraints, the surgeon can commence the operation. If a chemical peel will be undertaken, it should be completed first when the patient is still fully awake so that he or she can report inadvertent entry of peel solution into the eye. Also, the skin should be fully intact when a chemical peel is performed, so a skin pinch excision must always follow a peel. If a brow lift is entertained, a transconjunctival lower-lid blepharoplasty should be performed first, as the lower-lid skin is tightened considerably after a brow lift, making transconjunctival entry difficult.

2. With the patient sedated, 1 to 1.5 cc of 1% lidocaine mixed with 1:50,000 (or 1:100,000) epinephrine is infiltrated into the conjunctiva on each side. Care should be taken to instill sufficient local anesthesia both medially and laterally along the proposed incision line. After both sides have been injected, 10 minutes should be permitted to transpire for optimal hemostasis and anesthetic effect. During this time, the patient should have cold saline eye pads placed on the eyes to minimize postoperative bruising and swelling, and the surgical staff should assemble the required instrumentation for the operation. Of note, no sterile preparatory solution is required for a transconjunctival blepharoplasty.

3. The surgeon should be positioned comfortably in the sitting position above the patient's head, with the assistant situated to the right of both the patient and the surgeon for the entire operative case. Using headlight illumination, the surgeon gently retracts the lower eyelid downward and slightly upward with a wide, double-pronged hook, which is given to the assistant to hold. A Jaeger plate is then placed over the globe to apply countertraction on the conjunctiva and to protect the globe. Bipolar cautery is used to cauterize the arcade of superficial vessels that run anteroposteriorly along the proposed conjunctival incision line, which should fall just past the tarsal border (Fig. **10–29**).

4. A handheld, battery-operated, hot-tip cautery device is used to incise the conjunctiva medially to laterally, replacing the double-pronged hook as needed for proper retraction and exposure (Fig. **10–30**). To reiterate, the conjunctival incision should fall a millimeter or two past the tarsal border, as it is a common mistake to undertake the incision too far away from the ciliary margin,

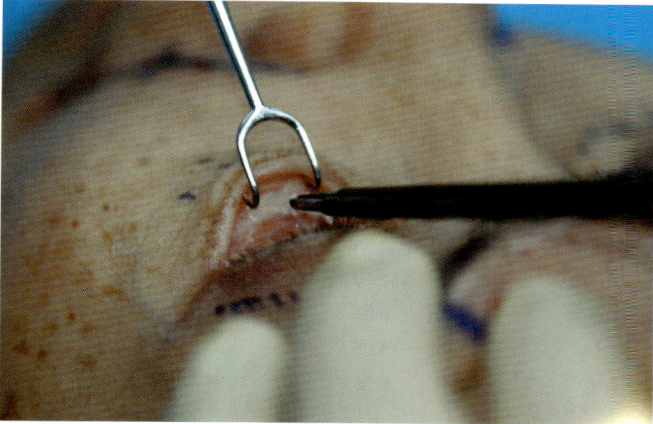

Figure 10–29 *Transconjunctival, Lower-Eyelid Blepharoplasty, Step 1:* Bipolar cautery is used to cauterize the superficial vascular arcade before conjunctival entry.

Figure 10–31 *Transconjunctival, Lower-Eyelid Blepharoplasty, Step 3:* Dissection should progress anteriorly toward the orbital rim to find the orbital fat. Gentle pressure on the globe will reveal the bulging of the fat below the orbital septum. Combination of conservative hot-tip cautery dissection and blunt cotton-tipped applicator dissection should be used to identify the fat pockets. The photograph shows the middle fat pocket (yellow color) and the medial fat pocket (pale color) exposed.

making a preseptal dissection (to be discussed) and identification of the fat pockets more onerous tasks.

5. After the conjunctiva is just superficially penetrated, a 6–0 silk suture is passed through the inferior but proximal (nearer to the surgeon) flap and pulled upward and held in place with a Mosquito clamp, which facilitates upward traction of the conjunctival flap and protection of the globe and rests on the patient's forehead.

6. The hot-tip cautery is used to deepen the incision further, aiming the instrument anteriorly (toward the bony orbital rim) so as to identify the preseptal plane, that is, the plane that divides the orbicularis oculi anteriorly from the orbital septum posteriorly.

7. Once this plane is initially developed, a cotton-tipped applicator should be used to expose the remaining plane in an atraumatic fashion. With gentle pressure on the globe, the fat to be removed should bulge through the overlying orbital septum.

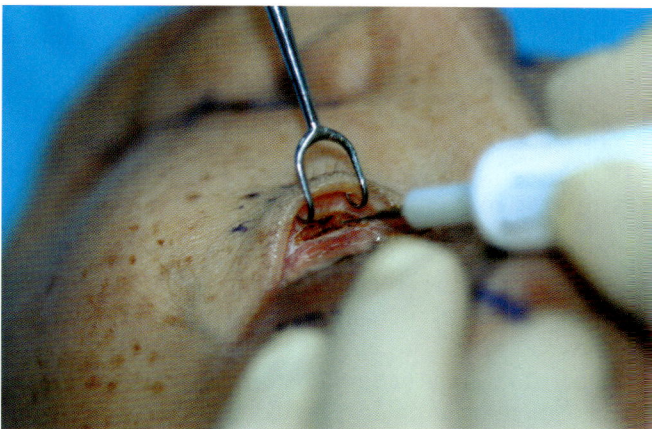

Working medially to laterally, the hot-tip cautery should be used to incise the orbital septum until the fat is fully visible. With a pair of toothed forceps, the fat can be gently teased out using a cotton-tipped applicator in the other hand. The pale, medial fat pad can be distinguished from the more yellow-colored middle fat pocket (Fig. **10–31**). The inferior oblique muscle that divides these two fat compartments can be (but need not be) identified, and injury should be avoided during fat removal.

8. With the medial fat pad exposed, 1% lidocaine *without* epinephrine can be injected into the fat pad to minimize discomfort during removal. The excess fat pad is clamped with a curved Mosquito instrument (Fig. **10–32**), and the bipolar cautery is passed

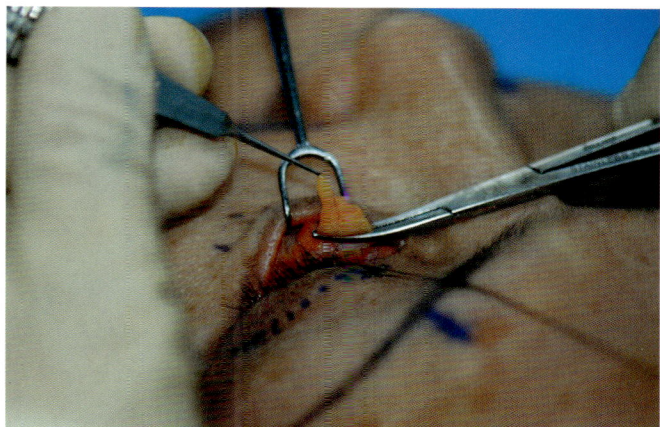

Figure 10–30 *Transconjunctival, Lower-Eyelid Blepharoplasty, Step 2:* A handheld, battery-operated, hot-tip cautery device is used to incise the conjunctiva medially to laterally.

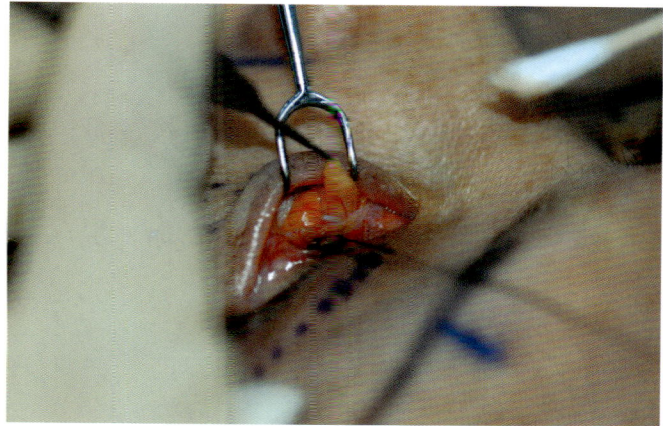

Figure 10–32 *Transconjunctival Lower-Eyelid Blepharoplasty, Step 4:* The excess fat pad is clamped with a Mosquito instrument, and bipolar cautery is passed over the clamp prior to fat excision.

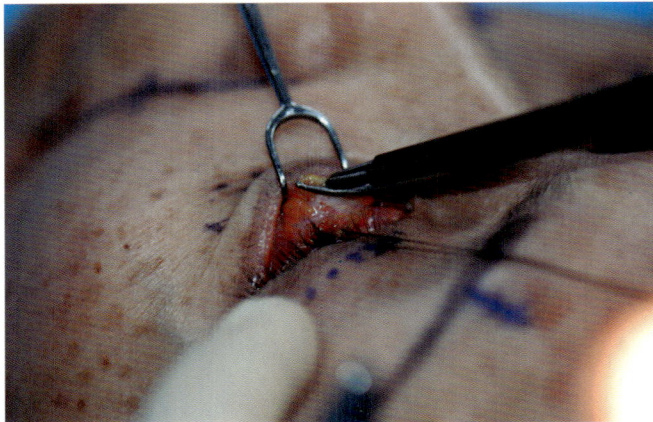

Figure 10–33 *Transconjunctival, Lower-Eyelid Blepharoplasty, Step 5:* The excess fat pad is excised, leaving a small cuff of fat over the clamp for additional bipolar cautery application.

over the clamp before fat excision. The excess, clamped fat is then trimmed with a pair of fine, sharp scissors, leaving a small cuff of fat over the clamp for additional bipolar cautery application (Fig. **10–33**).

9. When the cuff of fat appears to be thoroughly cauterized, the toothed forceps are used to hold the fat under the clamp while the clamp is gently removed (Fig. **10–34**). The fat is meticulously inspected for hemostasis prior to its release.

10. The same technique is used to remove the middle and lateral fat pockets. The patient's preoperative photographs should be prominently displayed in the operating room so that the surgeon can confirm how many fat pockets and how much fat should be removed. Oftentimes, only the medial and middle fat pockets need to be addressed. It is helpful to place the fat pads on the Mayo stand in a sequential

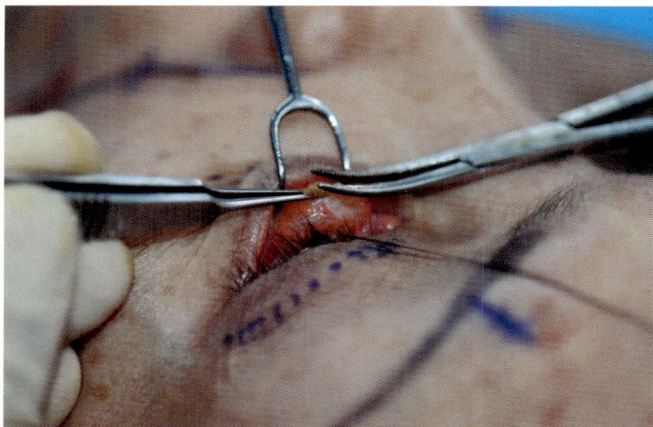

Figure 10–34 *Transconjunctival, Lower-Eyelid Blepharoplasty, Step 6:* When the cuff of fat appears to be thoroughly cauterized, the toothed forceps are used to hold the fat under the clamp while the clamp is gently removed. The fat is meticulously inspected for hemostasis prior to its release.

fashion to ensure that a symmetrical amount has been removed. No suture is needed to close the conjunctiva. Instead, the lower eyelid is gently tucked upwards to ensure that the conjunctival edges lie in good apposition. The same surgical sequence is undertaken in the contralateral eyelid.

11. If a skin pinch is planned, an Allis clamp can be used to grasp the redundant skin 1 mm below the ciliary margin until incipient eyelash eversion (as described for the upper-blepharoplasty technique). When the eyelashes appear to assume a perpendicular orientation, a sufficient amount of skin has been grasped. The tines of the Allis clamp are fully closed until an island of skin is pinched and remains heaped up after the removal of the Allis clamp. This technique is repeated along the entire length of the lower eyelid.

12. The excess skin is then carefully excised with a pair of fine scissors, taking note not to excise more skin than has been clamped. If the edges of the skin appear to be somewhat jagged, additional skin resection should not be undertaken because it is unnecessary and because this maneuver risks lagophthalmos. With the Allis clamp technique, only skin and no underlying muscle is resected. Accordingly, there should be minimal bleeding and less postoperative bruising. The muscle should not be transected, as this maneuver will result in a through-and-through eyelid defect after transconjunctival surgery.

13. The skin edges are approximated with a running, nonlocking 7–0 nylon suture from medial to lateral. The medial extent of the closure need not be tied off but should be affixed to the medial cheek with a Steri-Strip tape. The reader is reminded that no skin excision (or a very conservative amount) should be undertaken after a chemical peel to avoid potential vertical lid shortening.

14. Immediately after surgery, the patient should have ice packs placed over both eyes to lessen postoperative edema and bruising. The patient is then advised to apply these cold packs for the first 2 postoperative days and sleep in an inclined position for the first postoperative week.

Postoperative Remarks

If no skin pinch or chemical peel is done, then very little postoperative care is required. A topical antibiotic solution (e.g., tobramycin) and artificial teardrops can be used to minimize the chance of conjunctivitis and to reduce irritation in the first postoperative week, both of which can be used on an as-needed basis thereafter. If the patient has had a skin pinch, then the incision line should be cleansed two or three times daily for the first

A–C

D

E–G

H

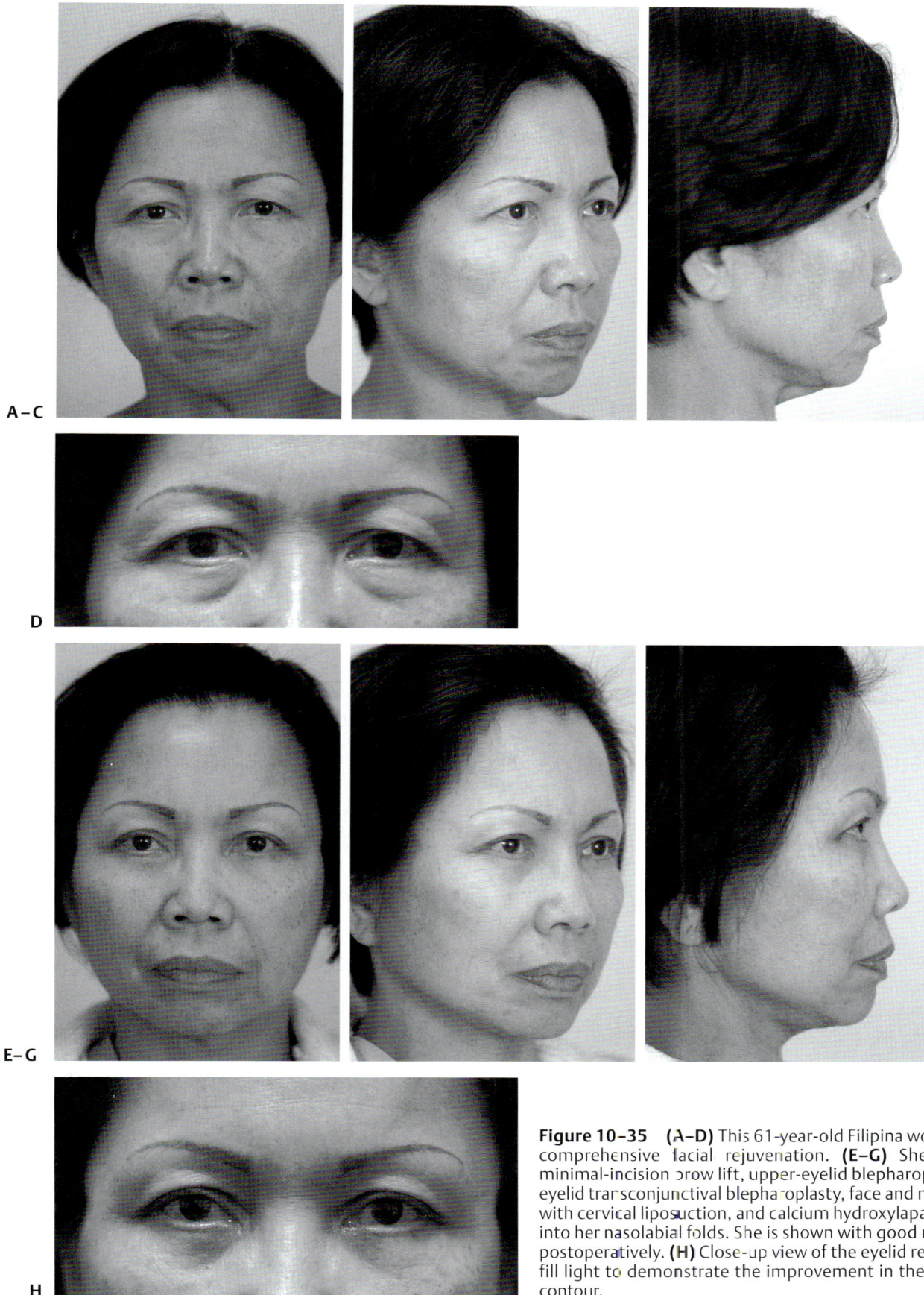

Figure 10–35 **(A–D)** This 61-year-old Filipina woman desired comprehensive facial rejuvenation. **(E–G)** She underwent minimal-incision brow lift, upper-eyelid blepharoplasty, lower-eyelid transconjunctival blepharoplasty, face and neck lift along with cervical liposuction, and calcium hydroxylapatite injection into her nasolabial folds. She is shown with good management postoperatively. **(H)** Close-up view of the eyelid region without fill light to demonstrate the improvement in the lower-eyelid contour.

postoperative week with hydrogen peroxide applied using a cotton-tipped applicator. Then, bacitracin ointment is applied to the incision line to optimize wound healing. The sutures can be removed 6 to 7 days postoperatively. For postpeel care instructions, the reader is referred to Chapter 14 for a more in-depth discussion. Contact wearers should abstain from use for the initial two weeks postsurgery to minimize irritation of the eye and to permit the conjunctival incision to heal properly.

◆ Rejuvenation of the Lower Face and Neck: SMAS Rhytidectomy

Preoperative Remarks

Generally speaking, Asians tend to exhibit a greater degree of upper than lower facial aging. The characteristic "turkey gobbler" deformity that arises from platysmal diastasis is much more commonly encountered in the fairer-skinned races than in Asian patients. Nevertheless, jowl formation is a relatively common phenomenon in Asian patients and can be readily addressed with a cervicofacial rhytidectomy. Unlike Caucasian patients, the amount of skin removal after superficial musculoaponeurotic system (SMAS) suspension also tends to be considerably less. Despite these anatomic differences, the technique that the author uses for lower facial rejuvenation is practically the same for all races. The technique is predicated on favorable incision lines that are well camouflaged, which is particularly important for the Asian, who tends to exhibit obvious incision lines if not properly fashioned (Fig. **10–35A–H**).

Surgical Technique

1. Prior to entering the operating room, the patient is appropriately marked out along the proposed incision lines, including the pre- to postauricular incision and the separate submental incision. Additionally, a line is drawn below the jawline and another along the cervicomental angle, which defines the inferior limit of dissection for the submentoplasty portion of the procedure.

2. The neck and the right side of the face are infiltrated with local anesthesia consisting of 1% lidocaine with 1:100,000 epinephrine, and 10 minutes should be allowed to transpire for adequate hemostasis and anesthetic effect.

3. A submentoplasty is always performed first. A no. 15 blade is used to make an incision immediately posterior to the submental crease for access to the neck (Fig. **10–36**).

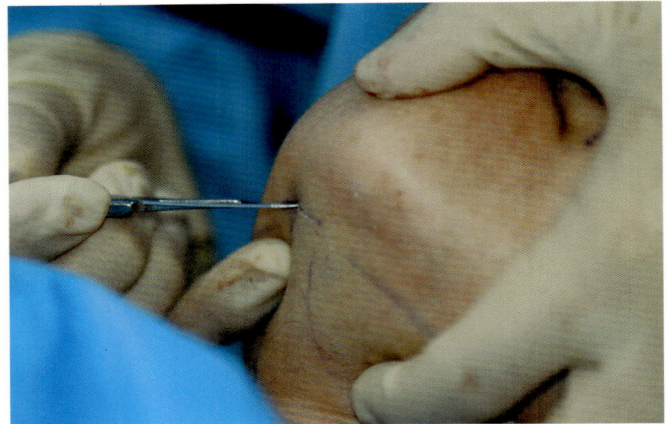

Figure 10–36   *Submentoplasty/Face Lift, Step 1:* The submentoplasty is performed first: a no.15 blade is used to make an incision immediately posterior to the submental crease.

4. Using the submental incision, wide undermining is performed with Metzenbaum scissors in the subcutaneous plane from jawline to jawline down to the line drawn through the cervicomental angle (Fig. **10–37A,B**). The scissors should not pass directly over the jawline to minimize risk to the marginal mandibular nerve, which becomes more superficial at this level.

5. A liposuction cannula is then inserted into the submental incision, and wide liposuction is performed with the suction set at the ideal setting of –29 Hg (Fig. **10–38A,B**). As per routine, the aperture of the liposuction cannula always faces the deep tissue and never the overlying flap to avoid creation of an uneven skin contour. Similarly, sharp scissor dissection precedes liposuction to avoid potential irregularity caused by the forceful tunneling of the liposuction cannula through undissected tissue.

6. After wide, even liposuctioning is performed across the entire expanse of the neck, additional treatment can be applied to the central aspect of the neck, where greater fat accumulation may be present. Selective open lipectomy can be performed as well in this region, but care should be taken not to overresect adipose tissue in this area, which may lead to a cobra deformity or an overskeletonized appearance.[8] Liposuctioning and lipectomy are critical to expose the platysmal bands that should be united next.

7. With direct visualization of the medial platysmal bands using a headlight, a 4–0 polydioxanone suture is secured inferiorly at the level of the desired cervicomental angle (Fig. **10–39A,B**). The suture is then loosely run in a nonlocking fashion up toward the submental incision. This suture should not be overtightened to avoid any bunching along the suture line.

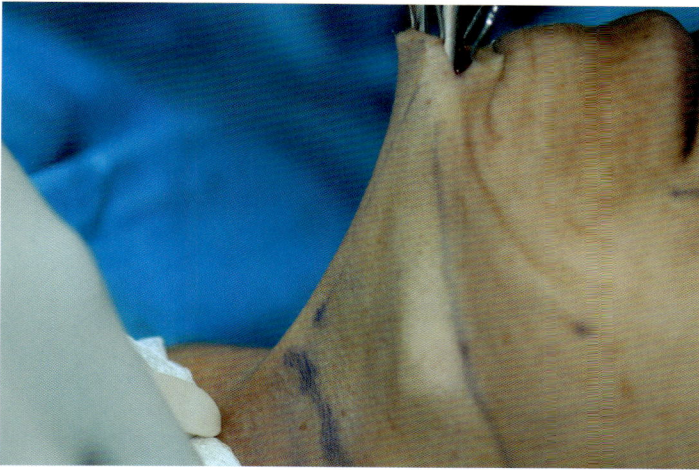

1. Dissection

A

B

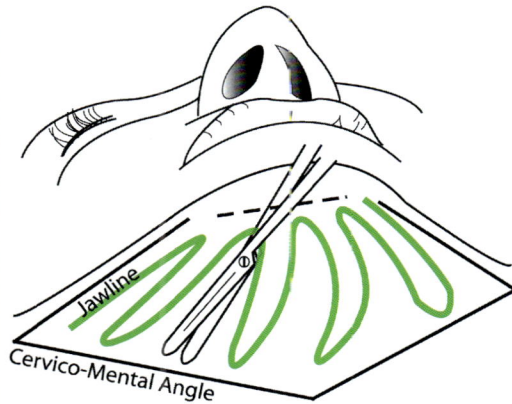

Figure 10–37 *Submentoplasty/Face Lift, Step 2:* **(A)** Metzenbaum or face lift scissors are used to undermine widely the preplatysmal flap from jawline to jawline down to the cervicomental angle. Wide, double-pronged hooks are used to retract the incision on either side. **(B)** Illustration shows the preplatysmal flap elevation with scissors. (From Williams EF, Lam SM. Comprehensive Facial Rejuvenation: A Practical and Systematic Guide to Surgical Management of the Aging Face. Philadelphia: Lippincott, Williams & Wilkins; 2004; with permission.)

8. The incision is then closed with a running, locking 6–0 polypropylene suture (Fig. **10–40**).

9. The right side of the face is approached next. A 2–0 silk suture is placed through the posterior aspect of the ear, which is then secured to a hemostat to provide retraction of the ear anteriorly when working on dissection of the postauricular territory.

10. A stab incision is made at the ear lobule–cheek interface with a no. 15 blade, and a single hook retractor is placed into this incision for inferior retraction.

11. With the ear retracted anteriorly and inferiorly, a no. 15 blade is used to incise the postauricular skin

from the lobular stab incision superiorly ~1 to 2 mm on the auricular surface rather than directly in the postauricular sulcus. (An incision directly in the sulcus will deepen and retract the ear farther back unnaturally over time.)

12. The incision is continued across the postauricular skin in a V-notched configuration toward the hairline to avoid a scar band in this region (Fig. **10–41**). The incision should traverse the postauricular skin as far superiorly as possible for optimal scar camouflage. The incision is then completed by continuing inferiorly along the hairline.

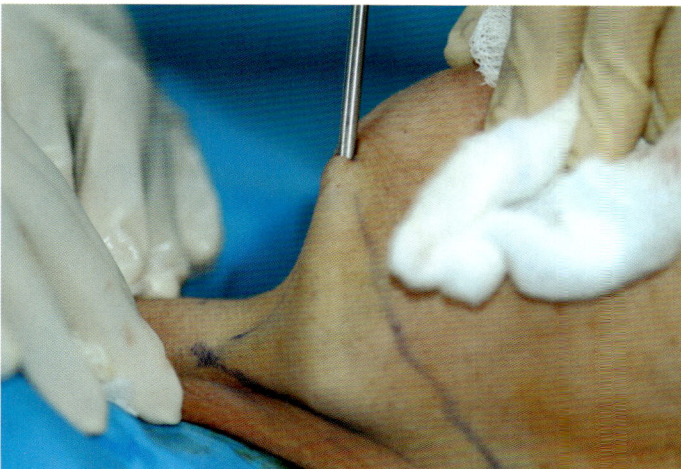

2. Liposuction

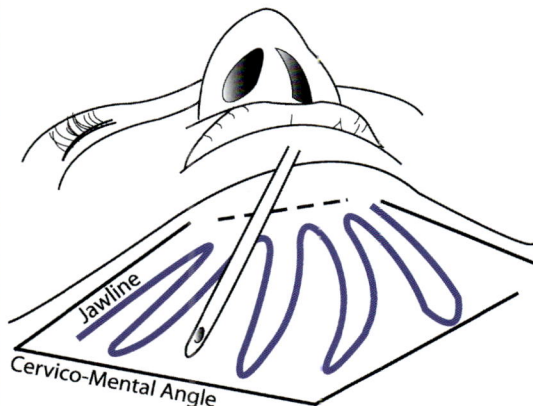

A

B

Figure 10–38 *Submentoplasty/Face Lift, Step 3:* **(A)** Liposuction cannula is then passed through this dissected preplatysmal plane from jawline to jawline, with attention paid as necessary to the submental area if a greater amount of adipose tissue is present in that region. **(B)** Illustration shows the path of the liposuction cannula. (From Williams EF, Lam SM. Comprehensive Facial Rejuvenation: A Practical and Systematic Guide to Surgical Management of the Aging Face. Philadelphia: Lippincott, Williams & Wilkins; 2004; with permission.)

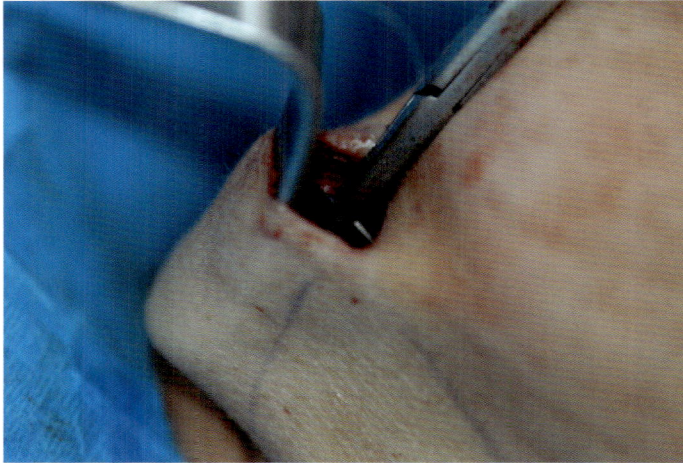

3. Platysmaplasty

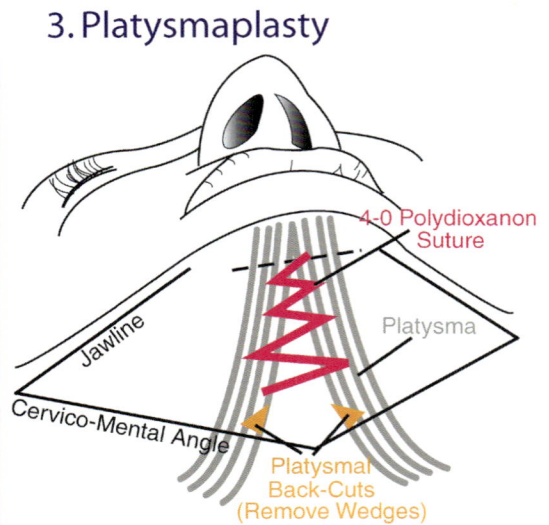

Figure 10–39 *Submentoplasty/Face Lift, Step 4:* **(A)** The exposed medial platysmal bands are then loosely approximated in a running fashion with 4–0 polydioxanone suture from the cervicomental angle to the incision. Back cuts can be made at the cervicomental angle to facilitate a more natural break at the cer- vicomental angle. **(B)** Illustration shows the closure of the platysma. (From Williams EF, Lam SM. Comprehensive Facial Rejuvenation: A Practical and Systematic Guide to Surgical Management of the Aging Face. Philadelphia: Lippincott, Williams & Wilkins; 2004; with permission.)

13. A tiny, double-hooked retractor is placed at the superior limit of the incision, and a no. 15 blade is used to initiate dissection of the postauricular flap inferiorly. The plane of dissection begins in the subcutaneous level and continues over the glistening sternocleidomastoid fascia. When the muscle is encountered, the greater auricular nerve may be injured, and the muscle may cause an undue amount of bleeding if transected. Dissection may proceed inferiorly to join the dissected neck pocket in a deliberate and careful manner using Metzenbaum or face lift scissors (Fig. **10–42**).

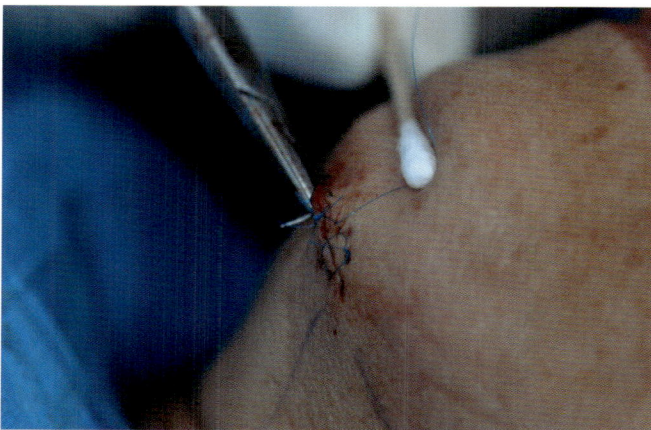

Figure 10–40 *Submentoplasty/Face Lift, Step 5:* The submental incision is closed with a running, locking 6–0 polypropylene suture.

14. A post-tragal incision is favored for optimal scar camouflage, especially in Asian patients. A no. 15 blade is used to dissect the skin inferiorly around the temporal hair tuft and continued in a curvilinear fashion around the helical crus toward the tragus. The incision is initiated again immediately inferior to the tragus toward the ear lobule to join the postauricular incision.

15. Tiny, double-hooked retractors are then used to retract the incision created immediately superior and inferior to the tragus forward while the surgeon purposefully joins the two incisions just behind the tragal cartilage. The no. 15 blade is used to continue dissection in the subcutaneous plane anteriorly until the flap is elevated across the entire preauricular expanse for a distance of several centimeters (Fig. **10–43A–C**).

16. Wide, double-pronged retractors then replace the tiny hooked retractors, and the face lift scissors are used to dissect the skin flap forward by pushing the scissor anteriorly with the tines held slightly open (Fig. **10–44A,B**). The flap is then joined with the neck and postauricular flaps. Dissection along the jawline should be limited to less than half of the distance toward the midline, as the marginal mandibular branch of the facial nerve and the facial vessels lie near the middle aspect of the jawline.

17. The wide double hooks are removed and replaced with Army-Navy retractors. Approximately a 2 to 3 cm path of SMAS tissue should be removed anterior to

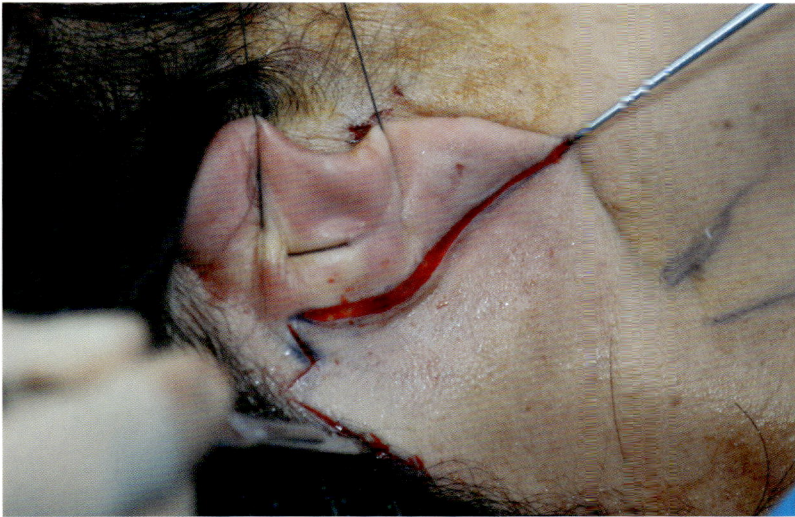

Figure 10–41 *Submentoplasty/Face Lift, Step 6:* The face lift begins with the postauricular incision. A 2–0 silk suture is used to retract the ear forward, and a single hook is placed into a stab incision at the ear lobule for retraction of the skin inferiorly, as seen. A no. 15 blade is used to incise the skin 1 to 2 mm on the ear along the postauricular sulcus and continued along the hairline. A V notch is created superiorly across the postauricular scalp when transitioning toward the hairline to avoid scar contracture in this region.

the ear to permit imbrication of the SMAS over this defect (Fig. **10–45A,B**).

18. The first SMAS-suspension suture is placed along the jawline to improve the descended jowl region (Figs. **10–45B, 10–46A,B**).

19. A CV-3 Gore-Tex suture is used to retract the neck tissue in a superoposterior vector to re-create the neckline. The suture should fall anterior to the sternocleidomastoid to avoid ensnaring the greater auricular nerve, which may lead to a painful neuroma (Figs. **10–45B, 10–47**).

20. Finally, one or two sutures are placed more superiorly to lift the cheek and facial tissues in a superoposterior vector (Figs. **10–45B, 10–48A,B**)

21. Trimming of redundant skin and suspension begins along the temporal tuft first. Two hemostats are

placed along the preauricular skin flap and drawn without tension in a posterosuperior vector. The redundant skin along the temporal tuft is resected in a tapering fashion anteriorly, and this incision is then closed with a running locking 5–0 nylon suture (Fig. **10–49A–E**).

22. Two hemostats are placed to draw the postauricular skin flap posterosuperiorly without tension, and the redundant skin is resected. The reader is reminded that the V-notch configuration should be re-created (Fig. **10–50**). Also, the amount of redundant skin in Asians may be considerably less than in Caucasian counterparts. The superior aspect of the flap is then secured with two or three interrupted 5–0 chromic sutures (Fig. **10–51**).

23. The incision along the hairline is then closed with surgical staples (Fig. **10–52**).

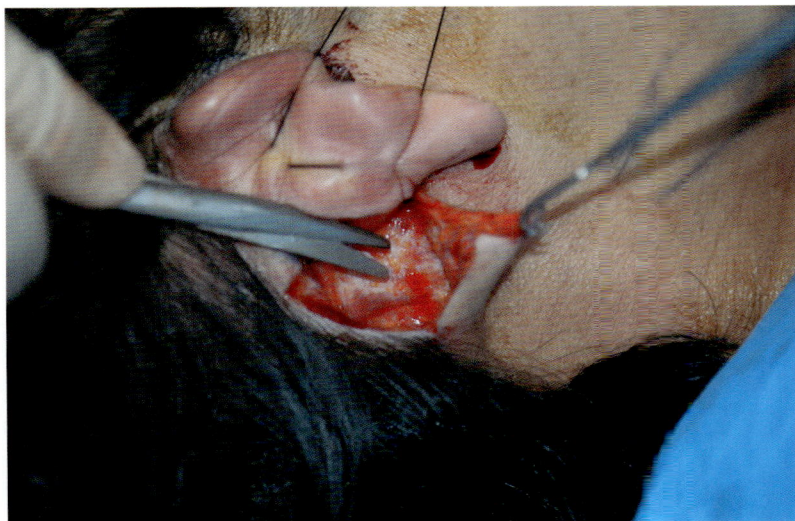

Figure 10–42 *Submentoplasty/Face Lift, Step 7:* Postauricular dissection is begun with a no. 15 blade, and Metzenbaum scissors are used to complete the postauricular flap inferiorly. Care is taken to remain over the glistening surface of the sternocleidomastoid fascia and to avoid inadvertent injury to the tail of the parotid and great auricular nerve in that area.

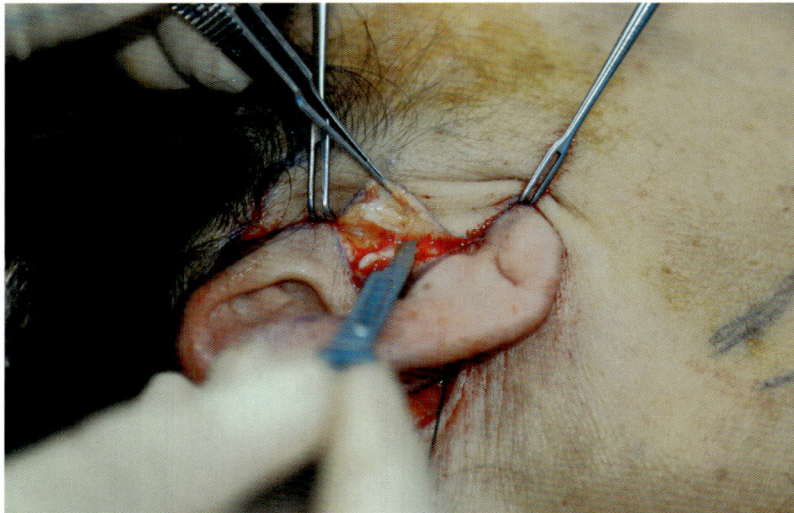

A

Female Face Lift Incisions

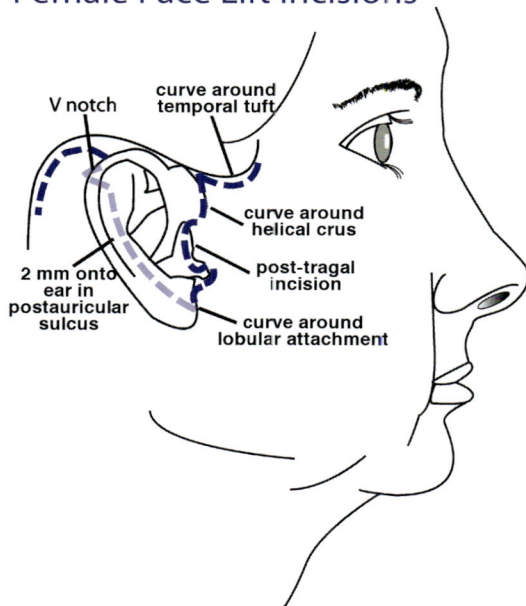

V notch

curve around
temporal tuft

curve around
helical crus

post-tragal
incision

curve around
lobular attachment

2 mm onto
ear in
postauricular
sulcus

Male Face Lift Incisions

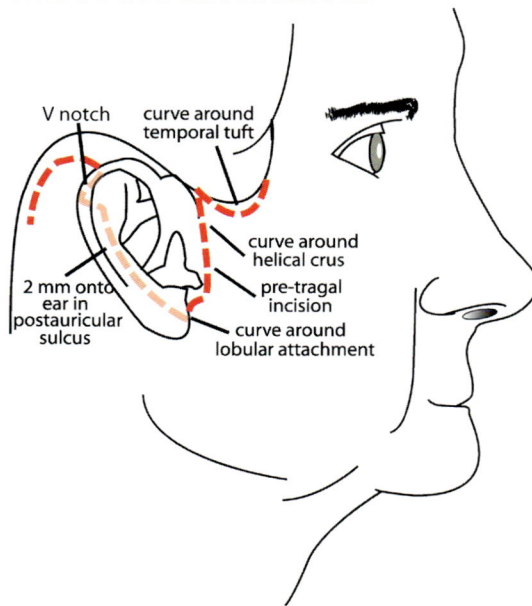

V notch

curve around
temporal tuft

curve around
helical crus

pre-tragal
incision

curve around
lobular attachment

2 mm onto
ear in
postauricular
sulcus

B

C

Figure 10–43 *Submentoplasty/Face Lift, Step 8:* **(A)** The preauricular incision is performed with a no.15 blade around the temporal tuft and toward the ear lobule, leaving the tragal skin uncut. Tiny double hooks are placed on either side of the tragus, and the no.15 blade is used to complete the post-tragal incision. The photograph shows the dissection in the subcutaneous plane with a no.15 blade in the area of the tragus. **(B)** A post-tragal incision is preferred in women, especially those who are darker complected, to avoid an obvious incision line. The incision is carried around the temporal tuft to preserve hair in this region. The postauricular incision is carried high into the postauricular sulcus to avoid a conspicuous incision, especially in an individual with a short or pulled-back hairstyle. **(C)** A pretragal incision is preferred in men to avoid the burden of shaving onto the tragus every day. The placement of the incision anteriorly is dependent upon the depth of the pretragal fold versus the location of where the natural beard distribution begins and how close the male patient is willing to shave near the ear. If the patient has very sparse or no beard near the ear area, a post-tragal incision may be performed.

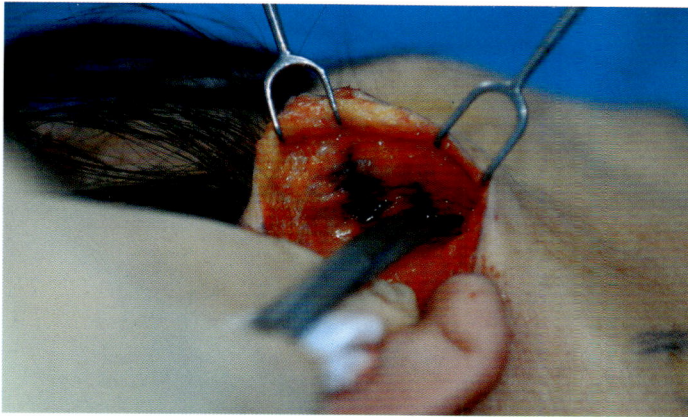

Figure 10–44 *Submentoplasty/Face Lift, Step 9:* **(A)** The wide, double-pronged retractors are used to replace the tiny hook retractors, as the flap is further elevated. A pair of Metzenbaum or face lift scissors is used to continue raising the remaining preauricular flap. Subcutaneous dissection should progress anteriorly until the underlying SMAS tissue can be easily mobilized: a pair of Brown-Adson forceps can be used to pull the SMAS back to determine whether further subcutaneous dissection is warranted. **(B)** Care should be taken not to pass the midpoint of the mandible to avoid injury to the marginal mandibular branch of the facial nerve. The marginal mandibular branch becomes relatively superficial ~2 cm posterior and inferior to the oral commissure; and the facial artery and vein lie proximal to the nerve in this region. Accordingly, care should be taken to cauterize any bleeding in this area.

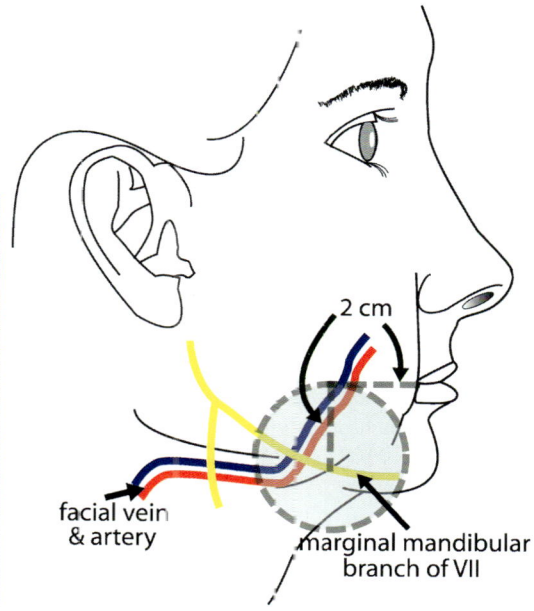

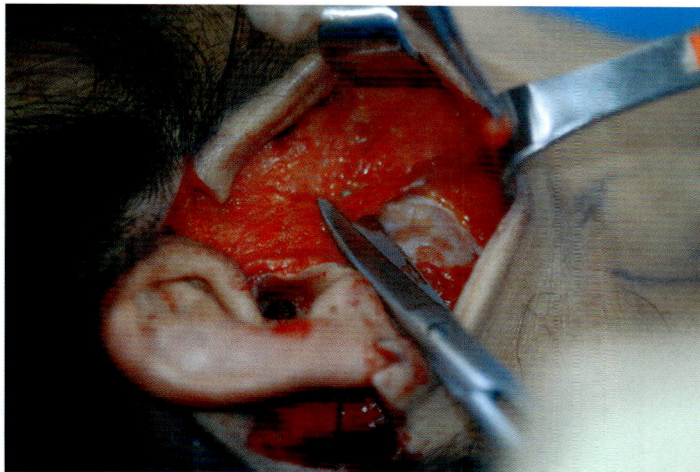

Figure 10–45 *Submentoplasty/Face Lift, Step 10:* **(A)** A strip of SMAS should be excised in the preauricular region to reduce the tissue redundancy when the SMAS is imbricated. **(B)** Illustration shows the area of SMAS excision as well as the three vectors of SMAS suture suspension. From Williams EF, Lam SM. Comprehensive Facial Rejuvenation: A Practical and Systematic Guide to Surgical Management of the Aging Face. Philadelphia: Lippincott, Williams & Wilkins; 2004; with permission.

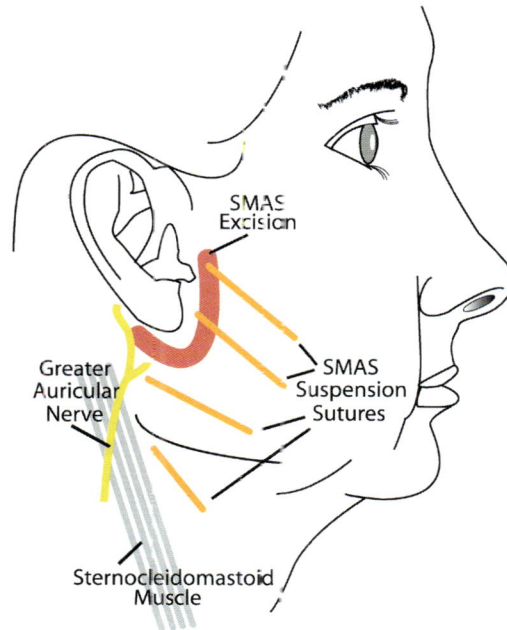

A   B

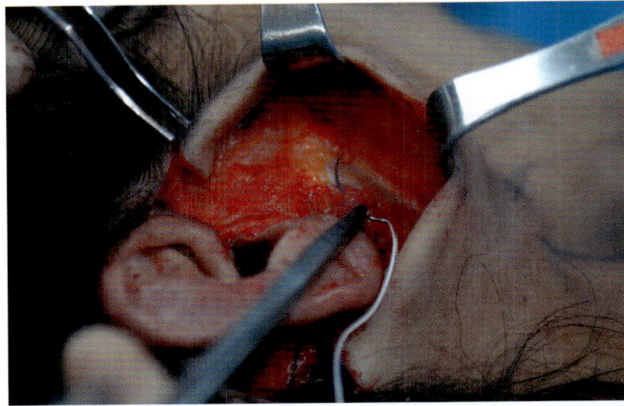

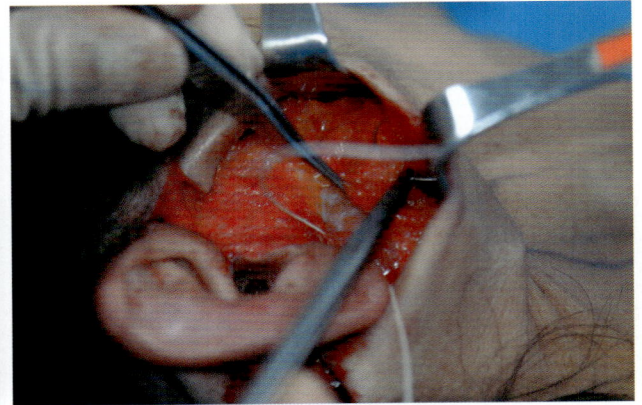

Figure 10–46   *Submentoplasty/Face Lift, Step 11:* **(A,B)** A CV-3 Gore-Tex suture is used to retract the jawline back, with the first suture placed nearer to the ear to bury the suture knot.

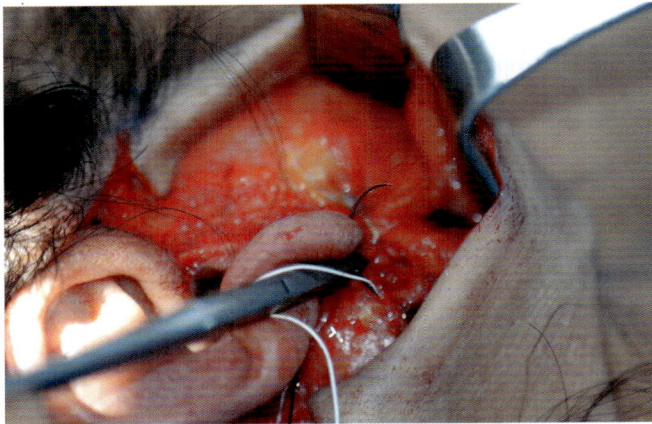

Figure 10–47   *Submentoplasty/Face Lift, Step 12:* The following suture is placed again near the ear inferiorly (shown) and then placed further anteroinferiorly (not shown) in the neck to restore the neckline. As the suture is cinched down, the surgeon should be able to observe the suspension of the neck tissue. Care should be taken to avoid placement of any suture behind the sternocleidomastoid muscle to circumvent injuring the greater auricular nerve and thereby cause a painful neuroma to arise.

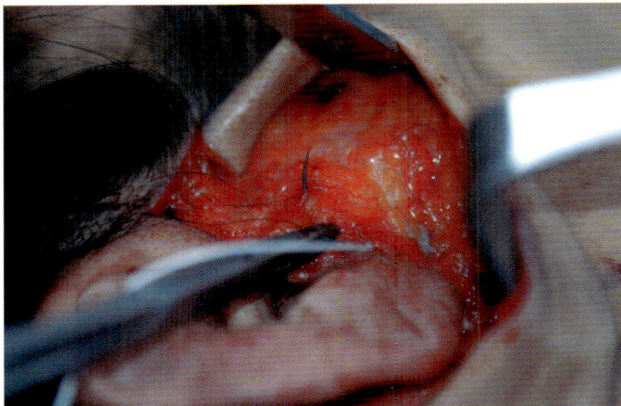

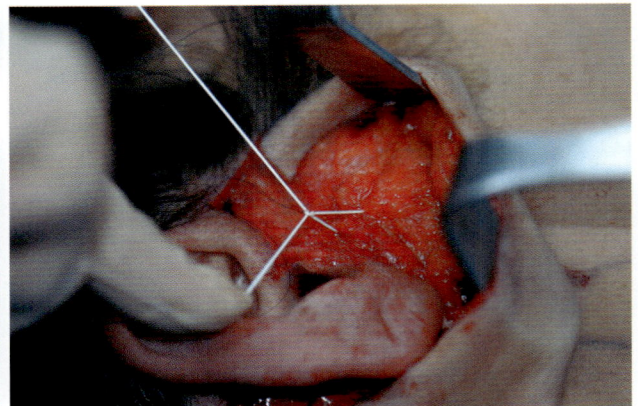

A   B

Figure 10–48   *Submentoplasty/Face Lift, Step 13:* **(A)** The final one or two sutures are placed higher to suspend the cheek tissue superoposteriorly, as illustrated in Fig. **10–45B**. **(B)** The photograph shows the correct manner of tying a Gore-Tex suture: a square knot should be thrown in midair and cinched down until the proper amount of tissue suspension is attained. Additional five or six knots should be placed to prevent slippage of the knot.

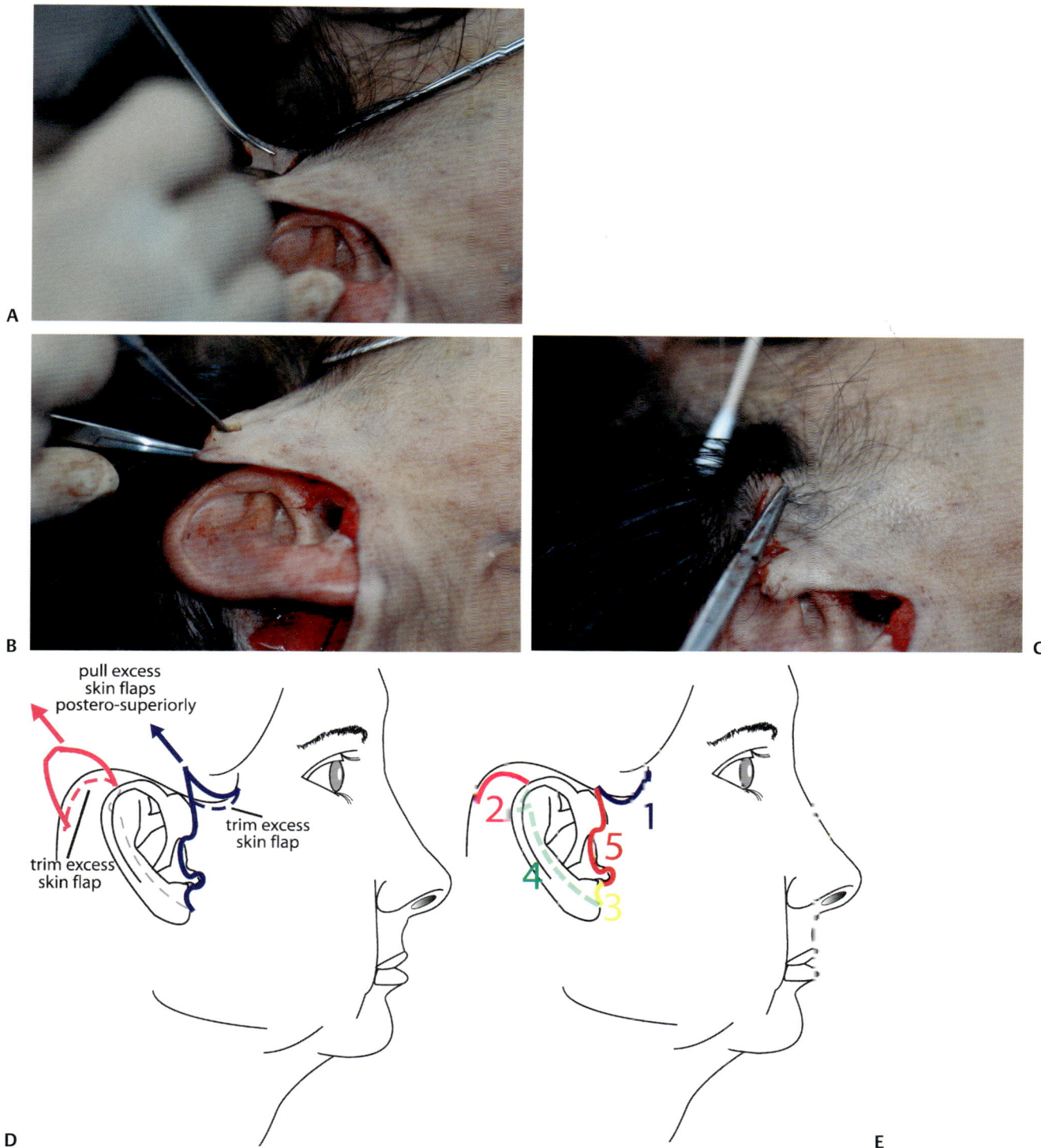

Figure 10–49 *Submentoplasty/Face Lift, Step 14:* **(A)** Trimming of redundant skin begins with the temporal tuft. Two hemostats are placed along the corners of the preauricular flap and gently drawn back without tension in a posterosuperior vector. A single-pronged hook is placed at the anterior limit of the temporal incision but not retracted with any degree of tension. The redundant skin is trimmed in a tapering fashion from anterior to posterior, with a greater amount of skin removed posteriorly and a smaller amount, removed anteriorly (Refer to Fig. **10–49D.**) **(B)** A small incision is made at the posterior limit of the temporal incision to indicate where the temporal suture should end. **(C)** A 5–0 nylon suture is used to close the temporal incision in a running, locking fashion. **(D)** The illustration shows the posterosuperior vector that the redundant skin should be drawn back for trimming in both the temporal tuft and postauricular flap regions. **(E)** The illustration shows the order in which the skin should be trimmed and reset: (1) temporal tuft, (2) postauricular hairline, (3) ear lobe, (4) postauricular sulcus, (5) preauricular area. (From Williams EF, Lam SM. Comprehensive Facial Rejuvenation: A Practical and Systematic Guide to Surgical Management of the Aging Face. Philadelphia: Lippincott, Williams & Wilkins; 2004; with permission.)

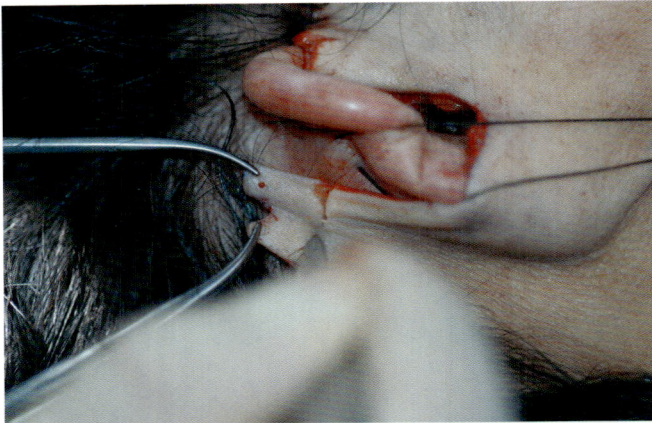

Figure 10–50 *Submentoplasty/Face Lift, Step 15:* The postauricular flap is then redraped and suspended next. Two hemostats are placed on two corners of the postauricular flap to draw it posterosuperiorly without any tension, and the redundant skin is resected in a V configuration.

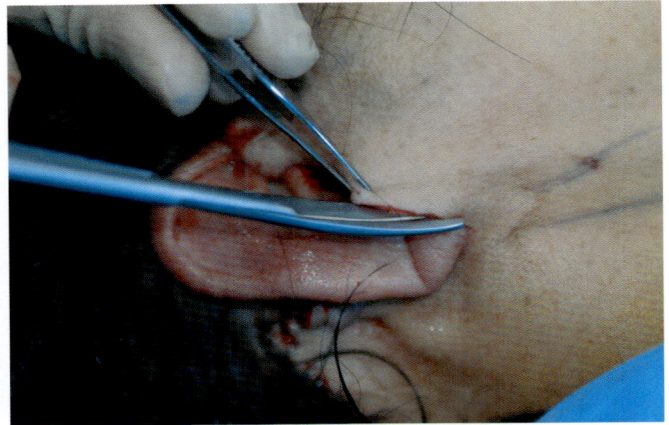

Figure 10–51 *Submentoplasty/Face Lift, Step 16:* The points of the V-shaped incision are approximated with interrupted 5–0 chromic sutures.

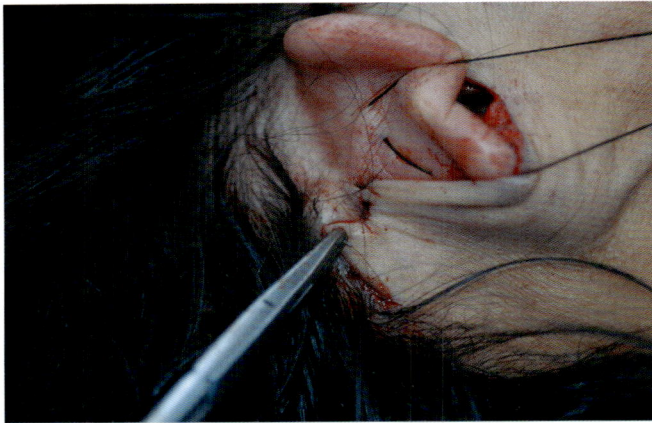

Figure 10–52 *Submentoplasty/Face Lift, Step 17:* The incision along the hairline is then closed with surgical staples.

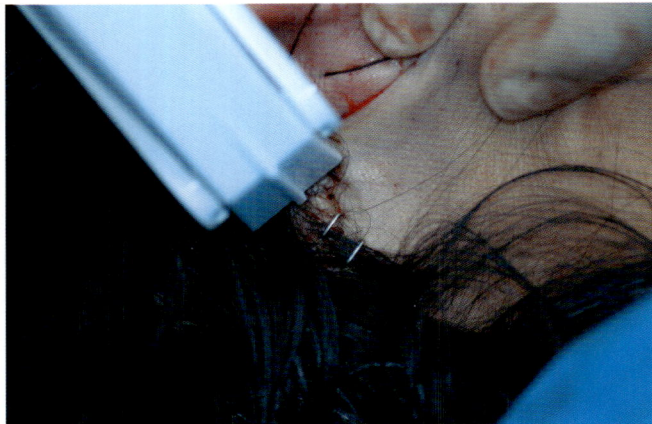

Figure 10–53 *Submentoplasty/Face Lift, Step 18:* At this point, the contralateral side should be infiltrated with local anesthesia. The ear lobule is then exposed with sharp Metzenbaum or face lift scissors. The surgeon should aim to be conservative when cutting down to expose the ear lobule to prevent the skin flap from drawing the lobule excessively downward, which would translate into a pixie-ear deformity. The ear lobule is then secured in its new position with a 5–0 chromic suture.

24. At this time, the surgeon should infiltrate the contralateral face with the same anesthetic regimen (1% lidocaine with 1:100,000 epinephrine) before completing work on the right side of the face.

25. Returning to the right hemiface, the surgeon should carefully transect the extra skin tissue toward the ear lobule until the lobule is fully exposed (Fig. **10–53**). Of note, the surgeon should always err on the conservative side when exposing the ear lobule because the eventual weight of the flap may draw the lobule farther down to cause a pixie-ear deformity. The exposed ear lobule is then secured to the transected skin flap with an interrupted 5–0 chromic suture.

26. The excess postauricular flap is trimmed away (Fig. **10–54**), and the postauricular incision is closed with a running, nonlocking 5–0 chromic suture. Halfway through this closure, half the length of an 8-French red rubber catheter is inserted into the incision as a drain that will be removed on the first postoperative day (Fig. **10–55**).

27. The preauricular flap is trimmed away to re-create the new tragus (Figs. **10–56, 10–57**), and the tragal portion of the flap is thinned by removing excessive subcutaneous adipose tissue to simulate the naturally thin tragal skin (Fig. **10–58**). To re-create the pretragal dimple, a single 5–0 chromic suture can be used in a buried fashion to draw the pretragal skin down.

28. The preauricular flap is approximated with a running, nonlocking 6–0 polypropylene suture (Fig. **10–59**).

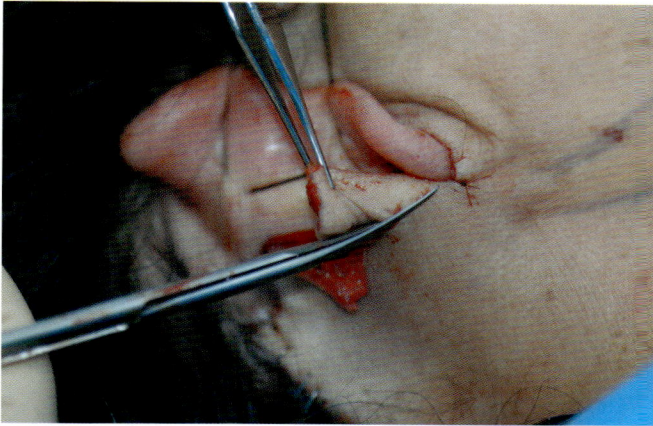

Figure 10–54   *Submentoplasty/Face Lift, Step 19:* The flap along the postauricular sulcus is trimmed away in preparation for closure with a running 5–0 chromic suture.

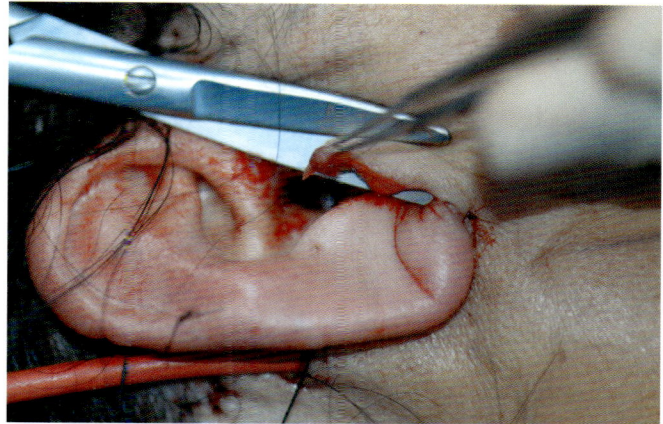

Figure 10–57   *Submentoplasty/Face Lift, Step 22:* The inferior half of the preauricular flap that encompasses the tragus to the ear lobule is removed with a slight curve that matches the tragal contour and a reverse curve that extends down the remaining distance to the ear lobule.

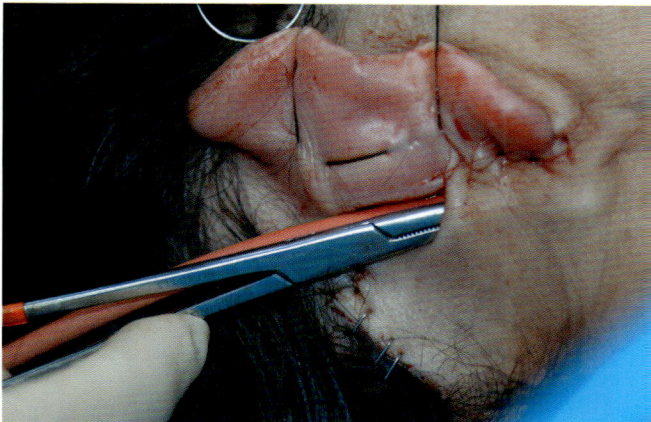

Figure 10–55   *Submentoplasty/Face Lift, Step 20:* Halfway through the closure of the postauricular sulcus, half the length of an 8-French red rubber catheter is inserted into the incision a a drain that will be removed on the first postoperative day.

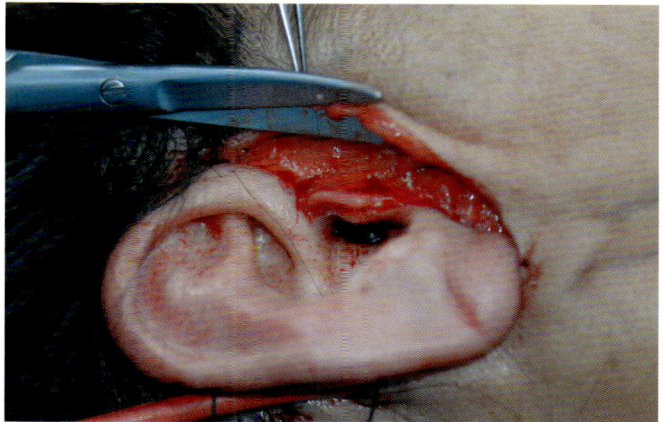

Figure 10–58   *Submentoplasty/Face Lift, Step 23:* The subcutaneous fat is trimmed away from the tragus to thin the flap sufficiently to mimic a normal tragal contour.

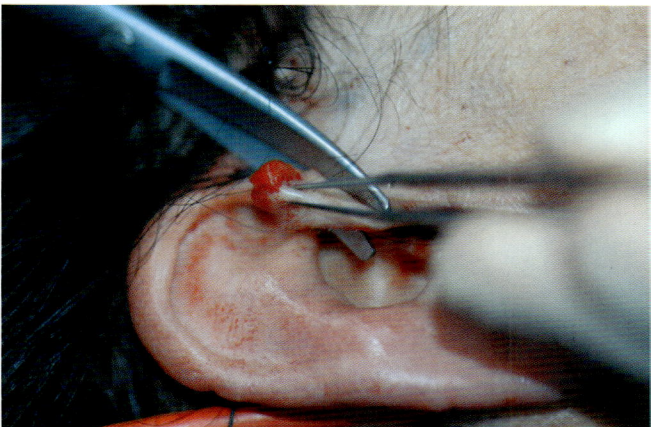

Figure 10–56   *Submentoplasty/Face Lift, Step 21:* The excess preauricular flap is then trimmed, starting with the curvilinear portion that extends around the helical crus from the tempora tuft down to the tragus.

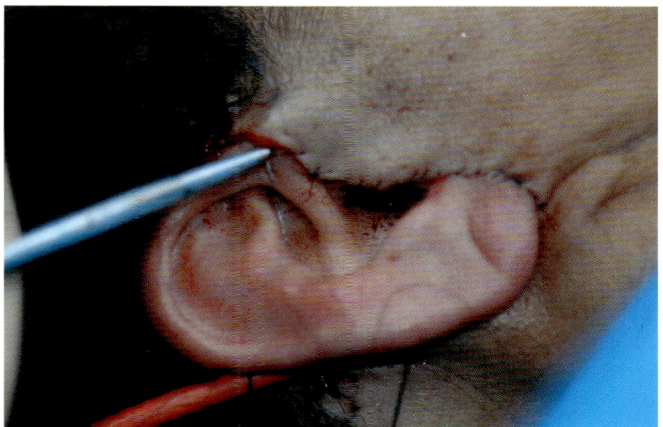

Figure 10–59   *Submentoplasty/Face Lift, Step 24:* The preauricular flap is then closed with a running, nonlocking 6–0 polypropylene suture. The contralateral side is approached in the same manner described above for the right face.

29. The contralateral side is approached in the exact same manner.

30. After bacitracin is applied to all of the incision sites, a pressure dressing is applied circumferentially around the head with a 3 inch conforming bandage (Kling) and 4 × 4 gauze.

Postoperative Remarks

The patient is seen the first postoperative day, and the heavy bandage is removed. The red rubber catheters that serve as postauricular drains are removed, and the incisions are cleaned with peroxide and redressed with bacitracin ointment. The patient has a lighter dressing reapplied, which the patient removes at home the following day. Showering can resume on the second postoperative day when the second, lighter dressing is removed. After the lighter dressing is removed, the patient should wear an Ace-style bandage (not wrapped very tightly) from the top of the head to under the chin for 1 to 2 weeks thereafter to minimize and expedite resolution of edema. For the first 2 postoperative days, the patient should be reminded to apply ice packs liberally to minimize edema and thereby expedite recovery. The patient is seen again on the seventh postoperative day to remove all of the sutures. The patient is reminded to avoid any hot packs, curling irons, or hair dryers during the first 6 weeks, when sensation may be compromised and the flap may thereby be thermally injured.

◆ Conclusion

Surgical strategies for management of the aging Asian face do not differ markedly from those that the author uses for the Caucasian face. However, incisions may remain conspicuous for a very long time in the Asian, and well-designed and executed incisions are a critical cornerstone for successful surgery in the Asian face. For instance, a transconjunctival blepharoplasty offers the advantage of a scarless surgical endeavor. Furthermore, insertion of augmentation materials into the smile lines through incisions in the central face should be undertaken only if the patient is fully cognizant that these incisions may remain noticeable for several weeks to months (see Chapter 11). Because Asian skin tends to heal poorly (prolonged erythema, hyperpigmentation, hypopigmentation, and risk of scarring), resurfacing techniques must be used selectively in the Asian face (see Chapter 14). Judicious application of surgical and dermatological procedures for the Asian face that limit the recovery period will ultimately yield a satisfied patient.

References

1. Shirakabe Y, Suzuki Y, Lam SM. A new paradigm for the aging Asian face. Aesthetic Plast Surg, 2003; 27:397–402
2. Williams EF, Lam SM. Comprehensive Facial Rejuvenation: A Practical and Systematic Guide to Surgical Management of the Aging Face. Philadelphia: Lippincott, Williams & Wilkins; 2004
3. Cook TA, Brownrigg PJ, Wang TD, Quatela VC. The versatile midforehead browlift. Arch Otolaryngol Head Neck Surg 1989;115:163–168
4. Knize DM. An anatomically based study of the mechanism of eyebrow ptosis. Plast Reconstr Surg 1996;97:1321–1333
5. Cook BE Jr, Lucarelli MJ, Lemke BN. Depressor supercilii muscle: anatomy, histology, and cosmetic implications. Ophthal Plast Reconstr Surg 2001;17:404–411
6. Lemke BN, Stasior OG. The anatomy of eyebrow ptosis. Arch Ophthalmol 1982;100:981–986
7. Lam SM, Williams EF. Midfacial rejuvenation via an endoscopic browlift approach: a review of technique. Facial Plast Surg 2003;19:147–156
8. Kamer FM, Minoli JJ. Postoperative platysmal band deformity: a pitfall of submental liposuction. Arch Otolaryngol Head Neck Surg 1993;119:193–196

11

Implants in the Asian Face

◆ General and Anatomic Considerations

Although nasal implants are a mainstay of Asian rhino plasty, facial implants elsewhere constitute a less customary desire for the Asian patient. A characteristic anatomic deficit that many Asians exhibit is maxillary and premaxillary hypoplasia. However, despite this skeletal deficiency, some Asian patients tend to be wary of augmentation in this region even if they concur that a higher malar eminence would be aesthetically pleasing. Their reservation stems partly from cultural unfamiliarity with this type of procedure, making it appear seemingly more ominous and even unnecessary. Interestingly many Asian cultures actually do not desire a prominent malar eminence. Unlike Western cultures that prize a well-defined cheekbone as an attribute of feminine beauty, Asian societies often perceive a high malar prominence as a masculine trait, which combined with a square jawline makes the face appear overly boxy (refer to Chapter 12). Furthermore, augmentation mentoplasty is oftentimes perceived as a superfluous undertaking in overall facial harmony, despite digital imaging that may contravene this notion. However, mounting assimilation of second- and third-generation Asians in Western society has encroached on traditional perspectives in favor of adoption of Western ideals and customs. Therefore, the role of facial implants (e.g., malar and chin) will probably continue to rise in popularity among Asians reared in the West.

Although malar and chin augmentations constitute familiar forms of implant surgery in the West, the unique Asian skeletal structure favors other types of alloplastic enhancement. Premaxillary retrusion is a common finding that is characterized by an acute nasolabial angle and contributes to a primate-like facies.

These implants serve as effective adjuncts to rhinoplasty or equally well as an independent procedure. A relative zygomatic prominence in the Asian face creates a hollowed appearance in the temporal fossa that may be deemed unappealing. Temporal implants have received some interest in Asia but have also met with complications involving instability and mobility due to the activity of the overlying temporalis musculature. The posteriorly inclined forehead has also been construed as an unattractive feature in some Asian women, and silicone implants have been advocated to address this undesirable contour. However, similar to temporal implants, forehead implants may suffer from displacement secondary to the active frontalis muscle.

As a general rule implants that succeed particularly well are anchored to a fixed underlying bony structure (malar, nasal, chin) and are not subject to mobile forces. For instance, lip augmentation with solid alloplasts (a relatively uncommon request by Asians) has a higher likelihood for extrusion, infection, and mobility than more stable sites. In addition to the lip, the nasolabial and labiomandibular folds have been increasingly more popular areas for facial rejuvenation with alloplastic implants and may suffer fewer complications than lip augmentation. Implants can soften these unappealing folds, which may be relatively more accentuated in the Asian patient owing to a substantial buccal fat pad and less defined malar skeletal framework. Despite the benefit that solid implants may afford the central facial region, incisions (even very short ones) may remain quite visible for a long time after surgery in the Asian patient, making this option less than ideal. For this reason, the author prefers to use injectable implants in the smile lines and marionette lines in Asian patients when possible unless the patient is willing to accept the likelihood of visible incision lines that may endure for several months, if not longer.

Currently, many options exist for soft-tissue or skeletal augmentation, of which solid implants constitute only one alternative. Liquid injectables may offer a viable solution for soft-tissue defects, but permanent injectable materials that cannot be easily removed following overinjection, infection, or late granuloma formation should be used with great caution. Various strategies for augmentation with injectable agents are reviewed in Chapter 13. This chapter focuses primarily on surgical methods of solid implantation. A versatile but potentially more invasive option for aesthetic augmentation is skeletal surgery that permits both reduction and augmentation and may also correct any orthognathic disharmonies. This type of surgery is covered in detail in Chapter 12, which is devoted to bony reduction and advancement procedures.

Many materials abound for solid-implant augmentation. Traditionally, silicone has proven to be a well-tolerated alloplast that achieves its stability by fibrous capsule formation. Softer versions of this material that have been developed facilitate a lower extrusion rate in the nose. Many forms of expanded polytetrafluoroethylene (Gore-Tex, Advanta, Ultrasoft, etc.) have also entered the marketplace and have proven to be a reliable method for augmentation in the chin, cheek, nose, and elsewhere. The limited fibrous ingrowth of surrounding tissue enhances stability but still permits ease of removal. Polyamide mesh (Mersilene) may be a relatively inexpensive, well-tolerated, and stable implant for the chin and premaxillary regions but may be difficult to extract if this occasion should arise. Surgical preference and experience dictate implant selection, but all of the above implants have withstood the test of time and merit inclusion in the surgical armamentarium. As mentioned before, the main limiting factor for the Asian patient when considering solid implantation is the risk of obvious incision lines in the central portion of the face that remain conspicuous for an extended period of time. A detailed preoperative consultation, weighing the risks and benefits of each surgical procedure for the patient, will minimize postoperative dissatisfaction.

◆ Premaxillary Augmentation

Although premaxillary augmentation may appear to be a subject worthy of inclusion in a broader treatment of Asian rhinoplasty, this type of implant may not always be combined with rhinoplasty. Therefore, a separate section has been dedicated to this type of implant as an independent procedure, and the reader is encouraged to use this implant as deemed indicated. Although

maxillary hypoplasia may not be considered an unfavorable trait in certain Asian cultures, premaxillary deficiency is more universally dismissed as an unpleasant feature.

The premaxilla describes the midline bony segment that is bordered by the incisive foramina. Therefore, this osseous region lies immediately below the nose and constitutes the central upper lip. Premaxillary hypoplasia can impact on the surrounding structures, rendering the nasal tip relatively ptotic, the nasolabial angle acute, and the upper lip incompetent (Fig. **11–1A,B**). The overall profile that results is reminiscent of a more simian appearance.[1] Besides prevalence of this condition in certain pathologic diseases (e.g., cleft lip deformity and Binder's syndrome), various ethnicities have a tendency toward premaxillary retrusion, namely, African, Hispanic, and Asian (Fig. **11–2A–D**).[2] Protuberant lips that also typify some of these ethnicities further compound the illusion of a retro-inclined nose-to-lip profile and may benefit from reductive surgery (see Chapter 13).

If concomitant malocclusion exists due to deficiency of the premaxillary segment, orthognathic correction may be a more suitable surgical option than simple implantation (refer to Chapter 12 for greater detail regarding skeletal surgery). However, if premaxillary retrusion represents only an unaesthetic attribute and not a functional deficiency, then an implant may be the better solution. Various implants have been advocated that include autogenous (cartilage and bone) and alloplast

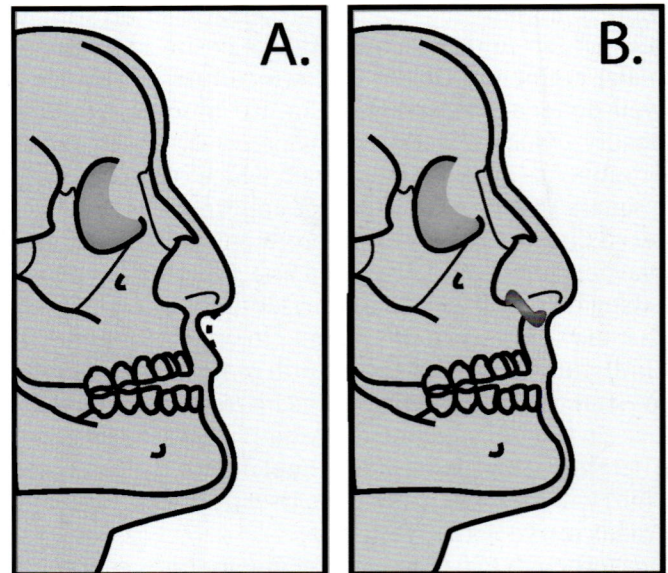

Figure 11–1 **(A)** Relative premaxillary hypoplasia may contribute to a simian-like appearance to the nasal and upper-lip profile: an acute nasolabial angle and ptotic nasal tip as well as a "gummy" smile and possibly incompetent upper lip. **(B)** A premaxillary implant placed either transnasally or transorally can enhance the nasal profile and upper-lip appearance.

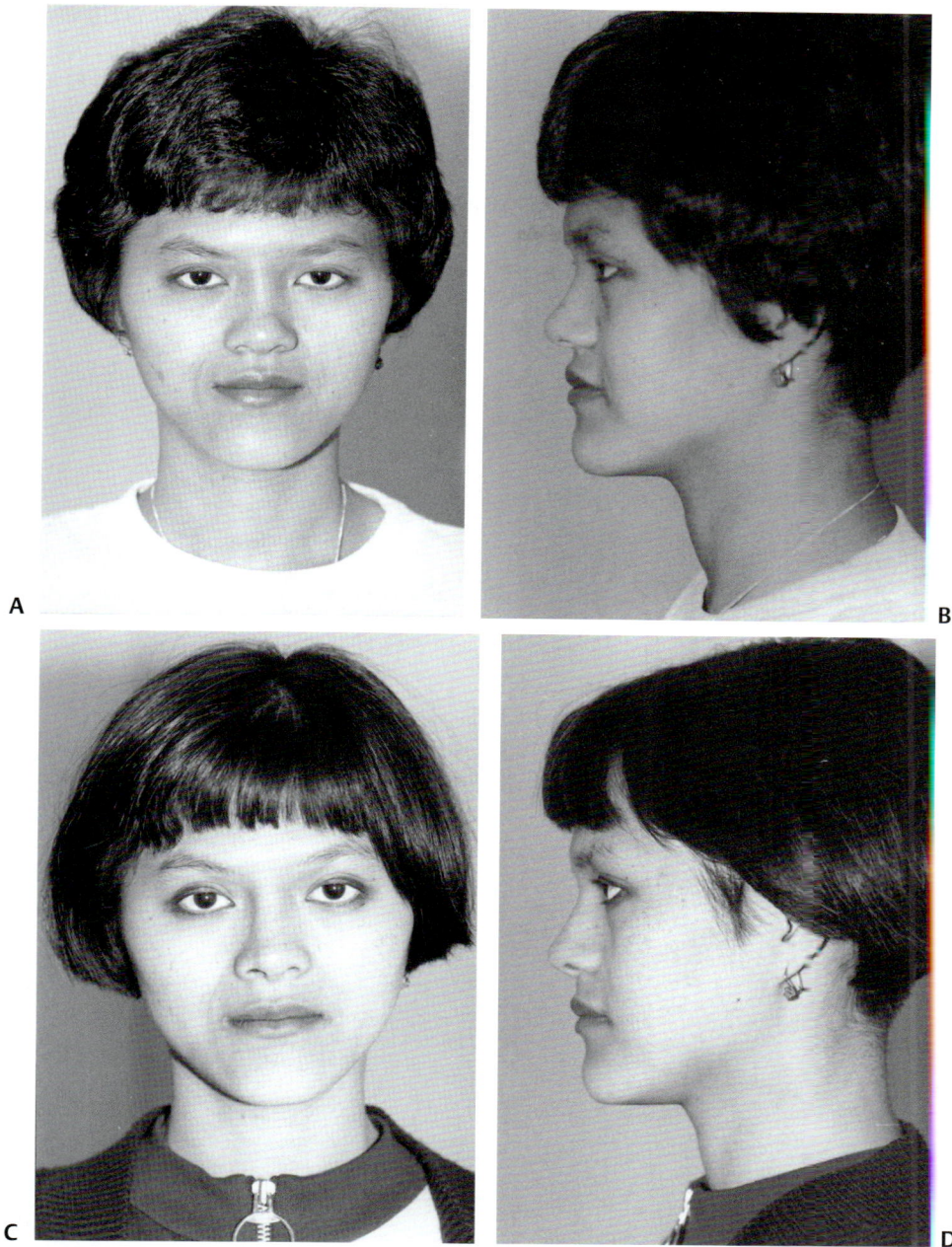

Figure 11–2 A 24-year-old Asian patient who underwent premaxillary augmentation and augmentation rhinoplasty and is shown 13 months after surgery. (From Fanous N, Yoskotovitch A. Premaxillary augmentation for central maxillary recession: an adjunct to rhinoplasty. Facial Plast Surg Clin N Am 2002;10:415–422, Figure 5; with permission.)

material (Mersilene mesh and silicone). Although autogenous materials have proven a reliable method of augmentation in the Caucasian population, the greater severity of premaxillary retrusion often mandates a more substantial alloplastic material. Both intranasal and sublabial techniques have been promoted using various configurations of implants, ranging from small silicone blocks to larger flared profiles. The intranasal approach permits placement of smaller implants for less pronounced augmentation, whereas the sublabial approach facilitates better visualization, potential sectioning of the depressor septi muscle (which may otherwise add tension to the nasal tip), and placement of a larger implant. Both approaches have been applied with success to achieve the desired degree and breadth of augmentation.

◆ Premaxillary Silicone Implant

Design and Method of Nabil Fanous

Design

A bat-, or V-shaped, silicone implant (Implantech, Ventura, CA) (Fig. 11–3) that spans the entire nasal base may be inserted either transnasally or transorally (Fig. 11–4).[3,4] The implant consists of a central component that modulates the degree of premaxillary projection and that is connected by two thinner arms to tapered winglike ends laterally. The implant measures ~38 to 40 mm in horizontal breadth, with the central component exhibiting a depth of 6 to 8 mm and a height of 6 to 7 mm, with 2 mm wide tapered arms that connect to 4 mm wide lateral, winged termini. The central component of the implant should not exceed the implant's specifications of 6 to 7 mm, which would risk a visible ridge during smiling. The implant is thickest in dimension superiorly (under the columella) and tapers inferiorly over the upper lip to avoid this problem of a visible ridge formation. Finally, a shallow cleft resides on the posterior aspect of the implant's midline to maintain the implant's position over the nasal spine. The implant comes in two sizes, regular and large, with the former suitable for 90% of patients and the latter reserved for the remaining 10% of patients.*

During the preoperative analysis, it is important to assess the nose–lip complex not only in repose but also during smiling. If the upper lip appears already long with poor dental show despite a retruded premaxilla,

the surgeon is advised to augment the premaxilla cautiously, as the consequent lengthening of the upper lip may further limit dental show. Larger implants may also be palpable by the patient during smiling, and preoperative consent should include discussion of this possibility. In any case, conservative augmentation will avoid the potential for complications.

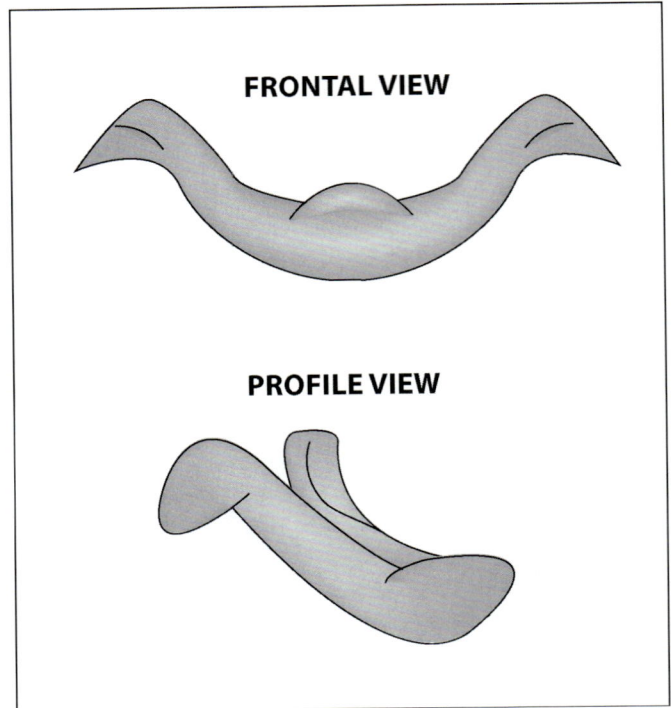

Figure 11–3   The bat-shaped silicone implant is used to augment the deficient premaxilla. The implant is designed to enhance the retrusion of the entire nasal base.

---

*The dimensions given for the implant refer to the regular size of the implant.

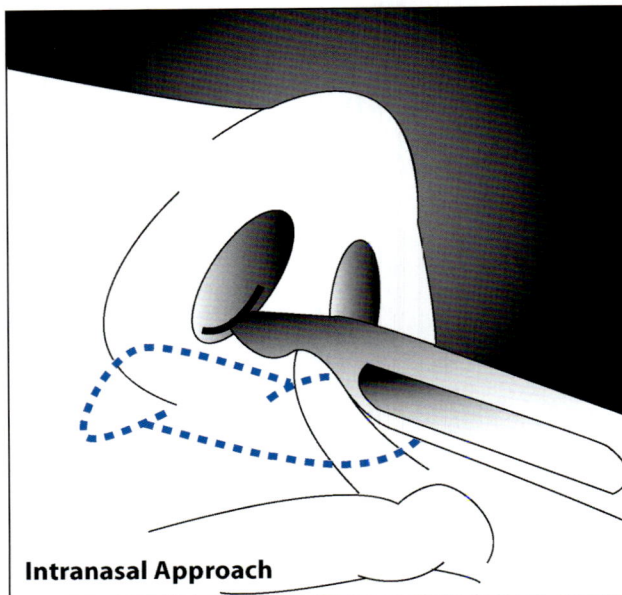

Intranasal Approach

A

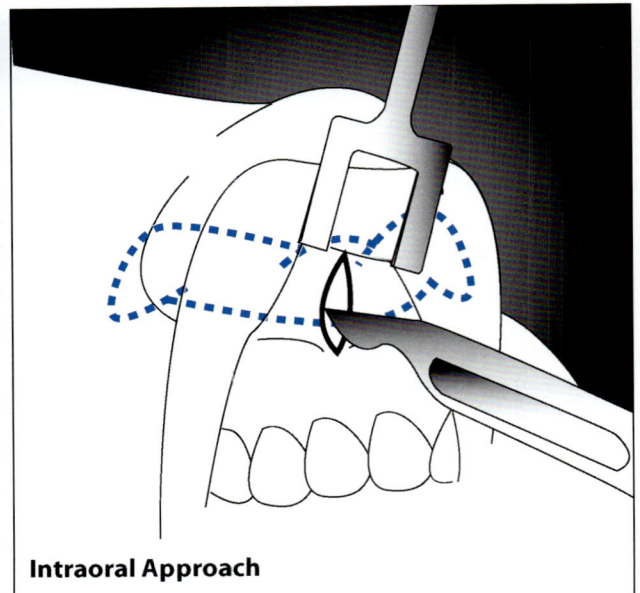

Intraoral Approach

B

Figure 11–4   The silicone implant can be inserted via an intranasal **(A)** or transoral approach **(B)**.

Surgical Technique: Intransal Route

1. The transnasal approach begins with a wide, 3 cm incision in the right nasal vestibule, with the medial half of the incision (1.5 cm) falling vertically in the membranous septum behind the columella and the other half of the incision falling horizontally in the medial part of the vestibular floor.

2. Using a nasal speculum for retraction, deepen the incision with the blade to the bone of the nasal spine in the midline.

3. Using the Joseph periosteal elevator, a subperiosteal pocket is dissected over the nasal spine and continued as left and right tracts that extend beneath the alar bases. The tip of the periosteal elevator is then used to enlarge a wider subperiosteal pocket immediately lateral to the nostrils to accommodate the flared ends of the implant. As a rule, the size of the dissected pocket should be larger than the size of the implant. However, the implant does partially reside lateral to the alar margin as well.

4. Place the implant over the upper lip and immediately below the nose to verify orientation of the left and right arms and how the implant will sit inside the surgical pocket.

5. Using a Senn retractor or thin malleable retractor to expose the dissected right pocket, a Brown-Adson forceps is used to introduce the right arm of the implant into the right pocket as far laterally as possible. The same technique is used to introduce the left arm of the implant as far laterally into the left subperiosteal pocket.

6. The central, grooved portion of the implant should be confirmed to rest against the prominence of the nasal spine.

7. Palpate the two lateral ends of the implant, which should feel like a small mound lateral and deep to the alar margin so as to ensure that the implant is not folded onto itself. A finger can be placed inside the nostril as well to verify that the implant contour appears to be appropriate along its medial extent.

8. The incision is closed with two, interrupted 4–0 chromic sutures.

Surgical Technique: Intraoral Route

Generally speaking, the intraoral route is less commonly used because it may predispose toward implant extrusion through the mucosal incision, as the implant is close to the mucosal surface. However, it can be reserved for implant removal if the surgeon should prefer this option.

1. The intraoral route is performed in a similar fashion. The incision is made in the midline oriented vertically, and the dissection is taken down to the anterior nasal spine.

2. Following the initial incision, the steps parallel those described above for the intranasal approach.

◆ Premaxillary Augmentation with Conchal Cartilage

Although a premaxillary implant that extends across the entire nasal base may aesthetically benefit the patient, an implant that resides simply below the central, columellar component oftentimes may suffice (Fig. 11–5A,B). Clearly,

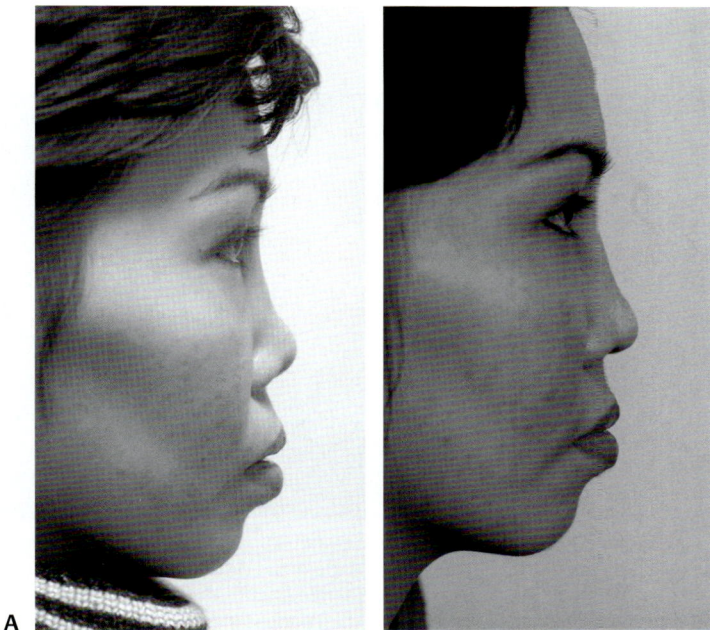

Figure 11–5 This 39-year-old Vietnamese woman, who had undergone two rhinoplasties in the past and had her implant removed over a year before due to infection, presented with notable contraction of the nasal tip. She underwent revision rhinoplasty with a silicone implant and premaxillary augmentation with conchal cartilage grafting.

use of autogenous materials is preferred whenever possible for the obvious reason of biocompatibility with a lower risk of infection and extrusion. Furthermore, the use of a morselized cartilage graft truly limits the chances of mobility and extrusion that could more likely occur with a larger implant style. However, use of this type of premaxillary type of plumping graft will fail to address a patient that requires significant premaxillary augmentation and the need for combined alar-base projection.

Septal and auricular cartilage provide useful graft sites for autogenous premaxillary augmentation. The author prefers auricular cartilage for premaxillary augmentation for several reasons. Almost all augmentation rhinoplasty endeavors are performed in the office setting under local anesthesia. Conversely, a formal septoplasty that is required to harvest septal grafting material should be performed in an operative suite with the patient under sedation. However, auricular harvesting can be undertaken quite readily with the patient fully awake. The author prefers to use a topical anesthetic cream (e.g., topical lidocaine or tetracaine) for both ear and nose surgery to minimize discomfort during infiltration of local anesthesia. Unlike in the Caucasian patient, a functional septoplasty is relatively rare in the Asian patient because septal deflections are uncommon and internal nasal valve compromise also are infrequent. Technically, septoplasty for the Asian nose is also more demanding, as the cartilaginous septum is considerably thinner than in the Caucasian and therefore much less abundant for grafting. For all of these reasons, auricular concha remains the mainstay of premaxillary augmentation material for the Asian patient in the author's practice.

Surgical Technique

1. The patient has a generous coat of topical anesthetic solution (EMLA, ELA-Max, tetracaine, etc.) applied over the anterior and posterior aspects of the auricular concha. (Generally speaking, the right-handed surgeon who remains seated for the procedure should elect to operate on the right ear for technical ease.) If augmentation rhinoplasty will be undertaken concurrently, the anesthetic solution is distributed over the entire external nasal skin as well as along the internal nares, where the right intranasal incisions (modified marginal and premaxillary incisions) will be executed. A minimum of 30 minutes to 1 hour is allowed to transpire to ensure that the topical anesthetic has achieved its effect, which can be confirmed by palpating the treated areas to determine adequate anesthesia.

2. One percent lidocaine mixed with 1:100,000 epinephrine is infiltrated into both the anterior and posterior aspects of the conchal bowl. Ten minutes should be allowed to elapse prior to surgical incision.

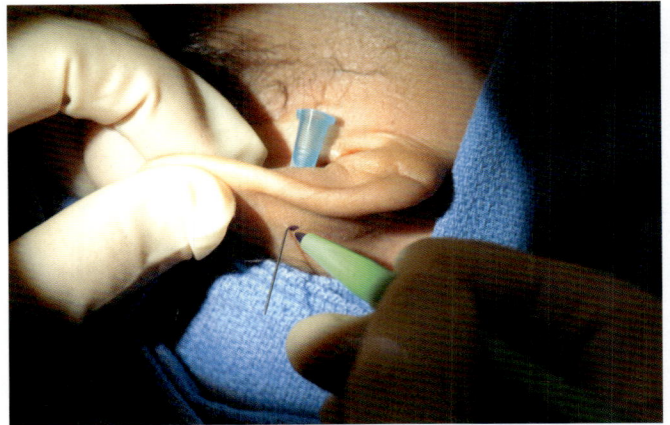

Figure 11–6 *Premaxillary Augmentation with Conchal Cartilage, Step 1:* The extent of the conchal bowl is identified postauricularly by driving a 25-gauge needle from the anterior to the posterior side of the ear and then marking this perimeter with a surgical marking pen.

During this time, the ear and nose should be thoroughly prepared with povidone-iodine solution.

3. A postauricular incision is preferred in the Asian patient due to the risk of unsightly scar formation in the darker-complected skin. Because the conchal border cannot be seen along the posterior aspect of the ear, a 25-gauge needle is driven through the perimeter of the conchal bowl from the anterior to the posterior side, and a marking pen is used to designate each point that the needle passes through on the posterior surface (Fig. **11–6**). This procedure is repeated until the perimeter of the concha can be estimated on the posterior surface of the ear by connecting all of the marked points.

4. A no. 15 Bard-Parker blade is used to incise the full thickness of the postauricular skin and a partial thickness of cartilage in a curvilinear fashion along the marked incision line (Fig. **11–7**).

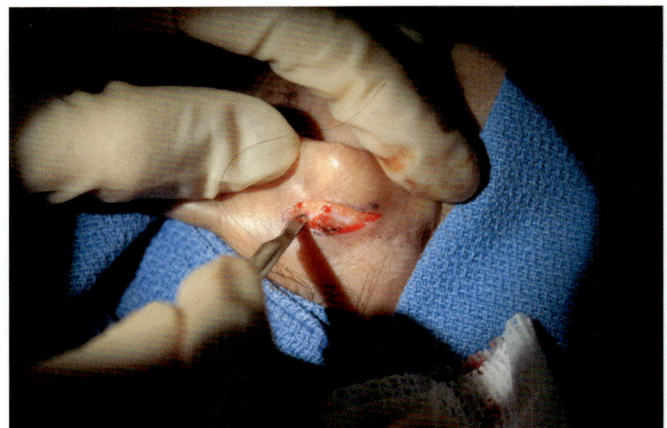

Figure 11–7 *Premaxillary Augmentation with Conchal Cartilage, Step 2:* A no. 15 Bard-Parker blade is used to incise the full thickness of the postauricular skin and a partial thickness of cartilage in a curvilinear fashion along the marked incision line.

A

B

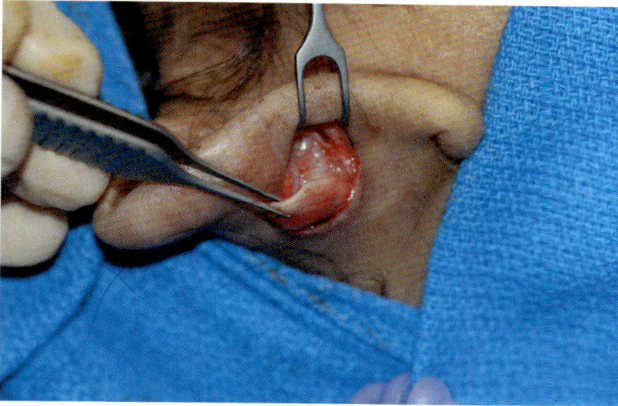

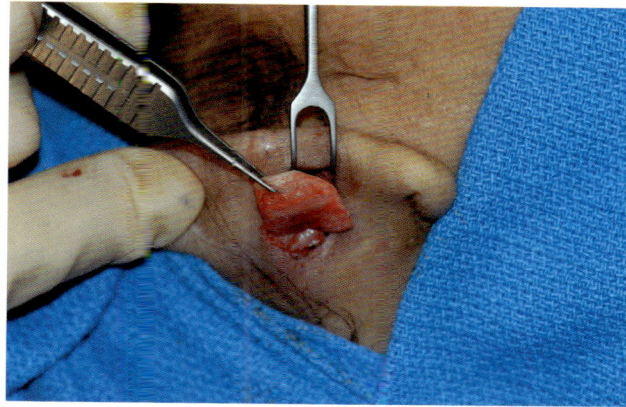

Figure 11–8 *Premaxillary Augmentation with Conchal Cartilage, Step 3:* **(A)** The transected cartilage graft is carefully dissected free from the anterior auricular skin without damaging the overlying skin. **(B)** The graft is removed and then placed into saline until time to morselize and insert the cartilage into the premaxillary soft-tissue pocket.

5. Tiny double-pronged hooks are used to retract the postauricular skin flap, while sharp dissecting scissors are used to elevate the skin from the underlying cartilage.

6. The cartilage that is already partially transected is fully incised, taking care not to pass through the anterior auricular skin. Dissection of the cartilage away from the anterior skin is performed in the same fashion described above (Fig. **11–8A**).

7. The cartilage piece is removed and placed into saline until insertion time (Fig. **11–8B**).

8. Hemostasis is achieved with bipolar cautery as needed before continuing.

9. If augmentation rhinoplasty will be performed concurrently, the nose is infiltrated with local anesthesia in preparation for both the rhinoplasty and premaxillary components of the procedure. If premaxillary augmentation will be undertaken alone, then anesthesia is infiltrated only into the premaxilla.

10. Attention is returned to the ear, and the incision is closed with a running, locking 5–0 chromic suture.

11. Two kidney bean–shaped Telfa pads that match the conchal size are fashioned as a pressure dressing. The Telfa pads are held with hemostats over the anterior and posterior aspects of the concha by the surgical assistant. The surgeon then places a 2–0 silk suture in a mattress fashion, passing through the anterior Telfa pad, concha, and posterior Telfa pad and then passing back through the posterior Telfa pad, concha, and anterior Telfa pad. The suture is tied down securely (Fig. **11–9**). At the end of the procedure, the patient should have a conforming bandage placed around the head to apply added pressure to the ear. The circumferential head bandage may be removed the following day, and the

Telfa dressing should be removed on the seventh postoperative day.

12. If augmentation rhinoplasty is elected, it should be undertaken at this point.

13. A right-sided intranasal incision is made down to the nasal spine along the caudal aspect of the columella that extends a short distance toward the nasal floor (Fig. **11–10**). Scissor dissection is taken down to the nasal spine until a recipient pocket is created for the premaxillary plumping graft (Fig. **11–11**)

14. After the pocket is prepared, the harvested conchal graft is morselized with a no. 15 Bard-Parker blade into 1 mm pieces (Fig. **11–12**), which are then inserted one at a time into the soft-tissue pocket (Fig. **11–13**)

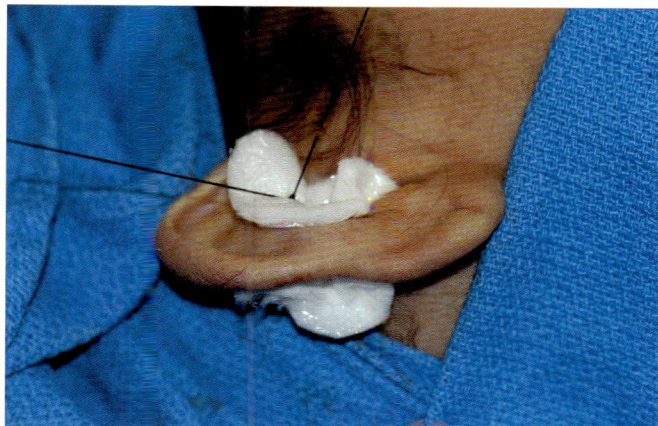

Figure 11–9 *Premaxillary Augmentation with Conchal Cartilage, Step 4:* An auricular hematoma is prevented by a Telfa pressure dressing secured into place with a 2–0 silk mattress suture. At the end of the procedure, a conforming bandage should also be applied circumferentially around the head to exert extra pressure on the dissected ear.

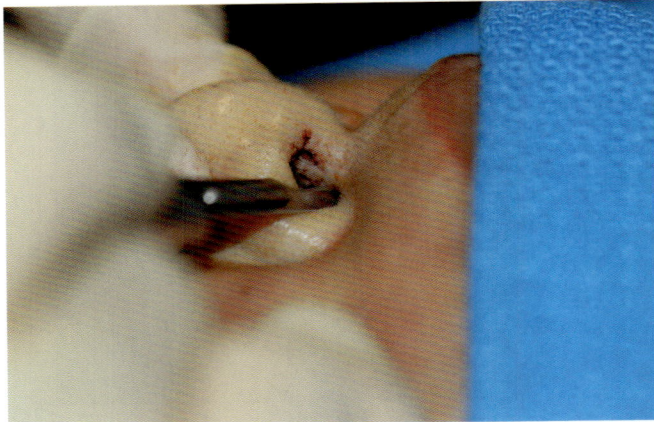

Figure 11–10 *Premaxillary Augmentation with Conchal Cartilage, Step 5:* A no.15 blade is used to dissect a pocket down to the nasal spine along the caudal aspect of the columella and a short distance toward the nasal floor.

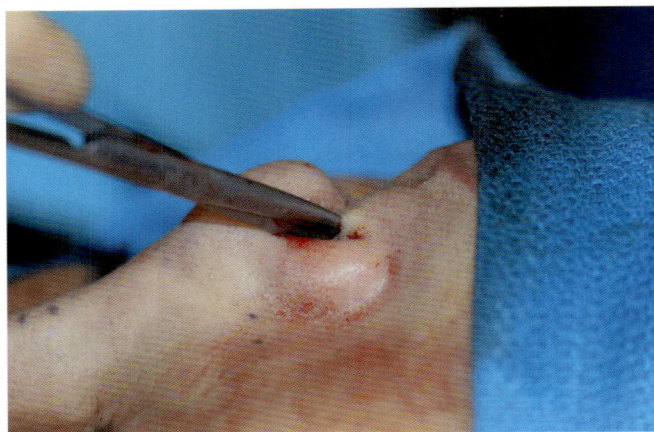

Figure 11–12 *Premaxillary Augmentation with Conchal Cartilage, Step 7:* After the pocket is prepared, the harvested conchal graft is morselized with a no.15 Bard-Parker blade into 1 mm pieces.

until the desired aesthetic improvement is observed. Use of fine-toothed forceps facilitates ease of insertion.

15. The incision is closed with interrupted 5–0 chromic suture, which can be trimmed or removed after 1 week.

◆ Malar Augmentation

As mentioned earlier, malar hypoplasia is a common attribute that typifies the Asian midface. Nasal augmentation surgery should always be tempered by the natural elevation of the malar eminence, as an overprojected dorsum looks particularly unnatural in the setting of a shallow midface. Despite the absence of a high malar bony prominence, traditional Asian immigrants are not troubled by this aesthetic deficiency and may express

confusion over the possibility of malar augmentation. Curiously, some Asians request reduction of the malar region via skeletal surgery when the malar bone appears too high for their cultural sensibility (see Chapter 12). Nevertheless, increasing influence of Western ideals of beauty and a greater proportion of a third-generation Asian population in the West have contributed to wider acceptance of this type of surgery.

Surgical Technique

1. The surgical technique begins with adequate anesthesia. The author prefers general endotracheal anesthesia to achieve the desired level of sedation.

2. Hemostasis is obtained with 1% lidocaine and 1:100,000 epinephrine infiltrated into the gingivobuccal sulcus bilaterally.

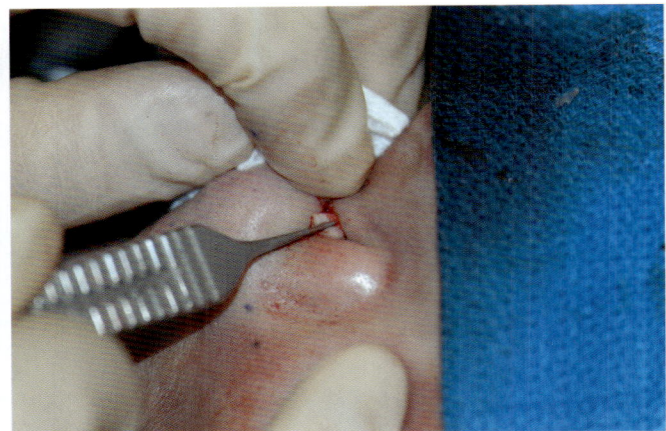

Figure 11–11 *Premaxillary Augmentation with Conchal Cartilage, Step 6:* Scissor dissection is taken down to the nasal spine until a recipient pocket is created for the premaxillary plumping graft.

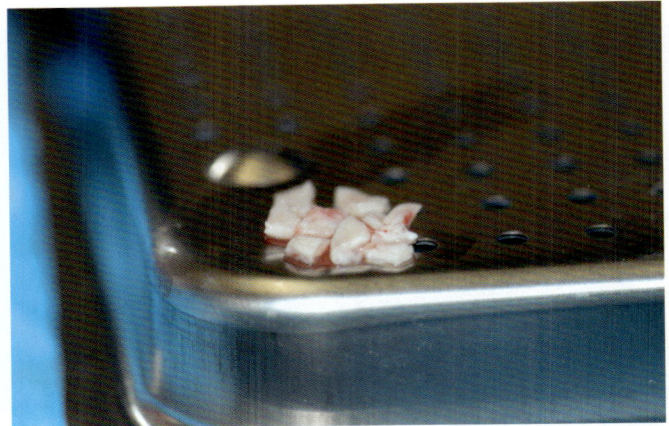

Figure 11–13 *Premaxillary Augmentation with Conchal Cartilage, Step 8:* The morselized pieces of conchal cartilage are inserted one at a time into the soft-tissue pocket until the desired aesthetic effect is achieved. The incision is then closed with interrupted 5–0 chromic sutures.

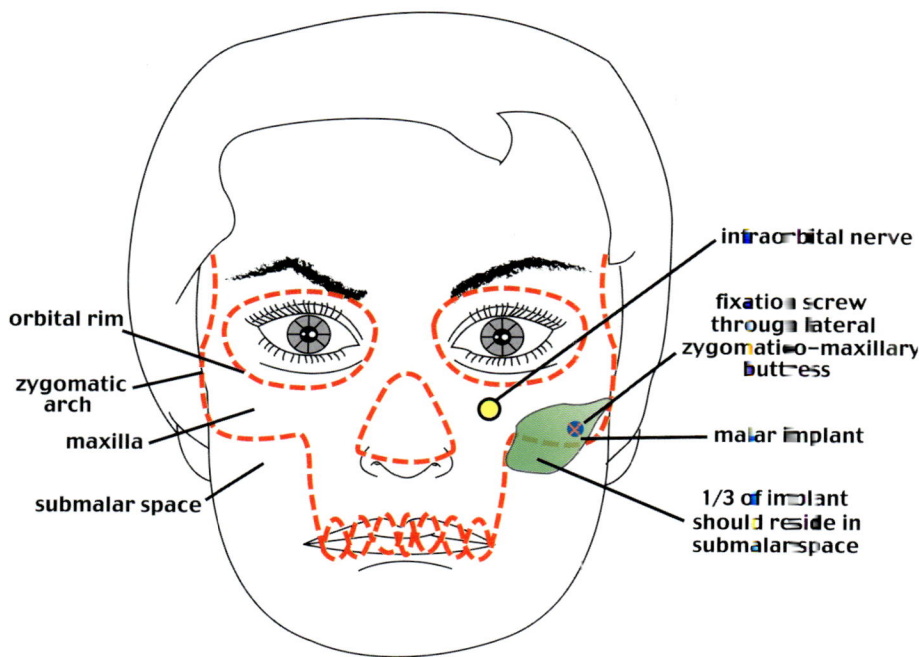

Figure 11–14 Illustration shows the relationship of the bony landmarks vis-à-vis the position of the malar implant. Note that the implant should be positioned with approximately one-third of its body over the submalar space. The closer the implant resides near the inferior orbital rim or zygomatic arch, the proportionately higher the risk that exists for potential postoperative asymmetry. (From Williams EF, Lam SM. Comprehensive Facial Rejuvenation: A Practical and Systematic Guide to Surgical Management of the Aging Face Philadelphia: Lippincott, Williams & Wilkins; 2004; with permission.)

3. The malar implant is then placed on the cheek skin where the desired position will be and outlined with a marking pen (Fig. **11–14**). Although many types of malar implants are available, a Gore-Tex implant is advocated for its biocompatibility, limited tissue ingrowth, and natural feel.

4. After 10 minutes, Army-Navy retractors are used to elevate the lip away from the gingiva. A monopolar cautery is used to enter the gingivobuccal sulcus, leaving a generous 1 cm cuff of buccal mucosa to the attached gingiva to facilitate easy mucosal approximation at the end of the case.

5. Dissection is taken straight down to the anterior face of the maxilla through the periosteum. A large periosteal elevator is used to dissect an adequate pocket to accommodate the implant. Generally, the direction of dissection should commence medially and be aimed upward while inspecting for the infraorbital nerve that may come into view. The dissection is then aimed laterally until the lateral zygomaticomaxillary (ZM) buttress is encountered.

6. The implant is placed into the pocket, and the overlying skin outline is used to confirm accurate positioning.

7. A drill hole is then created through the implant and the ZM buttress using a 1.5 mm × 10 to 12 mm hand drill.

8. A 2 × 12 mm screw is secured into position so that the malar implant is fixated at this point. The same technique is used for the contralateral placement of the implant.

9. Symmetry is confirmed by simultaneous, bilateral palpation and observation before closure.

10. The girgivobuccal incision is closed with a running 3–0 chromic suture.

◆ Nasolabial-Fold Augmentation

Although deepening of the nasolabial and labiomandibular folds are universal stigmata of the aging face, Asians may have a more pronounced proclivity to develop a deeper fold, given the relatively more abundant malar fat that descends and the lack of midfacial skeletal support. The nasolabial and labiomandibular folds are poorly treated with botulinum toxin (Botox) therapy, as these lines represent actual ptosis of tissue rather than wrinkles in animation. Instead, these lines can be augmented with a soft-tissue filler, whether a liquid injectable or a solid material, to soften these ptotic folds. The patient should be fully cognizant of the limitations in completely effacing these lines and understand that limited improvement is the goal and not the exception. Furthermore, the patient should realize that a liquid filler (e.g., collagen, Restylane, Radiesse) should be temporary, as permanent injectables may be a risky venture, and that a permanent solid filler (e.g., Gore-Tex) may be both palpable and visible and may risk extrusion and infection. If this anatomic area is the primary focus of grievance, then the patient should understand that a face lift, whether deep-plane or superficial musculoaponeurotic system (SMAS), will do little to improve this line and may actually worsen it on occasion.

If the patient elects to have a permanent soft-tissue filler, then Gore-Tex may be the most suitable option. Expanded polytetrafluoroethylene (ePTFE) comes in many brands, each touting an advantage based on porosity and pliability. However, in the author's experience with these different implants, these considerations remain squarely within the realm of theory and carry very little practical import. As mentioned, the limitations that concern this type of implant are palpability, particularly when smiling or during extreme animation of the lower face, and possibly visibility, extrusion, and infection. These latter three complications are relatively rare and can be managed by simple excision and removal of the implant if need be. Women tend to tolerate the issue of palpability much better than men, as is generally true for most cosmetic endeavors.

Alternatively, acellular dermis (Alloderm) may prove to be a favorable compromise between a permanent substance such as ePTFE and a temporary liquid injectable like collagen. Although touted as permanent, the author has found that Alloderm is semi-permanent to permanent, depending on the patient's biophysiologic ability to degrade the foreign material. The benefit of Alloderm is that usually the substance lasts considerably longer than collagen and is not as palpable (if at all) compared with Gore-Tex or other type of ePTFE. However, the degree of augmentation may be somewhat less than what may be achievable with Gore-Tex. The patient should be educated as to the derivation of Alloderm, namely, processed cadaveric dermis, and should understand the rigorous screening and mechanical process through which the material has been subjected. Based on these advantages and drawbacks, the surgeon and patient should arrive at a mutually agreed upon modality for intervention. One reminder that has already been stated throughout the text and that merits reiteration is the potential for visible incision lines in the central aspect of the Asian face for quite some time after surgery. The likelihood of this outcome should be carefully delineated for the patient when deciding on treatment strategy.

With this caution in mind and with the advent of longer-lasting biocompatible and biodegradable injectable fillers (e.g., Restylane and Radiesse), the author almost exclusively relies on these injectable fillers to manage the aging folds of the lower face. The merits, drawbacks, and techniques for these unique injectable fillers can be found in Chapter 13.

◆ Augmentation Mentoplasty

Facial harmony is predicated on a pleasing overall profile, and chin projection is an integral element in a balanced, lateral facial appearance. Although chin augmentation may be a more common procedure for Caucasians, increasing awareness and acceptance have arisen on the part of Asian patients as to the inherent value of this procedure.

For Caucasians, proper chin position can serve to balance and offset an overly prominent proboscis. For Asians, the more rounded profile created by the forward-sloping premaxillary segment and the backward-sloping chin can be balanced with premaxillary and chin implants, respectively. Anatomic differences of the chin area characterize the various races.[5] Caucasians demonstrate a more vertically oriented lateral profile, whereas Asians typically exhibit a more posterior inclination of the inferior chin aspect. Africans have an even more accentuated rounded chin appearance and posteriorly oriented lower chin area (Fig. **11–15**). Despite some of these subtle yet concrete differences, surgical implantation in the chin region differs little among the races.

An important consideration when considering chin augmentation is whether a coexisting malocclusion is present. If this condition exists, then orthognathic surgery may be a more appropriate avenue to pursue to correct this deformity. Depending on surgeon and patient preference, advancement genioplasty may represent a suitable alternative to augmentation mentoplasty with an alloplast. Sliding osseous genioplasty is a versatile surgical procedure that permits correction of vertical-height abnormalities and lateral asymmetries.[6] These skeletal-based surgical options are discussed in greater detail in Chapter 12.

Surgical Technique

Although many materials and methods abound for alloplastic insertion, only one technique will be reviewed here that has proven efficacy regarding stability, reproducibility, and longevity. An ePTFE (Gore-Tex) implant has been reliably used for augmentation mentoplasty in the author's experience, although other materials (e.g., silicone and Mersilene mesh) may be reasonable alternatives. Also, ePTFE provides optimal stability compared with silicone yet still remains easily removable compared with Mersilene mesh. A transcutaneous approach is advocated for several reasons: ease of insertion (especially for longer-style ePTFE implants), minimal morbidity, ability to combine the procedure with a submentoplasty, reduced exposure to contaminating oral flora, and excellent scar camouflage. The step-by-step approach for transcutaneous augmentation mentoplasty is explained as follows (Fig. **11–16**):

1. A line parallel and slightly posterior to the submental crease is outlined with a surgical marking pen that extends ~3 cm in length in the midline.

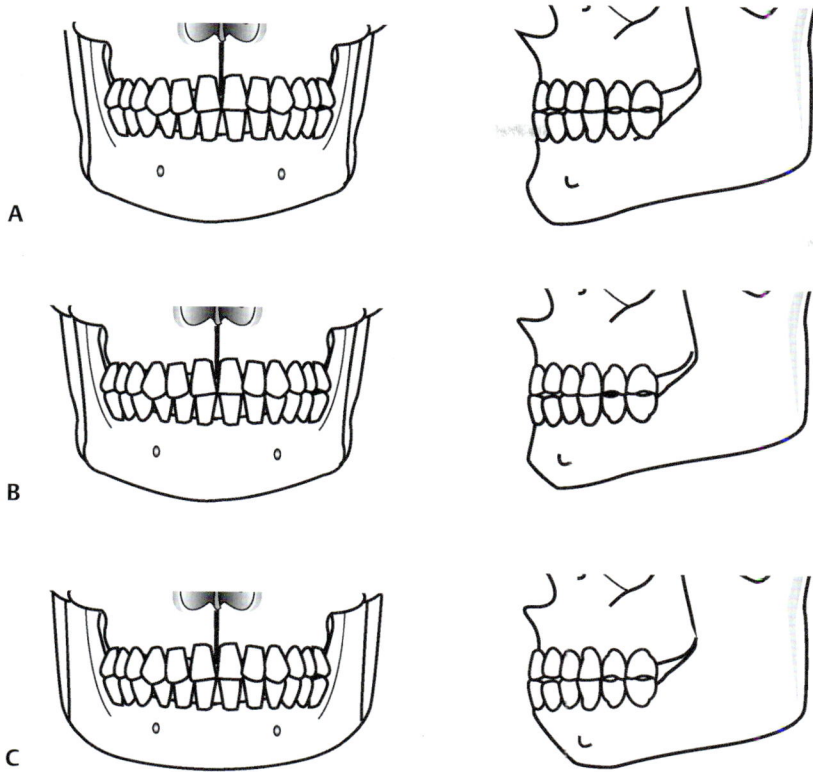

A

B

C

Figure 11–15 Various chin shapes typify the three major races: Caucasian, Asian, and African. **(A)** The Caucasian chin is characterized by a relatively prominent chin and longer vertical mandibular height. **(B)** The Asian chin shows some posterior inclination and less vertical height than that of the Caucasian. **(C)** These attributes are even more retruded in the African chin.

2. Local anesthesia with 1% lidocaine and 1:100,000 epinephrine is infiltrated along the line of incision. In addition, a regional nerve block should be administered to the mental-nerve bundles via bilateral transoral injections (Fig. **11–17**).

3. The center of the implant is marked with a modest V-shaped, incised notch if the center is not already indicated in some manner by the manufacturer.

4. A no. 15 Bard-Parker blade is used to incise the full thickness of the skin, and monopolar cautery

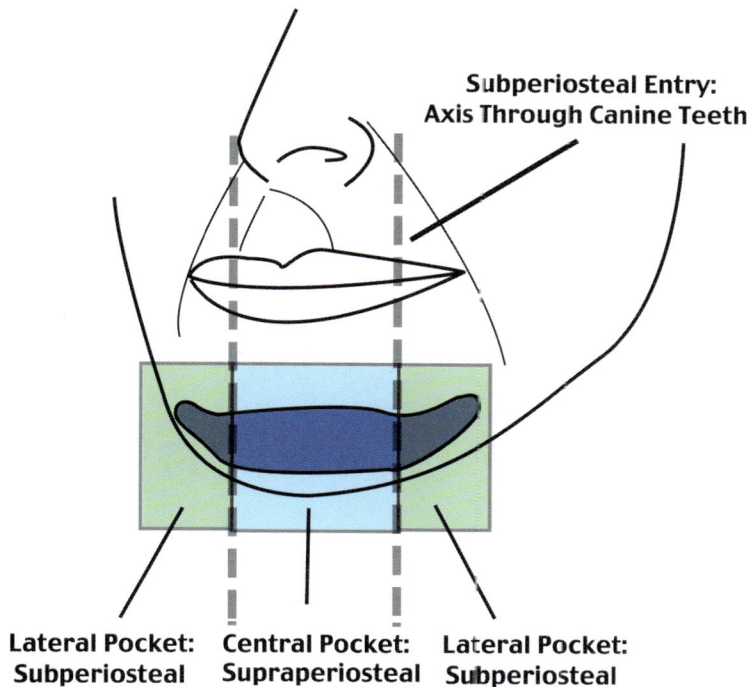

Subperiosteal Entry:
Axis Through Canine Teeth

Lateral Pocket: **Central Pocket:** **Lateral Pocket:**
Subperiosteal **Supraperiosteal** **Subperiosteal**

Figure 11–16 Illustration showing the ideal position of a chin implant (*in dark blue*), subperiosteal lateral pockets (*in light green*), and a supraperiosteal central pocket (*in light blue*) to ensure maximal fixation and projection along with minimal bone resorption. The point of entry into the subperiosteal plane should be performed at a point along the axis through the canine teeth. (From Williams EF, Lam SM. Comprehensive Facial Rejuvenation: A Practical and Systematic Guide to Surgical Management of the Aging Face. Philadelphia: Lippincott, Williams & Wilkins; 2004; with permission.)

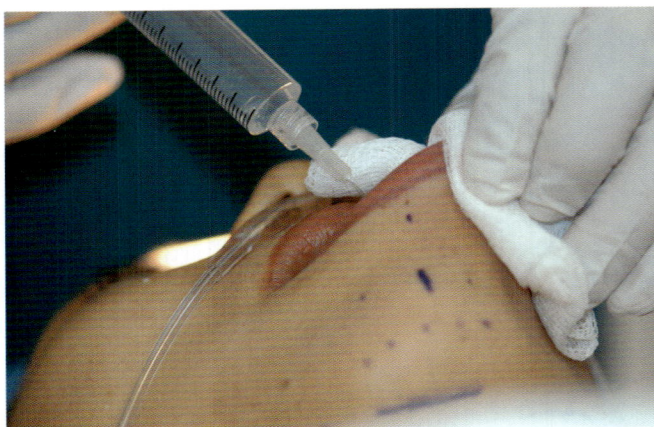

Figure 11–17 *Chin Implantation, Step 1:* In addition to infiltration of the proposed incision line with local anesthesia, a mental nerve block can be performed.

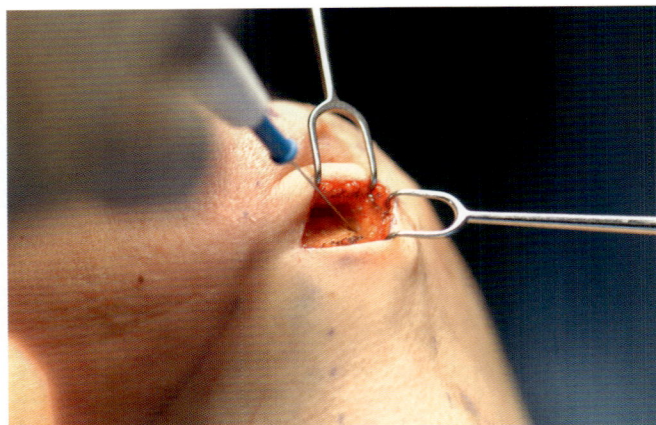

Figure 11–19 *Chin Implantation, Step 3:* With proper retraction, monopolar cautery is used to incise the periosteum in a parasagittal plane along the inferior border of the mandible.

permits dissection down to the periosteum as well as over the mental prominence in a supraperiosteal plane toward the midline (Fig. **11–18**).

5. The cautery may then be used to score the periosteum 2 to 3 cm lateral to the midline in a vertical fashion so that lateral subperiosteal pockets may be fashioned for implant placement (Fig. **11–19**).

6. Wide double-hooked retractors are used to expose the incision during this dissection. The laterally based subperiosteal pockets are created with a Joseph elevator to accommodate the ends of the implant (Fig. **11–20**).

7. The implant should be situated over the pogonion, or mental prominence, but not so high that it rests near the mental nerves and dental roots nor so low that it may ride inferiorly over the chin. To

ensure that the implant does not inadvertently fall inferiorly over the chin, sufficient soft-tissue dissection should be carried superiorly to accommodate the implant centrally. The implant is inserted into the subperiosteal pockets one side at a time with a long, curved tonsil clamp (Fig. **11–21**). After insertion, bilateral palpation ensures that the implant is properly situated and not kinked. The implant should also be confirmed to be in the midline by visually noting the midline previously marked on the implant (Fig. **11–22**).

8. The implant is secured to the periosteum inferiorly with a buried 4–0 polydioxanone suture to minimize the risk of its slipping inferiorly (Fig. **11–23**).

9. The overlying mentalis and soft tissue are then oversewn with a single buried 4–0 polydioxanone

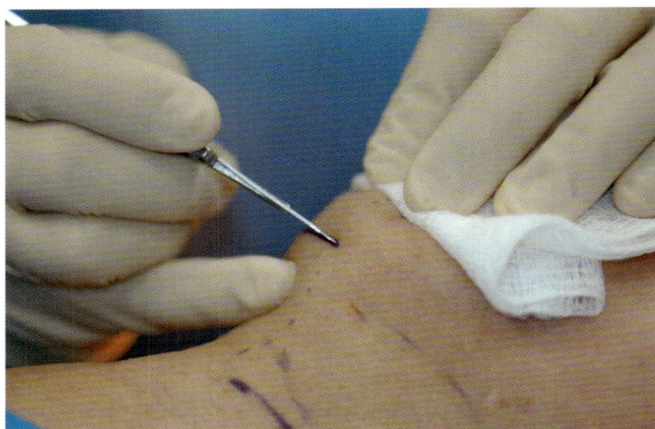

Figure 11–18 *Chin Implantation, Step 2:* A no.15 blade is used to incise the submental incision, which should fall at or slightly behind the submental crease. An incision made too far anteriorly may ride forward over the chin after the implant is inserted.

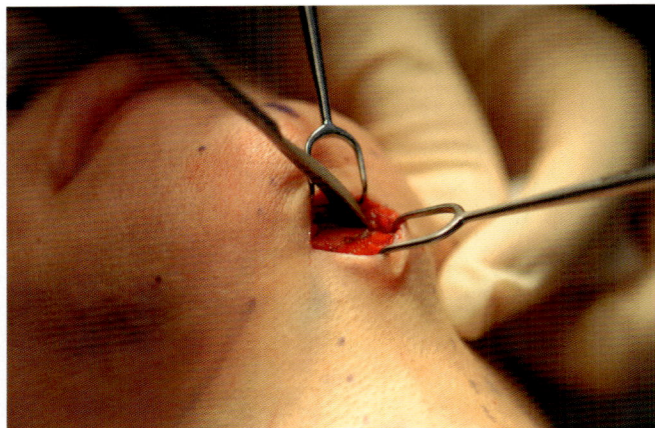

Figure 11–20 *Chin Implantation, Step 4:* A Joseph elevator is used to elevate the periosteum laterally for a distance of 4 to 5 cm, taking care to stay precisely along the inferior border of the mandible. The mental nerves that reside superiorly are often not identified during the procedure. The contralateral side is approached in the same fashion.

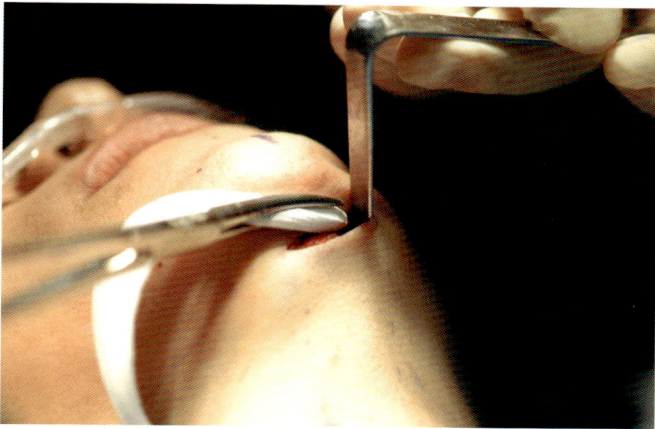

Figure 11–21 *Chin Implantation, Step 5:* The implant is inserted into the subperiosteal pocket laterally using a long, curved tonsil clamp. The clamp should extend all the way to the end of the implant to avoid kinking. After insertion bilaterally, the implant should be confirmed to be in the midline and without any kinking along its lateral extent.

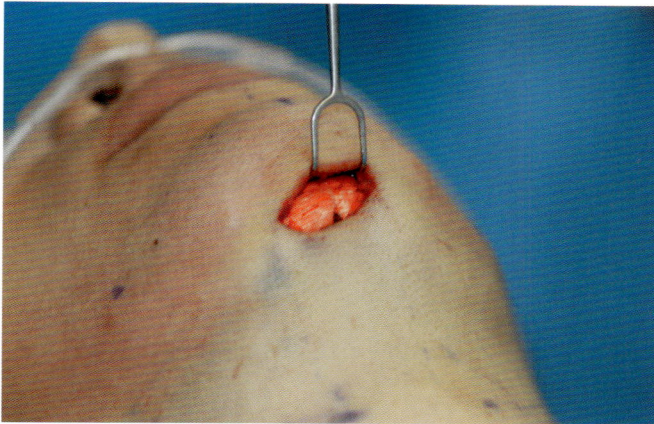

Figure 11–22 *Chin Implantation, Step 6:* The photograph shows the implant resting in the midline as confirmed by the alignment of the V-notch (created at the beginning of the case) and the midline mark drawn on the patient's skin.

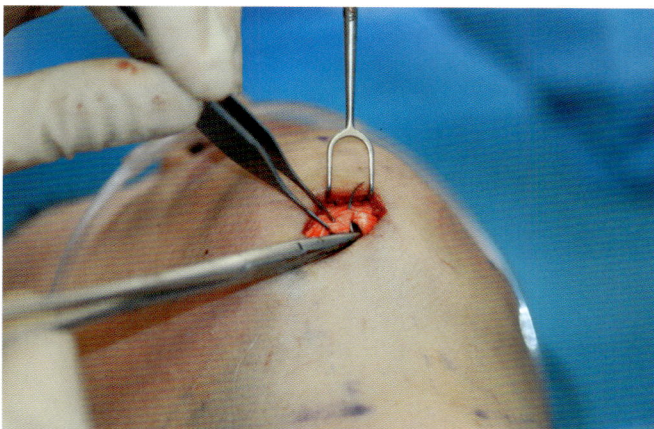

Figure 11–23 *Chin Implantation, Step 7:* The inferior aspect of the implant is secured to the periosteum in the midline with a 4–0 polydioxanone suture to prevent the implant from riding inferiorly over the mandibular border. The suture is placed in an inverted, buried fashion.

suture in an inverted fashion in the midline (Fig. **11–24**), and the skin is approximated with a running, locking 6–0 polypropylene suture (Fig. **11–25**).

10. The implant is further secured with adhesive tape that spans the anterior and inferior aspects of the mentum and is left in place for 1 week postoperatively.

◆ Temporal Augmentation

Largely as a consequence of zygomatic prominence, Asian faces often demonstrate a relative depression of the temporal region, and requests for augmentation of this region are becoming more frequent (Fig. **11–26**). Although silicone implants are commonly used, lack of stability secondary to activity of the temporalis muscle results in a high incidence of discomfort and displacement, often necessitating removal of the implant. Placement of the implant in the subperiosteal plane reduces but does not eliminate these problems.

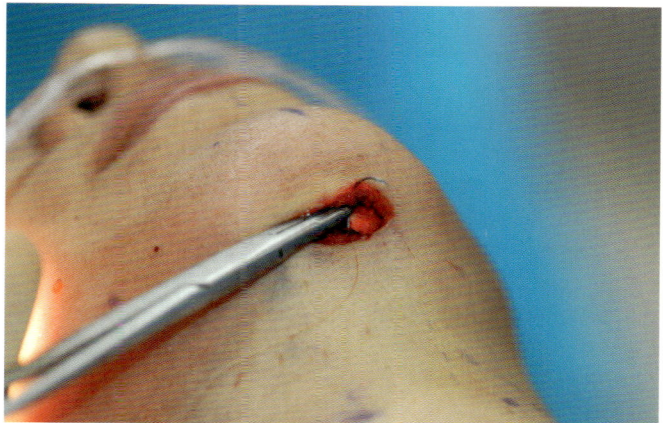

Figure 11–24 *Chin implantation, Step 8:* Unlike a simple submentoplasty, the mentalis and subcutaneous soft tissue are closed with an additional single buried 4–0 polydioxanone suture.

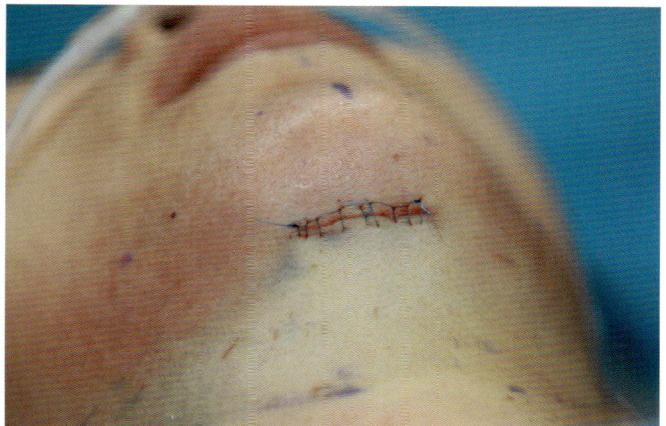

Figure 11–25 *Chin Implantation Step 9:* The skin is closed with a running, locking 6–0 polypropylene suture. A single interrupted suture is placed in the midline as insurance against the suture unraveling.

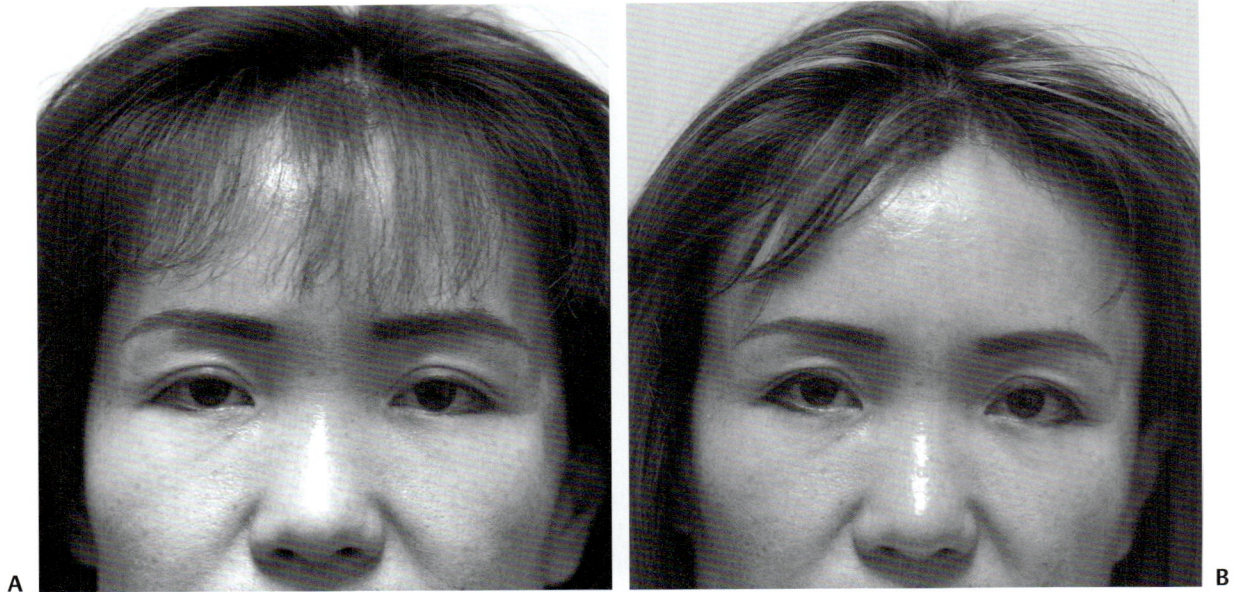

Figure 11–26   (A,B) This Korean patient complained of her relative temporal depression. She underwent temporal augmentation with acellular dermis (Alloderm) and is shown 6 months after the procedure with notable aesthetic improvement in her temporal area.

Fat grafting offers an alternative to solid prosthesis, but variable resorption of fat should be recalled if this technique is considered. Use of "tissue clay" (Avitene [Danol, Inc., Cranston, RI] plus autogenous blood) offers an interesting alternative to fat grafting because of the low absorption rate of this material. Many patients, however, object to the often palpable lumpiness of this material, even though the augmented temporal region is rarely visually abnormal, and the lumpiness resolves within 10 to 12 weeks. Silicone temporal prostheses of various sizes are manufactured in Asia.

An alternative that may work well for the Asian patient with a notable temporal depression is acellular dermis in its solid form (Alloderm). Although the material should be slightly overcorrected by ~25% to compensate for eventual resorption, it has less chance of mobility than other solid implants, especially when fixated to the underlying temporalis fascia. The patient should be aware of the nature of acellular dermis and that some overcorrection is justified and some resorption will occur in a variable fashion. The patient's temporal region should be measured preoperatively to determine how much acellular dermis would be required (Fig. **11–27**): generally speaking, two layers of acellular dermis will be sufficient, and the surgeon should account for this double layer when ordering the material. The second, stacked layer of acellular dermis should measure approximately 1 cm smaller than the basal layer along the anterior and lateral borders so that the implant edges will be less visible after insertion. Because acellular dermal sheets come in varying thicknesses, the author prefers to order the thickest configuration for augmentation. For each side of the patient's head, a single sheet of acellular dermis that is large enough to be cut into the prescribed two layers should be obtained. Depending on the degree of temporal recession, a greater number of layers can be stacked, but the reader is cautioned that the edge of the implant near the orbital rim may be visible in cases with significant augmentation.

Surgical Technique

1. Prior to entry into the operative suite, the patient's hair is bundled with $^1/_2$ inch Micropore tape to expose an incision line that will fall approximately

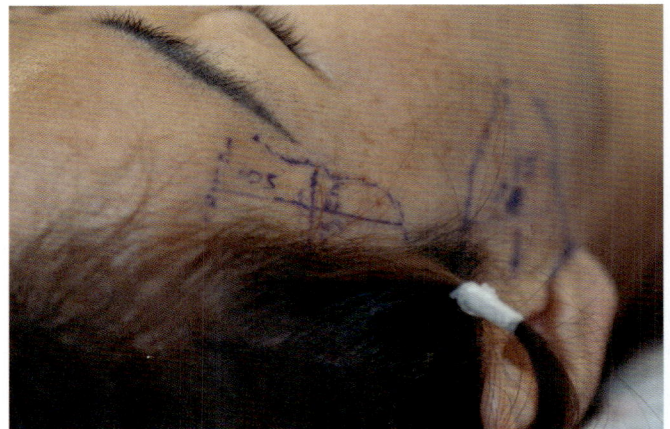

Figure 11–27   *Temporal Augmentation with Acellular Dermis, Step 1:* The area of temporal deficiency is measured and marked out preoperatively.

two finger breadths behind the temporal hairline—the same incision that is used for brow lifting. (A concurrent brow lift may be undertaken, and brow-suspension sutures should be placed prior to temporal implant placement.)

2. The patient is administered intravenous sedation or general anesthesia. After the patient has been sedated, 1% lidocaine with 1:100,000 epinephrine is infiltrated into the incision lines and along the orbital rim (arcus marginalis) in the temporal region.

3. While the anesthetic is taking effect, the acellular dermis should be rehydrated according to the package instructions in preparation for intraoperative use.

4. A no. 15 Bard-Parker blade is used to transect the skin and subcutaneous tissues down to the glistening layer of the true temporalis fascia. As mentioned in Chapter 4, the surgeon should be absolutely certain that he or she is below the temporoparietal fascia before continuing (see Chapter 10 for details).

5. A brow elevator should be used to dissect down toward the orbital rim, and the arcus marginalis at the orbital rim can be released, depending on the implant size (Fig. 11–28). If the implant extends closely toward the orbital rim, the arcus should be released to avoid bunching of the implant edges in this area. Similarly, the conjoined tendon may require release to prevent any buckling or implant show medially.

6. The acellular dermis should be prepared at this point for insertion: the rehydrated piece is trimmed to fit the proposed defect and divided into the two

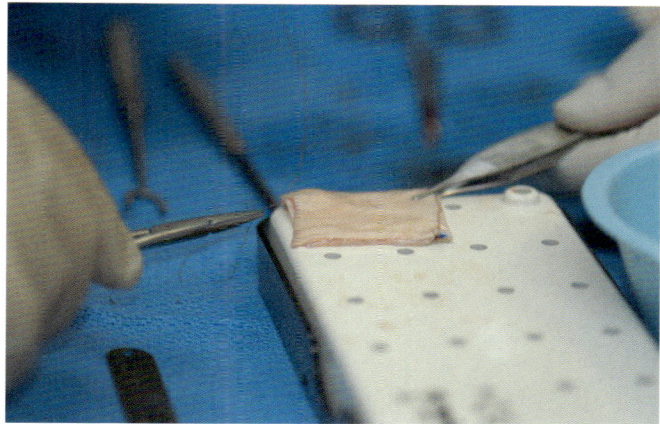

Figure 11–29 *Temporal Augmentation with Acellular Dermis, Step 3:* The reconstituted and trimmed pieces of acellular dermis are stacked and sutured together with 4–0 polydioxanone suture.

layers mentioned earlier. The layers are then held together with two or three mattress sutures of 4–0 polydioxanone (Fig. **11–29**).

7. With two atraumatic forceps, the implant is inserted and the surgeon confirms externally and internally that no buckling or folding has taken place.

8. The posterior corners of the implant are then secured with 4–0 polydioxanone suture to the underlying temporalis fascia (Fig. **11–30**). (The parachuting technique described in the following section on forehead augmentation can also be used to position and temporarily secure the implant into position.)

9. Skin incisions are then closed with surgical staples, which will be removed on the seventh postoperative day.

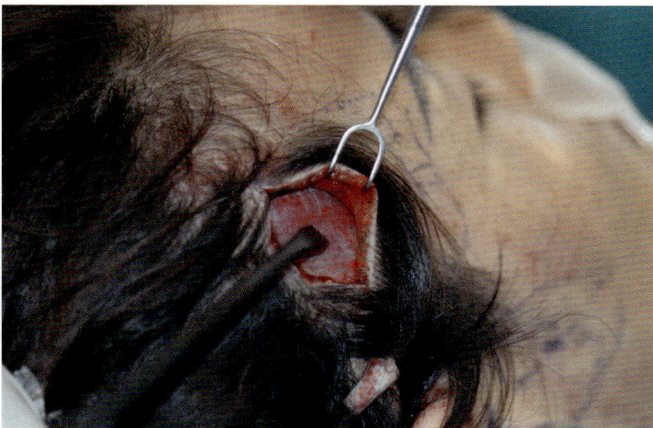

Figure 11–28 *Temporal Augmentation with Acellular Dermis, Step 2:* Dissection is performed in the standard endobrow plane: between the temporoparietal fascia and the true temporalis fascia.

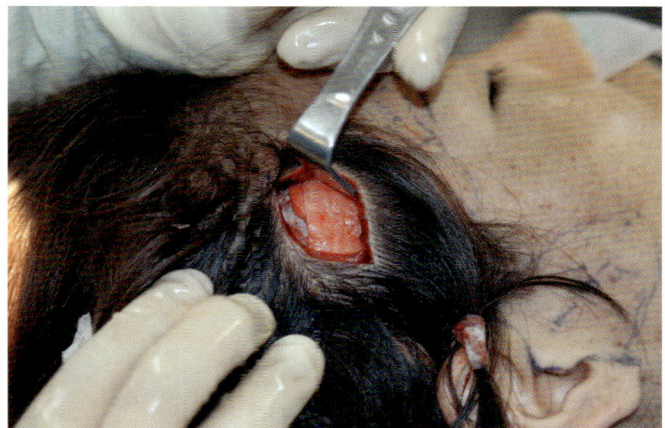

Figure 11–30 *Temporal Augmentation with Acellular Dermis, Step 4:* The layered implant is shown after it has been placed into the temporal pocket and sutured to the temporalis fascia with 4–0 polydioxanone suture.

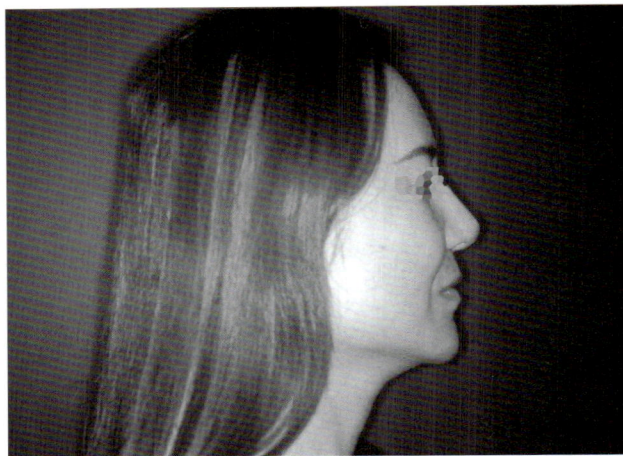

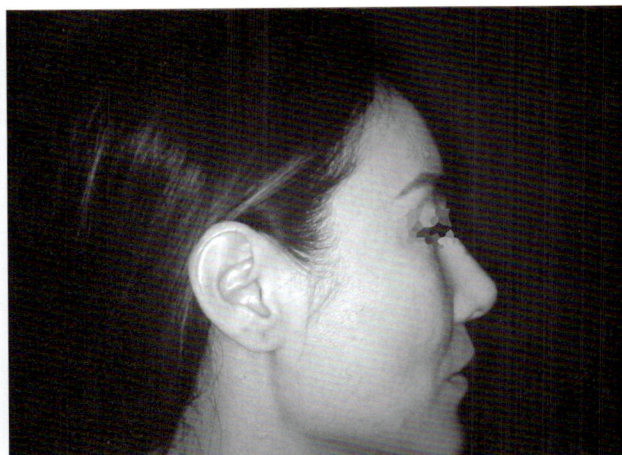

Figure 11–31   (A,B) This 38-year-old Asian female underwent forehead augmentation with a 4 mm silicone implant and is shown after surgery with a favorable aesthetic improvement. (Courtesy of Joseph K. Wong, M.D.)

10. The contralateral side is addressed in the same fashion, and a circumferential pressure-style dressing is applied to the head for 1 day. No drains are needed.

◆ Forehead Augmentation

Method of Joseph K. Wong

Relative depression or posterior inclination ("sloping") of the forehead is a concern to some Asian women and men (Figs. **11–31, 11–32**). Silicone implants of varying sizes are available in Asia for correction of this aesthetic defect, but, as in the temporal region, constant activity of the frontalis muscle may predispose to implant displacement. Subperiosteal placement may enhance

overall stability but not entirely prevent mobility. Custom-made silicone implants are available in North America, being fabricated from facial moulage kits that are reliable and easy to use. Surgeons contemplating augmentation of the frontal region with a silicone implant should consider this option.

Augmentation of the forehead/brow region begins with a careful preoperative consultation in which the precise anatomic deficit is identified and a suitable implant is selected. Implants may vary from smaller regional variants to full-sized implants that span the entire forehead region. Oftentimes, verbal dialogue will not suffice to communicate with the patient the intended aesthetic objective. Rather, digital imaging and a preoperative template are required to establish more effectively the exact dimensions of the implant that will fulfill the patient's cosmetic concerns. Digital imaging

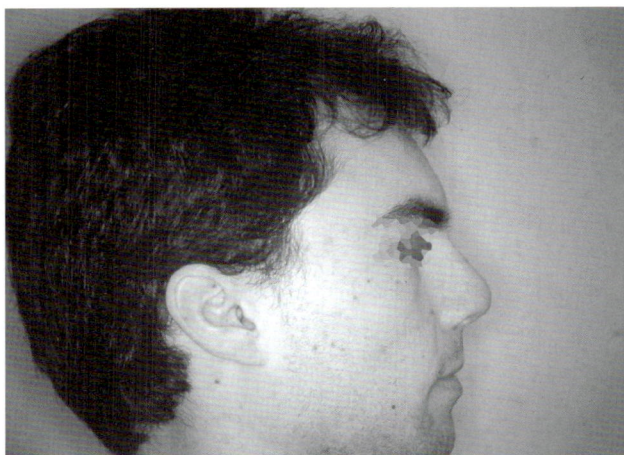

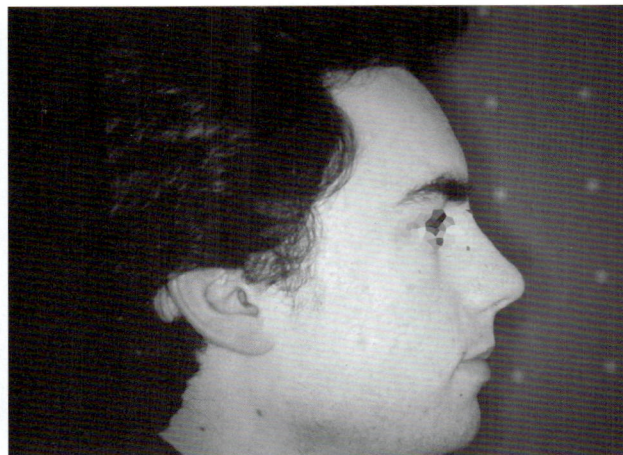

Figure 11–32   (A,B) This 25-year-old Caucasian patient underwent forehead augmentation with a 3 mm silicone implant and rhinoplasty and is shown after surgery with favorable aesthetic improvement. (Courtesy of Joseph K. Wong, M.D.)

and morphing manipulation of the patient's profile will enable the surgeon to show how the implant will improve the patient's brow contour more effectively than a frontal view. An isolated temporal deficiency may be better perceived, however, on a frontal or oblique view, and digital morphing is more difficult and less necessary than the larger forehead/brow implant. After a consensus is achieved between the surgeon and patient regarding what look the patient would like, a template can be fashioned to simulate the aesthetic appearance that will occur after implantation and which can serve as a model for further physician–patient dialogue and for construction of the silicone implant.

The model discussed here was developed by Joseph K. Wong.

Template Fabrication and Silicone Implant Creation

Fabrication of a template is a multistep process and can be undertaken from simple materials found in a dental office (dental alginate, dental plaster, and dental wax). In overview, a negative template is created using fast-setting dental alginate, which is then used to create a positive template plaster mold of the patient's forehead. A wax template is then sculpted onto the plaster template that will be used to create the silicone implant.

1. First the area of the patient's forehead that requires augmentation is outlined with a surgical marking pen, and the measurements of the horizontal and vertical dimensions are recorded (Fig. **11–33A,B**).

2. A fast-setting dental alginate is combined with water in a mixing bowl to form the negative template of the forehead (Fig. **11–34A,B**). Before the alginate completely dries, the paste is applied directly to the patient's forehead and sculpted to encompass the entire area that requires augmentation (Fig. **11–35A**).

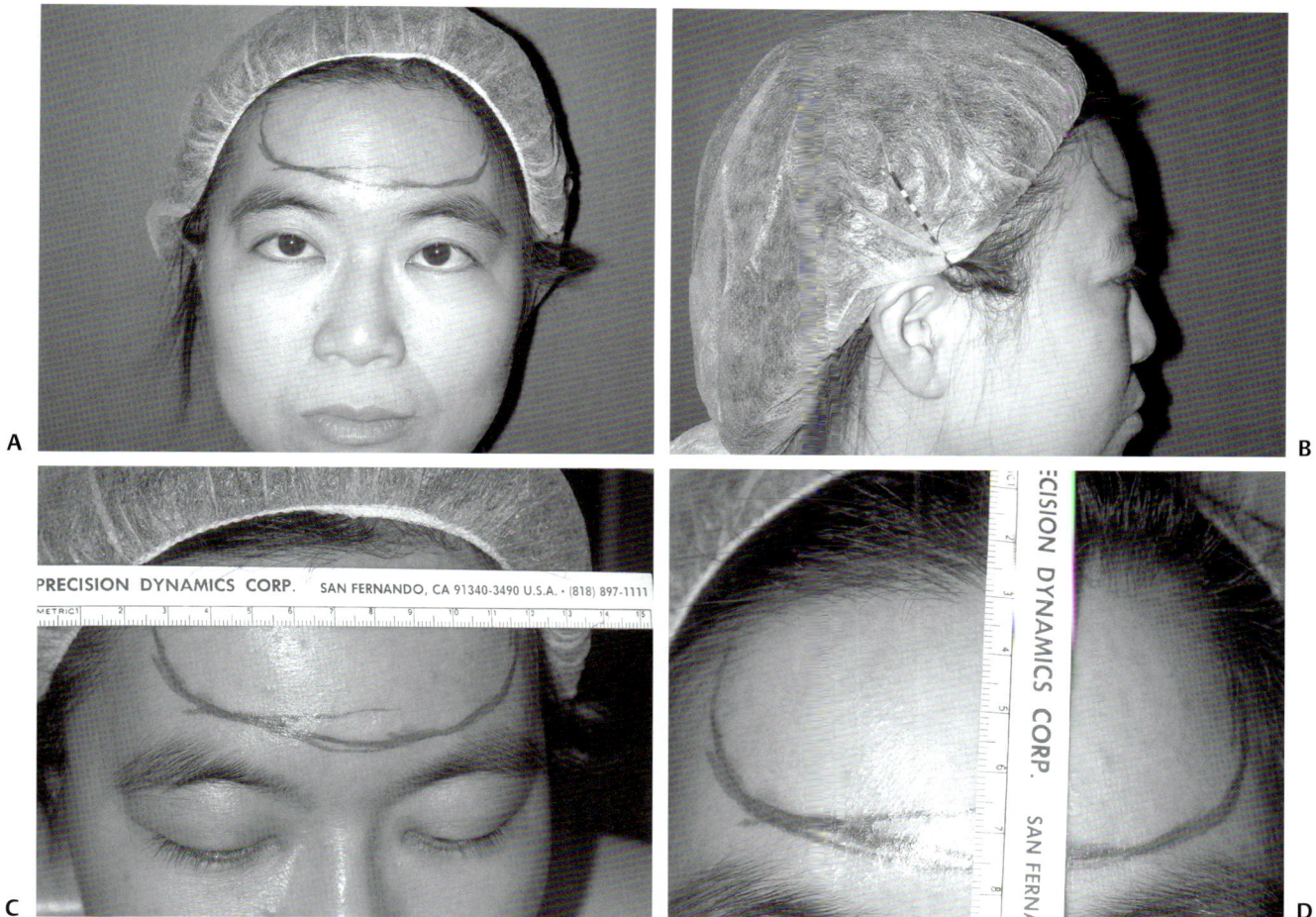

Figure 11–33 *Fabrication of the Template and Implant for Forehead Augmentation, Step 1:* **(A,B)** The area of the patient's forehead that requires augmentation is outlined with a surgical marking pen. **(C,D)** The measurements of the horizontal and vertical dimensions are recorded. (Courtesy of Joseph K. Wong, M.D.)

A   B

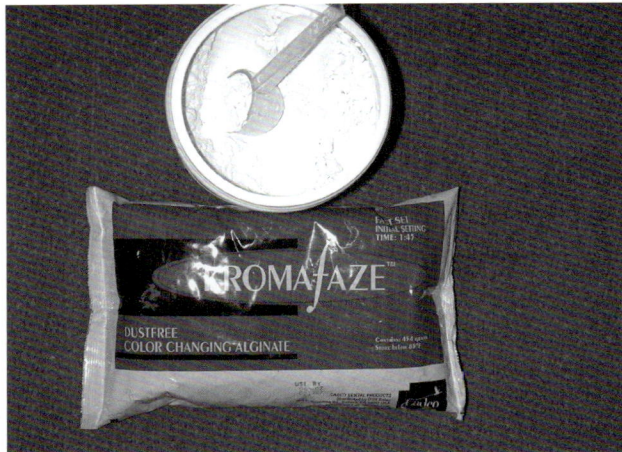

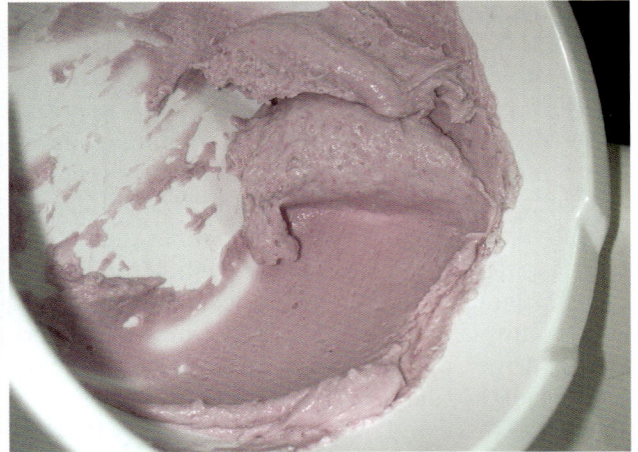

Figure 11–34   *Fabrication of the Template and Implant for Forehead Augmentation, Step 2:* **(A,B)** Fast-setting dental alginate is mixed with water until a thick, uniform paste develops and applied to the forehead quickly before the alginate mix hardens. (Courtesy of Joseph K. Wong, M.D.)

3. A firm base plate is affixed to the backside of the alginate template as a backing material. After the alginate fully hardens in several minutes, it is gently removed from the patient's forehead (Fig. **11–35B**). The remainder of the process can be performed at a later time without the patient being present.

4. A dental plaster mold is formed by pouring the plaster carefully onto the negative alginate template. A cardboard backing can be affixed to the plaster before it dries to provide a flat surface that will aid in the next step of fabricating the wax template (Figs. **11–36, 11–37A,B**).

5. Using digital-imaging analysis as a guide, the surgeon can estimate approximately how large the wax template (and ultimately the silicone implant) should be. A dental base plate wax can be heated in hot water until it softens and then placed onto the set plaster mold to sculpt the precise dimensions of the template that will serve as a guide for the silicone implant (Fig. **11–38A,B**). Typically, a thickness of 3 to 4 mm will be necessary to accomplish the task, and no greater than a 5 mm thick implant has been clinically necessary. The template should be designed with a thicker central region that tapers laterally in the temporal areas. Inferiorly, the im-

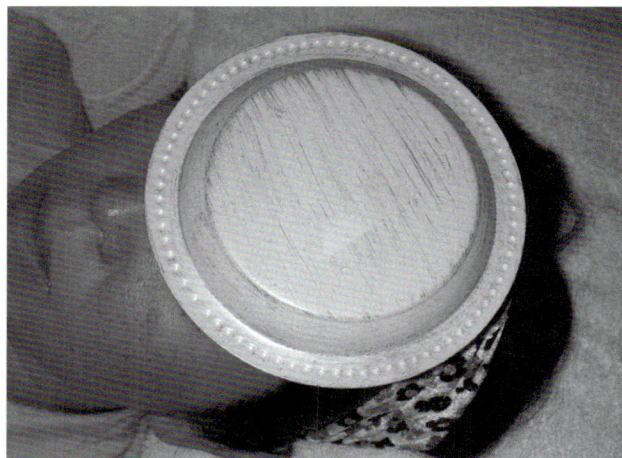

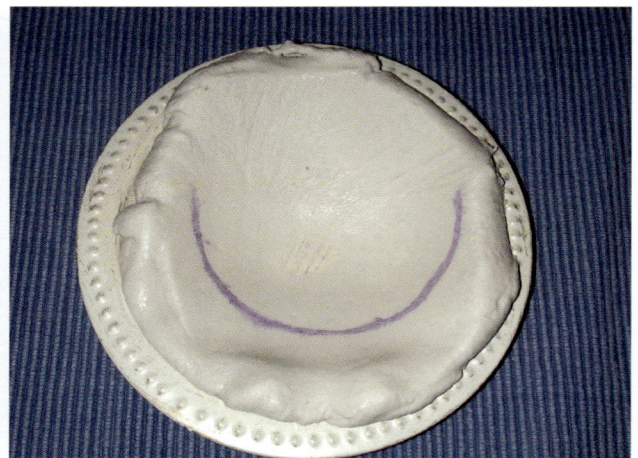

A   B

Figure 11–35   *Fabrication of the Template and Implant for Forehead Augmentation, Step 3:* **(A)** Before the alginate completely dries, the paste is applied directly to the patient's forehead and sculpted to encompass the entire area that requires augmentation. A firm base plate is affixed to the backside of the alginate template as a backing material. **(B)** After the alginate fully hardens in several minutes, it is gently removed from the patient's forehead. The photograph shows the impression of the forehead and the outline of the proposed implant seen on the negative alginate template. (Courtesy of Joseph K. Wong, M.D.)

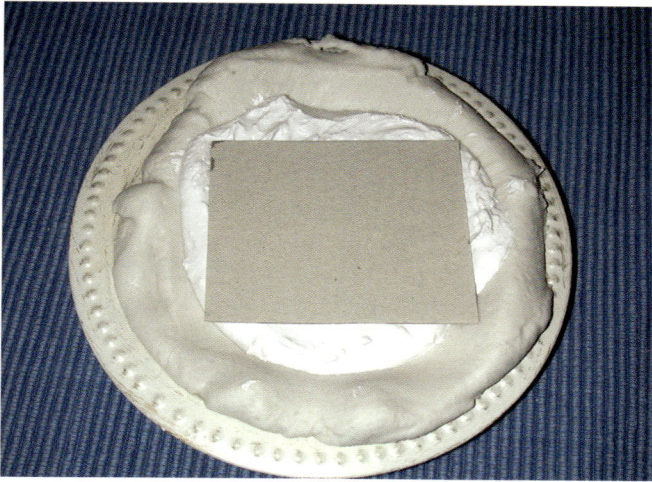

Figure 11–36 *Fabrication of the Template and Implant for Forehead Augmentation, Step 4:* A dental plaster mold is formed by pouring the plaster carefully onto the negative alginate template. A cardboard backing can be affixed to the plaster before it dries to provide a flat surface that will aid in the next step of fabricating the wax template. (Courtesy of Joseph K. Wong, M.D.)

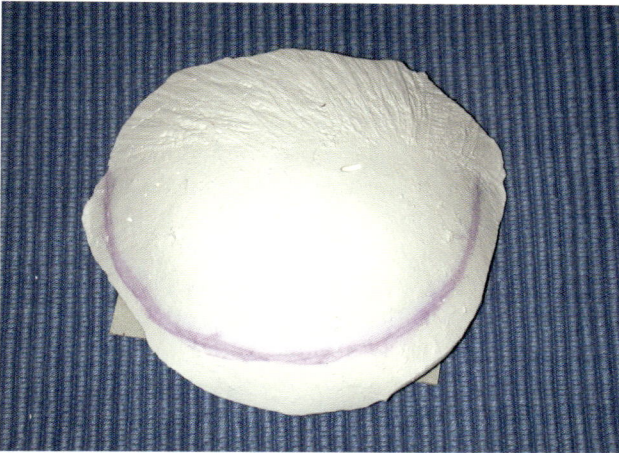

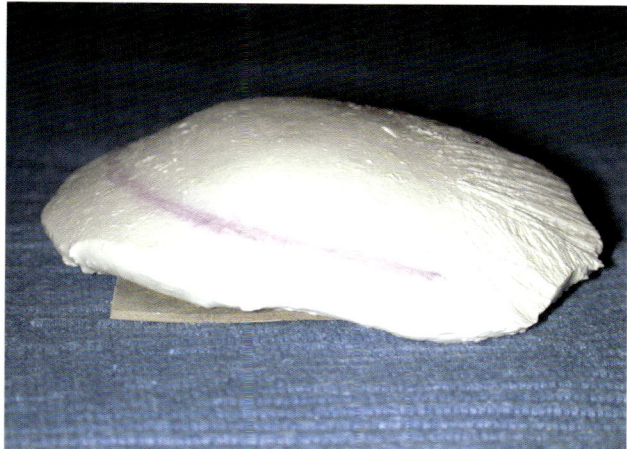

A   B

Figure 11–37 *Fabrication of the Template and Implant for Forehead Augmentation, Step 5:* **(A,B)** The plaster mold is removed from the alginate template and is shown with the proposed implant outline visible on its surface. The plaster mold now serves as a positive template of the forehead for creation of the wax template. (Courtesy of Joseph K. Wong, M.D.)

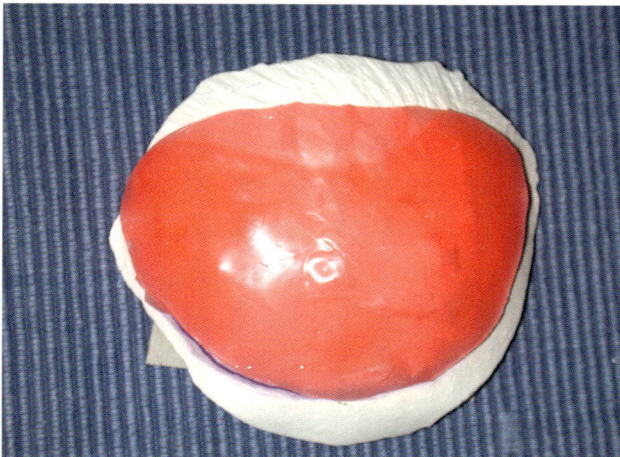

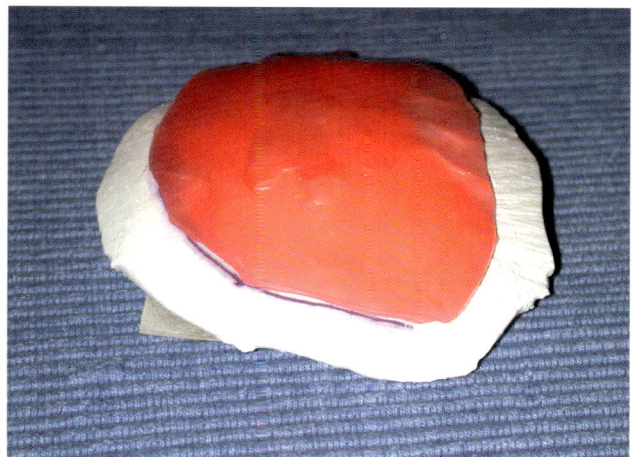

A   B

Figure 11–38 *Fabrication of the Template and Implant for Forehead Augmentation, Step 6:* **(A,B)** A dental base plate wax is heated in hot water until it becomes soft; then the wax is sculpted onto the plaster mold to the precise dimensions that will match the patient's wishes for forehead augmentation. The patient will try on the wax template and have the desired contour and height confirmed; the wax template will be used to model the final silicone implant. (Courtesy of Joseph K. Wong, M.D.)

plant should taper toward the superior aspect of the suprabrow ridge, or bony prominence, that typically begins several centimeters above the orbital rim. The base plate wax is packaged in sheets, which can be layered and sculpted when soft until the desired size and shape have been attained according to the above specifications.

6. With one or two wax templates created, the patient can then return for a second visit and at that time don the wax template to see if the dimensions conform to his or her aesthetic expectations. After the template has been applied to the patient's forehead, the patient can be asked to view his or her brow obliquely using a handheld mirror to confirm the suitability of the design. Digital imaging of the profile view with the template in place can help the patient better appreciate whether the implant will meet the patient's aesthetic criteria. The wax template can be further refined during this session by heating it again and/or sculpting it more until the patient expresses satisfaction.

7. The silicone implant is carved from a standard solid rectangular block (usually 15 × 8 cm of soft silicone) that matches as precisely as possible the dimensions of the carved wax template. (The surgeon may elect to have the carved wax template and plaster mold forwarded to a silicone manufacturer for fabrication and returned to obviate the burden of carving the implant himself or herself. Nevertheless, acquired proficiency will often permit carving the implant within 30 minutes.) A no. 10 or 15 Bard-Parker blade can be used to refine the silicone block until the shape and size conform to the proposed wax template design (Fig. **11–39A,B**). The very nature of carving the silicone block will lead to an imprecise and rough-hewn contour, which not only is acceptable but leads to better protection from site dislodgement after implantation. The general shape of the implant should approximate a crescent on profile view, with the thickest section in the midforehead that tapers gradually toward the temporal edges, as described for the wax template. This crescentic shape permits a smooth transition from the augmented to the nonaugmented regions. Because of the aforementioned surface irregularities that arise after carving, it is not recommended to show the patient the carved implant for fear that he or she might misinterpret the accuracy of the design. Eight to 10 holes are then created in a uniform distribution across the implant that will facilitate tissue ingrowth and add to implant stability; a 3 or 4 mm round punch biopsy instrument can expedite creation of these holes. In addition, V-shaped wedges should be removed along the entire perimeter of the implant: the triangular excisions can measure ~3 to 4 mm in size and be distributed roughly every centimeter across the entire perimeter. These V-shaped excisions permit the edges of the implant to conform to the rounded contour of the forehead more easily and minimize the risk of buckling that may otherwise occur. After carving, the implant can be autoclaved in preparation for surgical implantation.

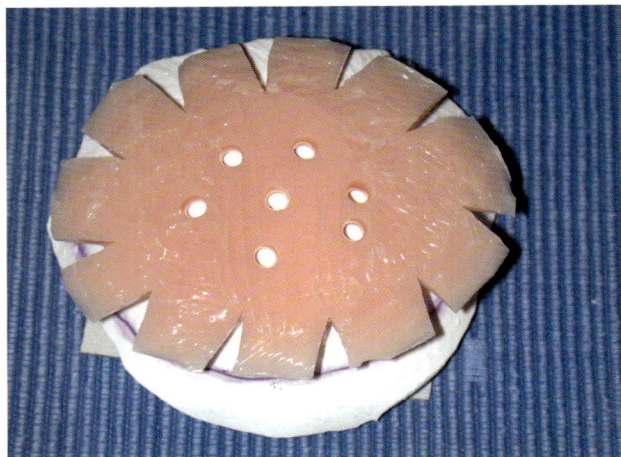
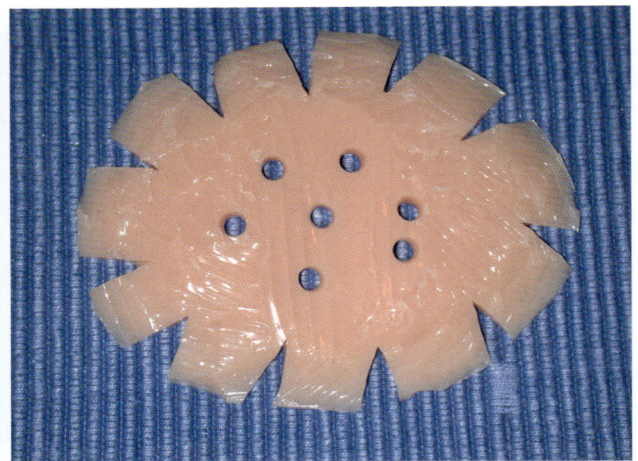

A   B

Figure 11–39 *Fabrication of the Template and Implant for Forehead Augmentation, Step 7:* **(A,B)** When the patient confirms the exact specifications of forehead augmentation based on the wax template, the surgeon can then fashion the silicone implant based on these prescribed dimensions. The soft silicone implant has holes punched centrally to provide a route for tissue ingrowth and wedges excised along its perimeter to allow the implant to curve easily to the forehead's rounded contour. (Courtesy of Joseph K. Wong, M.D.)

Surgical Technique

1. In the preoperative surgical room, the patient has three incisions marked out that closely match three of the five standard incisions for an endoscopic, or minimal-incision, brow lift: one vertical incision that measures ~2 cm is placed centrally immediately behind the hairline, and two temporal incisions are designed that extend ~4 cm in length behind the hairline. The hair can be secured with paper tape to expose the proposed incision lines to facilitate surgery. Note: a minimal-incision brow lift can be undertaken concurrently with a forehead implant in a patient who would benefit from this rejuvenative procedure. The implant would be inserted and secured into proper position (see below) before brow-suspension sutures would be placed.

2. The patient is administered intravenous sedation or general anesthesia, and 1% lidocaine with 1:100,000 epinephrine is infiltrated into the incisions directly and along the arcus marginalis.

3. A no. 15 Bard-Parker blade is used to incise the central incision down through the periosteum, and a brow elevator is used to dissect downward to release the arcus marginalis along the orbital rim, carefully avoiding the supraorbital neurovascular bundles. A "smart hand" dissection (see Chapter 10 for details) or endoscopic guidance can be used. The arcus marginalis should be completely released for implants that extend to the immediate suprabrow position so that the implant can freely rest in the intended position without buckling inferiorly or being restricted from proper positioning.

4. The two temporal incisions are then made, and dissection is performed in the subtemporoparietal fascia plane as undertaken in a standard endoscopic, or minimal-incision, brow lift. The conjoined tendons that separate the lateral temporal from the medial subperiosteal pockets are completely severed from a lateral to medial direction, as per routine for a brow lift.

5. A surgical marking pen is used to mark out two dots that are separated a distance of 1.0 to 1.5 cm and that are located along the central aspect of the forehead. The clear implant is then laid over the forehead where the surgeon would like it to be placed, and two dots are drawn onto the implant exactly over the two dots that were made on the skin below.

6. A 3–0 nylon suture is passed through one of the marked dots on the skin, and the needle is pulled out through one of the temporal incisions.

7. The same needle is placed through one of the marked dots on the silicone implant (the dot that corresponds with the outer skin dot that was pierced initially) from the superficial to deep surface and passed back through the other dot on the implant from deep to superficial.

8. The needle is driven back through the remaining dot on the skin, and the suture is gently pulled through.

9. A hemostat can be placed on both ends of the suture to prevent one end of the suture from falling through the skin inadvertently.

10. The implant is inserted into the subperiosteal pocket via one of the two temporal pockets, using the 3–0 nylon suture as a guide. The implant can be rolled for ease of insertion, as the implant oftentimes will be larger than the temporal incision length.

11. The implant is then unfurled in situ, and the edges are inspected carefully to ensure that there is no buckling or folding. The implant can be palpated carefully through the skin to ensure that it is properly positioned, and endoscopic confirmation can also be beneficial.

12. After the implant resides in perfect orientation and position, the 3–0 nylon suture can be tied down over a cotton bolster, which remains for 3 to 4 days postoperatively.

13. A 15-French Jackson-Pratt-style drain can be inserted and passed through a separate temporal stab incision behind the hairline, which is left in place overnight to be removed the following day if only a small amount of drainage is present.

14. The skin incisions are approximated with surgical staples, which can be removed on the seventh postoperative day. No compressive dressing is necessary.

◆ Facial Liposuction and Lipotransfer

Method of Tetsuo Shu

As mentioned, the Asian face has a unique set of characteristics that should guide liposurgery. The malar region tends to exhibit greater fat accumulation, heavier soft tissue, and weaker skeletal support. Because of the disproportionate fat deposition in the malar region and the unaesthetic appearance of a prominent cheek in Asian aesthetic standards, facial liposuction is a more common enterprise than in the Caucasian counterpart. The submental region demonstrates less fat deposit in the younger patient but more substantial accretion as the patient matures. Part of the reason for the appearance of fat accumulation over time is a receded chin that provides weak skeletal support and heavier soft tissue than the Caucasian that undergoes gravitational descent. For these reasons, cervicofacial liposuction may be indicated.

Although liposuction has proven to be an established method of cervical and body contouring, autologous lipotransfer has been met with greater circumspection. The belief that all of the fat that is transferred becomes ultimately reabsorbed is a fallacy. Furthermore, various methods of fat harvesting, separation, and transfer have been advocated. The technique that will be explained in this narrative is based on 23 years of clinical experience with this method and has proven to be a reliable procedure for facial aesthetic enhancement.[7] The originator of this technique, Dr. Tetsuo Shu, has documented that the persistence of fat is contingent upon gentle handling (no centrifugation) and the prevalence of fibrous adipose tissue. The other type of adipose tissue is known as fatty adipose tissue, which is more susceptible to resorption and appears as a liquefied, oilier substance during the collection process.

Lipotransfer to the face may provide a very narrow or gaunt face some bulk either in the submalar, malar, temporal, or upper-lid region. Some Asian patients desire malar augmentation, but this is a far less frequent request than malar reduction. Rather than malar reduction, the submalar region can be filled with lipotransfer to lessen the disparity between the two areas and thereby create the illusion of less malar height. The temporal region also may appear quite depressed in the Asian patient due to a relatively arched zygomatic prominence. Autologous fat transfer to this region can facilitate a more balanced facial contour. As previously mentioned, a hollow upper lid may be a stigma of advanced aging and can follow an overzealous upper-lid blepharoplasty. Lipotransfer is a reliable method to restore a more youthful countenance and to camouflage a prior surgical resection. For all these reasons, lipotransfer has proven to be an effective method that permits ~60% augmentation of the soft tissue that persists indefinitely—if the correct surgical technique is applied. Although lipotransfer can be accomplished with the use of cervicofacial adipose reserves, the amount and quality of fat are generally insufficient. Therefore, body liposuction provides an ample supply of harvested fat for transplantation.

Surgical Technique for Facial Liposuction

1. To accomplish cervicofacial liposuction, a tumescent solution of 1% lidocaine and 1:100,000 epinephrine is mixed with normal saline in a 1:4 ratio

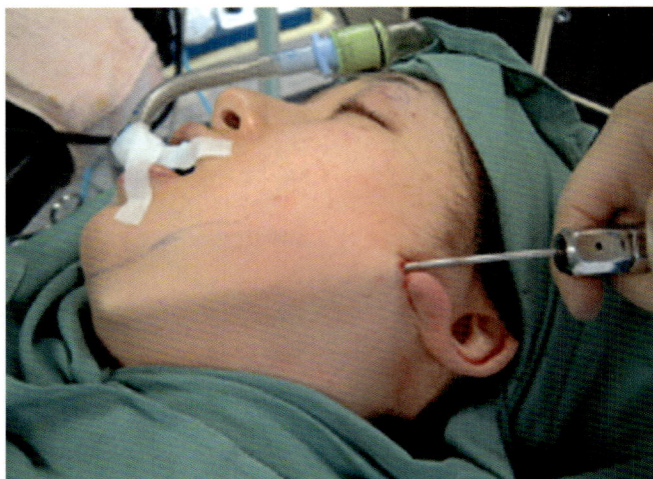

Figure 11–40 Cervicofacial liposuction is performed with a cannula inserted through the lobular-facial junction after tumescent infiltration. (From Shu T, Lam SM. Liposuction and lipostransfer for facial rejuvenation in the Asian patient. Int J Cosm Surg Aesthetic Dermatol 2003;5:165–173; with permission.)

and infiltrated into the targeted tissues for hemostasis, anesthesia, and ease and uniformity of liposuction. The infiltration is undertaken with a long 22-gauge spinal needle on a 25 cc syringe, which is injected in a radial fashion across the tissue bed from the ear lobule–facial interface.

2. A no. 11 Bard-Parker blade is used to make a stab incision at the same lobule-facial junction, and a 3 mm liposuction cannula is inserted via this incision. Liposuction is performed by passing the cannula in the subcutaneous plane from a deeper to a more superficial plane while rotating the cannula.[†] The cannula can be passed into the cervical, submental, and facial regions all from the one incision site in a radial manner (Fig. **11–40**). This technique avoids any conspicuous facial incisions that may leave a hyperpigmented or hypertrophic scar in the Asian skin. The stab incision need not be closed at the end of the case.

Surgical Technique for Facial Lipotransfer

1. The technique for body liposuction follows the method outlined for facial liposuction in that tumescent infiltration is used and the prescribed minimal-incision, radial technique is undertaken.

2. After the fat has been harvested, the collected speci-

[†]The liposuction cannula described in this text is a proprietary design in which the aperture of the cannula is located on the side, and the instrument can be rotated circumferentially at the base to permit uniform liposuctioning.

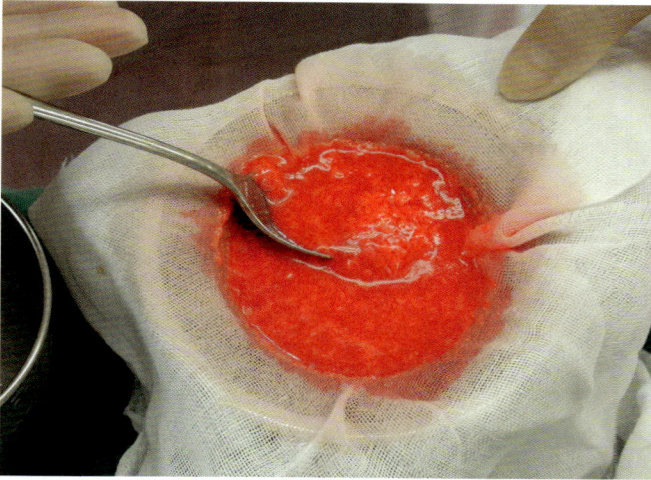

Figure 11–41   *Liposuction and Lipotransfer, Step 1:* The harvested adipose tissue is strained through a cotton gauze with saline. (From Shu T, Lam SM. Liposuction and lipostransfer for facial rejuvenation in the Asian patient. Int J Cosm Surg Aesthetic Dermatol 2003;5:165–173; with permission.)

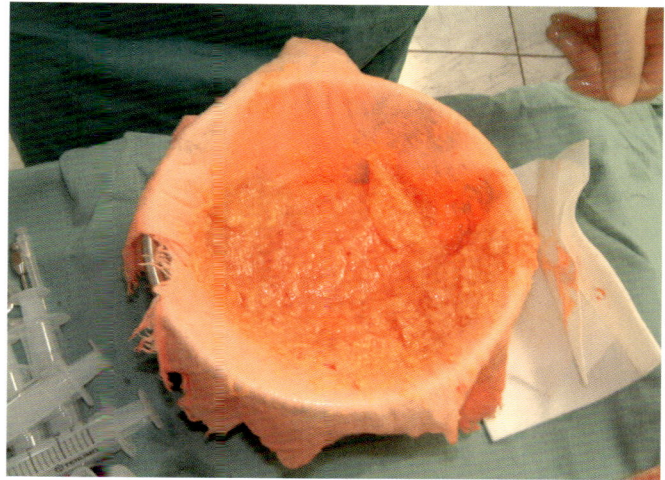

Figure 11–43   *Liposuction and Lipotransfer, Step 3:* The harvested fat has been dried and has assumed a yellow to orange color, and it is ready for transplantation. (From Shu T, Lam SM. Liposuction and lipostransfer for facial rejuvenation in the Asian patient. Int J Cosm Surg Aesthetic Dermatol 2003;5:165–173; with permission.)

men is placed on top of a cotton gauze, which rests in turn over an empty pitcher (Fig. **11–41**). Sterile iced saline is poured over the fat to filter the excess blood and liquefied fat through the cotton gauze. The saline and fat should be stirred to facilitate the passage of the saline through the gauze. When the mixture is semi-dry, the gauze should be picked up and squeezed dry to remove any remaining liquid (Fig. **11–42**). This process is repeated three or four times until the collected fat is dry and assumes a yellow to orange color (Fig. **11–43**).

3. The harvested fat can then be placed into the appro-

priate syringes for facial transplantation. Of note, the recipient site for fat transplantation is not infiltrated with local anesthesia so as to prevent tissue distortion, and the patient is anesthetized with intravenous sedation only.

4. For the upper lid, a 1 cc syringe with an 18-gauge needle can be used to inject fat into the subcutaneous plane, working from deep to more superficial, from an entry point under the lateral brow (Fig. **11–44**). The 2.5 or 5 cc syringe with a 2 mm cannula facilitates transfer of larger volumes that are required for the cheek and temporal regions. For the

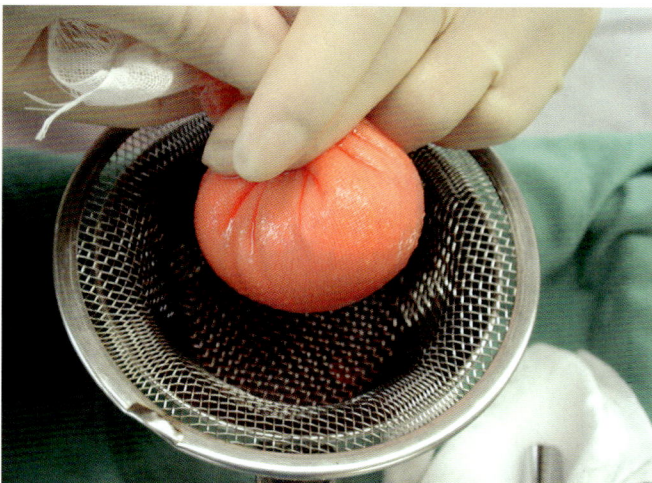

Figure 11–42   *Liposuction and Lipotransfer, Step 2:* After most of the saline has been filtered through the cotton gauze, the cotton gauze is picked up and the remaining saline is squeezed through the gauze. (*From* Shu T, Lam SM. Liposuction and lipostransfer for facial rejuvenation in the Asian patient. Int J Cosm Surg Aesthetic Dermatol 2003;5:165–173; with permission.)

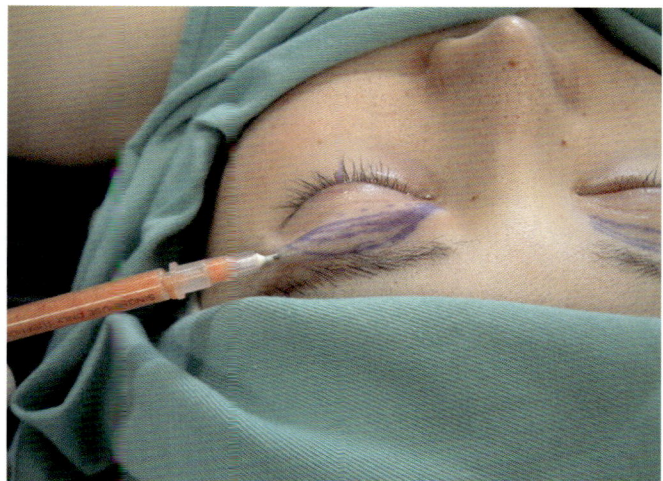

Figure 11–44   *Liposuction and Lipotransfer, Step 4A:* Eyelid fat injection using an 18-gauge needle and a 1 cc syringe. (From Shu T, Lam SM. Liposuction and lipostransfer for facial rejuvenation in the Asian patient. Int J Cosm Surg Aesthetic Dermatol 2003;5:165–173; with permission.)

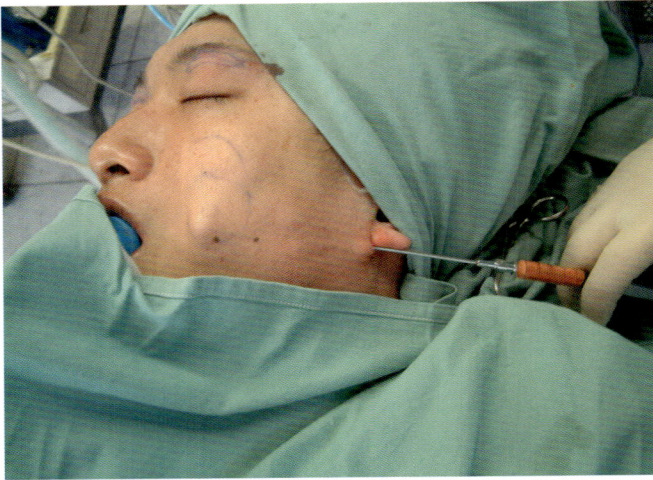

Figure 11–45 *Liposuction and Lipotransfer, Step 4B:* Cheek fat injection using a 2 mm cannula and a 5 cc syringe. (From Shu T, Lam SM. Liposuction and lipostransfer for facial rejuvenation in the Asian patient. Int J Cosm Surg Aesthetic Dermatol 2003;5:165–173; with permission.)

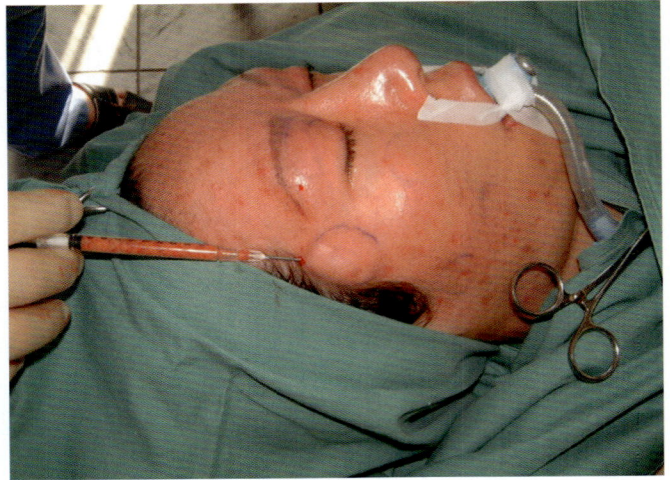

Figure 11–46 *Liposuction and Lipotransfer, Step 4C:* Temporal fat injection using an 18-gauge needle and a 1 cc syringe. (From Shu T, Lam SM. Liposuction and lipostransfer for facial rejuvenation in the Asian patient. Int J Cosm Surg Aesthetic Dermatol 2003;5:165–173; with permission.)

cheek, the cannula is inserted through a stab incision through the lobular-facial junction and passed in a similar manner as described for cheek liposuction (Fig. **11–45**). However, the cannula is not rotated, and the fat is dispersed only during cannula withdrawal. The temporal area can be accessed from the hairline, and the blunt cannula used to distribute the fat in the subcutaneous plane in a radial fashion from deep to superficial (Fig. **11–46**). It is imperative that a blunt device be used for lipotransfer to avoid

inadvertent passage of a needle through the temporoparietal fascia with resultant nerve injury. In addition, the 2.5 or 5 cc syringe should not be equipped with an 18-gauge needle, as the increased pressure achieved by delivery from a larger syringe into a smaller needle may traumatize the adipocytes excessively. An important step after fat transplantation that should not be overlooked is molding the transplanted fat between one's fingers to ensure a more uniform distribution. The fat can be pinched

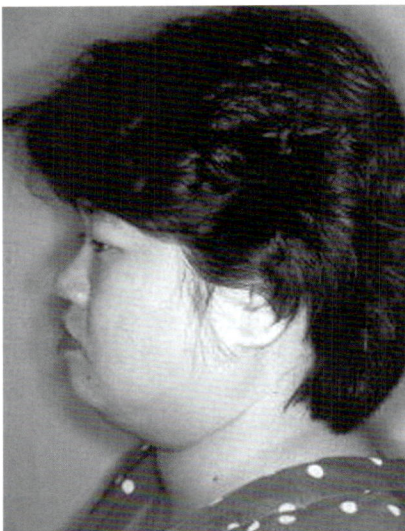
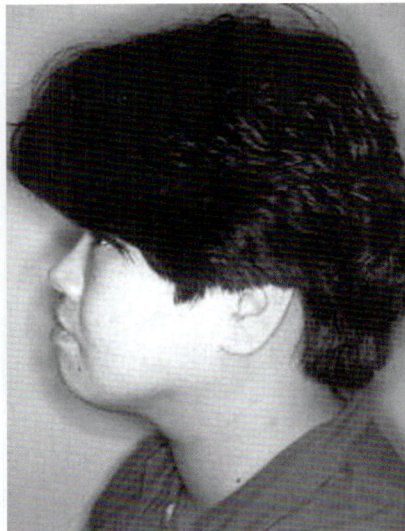

A   B

Figure 11–47 **(A,B)** This 21-year-old woman who has significant cheek and neck adipose accumulation underwent a cervicofacial liposuction via the tumescent technique and presents 1 month postoperatively. (From Shu T, Lam SM. Liposuction and lipostransfer for facial rejuvenation in the Asian patient. Int J Cosm Surg Aesthetic Dermatol 2003;5: 165–173; with permission.)

between two fingers and gently massaged until the contour feels smooth and even.

Asian aesthetics and anatomy should always be recalled when considering facial liposuction and lipotransfer (Figs. **11–47, 11–48, 11–49, 11–50**). If fat is

properly harvested, processed, and transplanted, then fat viability is ensured. Approximately 60% should permanently persist, and multiple procedures can be performed to arrive at the optimal degree of augmentation.

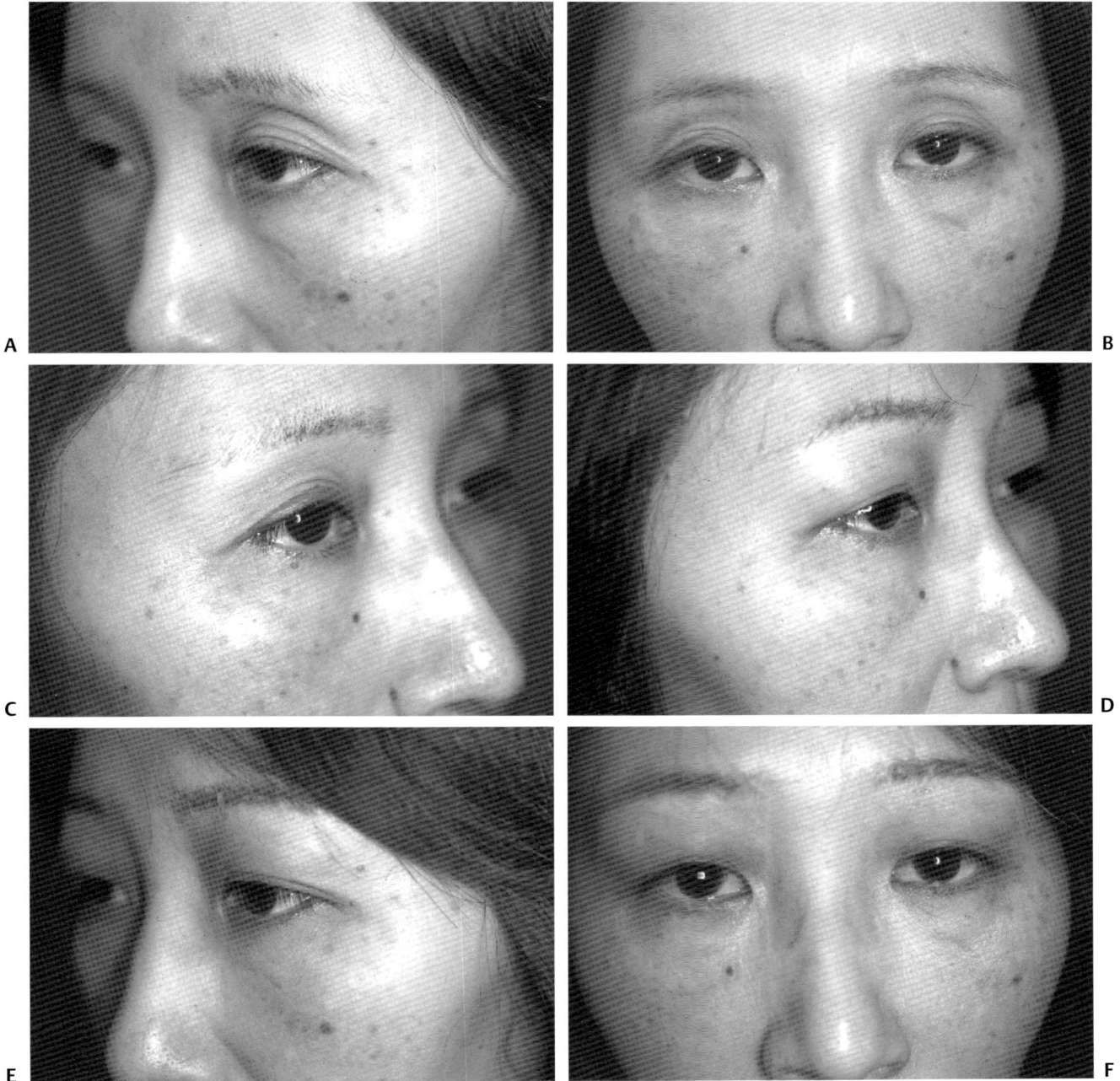

Figure 11–48 (A–C) This 48-year-old woman who exhibits an aged sunken eye appearance underwent a single session of lipotransfer to the upper-lid region and presents 7 months postoperatively. **(D–F)** (From Shu T, Lam SM. Liposuction and lipostransfer for facial rejuvenation in the Asian patient. Int J Cosm Surg Aesthetic Dermatol 2003;5:165–173; with permission.)

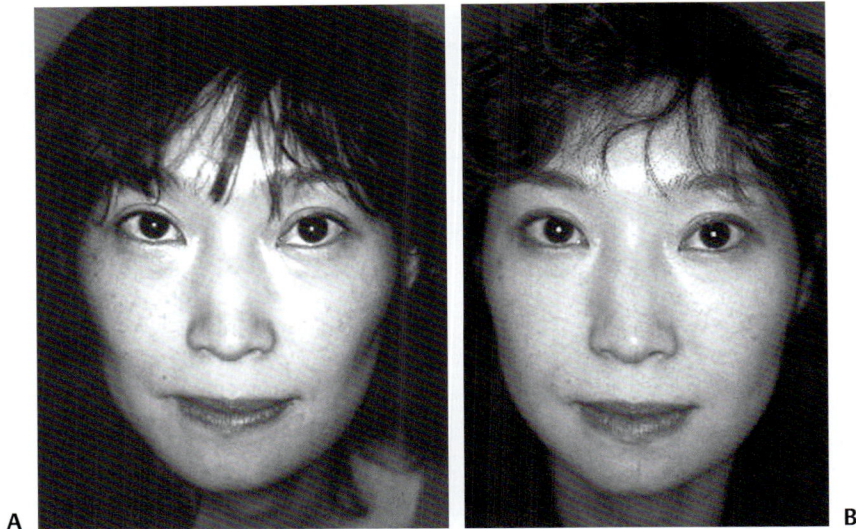

Figure 11–49 (A,B) This 22-year-old woman who underwent cheek (malar and submalar) fat transplantation is shown 7 years postoperatively. (From Shu T, Lam SM. Liposuction and lipostransfer for facial rejuvenation in the Asian patient. Int J Cosm Surg Aesthetic Dermatol 2003;5:165–173; with permission.)

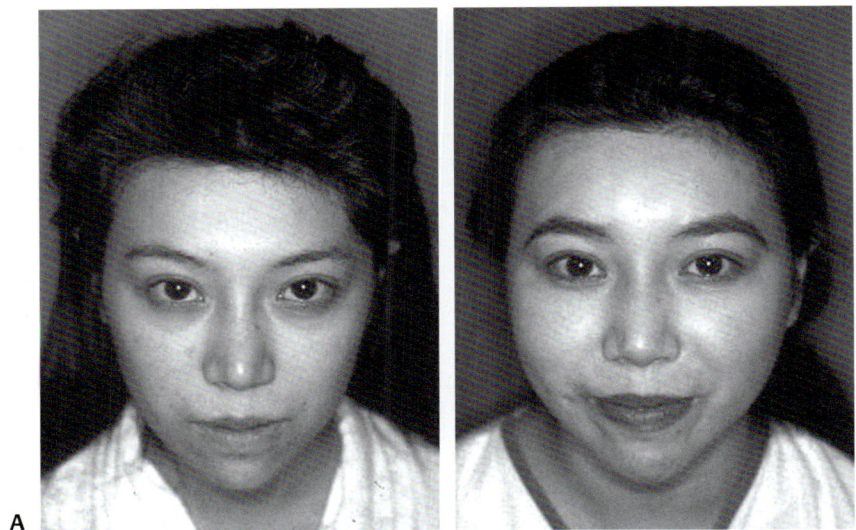

Figure 11–50 (A,B) This 19-year-old woman who underwent cheek, temporal, and forehead fat transplantation is shown 12 years postoperatively. (From Shu T, Lam SM. Liposuction and lipostransfer for facial rejuvenation in the Asian patient. Int J Cosm Surg Aesthetic Dermatol 2003;5: 165–173; with permission.)

References

1. Lam SM, Ahn JM. Rhinoplasty, premaxillary augmentation. Available at: www.emedicine.com.
2. Giunta SX. Premaxillary augmentation in Asian rhinoplasty. Facial Plast Surg Clin North Am. 1996;4:93–102[x1]
3. Fanous N, Yoskovitch A. Premaxillary augmentation: adjunct to rhinoplasty. Plast Reconstr Surg 2000;106:707–712
4. Fanous N, Yoskotovitch A. Premaxillary augmentation for central maxillary recession: an adjunct to rhinoplasty. Facial Plast Surg Clin North Am 2002;10:415–422
5. Giunta SX. Augmentation mentoplasty in Asian men and women. Facial Plast Surg Clin North Am 1996;4:117–128
6. Chang EW, Lam SM, Karen M, Donlevy JL. Sliding genioplasty for correction of chin abnormalities Arch Facial Plast Surg 2001;3:8–15
7. Shu T, Lam SM. Liposuction and lipostransfer for facial rejuvenation in the Asian patient. Int J Cosm Surg Aesthetic Dermatol 2003;5:165–173

12

Skeletal Surgery in the Asian Face

◆ General and Anatomic Considerations

The ideals of beauty are not always consistent across cultural divides. This truism is well exemplified by the unique skeletal-reduction surgeries that are fashionable in Asia. For instance, malar convexity that is a hallmark of Western allure is oftentimes considered an unattractive attribute for the Asian face. Despite the deluge of periodicals, posters, and other media that extol Western beauty, a fundamental desire to maintain one's distinct ethnicity informs many a decision to undergo cosmetic surgery. This trend has become increasingly evident over the past decade. However, certain Asian skeletal features, for example, relatively lower facial convexity, are deemed universally unaesthetic and transcend these peculiar cultural differences. The Western surgeon should always be cognizant of and sensitive toward these distinctive cultural and anatomic traits.

Before a careful review of surgical options for skeletal modification can be embarked upon, the reader should understand the particular skeletal features that serve as the structural underpinning of the Asian face. The forehead and brow region exhibit a narrow expanse and flat contour, with a posterior inclination superiorly. The temple region may appear more hollowed due to the relative protuberance of the zygomatic arch. The orbits are shallower due to both a less recessed bony orbital cavity and a fuller eyelid. The midfacial skeleton is often hypoplastic and extends to the central aspect of the face (i.e., a less prominent nasal spine and a deficient premaxillary segment). The straight brow contour, the shallower orbit, and the hypoplastic midface all contribute to the overall flatter appearance of the upper and midface. However, the lower face is typically more

convex due to several factors. The premaxillary deficiency is notable below the nose, but the bone tends to curve outward toward a prominent incisor show, which contributes to the perceived convexity. This bony configuration affects the overlying soft tissue with an acute nasolabial angle, potential labial incompetence, and "gummy" smile. This convexity is accentuated by the mandibular prognathism that often predominates in the Asian face. In addition, the inferior aspect of the chin tends to recede posteriorly, which further exacerbates the convex profile.

The subject of skeletal surgery of the Asian face is broad and complex. The topic embraces diverse disciplines, including craniofacial surgery, facial plastic surgery, and oral and maxillofacial surgery. The focus of this chapter as the title aptly declares, is confined to cosmetic facial endeavors. Reconstructive and orthognathic surgery procedures lie beyond the scope of the text. However, elective bony surgery that directly affects cosmesis will be included even if functional orthognathic proficiency is integral to the procedure. The reader is advised to undertake these more advanced surgical techniques after appropriate completion of formal training.

The following discussion will be broadly classified according to advancement (augmentation) and reduction procedures. The former category is more familiar in the West in that maxillary, mandibular, and chin advancements are staple procedures for the oral and maxillofacial surgeon and at times the facial plastic surgeon. Accordingly, any analogous bony reductions that involve the same technique as the described advancement will be considered the same procedure and not be further elaborated upon in a separate section. Several bony reduction-type surgeries are unique to the Asian

Le Fort I Advancement

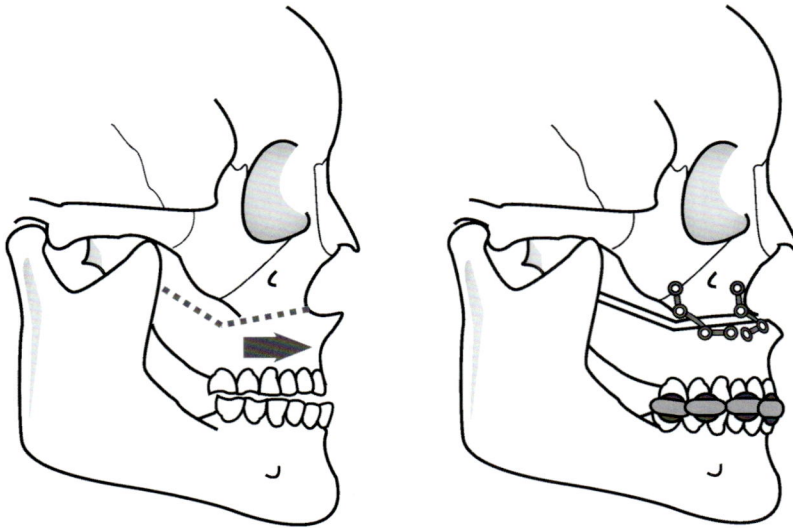

Figure 12–1 A Le Fort I advancement or recession can improve maxillary position and thereby correct occlusal disharmony and enhance cosmesis. The osteotomy is undertaken from the pyriform aperture back to the pterygomaxillary fissure bilaterally and more medially to separate the lateral nasal walls and septum from the maxilla and finally between the maxillary tuberosity and the pterygoid process.

patient and include both malar and mandibular-angle resections.

◆ Advancement and Recession Surgeries

Maxillary Advancement/Recession

Surgical Technique for a Le Fort I Osteotomy

Although a Le Fort III osteotomy has been advocated for midfacial advancement, traditionally a Le Fort I osteotomy is a more popular option (Fig. **12–1**). During the preoperative phase, the patient must be subjected to photographic, cephalometric, and occlusal analysis before embarking on the surgical enterprise. Precise preoperative dental models are used to plan the surgical procedure and to determine the degree of advancement or recession that should be undertaken. An occlusal wafer is fabricated based on these models that will serve as an intraoperative guide for alignment of the mobilized maxillary and mandibular segments.

1. The surgery commences with a generous gingivobuccal incision that exposes the entire face of the maxilla, and dissection is continued in a subperiosteal plane.

2. The first osteotomy that is created lies in a horizontal axis that spans from the pyriform aperture to the pterygomaxillary fissure bilaterally, at a distance of ~5 mm above the most inferior aspect of the pyriform aperture to ensure that the dental roots are not inadvertently transected.

3. Next, the maxillary complex must be freed from the nasal cavity and septum: the cartilaginous nasal septum is separated from the underlying bony

maxillary crest after mucoperiosteal flaps have been elevated. The medial nasal wall is similarly divided inferiorly using an osteotome.

4. The final bony release is achieved with a large curved Kawamato osteotome aimed between the maxillary tuberosity and the pterygoid process, with judicious regard for the vascular pterygoid plexus and the greater palatine neurovascular bundle in the vicinity (Fig. **12–2**).

5. The remaining soft-tissue attachments must then be gently teased free with blunt periosteal elevation

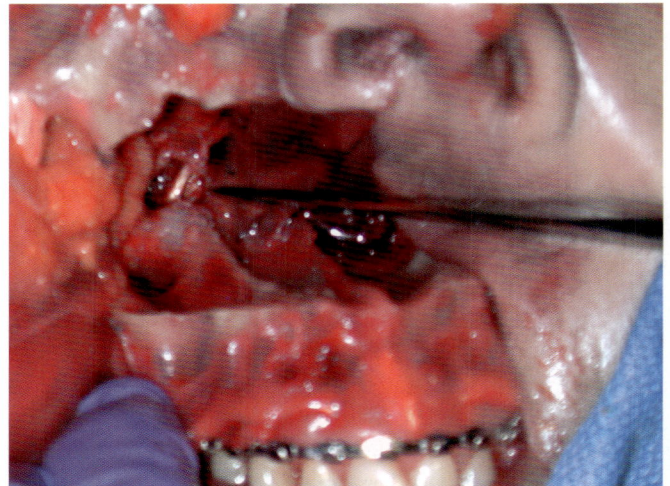

Figure 12–2 Cadaveric photograph shows the exposed greater palatine neurovascular bundle that must be carefully preserved during osteotomy. The lateral and medial osteotomies are executed with a reciprocating saw, whereas the final bony release near the neurovascular bundle should be judiciously undertaken with elevators and rongeurs. (Courtesy of Edward W. Chang, M.D., D.D.S.)

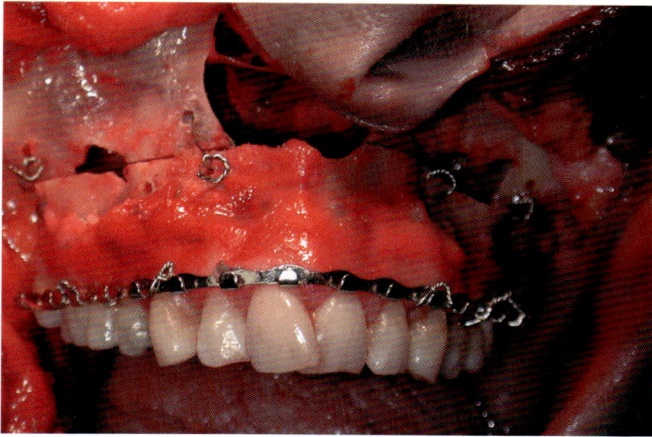

Figure 12–3 Cadaveric photograph shows wire fixation placed prior to miniplate fixation to secure the maxilla in its new position. Erich arch bars are shown that would normally be secured to the mandible to set proper occlusion before placement of maxillary wire fixation, using the interim occlusal wafer as a guide. (Courtesy of Edward W. Chang, M.D., D.D.S.)

and with a deliberate anterior force of distraction on the maxillary tuberosity rather than applied leverage.

6. Using the occlusal wafer as a guide, the maxillary segment is advanced to the proper position and secured with wire and/or miniplate fixation (Fig. 12–3). An alar-base cinch suture can be passed before final mucosal closure to preclude any undesirable alar flare.

Various combinations of osteotomies and bone grafting may be employed to achieve the optimal outcome. As the incidence of mandibular prognathism is relatively high in the Asian population, a combined mandibular setback and maxillary advancement may be accomplished for improved skeletal harmony. Premaxillary hypoplasia may be addressed with a Le Fort II advancement osteotomy. Alternatively, a Le Fort I osteotomy may be supplemented with a central premaxillary bone graft or alloplastic implantation, which may be preferred to the more morbid Le Fort II advancement. As alluded to in the opening portion of this chapter, maxillary setbacks will not be reiterated in a separate section, as the procedure mimics the described procedure except with retrograde displacement of the bony segment. However, it may be noted that posterior bony translocations may be unstable and less predictable.

Surgical Technique for Maxillary Anterior Segmental Osteotomy

Rather than advance the entire maxillary complex via a Le Fort I osteotomy, an anterior segmental osteotomy

may be undertaken to mobilize only the central, anterior dentoalveolar segment if that is the only bony region that merits repositioning. Bimaxillary protrusion (simianism) is characteristic of some Asians and may benefit from bimaxillary recession via combined maxillary and mandibular anterior segmental osteotomies (Fig. 12–4A–F). Rigid fixation of the mobilized maxillary and mandibular segments to their respective bony framework can facilitate an early return to social and professional life that would not be possible with traditional maxillomandibular wire fixation.

1. The maxillary first premolars must be extracted at the outset to facilitate proper alignment of bony segments and reorientation of teeth in a more vertical plane (Fig. 12–5 A,B).
2. Vertical mucoperiosteal incisions are then made in the region of the extracted first premolar and connected with a horizontal incision 3 to 5 mm above the labiogingival sulcus.
3. Dissection is carried along superiorly in a subperiosteal plane until the pyriform aperture is exposed and the nasal septum is encountered.
4. The nasal septal cartilage is mobilized from the bony vomer framework with a small osteotome back to the point where the posterior osteotomy through the palatine bone and vomer will be undertaken.
5. A subperiosteal pocket is tunneled from the region of the extracted maxillary first premolar back to the palatal midline along the proposed osteotomy line. The overlying palatal mucosa is separated so that it will not be injured during the osteotomy.
6. The osteotomy is performed with an oscillating saw that extends from the region of the extracted first premolar toward the pyriform aperture bilaterally, as indicated in Fig. 12–5.
7. The osteotomy is then continued to separate the maxillary attachment along the hard palate while protecting the mucosa with a thin, malleable retractor ensconced between the mucosa and bone in the created subperiosteal tunnel.
8. The necessary amount of palatal and alveolar bone is resected to permit recession of the mobilized segment, as determined by preoperative occlusal models.
9. The mobilized anterior bony segment is repositioned and guided by an interim occlusal wafer. The bony segment is held in place with miniplate fixation and interdental wiring between the canines and second premolar teeth. Intermaxillary (maxillomandibular) fixation is typically not required.

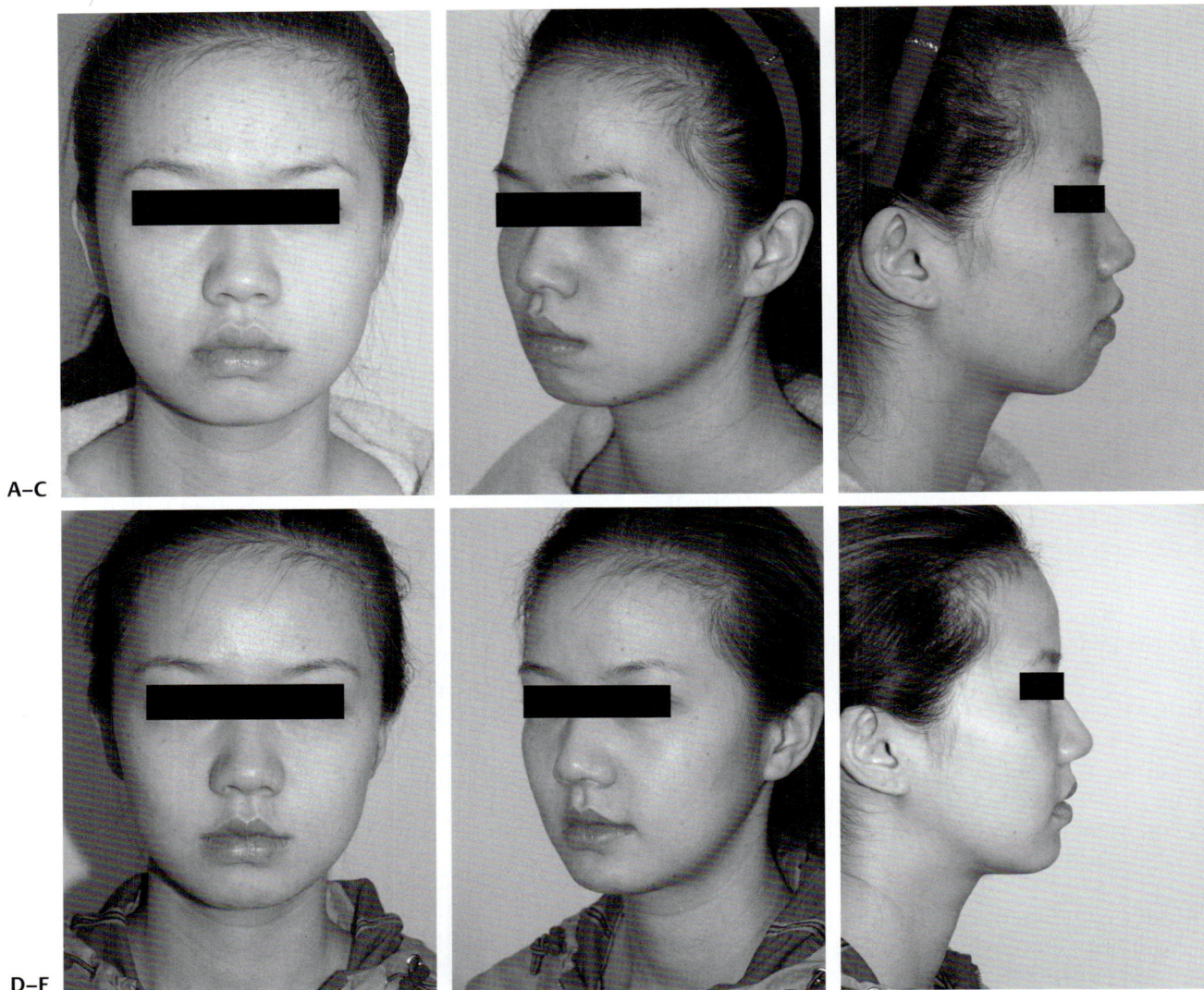

Figure 12–4 **(A–C)** This 23-year-old Korean woman underwent bimaxillary anterior segmental osteotomy with 4 mm recession and 3 mm downward movement of her maxillary segment and with 4.2 mm recession and 3 mm impaction of her mandibular segment. (The vertical reorientation of the bony segments was undertaken to show more of her teeth during smiling.) She also underwent concurrent mandibular contouring surgery. **(D–F)** She is shown 6 months postoperatively. (Courtesy of Jung Soo Lee, M.D.)

Mandibular anterior segmental osteotomy follows the same principles outlined above, but with the added attention that should be paid to avoid injury to the inferior alveolar nerve (IAN). The mandibular first premolars are extracted at the outset, and the two vertical mucoperiosteal incisions are made in the region of the extracted teeth. The horizontal incision is then made to join the vertical incisions below the dental roots. The osteotomy line is exposed, taking care not to injure the mental nerves. The oscillating saw is used to fashion the osteotomy cuts and to mobilize the anterior mandibular segment. The segment is repositioned to the desired position and guided into position with an occlusal wafer splint and fixed with miniplate and interdental wiring, as described above for maxillary anterior segmental osteotomy.

Mandibular Advancement/Recession

Preoperative Remarks

Preoperative evaluation of mandibular position follows the prescribed analyses for maxillary surgery (i.e., cephalometric, photographic, and occlusal studies). An overprojected mandible may be retrodisplaced via two principal methods—vertical-subcondylar and sagittal-split osteotomies—the latter of which represents the more common surgical technique. For a retruded mandible, a sagittal-split osteotomy, sliding genioplasty (*vide infra*), and placement of an alloplastic implant are all viable methods for advancement depending on the presence of a malocclusion (sagittal-split technique) or absence thereof (sliding genioplasty or alloplastic insertion).

Anterior Segmental Osteotomy

A. Maxillary

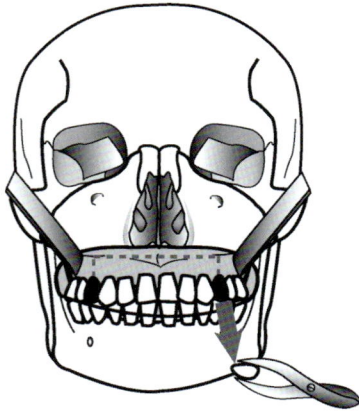

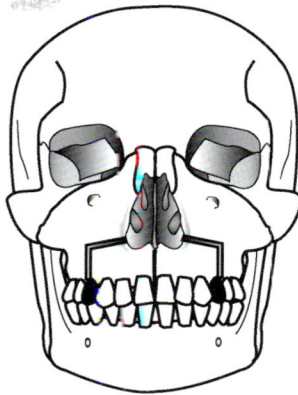

B. Mandibular

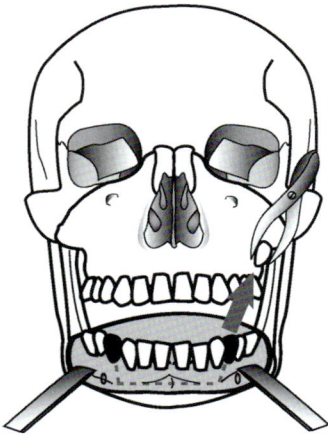

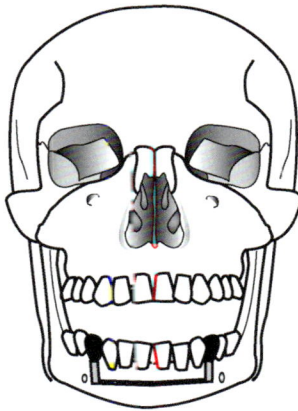

Figure 12–5 (A,B) As an alternative to advancement or recession of the entire malar or mandibular complex, the central dentoalveolar segment can be mobilized to improve occlusion and aesthetic appearance with an anterior segmental osteotomy. As part of both a maxillary and mandibular anterior segmental osteotomy, the first premolar must be extracted to facilitate alignment. Vertical osteotomy cuts are made in the region of the extracted teeth and joined with a horizontal osteotomy that resides just beyond the dental apices. Mobilization of the bony maxillary segment is more involved compared with mandibular anterior segmental osteotomy, and the details are elaborated in the text. Removal of any bone that restricts movement of the mobilized segment is proportionately undertaken. The mobilized segment is guided into position with an interim occlusal splint and fixed with a combination of miniplates and interdental wiring. Intermaxillary (maxillomandibular) fixation is generally not required.

Surgical Technique for the Vertical-Subcondylar Osteotomy

The vertical-subcondylar technique (Fig. **12–6**) for mandibular prognathism touts the major advantage of more infrequent inferior alveolar nerve injury than the sagittal-split method. The osteotomy may be approached either intraorally, which avoids an external incision and reduces marginal-mandibular nerve injury, or extraorally, which may be technically less demanding but may result in a conspicuous cutaneous scar. However, the greater obliquity of the mandibular rami in relation to the sagittal axis affords easier intraoral exposure.

1. The intraoral approach begins with a gingivobuccal incision that exposes the coronoid to the second bicuspid immediately posterior to the exit of the mental nerve. (The mental nerve usually exits between the second bicuspid teeth.)

2. The periosteum is then reflected posteriorly, and the lingular process is identified that corresponds to the medial entry of the IAN at the lingula.

3. Osteotomies are fashioned from the sigmoid notch down to the mandibular angle behind the antilingular process to avoid IAN injury. Care should be taken to avoid injury to the internal maxillary artery that travels in the vicinity of the sigmoid notch. The extraoral route may represent an alternative course for setbacks that exceed 10 mm as well as for asymmetric cases.

Surgical Technique for the Sagittal-Split Osteotomy

As mentioned, the sagittal-split technique (Fig. **12–7**) offers the versatility of bidirectional mandibular repositioning (advancement or recession) (Fig. **12–8A,B**). However, this technique suffers from three known potential complications: IAN injury (as high as a reported 45%), proximal-segment necrosis (a rare entity), and dental avulsion.

Vertical-Subcondylar Osteotomy

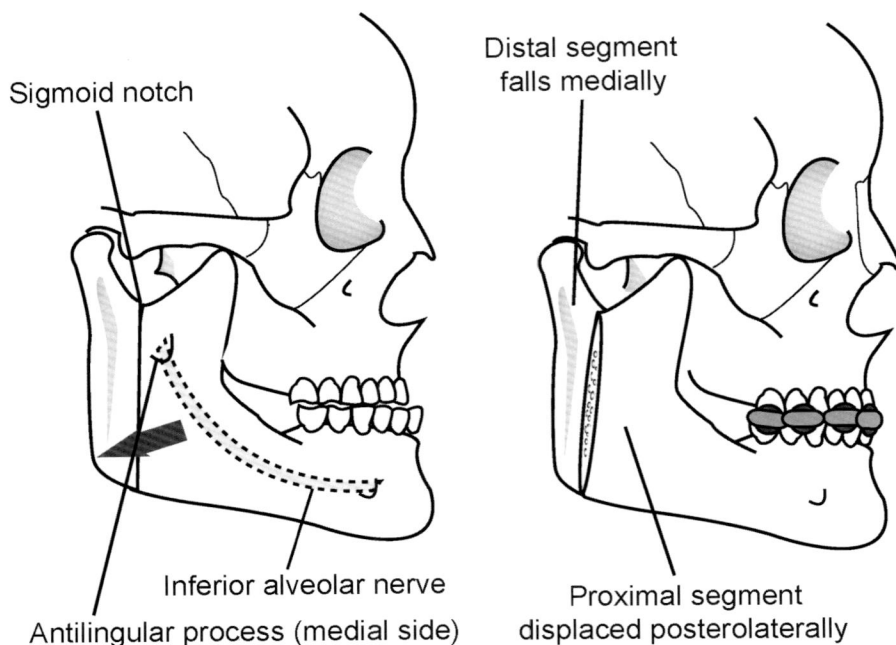

Sigmoid notch

Distal segment falls medially

Inferior alveolar nerve

Antilingular process (medial side)

Proximal segment displaced posterolaterally

Figure 12–6 The vertical-subcondylar method permits mandibular advancement or recession and is an alternative to the sagittal-split method. Osteotomies are fashioned from the sigmoid notch down to the mandibular angle behind the antilingular process to avoid IAN injury.

Sagittal-Split Osteotomy

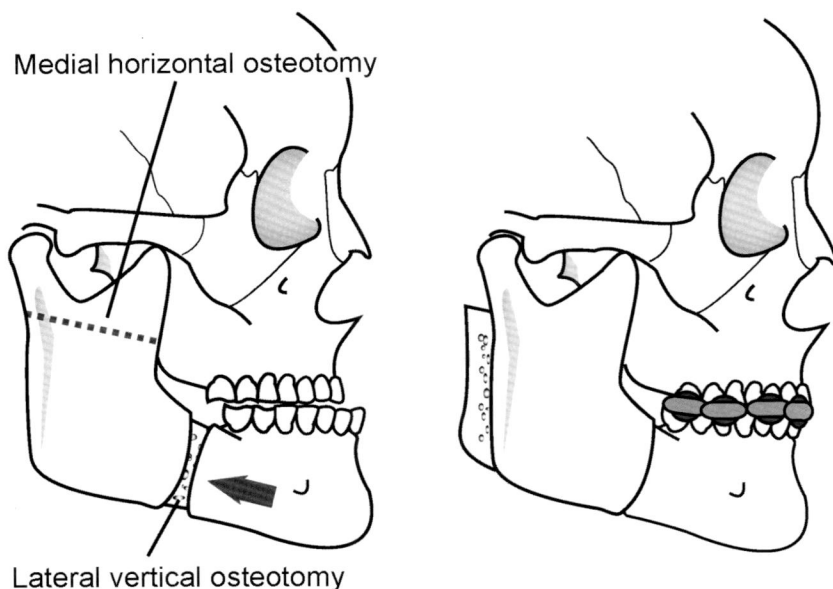

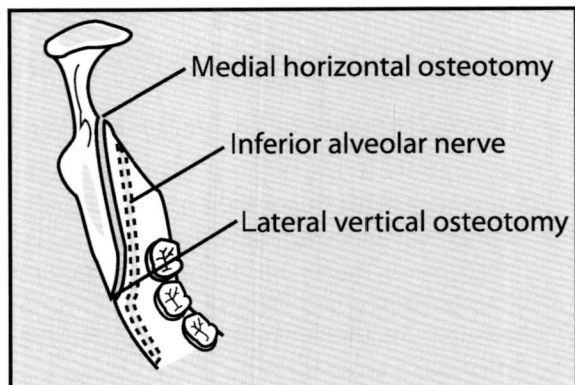

Medial horizontal osteotomy

Lateral vertical osteotomy

Medial horizontal osteotomy

Inferior alveolar nerve

Lateral vertical osteotomy

Figure 12–7 The sagittal-split method permits mandibular advancement or recession and is an alternative to the vertical-subcondylar method. A horizontal osteotomy is commenced 5 mm superior to the lingula through the medial cortex, whereas a vertical osteotomy is committed at the level of the first molar through the lateral cortex. The two osteotomies are joined at the oblique line, and the IAN remains with the distal, medial segment. An intervening block of bone is removed from the anterior aspect of the proximal (lateral) segment if the mandible is intended to be retropositioned. Contralateral osteotomies are conducted in a similar fashion, and the degree of advancement or recession is adjusted as dictated by the occlusal wafer.

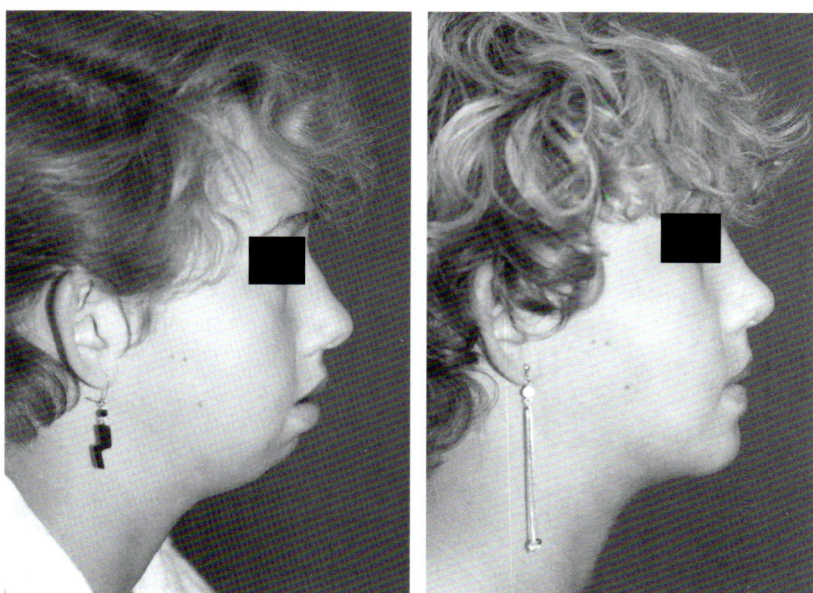

Figure 12–8   (A,B) This 18-year-old Caucasian woman underwent orthognathic surgery. She was jaw deficient and required a sagittal-split osteotomy with a sliding genioplasty to address the lower aspect of her facial skeletal disharmony. (Courtesy of Edward W. Chang, M.D., D.D.S.)

1. A horizontal osteotomy is commenced 5 mm superior to the lingula through the medial cortex, whereas a vertical osteotomy is committed at the level of the first molar through the lateral cortex.

2. The two osteotomies are joined at the oblique line, and the IAN remains with the distal, medial segment (Fig. **12–9**). Mobilization of the IAN may be necessary after the osteotomies are completed.

3. An intervening block of bone is removed from the anterior aspect of the proximal (lateral) segment if the mandible is intended to be retropositioned.

4. Contralateral osteotomies are conducted in a similar fashion, and the degree of advancement or recession is adjusted as dictated by the occlusal wafer (Fig. **12–10**).

Sliding Genioplasty

Preoperative Remarks

The sliding osseous genioplasty offers the distinct advantage over alloplastic mentoplasty in its versatility: a bony segment can be advanced or recessed and vertically or laterally repositioned (Fig. **12–11A–C**).[1] Although mandibular prognathism is a more prevalent condition in the Asian population, a posteriorly positioned mentum mandates more frequently advancement rather than reduction to minimize the undesirable convex profile (Fig. **12–12A,B**). Although occlusal imbalances are not addressed by this technique, proper cephalometric and photographic analyses are integral to preoperative assessment.

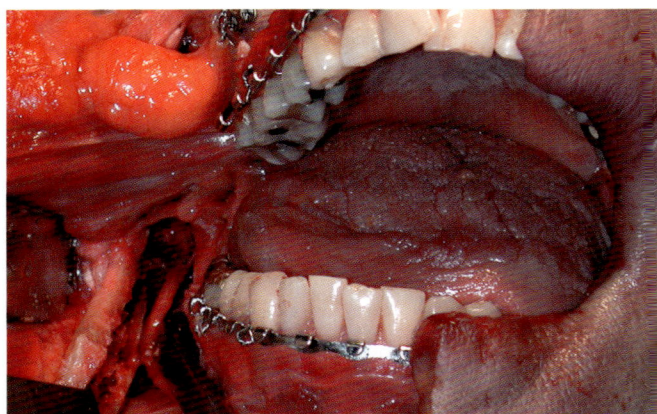

Figure 12–9   Cadaveric photograph shows the inferior alveolar nerve at risk during sagittal-split osteotomy. (Courtesy of Edward W. Chang, M.D., D.D.S.)

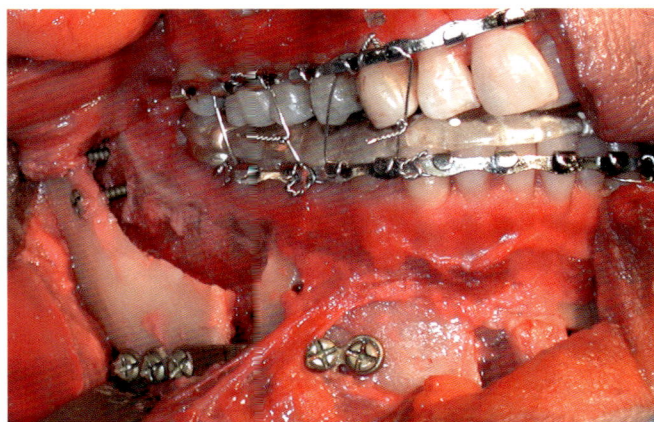

Figure 12–10   Cadaveric photograph shows miniplate fixation of the osteotomized segments during the sagittal-split technique. (Courtesy of Edward W. Chang, M.D., D.D.S.)

Sliding Genioplasty

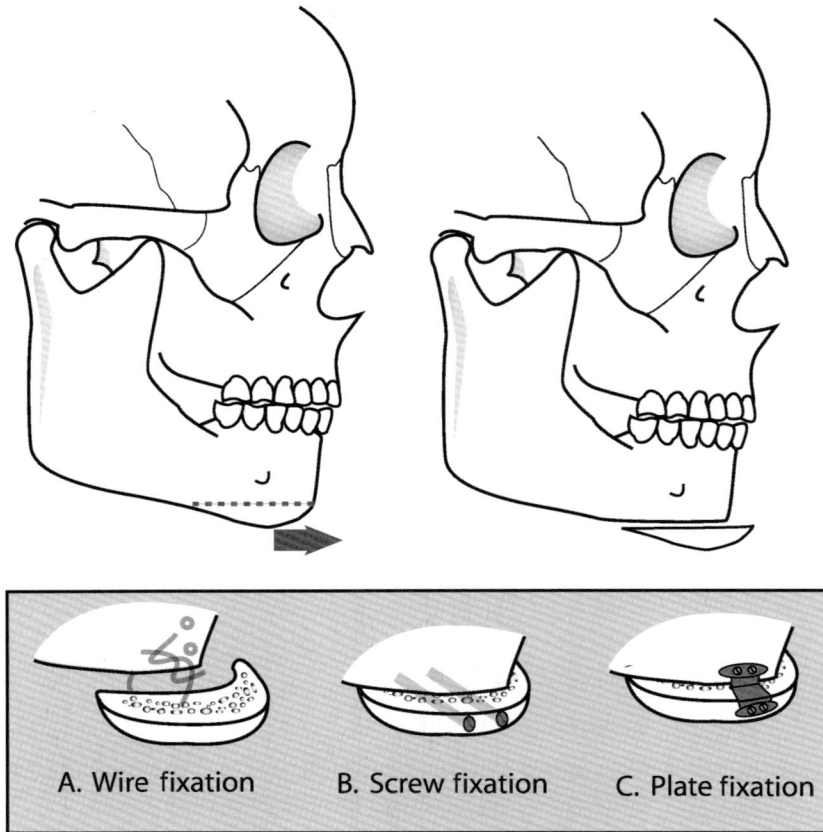

Figure 12–11   Illustration shows the horizontal osteotomy undertaken for a sliding genioplasty. The mobilized segment can then be advanced, recessed, or translocated side to side to match the desired aesthetic goal. Vertical excess or deficiency can be corrected with removal of an intervening bony segment or placement of an intervening bone graft. Because the technique does not involve movement of dentition, occlusion is not adjusted. The mobilized segment can then be secured with **(A)** wiring, **(B)** screws, or **(C)** miniplate fixation.

A. Wire fixation   B. Screw fixation   C. Plate fixation

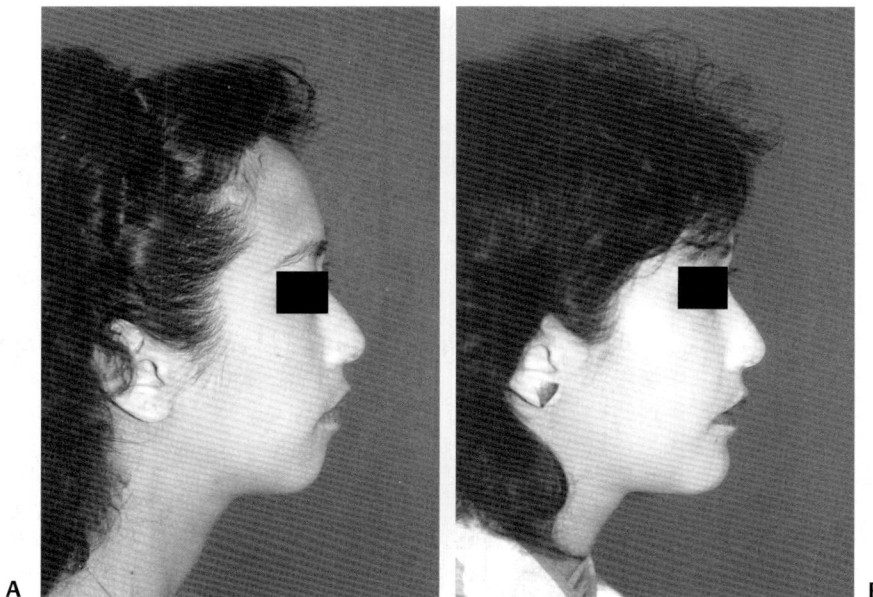

Figure 12–12   This 32-year-old Filipina woman underwent a sliding genioplasty under local anesthesia and monitored anesthetic care. She is shown postoperatively with a notable aesthetic improvement. (Courtesy of Edward W. Chang, M.D., D.D.S.)

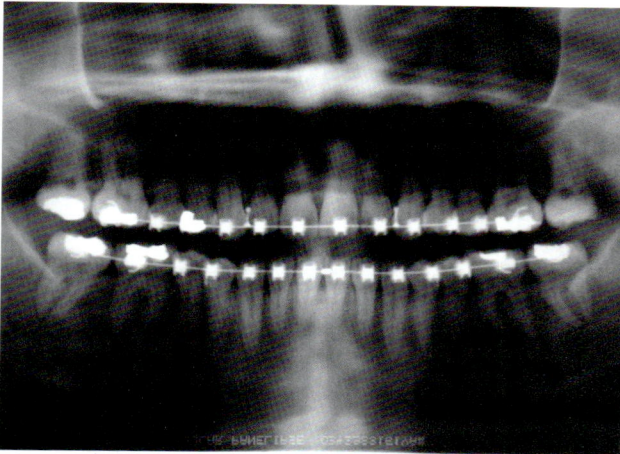

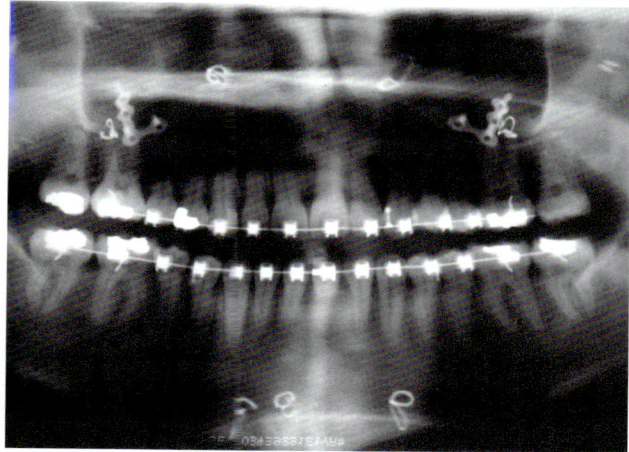

Figure 12–13 **(A)** Panoramic radiograph that shows orthodontic hardware that was placed 2 years prior to planning for orthognathic surgery. The preoperative Panorex is used in preparation for the sliding genioplasty to assess the length of the dental roots as well as to determine the path of the inferior alveolar nerve and the location of the mental nerves (which are shown located between the first and second premolars, with the right side more evident on the radiograph). **(B)** The postoperative Panorex shows the mobilized bony segment of the genioplasty secured with wire fixation. The patient also underwent a concomitant Le Fort I osteotomy that is secured with wire and miniplate fixation. (Courtesy of Edward W. Chang, M.D., D.D.S.)

Surgical Technique

1. The procedure begins with a gingivobuccal incision that extends from one cuspid to the other, with dissection continuing in a subperiosteal plane. A cuff of mucosa should be left along the superior aspect to facilitate wound closure at the end of the case.

2. Periosteal release should avoid injury to the mental nerves but should extend around and below the aforementioned nerves to develop a wide pocket for exposure.

3. As guided by the panoramic radiograph, a horizontal osteotomy is fashioned that extends medially from 25 mm below the superior aspect of the central incisor to more laterally 4 to 5 mm below the mental foramina and continued laterally until the segment is mobile (Fig. **12–13A,B**). The surgeon should be cautious laterally, as the facial artery resides near the lateral extent of the osteotomy. Typically, a 6 to 7 mm advancement may be achieved with the above-described maneuver (Fig. **12–14A**). More complicated and multiple osteotomies may be required to effect vertical movements.

4. The proximal segment can then be affixed to the remaining mandibular body with wires, screws, or plates (Figs. **12–14B**).

5. The mentalis muscle is approximated along with the mucosa to avoid a "witch's chin" deformity.

◆ Reduction Surgeries

The foregoing section is broadly applicable to both Caucasian and Asian patients alike, and the orthognathic procedures outlined are familiar, at least in concept if

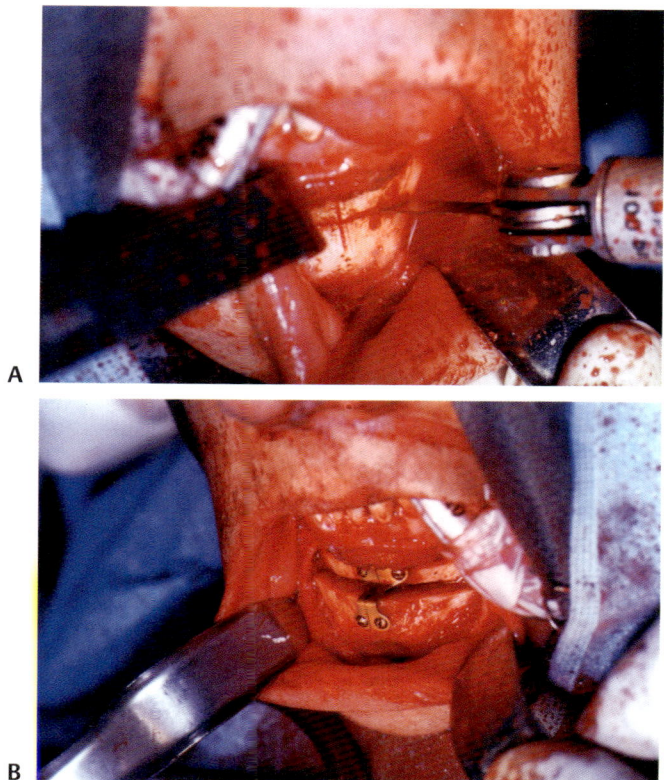

Figure 12–14 **(A)** The photograph shows the horizontal osteotomy created by a sagittal saw during sliding genioplasty. Prior to the osteotomy the midline is marked with a vertical bone score. Care should be taken to ensure that the osteotomy is continued with a smooth transition laterally and that soft-tissue injury is avoided laterally. Bone forceps are used to advance the bone segment. **(B)** Intraoperative photograph shows the specialized miniplate designed for sliding genioplasty (Stryker Leibinger Corp., Kalamazoo, MI) that has been secured into position. (Courtesy of Edward W. Chang, M.D., D.D.S.)

not in practice, to many Western surgeons. Certain skeletal patterns, for example, midfacial hypoplasia and lower facial convexity, are more prevalent in Asian populations; and these anatomic differences have been underscored to enlighten the surgeon as to the particular aesthetic deficits that require attention.

Unlike these more universal skeletal operations, a few notable osseous reduction surgeries have been developed and promulgated in Asia. These procedures have emerged in popularity due to the unique skeletal structure and cultural aesthetics in that region. In particular, Korea has led the vanguard in this regard partly due to

the more pronounced bony features that warrant this type of intervention, namely, a prominent mandibular angle and accentuated malar projection. What further distinguishes these types of surgeries from Western orthognathic/osseous translocation surgery is the sole objective of bony reduction as compared with the capacity for advancement or reduction of the latter.

Mandibular Angle Reduction

Prominent mandibular angles are a more prevalent condition in Asia, particularly in patients of Korean descent (Figs. **12–15A–D, 12–16A–G**). Koreans, who tend to have

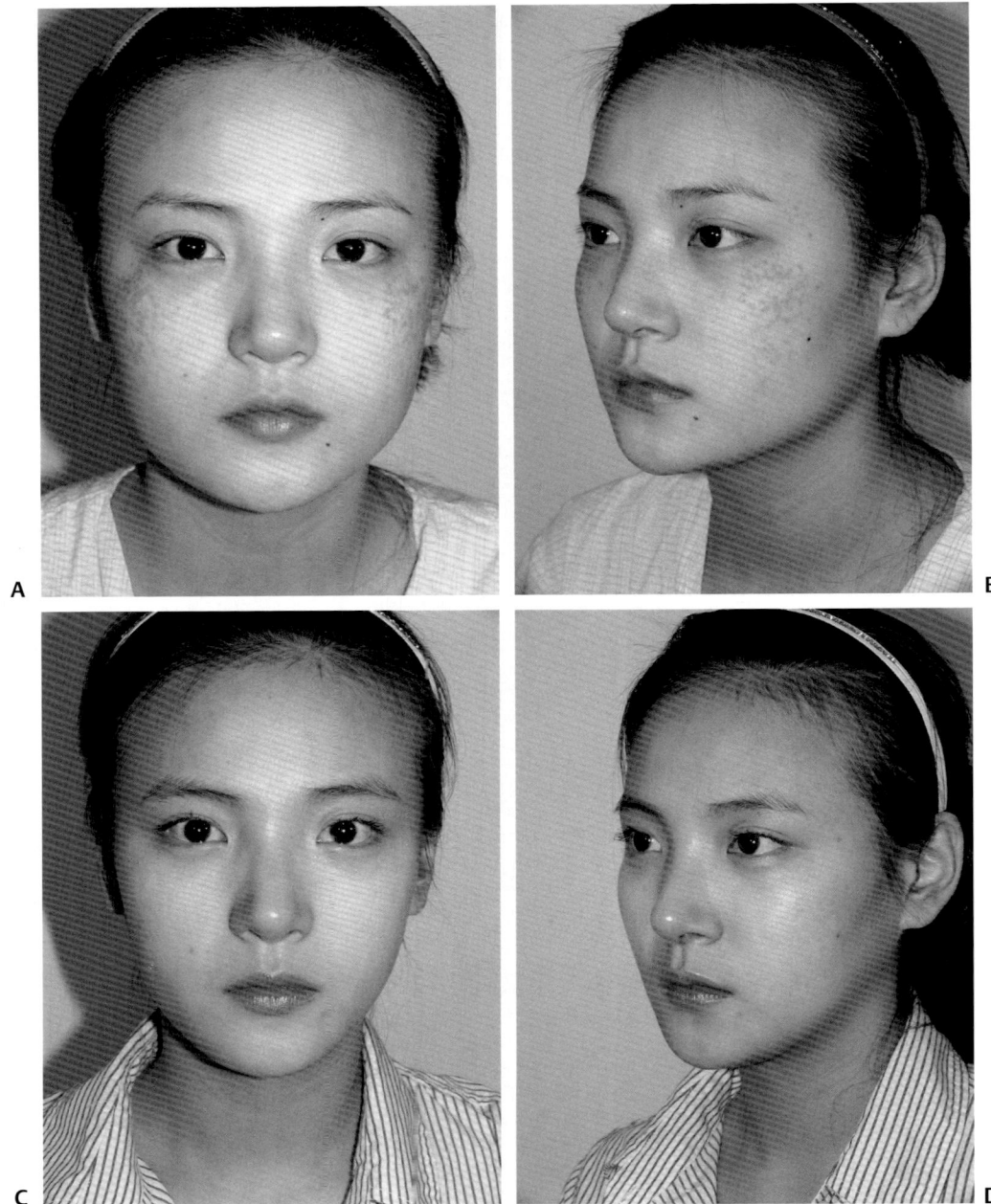

Figure 12–15 **(A,B)** This 23-year-old Korean woman underwent contouring of her mandible from the angle to the mental tubercle. **(C,D)** Patient shown 9 months after surgery. (Courtesy of Jung Soo Lee, M.D.)

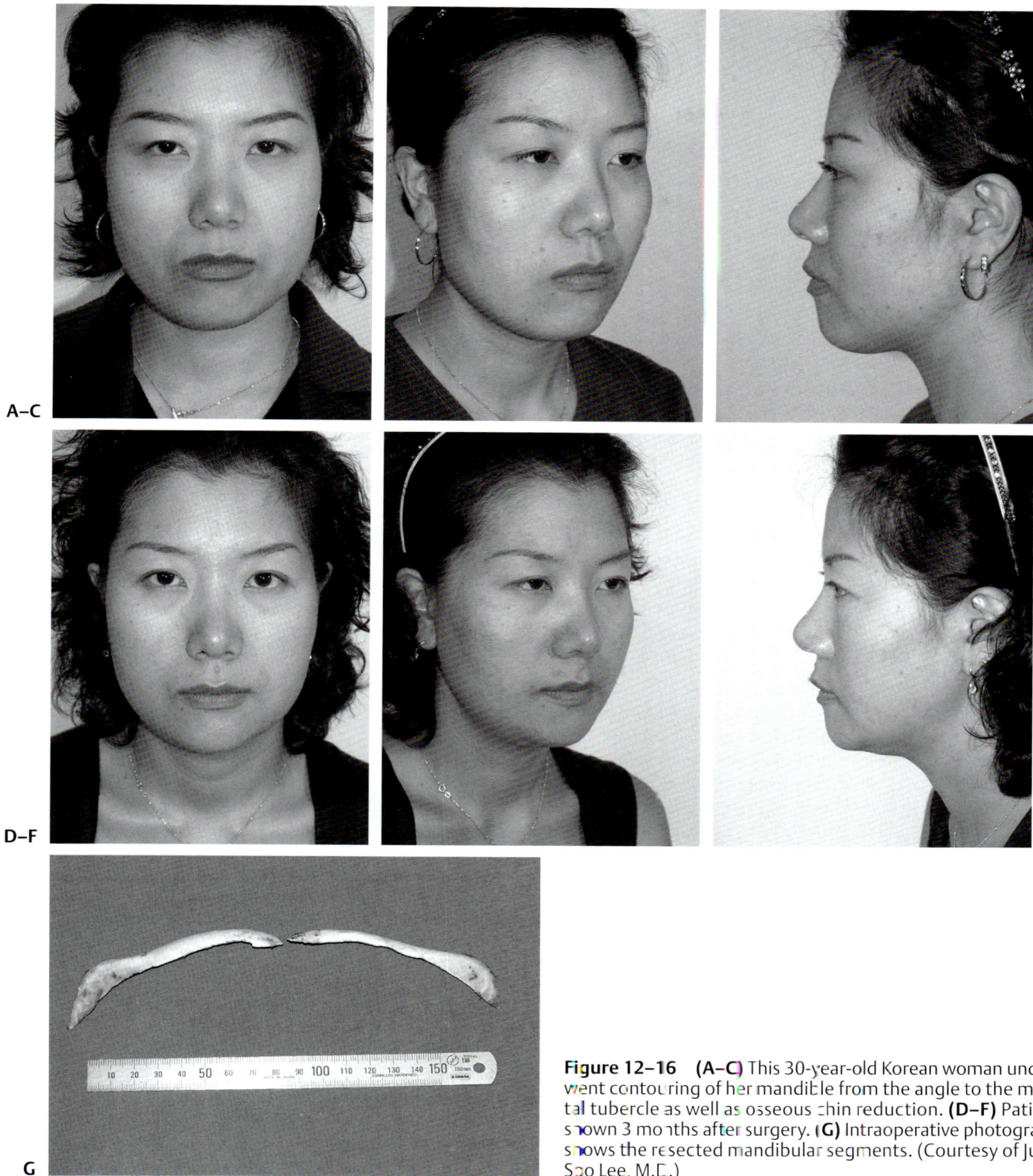

Figure 12–16 **(A–C)** This 30-year-old Korean woman underwent contouring of her mandible from the angle to the mental tubercle as well as osseous chin reduction. **(D–F)** Patient shown 3 months after surgery. **(G)** Intraoperative photograph shows the resected mandibular segments. (Courtesy of Jung Soo Lee, M.D.)

a broader face than their East Asian counterparts, may exhibit yet a wider facies by virtue of strong mandibular angles. A pronounced mandibular angle can render a harsh, flat, masculine appearance to the face as opposed to the desired feminine oval shape for which many Asian women yearn. Although benign masseteric hypertrophy, possibly due to paranormal behavior such as bruxism, has been viewed as the culprit for an accentuated, flared jawline in the Caucasian, the Asian may suffer from a prominent bone, a hypertrophied masseter muscle, or a

Mandibular Reduction

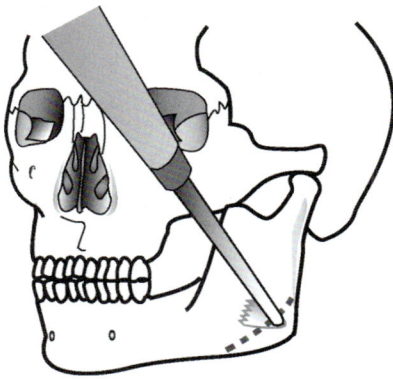

A. Curved osteotomy

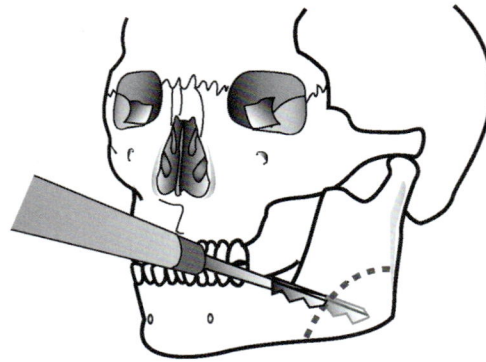

B. Tangential osteotomy

Figure 12–17   Two types of osteotomy cuts may be used to resect a prominent mandibular angle. **(A)** A curved saw is ideal for a mandibular angle that is principally projected posteriorly.

(B) A tangential saw may be preferred for a mandibular angle that primarily exhibits more lateral flaring.

combination of both. Careful physical examination will dictate whether botulinum toxin therapy alone will suffice for masseteric hypertrophy (refer to Chapter 13 for details) or if skeletal reduction surgery with or without surgical masseteric reduction is warranted.[2,3]

Like all bony surgical work, cephalometric and photographic analyses are integral to operative success. Panoramic radiography lucidly reveals the precise bony pathology: excessive lateral flaring and/or posterior overprojection. The degree and type of bony excess will dictate the optimal surgical treatment plan. After careful photographic review, the surgeon's and patient's objectives are enforced and aligned before operative embarkation.

Surgical Technique

1. A transoral approach via a gingivobuccal incision is the preferred route of access.

2. After proper hemostasis is achieved with local anesthesia, the anterior face of the mandibular ramus is exposed down to the second mandibular molar. Subperiosteal dissection is continued to the proposed osteotomy site along the posteroinferior aspect of the mandibular angle.

3. Selective burring of the anterolateral aspect of the mandibular angle may expand a restricted view of the targeted osteotomy site.

4. Two types of osteotomy cuts are advocated, curved and tangential, depending on the bony pathology (Fig. **12–17A,B**). A curved osteotome should be used to resect a posteriorly projected mandibular angle along the entire expanse of the angle from the ramus to the body to yield a smooth, rounded contour. However, a

tangential osteotome is preferred if lateral flaring of the mandibular angle is the principal pathology. The tangential osteotome cleaves the bone obliquely in a fashion similar to a sagittal-split transection. A combination of bony flare and posterior projection mandates judicious, proportionate application of both osteotomy techniques. Care must be taken to avoid injury to the inferior alveolar nerve (Fig. **12–18**). A

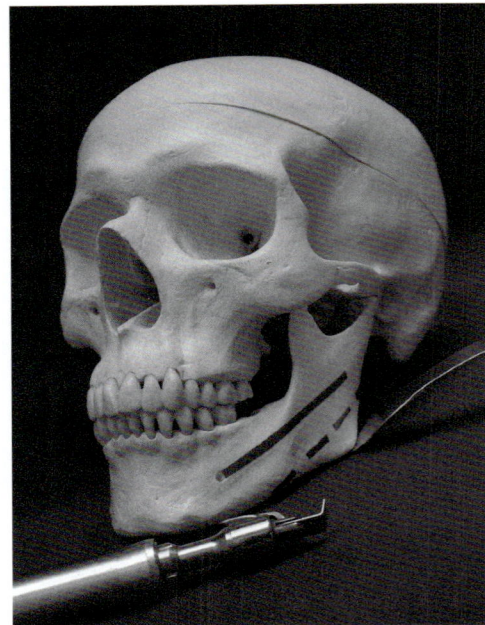

Figure 12–18   Skull model that depicts the track of the inferior alveolar nerve (solid line) and the proposed osteotomy line for mandibular angle reduction (dashed line). (Courtesy of Edward W. Chang, M.D., D.D.S.)

preoperative, panoramic radiograph can be reviewed before and during the operative case to ensure that a safe distance is maintained between the osteotomy line and the inferior alveolar nerve.

5. The gingivobuccal incision is approximated with absorbable suture, and a pressure dressing is designed to remain in place for several days.

Postoperative Remarks

Dietary advancement from liquid to semi-solid is taken as tolerated. Postoperative edema may be marked for several weeks to several months, and the patient should be reassured that notable improvement might not be evident for 3 to 6 months.

Besides hematoma and infection, unique complications that may arise include facial nerve injury, inferior alveolar nerve injury, asymmetry, and through-and-through mandibular fracture. Although these troublesome outcomes remain rare in properly trained surgical hands, they can be a source of extreme distress if they arise. Avoidance of masseteric dissection and conservative bony resection can help navigate a safe surgical course.

Malar Reduction

Preoperative Remarks

As stated, aesthetic concepts between the East and West do not always coincide. High cheekbones, an alluring feminine attribute by Western standards, may intimate conversely a masculine assertiveness in Asia. Accordingly, malar reduction surgery is more frequently requested than augmentation and constitutes a unique surgical preference in Asia. Malar prominence and mandibular angle protuberance jointly may outline a square, manly facial configuration that is deemed objectionable. This type of surgery has mainly been practiced in Korea, which may owe in part to cultural taste and to anatomic predisposition. Interestingly, the malar hypoplasia that characterizes the typical Asian facies does not restrain the popularity of malar reduction surgery.

Numerous techniques have been proposed to address the prominent malar complex. Onizuka et al were the first to report a technique for malar reduction, using an exclusively intraoral method.[4] Whitaker advocated burring the malar prominence down to a paper-thin depth of 1 mm, but this technique may suffer from a few major drawbacks: insufficient reduction, a flattened contour, and potential asymmetry.[5] Although many variations exist, osseous malar reduction methods may be broadly classified into four principal approaches: temporal, coronal, intraoral, and combined intraoral/preauricular. Each of these techniques will be reviewed in detail.

Every patient should receive proper preoperative consultation regarding the potential morbidity of bony reduction surgery. If the surgeon and patient have arrived at a mutual regard of the risks and benefits attendant with the procedure, then surgical planning may commence. As part of the preparatory phase, the patient must complete a full set of radiographic evaluations, including frontal, bilateral profile, submentovertex, and cephalometric perspectives.

Surgical Techniques

Method of Jung-Soo Lee: Temporal Approach with Endoscopic Guidance   This technique involves an abbreviated temporal incision with osteotomies performed under endoscopic guidance. In skilled hands, total operative time may be only 20 to 30 minutes. However, this operative method is suitable only for patients with select inclusion criteria: (1) severe zygomatic arch prominence and a normal zygomatic body prominence, (2) desire for reduction only of the lateral prominence, and (3) desire for a less invasive surgical procedure (Figs. **12–19A–F, 12–20A–H**).[6] With these limitations in mind, this method can offer a targeted approach to address the lateral flare of the zygomatic arch.

1. After the patient has been placed under general anesthesia, a 2 cm incision is made behind the temporal hairline, and dissection is taken down through the temporoparietal fascia to the level of the true temporalis fascia (Figs. **12–21, 12–22**).

2. Dissection is continued in this plane between the temporoparietal fascia and the temporalis fascia down to the superior margin of the zygomatic body under endoscopic guidance.

3. As the zygomatic body is approached, the lateral zygomaticotemporal artery and vein are cauterized to avoid any bleeding that can obscure endoscopic dissection. Care should be taken during cauterization, as the facial nerve typically lies in proximity to the vessel at a more superficial plane.

4. With the superior aspect of the zygomatic body in view, a periosteal elevator is used to elevate the periosteum to expose the zygomatic body fully.

5. A reciprocating saw outfitted with a 2.5 cm blade is used to make an *incomplete* osteotomy through the exposed zygomatic body.

6. More posteriorly, the zygomatic arch is then approached. A periosteal elevator is used to elevate

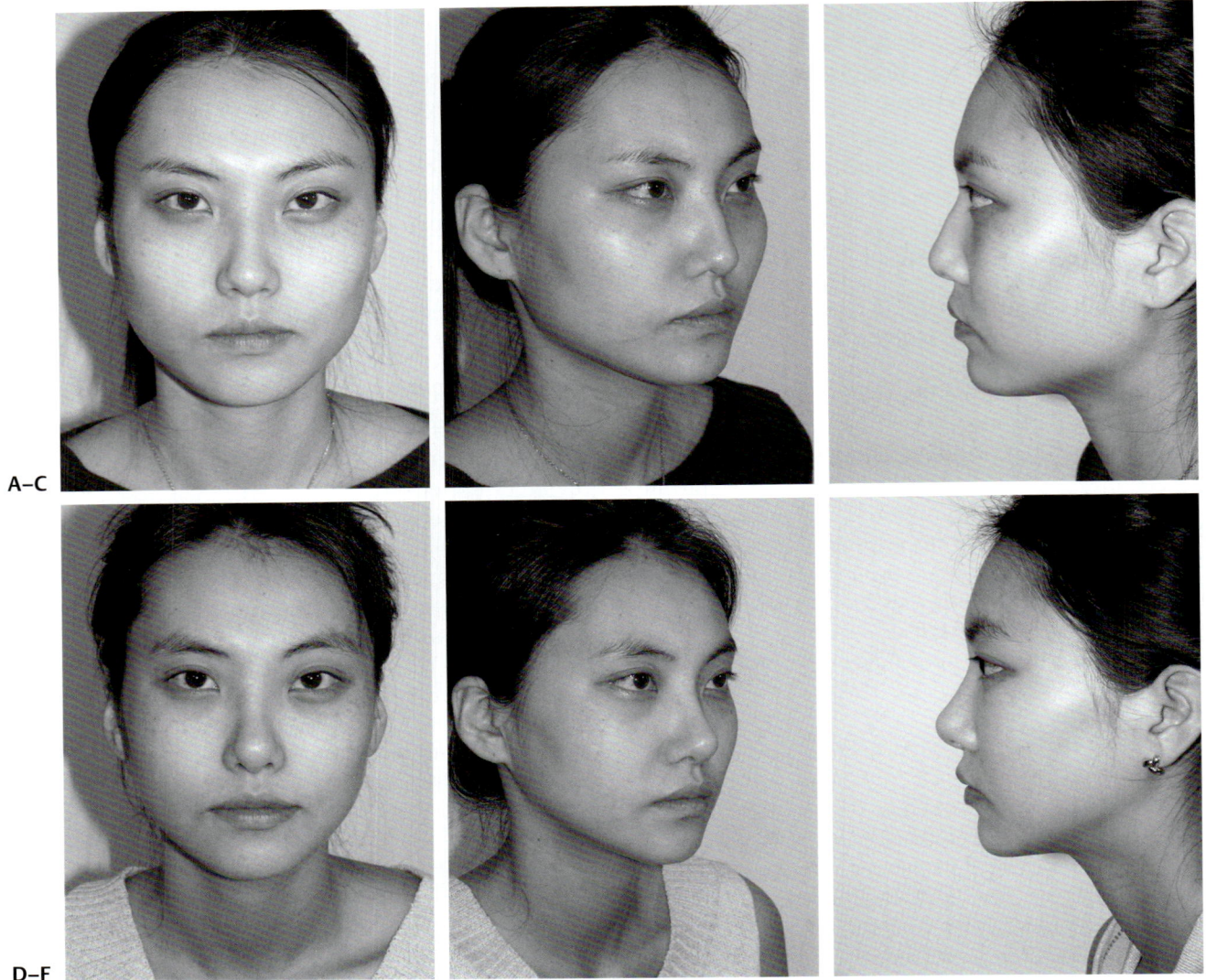

A–C

D–F

Figure 12–19 (A–C) This 25-year-old Korean woman underwent endoscopic malar bone reduction via an endoscopic temporal approach and mandibular contouring as well as rhinoplasty (dorsal hump reduction and cartilage tip augmentation). **(D–F)** Patient shown 6 months postoperatively. (Courtesy of Jung Soo Lee, M.D.)

the inner periosteal lining of the zygomatic arch, and a reciprocating saw with a 1.5 cm blade is used to create a *complete* osteotomy from inner to outer aspect of the bony arch, traversing this distance in an oblique fashion.

7. The zygomatic arch is infractured by external manual pressure so that the bony segments align in a Z configuration (Fig. **12–21**). The oblique nature of the osteotomy ensures that the bony segments will not return to their preoperative state after surgery.

8. Any remaining bony irregularities are addressed with a long, narrow rasp before closure.

The patients are discharged on the same operative day and may return to a normal diet immediately. They are advised to avoid any pressure or trauma to the surgical area for a period of 6 weeks.

Method of Yong-Ha Kim: Intraoral Approach The benefit of the intraoral approach is clearly the lack of any need for external incisions. Operative time may be reduced, but exposure may be more difficult. This method involves an L-shaped osteotomy (two vertical and one tranverse cut) through the medial zygomatic body with removal of the osteotomized segment, followed by an incomplete osteotomy of the lateral zygomatic arch from

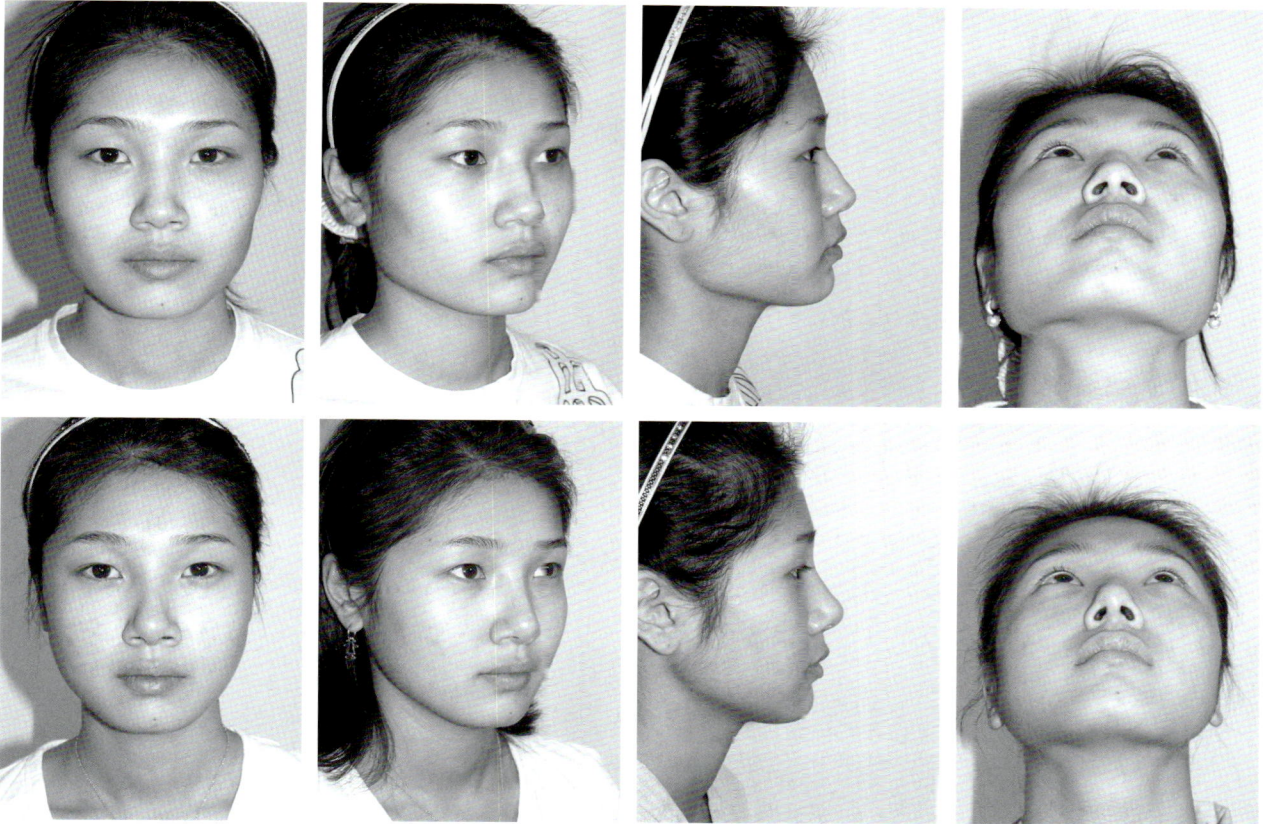

A–D

E–H

Figure 12–20 **(A–D)** This 25-year-old Korean woman underwent endoscopic malar bone reduction via an endoscopic temporal approach and mandibular contouring as well as rhinoplasty (dorsal augmentation with an expanded polytetrafluoroethylene (ePTFE) implant and cartilage tip augmentation). **(E–H)** Patient shown 5 months postoperatively. (Courtesy of Jung Soo Lee, M.D.)

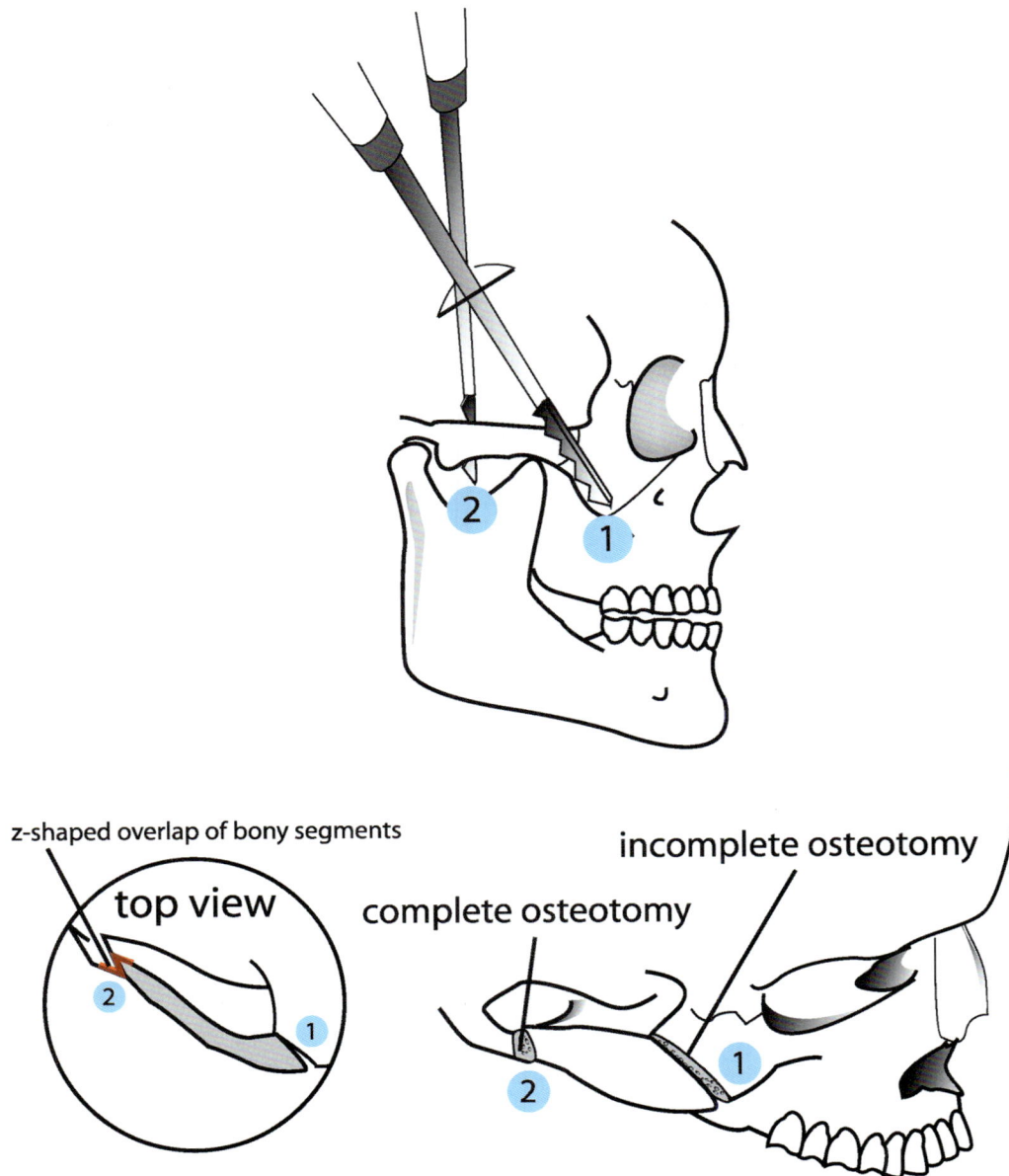

Figure 12–21   The endoscopic temporal approach for malar reduction is undertaken through a 2 cm temporal incision. **(1)** The first osteotomy is incomplete and undertaken with a 2.5 cm blade anteriorly on the zygomatic body. **(2)** The second osteotomy is complete and is made more posteriorly along the zygomatic arch from the inner to the outer bony cortex in an oblique fashion using a 1.5 cm blade. The zygomatic arch is then infractured by external manual pressure so that the bony segments align in a Z-configuration (*top view*).

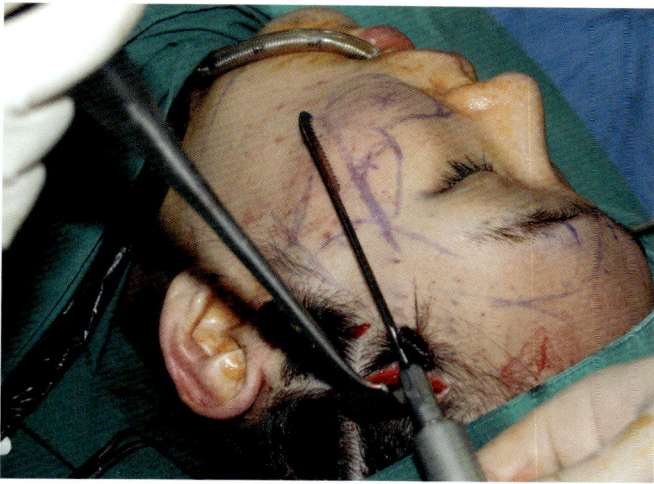

Figure 12–22 Intraoperative photograph showing the re-tracted temporal incision used for the endoscopic temporal approach for bony malar reduction. The "J saw" is shown overlying the skin in the orientation required to make the first osteotomy that is located anteriorly on the zygomatic body. The cutaneous markings with gentian violet outline the contour of the zygomatic body and arch, and the two proposed osteotomy sites are also drawn. (Courtesy of Jung Soo Lee, M.D.)

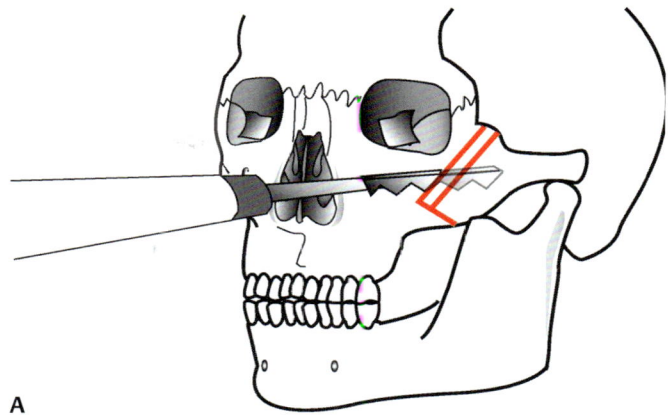

A

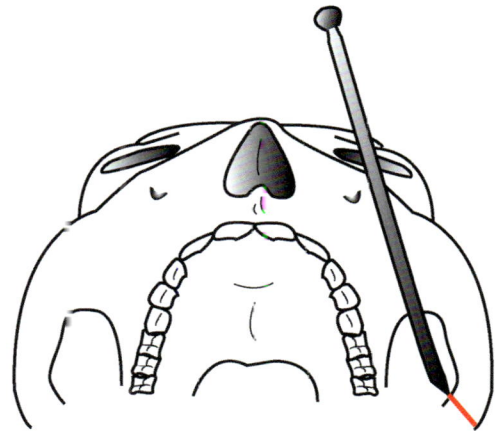

B

Figure 12–23 The illustration shows the basic steps to perform an intraoral malar reduction. **(A)** An L-shaped osteotomy is created that consists of two parallel vertical osteotomies and one transverse osteotomy. **(B)** The intervening bone segment is then removed, and a curved osteotome is inserted through this defect to access the lateral zygomatic arch from the medial aspect to commit a greenstick fracture.

the medial side (Fig. **12–23**).[7] After repositioning, the bony segments are secured with a miniplate and screws. Unlike the method described above for lateral zygomatic arch reduction, the intraoral method is primarily intended to reduce the more medial zygomatic body prominence (Figs. **12–24A–D, 12–25A,B, 12–26A–D 12–27A,B**).

1. After the patient undergoes general anesthesia via nasotracheal access, a 3 cm gingivobuccal incision is created on each side, and dissection is taken down to the underlying periosteum.

2. Through this mucosal window, subperiosteal dissection can be performed to expose the zygomatic body, anterior zygomatic arch, the anterior wall of the maxillary sinus, and inferior and lateral portions of the orbital rims. Medial dissection terminates at the infraorbital foramen.

3. A transverse osteotomy is created that extends from the zygomaticomaxillary buttress to the anterior maxillary sinus wall using a reciprocating saw.

4. Two parallel oblique vertical osteotomies are then made from the lateral orbital rim to the maxillary sinus to join the transverse osteotomy (Fig. **12–28**).

5. After all of the osteotomies are completed, the bony segment is removed (Fig. **12–29**). The size of the bony segment that is removed is directly proportional to the degree of bony reduction desired and generally ranges from 3 to 8 mm, with a mean of 5.5 mm.

6. A sharp, curved osteotome is inserted through this defect and aimed at the lateral zygomatic arch from the medial side. The arch is then greenstick fractured; that is, an incomplete osteotomy is made. More precisely, the point where the osteotomy is made falls at the anterior part of the zygomatic tubercle, which corresponds externally with the anterior sideburn.

7. The reduced zygomatic body segment is secured with miniplate fixation (Fig. **12–30**), and any residual bony irregularities are recontoured with a burr under direct vision.

8. The incision is closed with absorbable sutures, and the patient maintains a pressure-style dressing for 2 to 3 days.

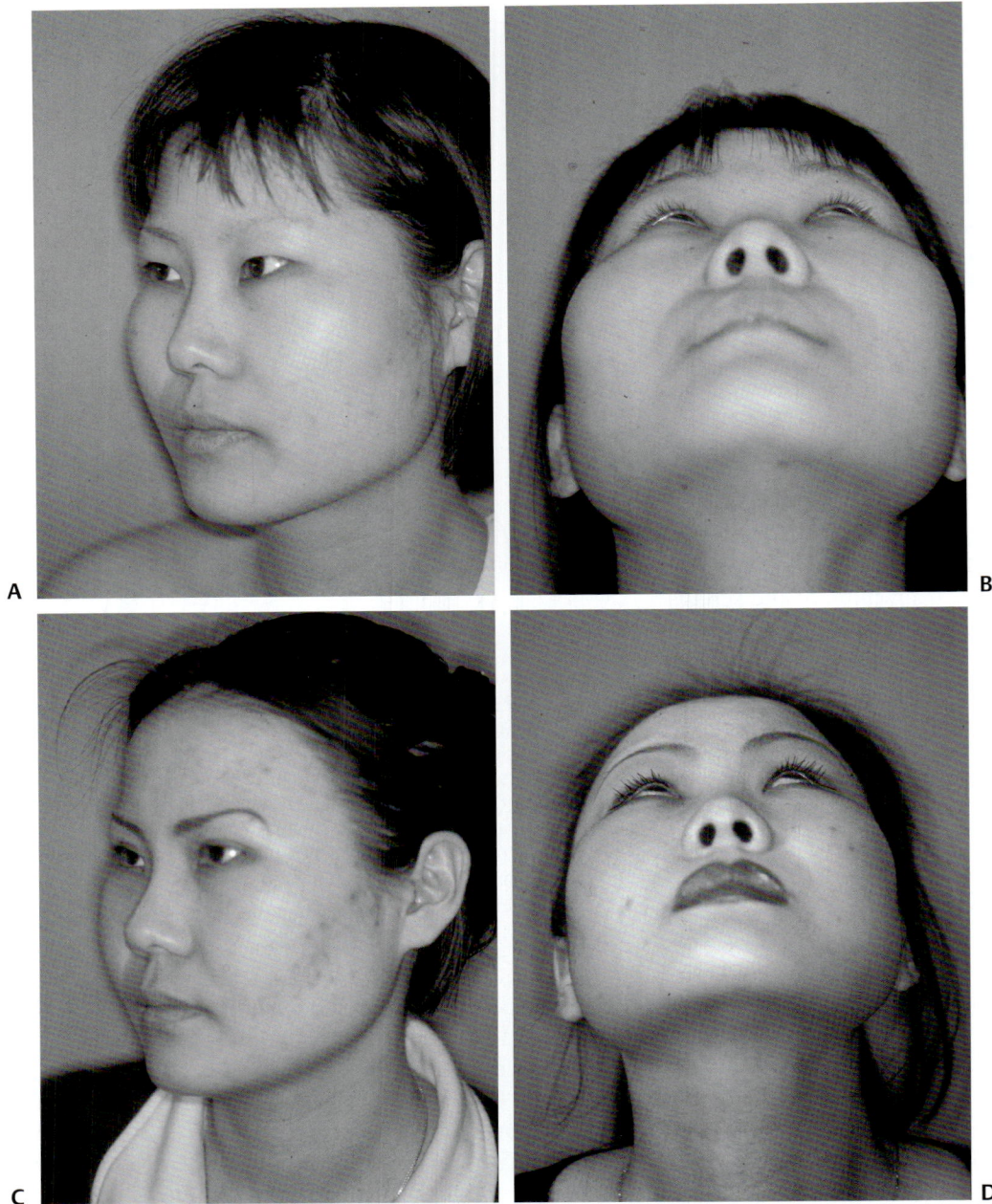

Figure 12–24   (A,B) This 23-year-old Korean woman underwent an 8 mm reduction malarplasty using an intraoral approach. **(C,D)** Patient shown 8 months postoperatively. (From Kim YH, Seul JH. Reduction malarplasty through an intraoral incision: a new method. Plast Reconstr Surg 2000;106:1514; with permission.)

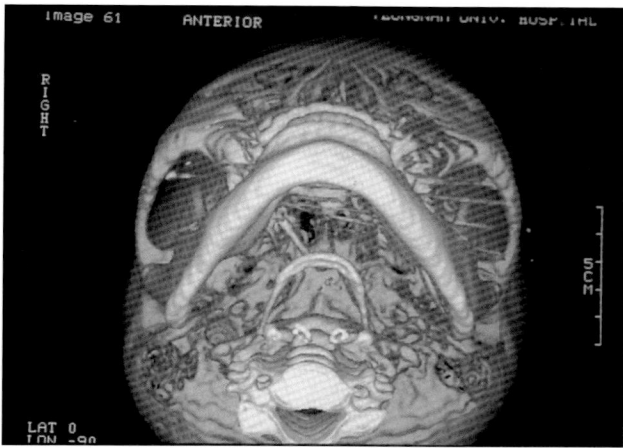

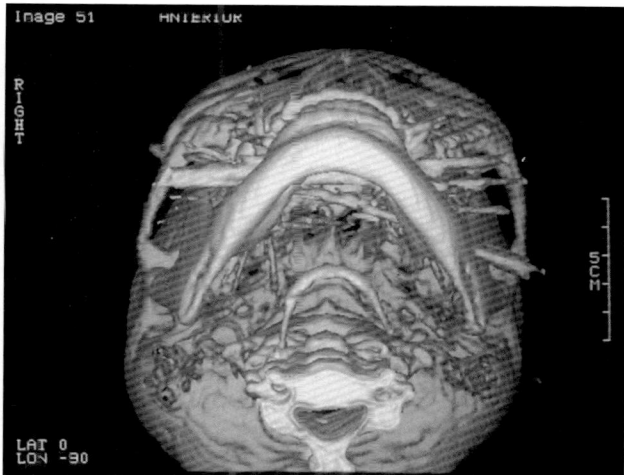

Figure 12–25 **(A)** Preoperative, three-dimensional computed tomography (CT) of the patient shown in Fig. **12–24**. **(B)** Postoperative CT showing the greenstick-fractured zygomatic arches. (From Kim YH, Seul JH. Reduction malarplasty through an intraoral incision: a new method. Plast Reconstr Surg 2000;106:1514; with permission.)

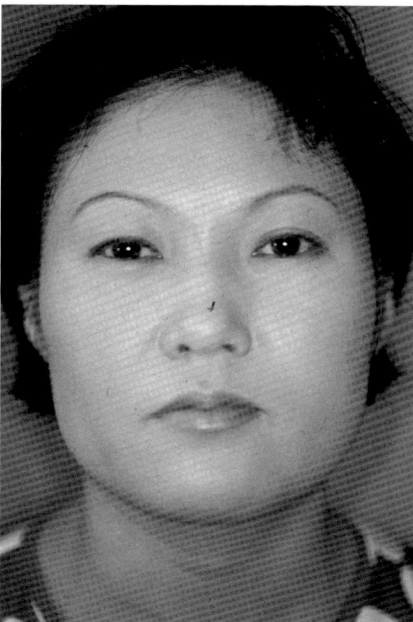

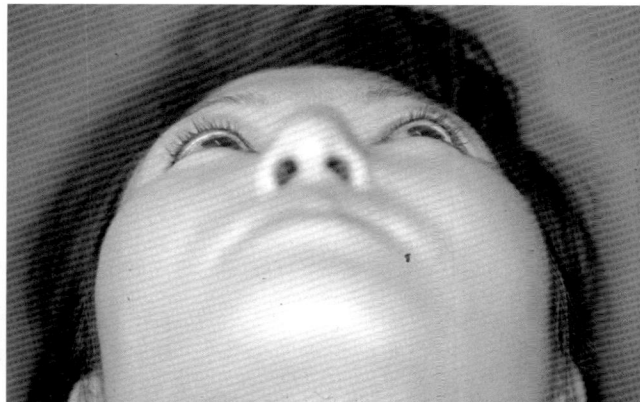

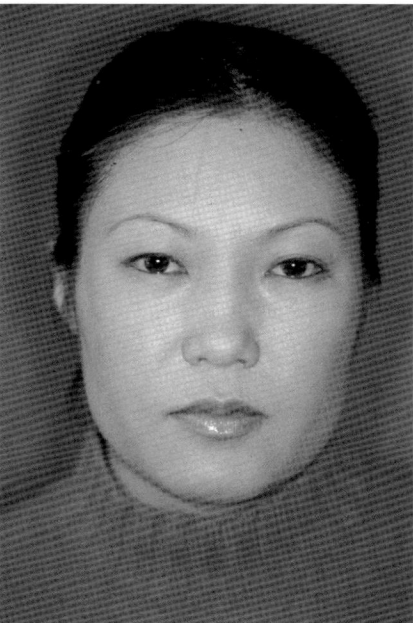

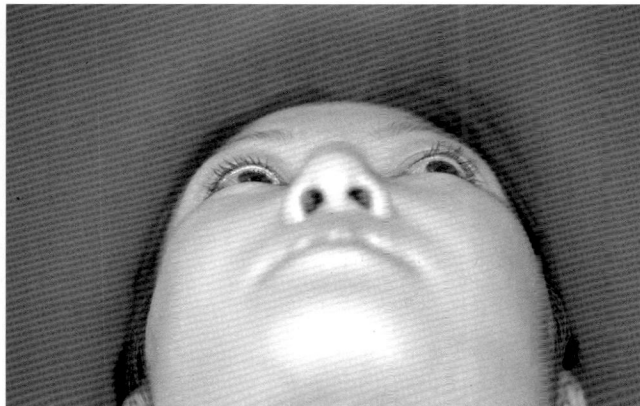

Figure 12–26 **(A,B)** This 34-year-old Korean woman underwent a 5 mm reduction malarplasty using the intraoral technique. **(C,D)** Patient shown 12 months after bony reduction. (From Kim YH, Seul JH. Reduction malarplasty through an intraoral incision: a new method. Plast Reconstr Surg 2000;106: 1514; with permission.)

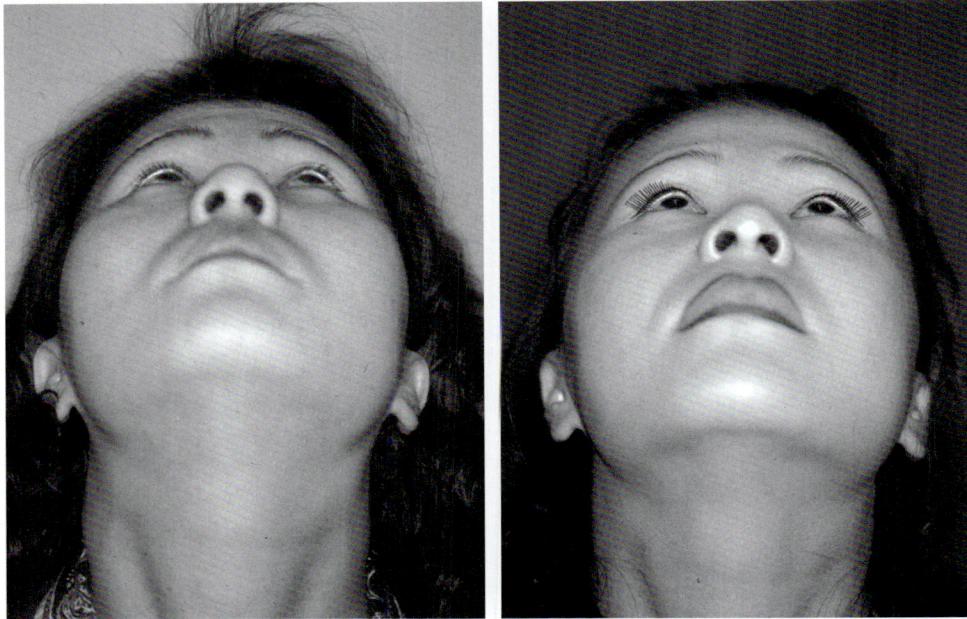

Figure 12–27 **(A)** This 29-year-old Korean woman underwent a 6 mm reduction malarplasty using the intraoral technique. **(B)** Patient shown 18 months after surgery. (From Kim YH, Seul JH. Reduction malarplasty through an intraoral incision: a new method. Plast Reconstr Surg 2000;106:1514; with permission.)

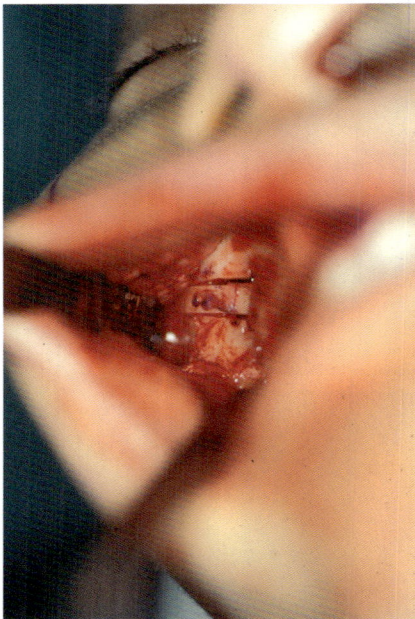

Figure 12–28 Intraoperative view shows the two parallel osteotomies that are illustrated in Fig. 12–23. The transverse osteotomy is not clearly shown in this photographic view. (Courtesy of Yong-Ha Kim, M.D., Ph.D.)

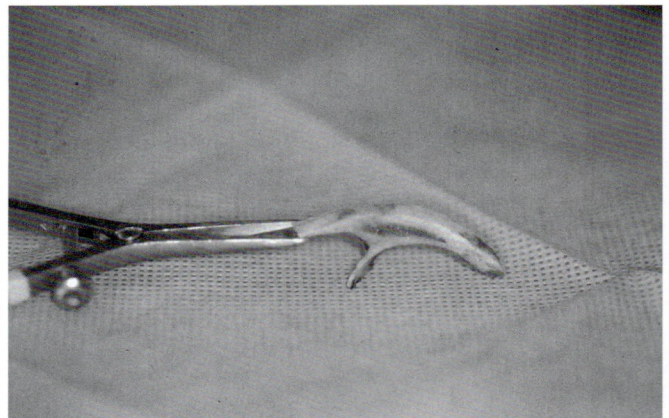

Figure 12–29 The intervening bone segment between the parallel osteotomies is removed and is shown. (Courtesy of Yong-Ha Kim, M.D., Ph.D.)

Method of Noriyoshi Sumiya: Combined Intraoral and Preauricular Approach The combined approach using intraoral and preauricular incisions permits direct access to the medial zygomatic body and lateral zygomatic arch, respectively (Fig. **12–31**).[8] Unlike the intraoral approach, an external facial incision is required. However, the length of the incision is rather abbreviated when compared with the coronal incision technique.

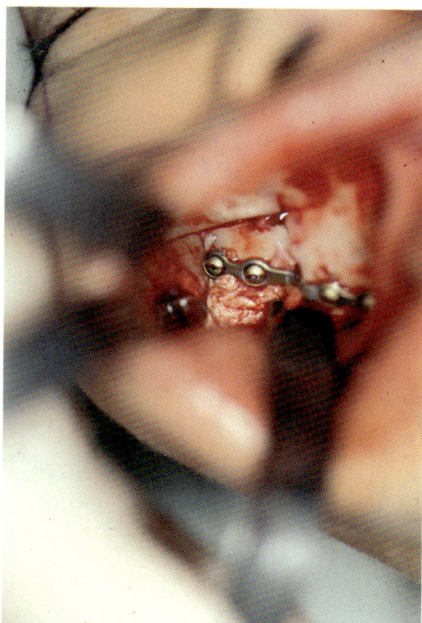

Figure 12–30   After greenstick fracture of the lateral zygomatic arch, the medial osteotomy site is secured with miniplate fixation, as illustrated in Fig. 12–23. (Courtesy of Yong-Ha Kim, M.D., Ph.D.)

1. The zygomatic body is first accessed through the intraoral route through a standard gingivobuccal incision. Dissection is performed in the subperiosteal plane to expose the superolateral orbital rim so that a thin retractor and a reciprocating saw can be inserted easily into this area.

2. The external landmarks of the orbital rim and zygoma are palpated, and a reciprocating saw is used to create an osteotomy through the zygoma ~5 mm away from the orbital rim (Fig. **12–32**). The osteotomy should be made at an angle directed away from the maxillary sinus so that inadvertent entry into the sinus is avoided.

3. A second osteotomy should be made lateral and parallel to the first bone cut ~3 mm away from the first osteotomy site so that a 2 mm bone island is removed. (The osteotomy width totals 1 mm, which accounts for the 1 mm difference between the measured 3 mm value and the actual 2 mm size of bone segment removed.)

4. A thin miniplate is then secured to the zygomatic body.

5. The preauricular area is incised a distance of 2 cm lying over the zygomatic arch behind a line drawn for the path of the temporal branch of the facial nerve (Fig. **12–33**). An osteotomy is then performed for the zygomatic arch with a reciprocating saw through this incision (Figs. **12–34, 12–35**). The saw blade should be oriented so that the osteotomy

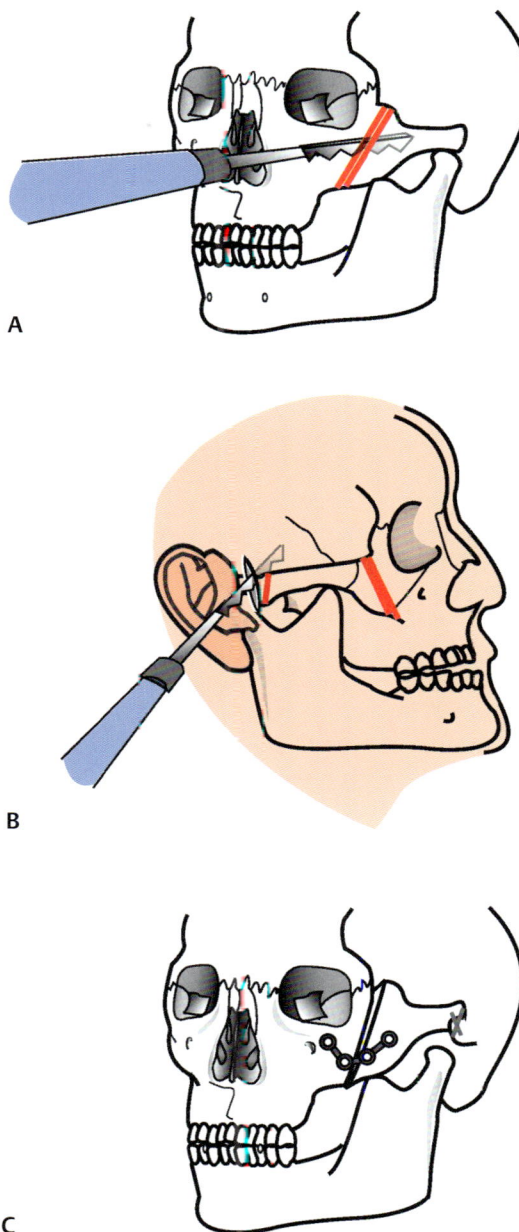

Figure 12–31   (A) The zygomatic body is cut with a reciprocating saw ~5 mm lateral to the orbital rim in an oblique fashion away from the maxillary sinus via an intraoral route. An additional parallel cut is made 3 mm lateral to the initial osteotomy so that a 2 mm wide portion of bone is removed (with the second cut accounting for the 1 mm difference). A miniplate is applied to the lateral side of the transected zygomatic body (not shown) in preparation for miniplate fixation at the end of the procedure. (B) The 2 cm incision is made in the preauricular area to access the lateral zygomatic arch, and an osteotomy is performed with a reciprocating saw anterior to the mandibular joint. (C) The mobilized arch segment is then moved inward and upward and wired into position. A miniplate is then fixed to the maxillary side of the transected zygomatic body.

permits easy translocation of the zygomatic arch inward and upward. Care should be heeded to avoid transection of the superficial temporal artery and entry into the temporomandibular joint.

6. After appropriate translocation of the zygomatic arch, the segments are wired together.

7. The zygomatic position is confirmed externally before securing the maxillary side of the miniplate via the intraoral incision (Fig. **12–36**).

8. All incisions are then closed.

Method of Se-Min and Rong-Min Baek: Coronal Approach
The coronal approach provides the most panoramic view of the malar bone and may afford a more accurate assessment of symmetric reduction.[9] In addition, ancillary procedures may be undertaken, for example, a concurrent

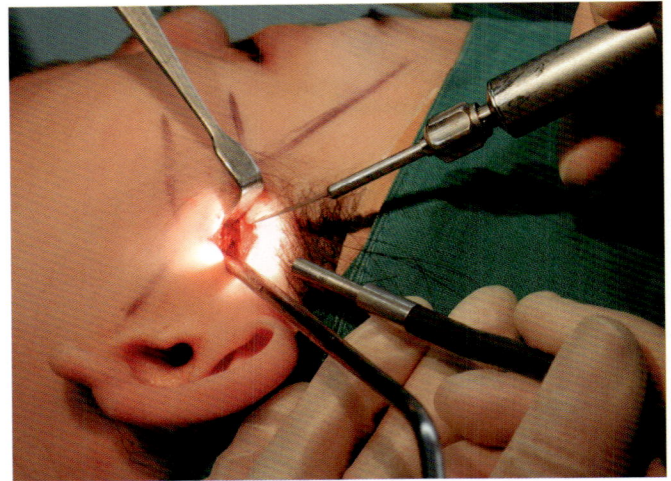

Figure 12–32 The first osteotomy is made via transoral approach, with the reciprocating saw beveled laterally and the osteotomy site made ~5 mm lateral to the lateral orbital rim. (Courtesy of Shin Kyu Lee, M.D.)

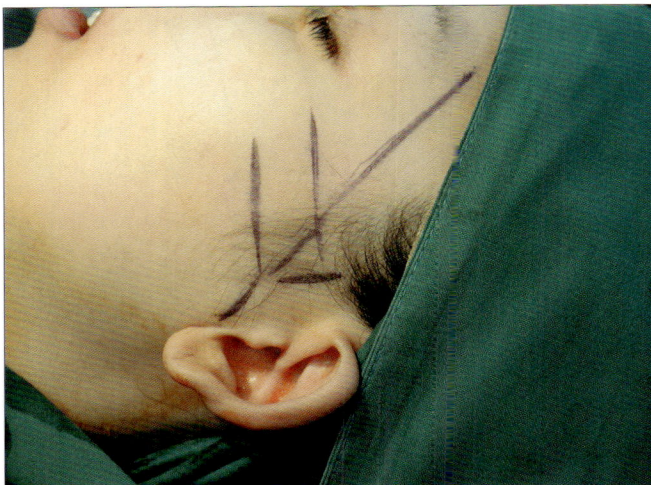

Figure 12–33 The 2 cm vertical preauricular incision is made behind the path that defines the facial nerve, as indicated by the diagonally drawn line extending from the base of the ear. The outline of the zygomatic arch is also drawn. (Courtesy of Shin Kyu Lee, M.D.)

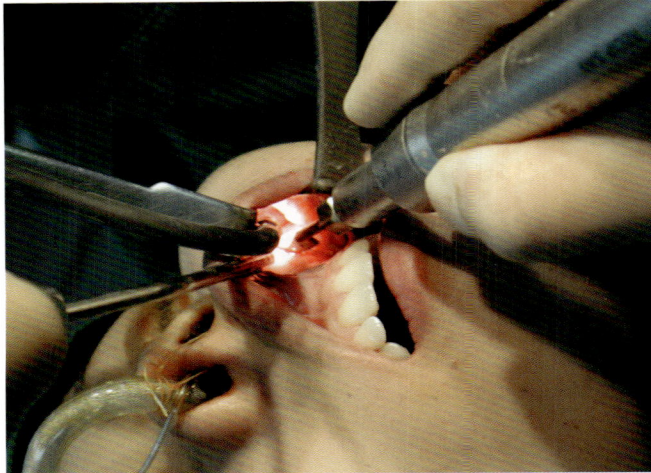

Figure 12–34 A reciprocating saw is used to create the osteotomy at the zygomatic arch in an oblique fashion to permit easy translocation of the arch inward and upward. (Courtesy of Shin Kyu Lee, M.D.)

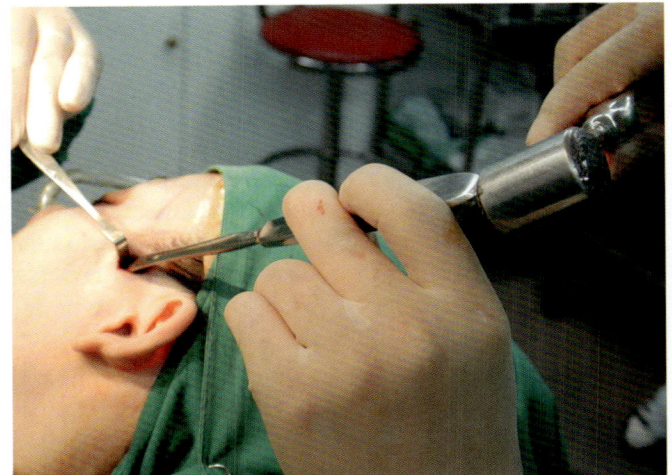

Figure 12–35 A mallet and osteotome can be used to complete an incomplete transection of the zygomatic arch. (Courtesy of Shin Kyu Lee, M.D.)

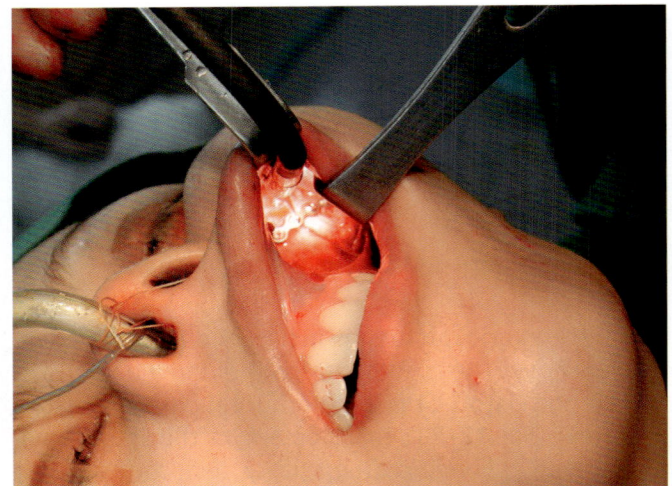

Figure 12–36 After zygomatic arch reduction, the zygomatic body is secured into its new position with a miniplate. (Courtesy of Shin Kyu Lee, M.D.)

brow lift, temporal fat pad resection, and forehead implantation (Figs. **12–37A–K, 12–38A–F**). Nevertheless, the potential morbidity involved with a longer incision and more involved surgical dissection will most likely predispose toward a longer recovery period for the patient.

1. The coronal incision is marked out ~8 cm posterior to the hairline to meet the superior helical crus laterally (Fig. **12–39**).

2. Subgaleal dissection is taken down to the supraorbital-rim level, at which point the subperiosteal plane is entered and developed over the malar complex to include the malar bone, zygomatic arch, lateral orbital wall, and anterolateral maxillary wall. Temporalis and masseteric attachments to the zygomatic bone are retained to preserve the vascular supply and the stabilizing forces, except where per force violated over the immediate osteotomy site.

3. The medial osteotomy is begun at the maxillary notch, a point that lies 5 to 8 mm medial to the inferior extent of the zygomaticomaxillary suture line (Fig. **12–40**) and traverses upward to terminate

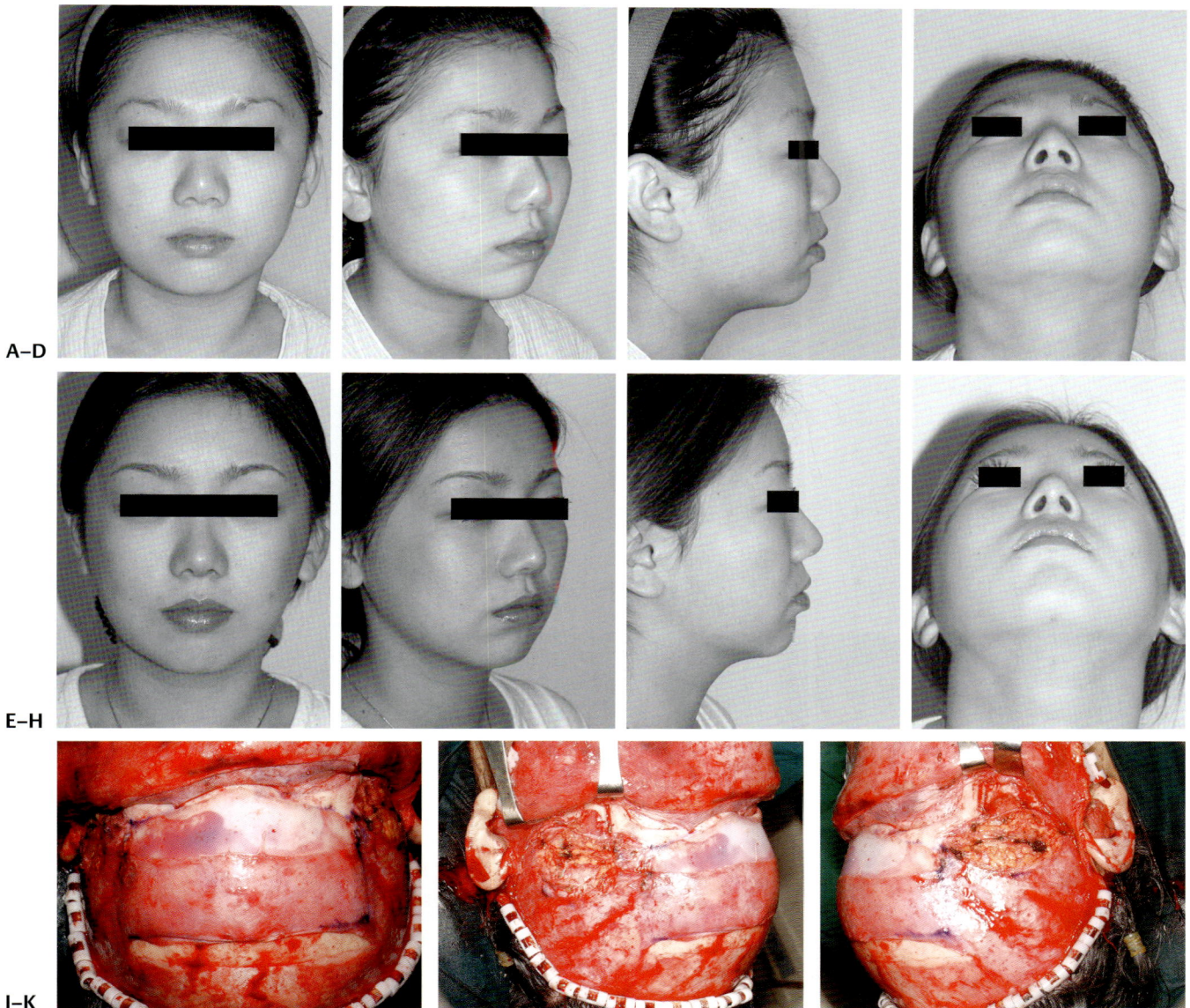

A–D

E–H

I–K

Figure 12–37 **(A–D)** This 21-year-old Korean woman underwent reduction malarplasty through a bicoronal incision and had concurrent resection of her superficial temporal fat pad, forehead augmentation with a prefabricated silicone implant, and rhinoplasty (dorsal augmentation with ePTFE graft, ePTFE strut graft, and tip-plasty with ear cartilage). **(E–H)** Patient shown 6 months after surgery. **(I)** Intraoperative view shows silicone implant for forehead augmentation placed via the bicoronal incision. The implant is positioned under a bipedicled periosteal flap closed with 4–0 polyglactic acid suture (Vicryl, Ethicon, Somerville, NJ). **(J)** The superficial temporal fat pad is partially resected to reduce bitemporal distance, and the malar complex can be seen reduced (*left view*). **(K)** Right view of what is depicted in J. (Courtesy of Jung Soo Lee, M.D.)

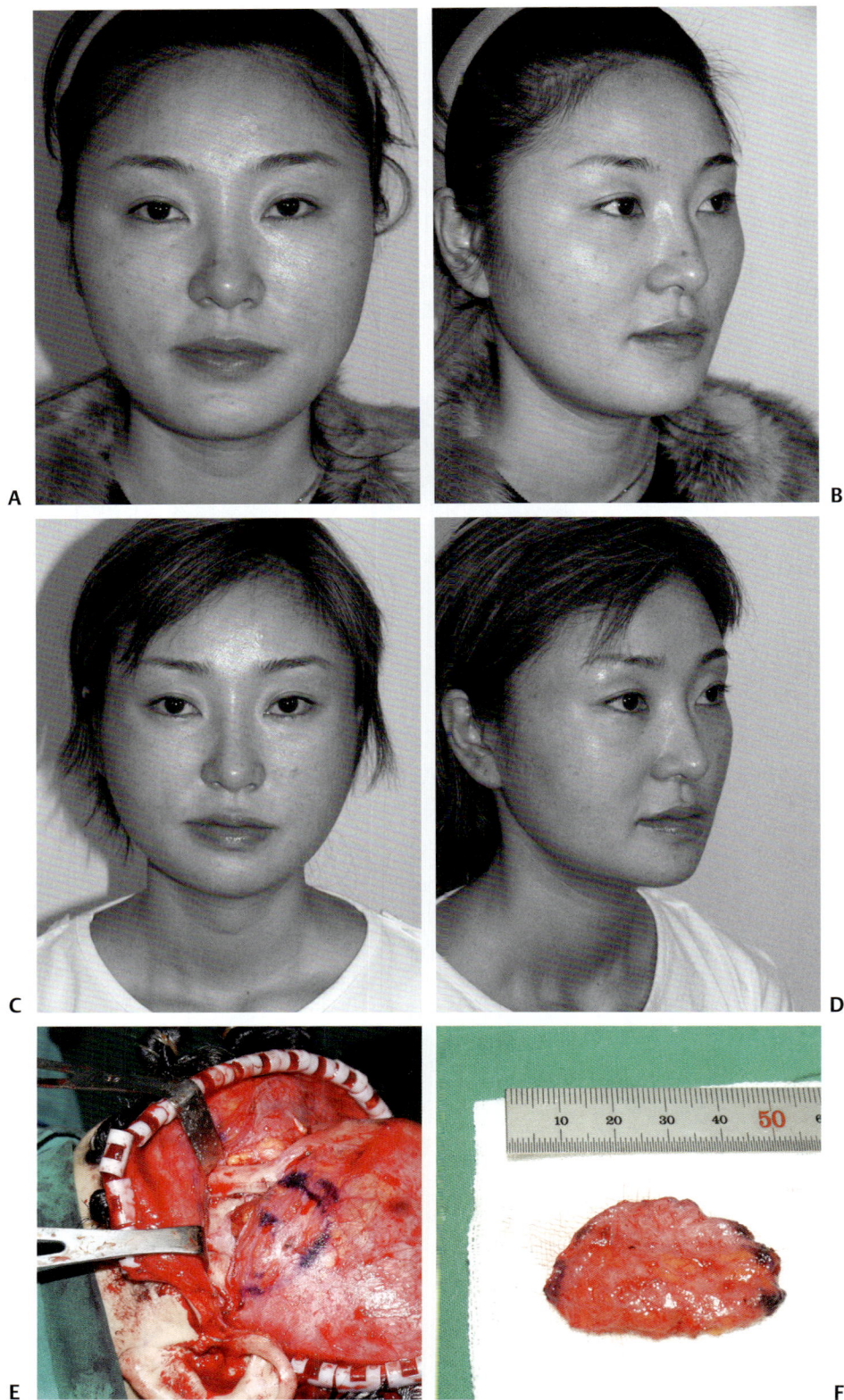

Figure 12–38 **(A,B)** This 32-year-old Korean woman underwent reduction malarplasty via a bicoronal incision as well as superficial temporal fat pad resection, revision mandibular contouring, osseous chin reduction, and cervical liposuction. **(C,D)** Patient shown 8 months postoperatively. **(E)** Intraoperative view shows infracture of the left osteotomized zygoma. **(F)** Intraoperative view of the resected superficial temporal fat pad. (Courtesy of Jung Soo Lee, M.D.)

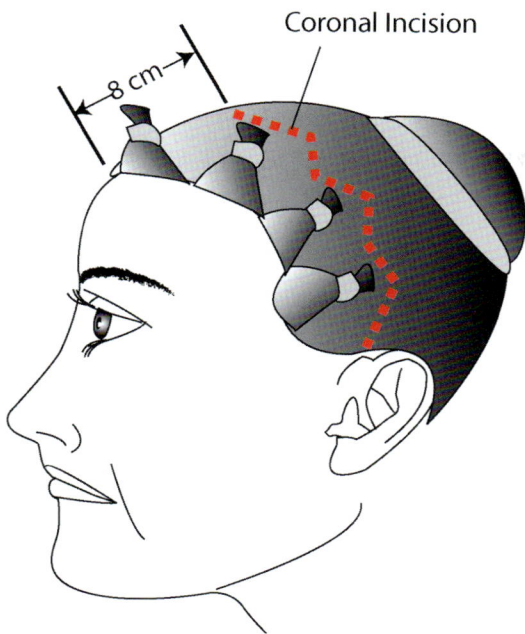

Coronal Incision

8 cm

Figure 12–39 Coronal incision is made approximately 8 cm behind the hairline extending to the superior helical crus on each side of the head as part of the approach to coronal-based reduction malarplasty.

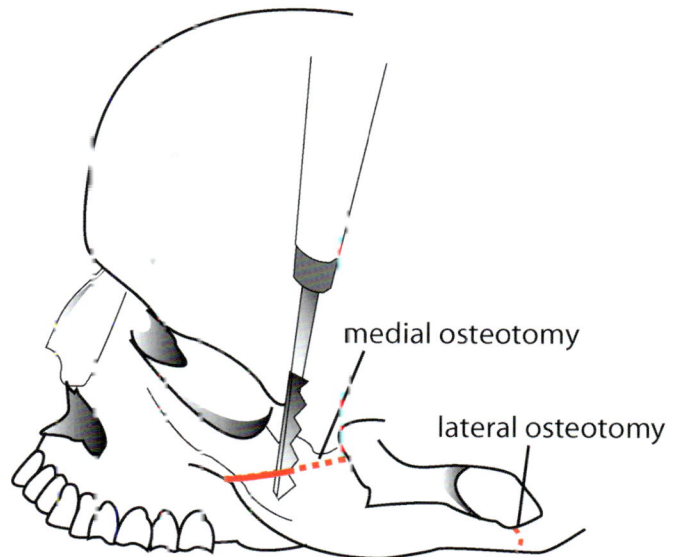

medial osteotomy

lateral osteotomy

Figure 12–40 The medial and lateral osteotomies used for coronal-based reduction malarplasty are shown.

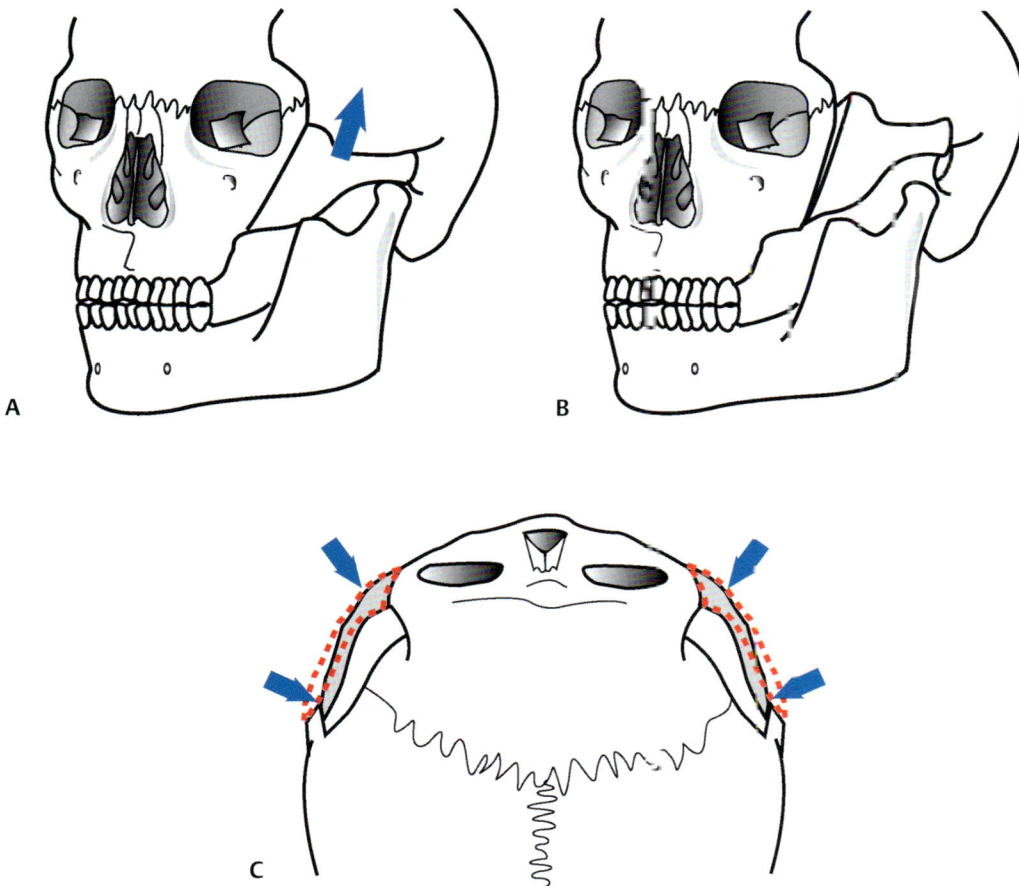

A

B

C

Figure 12–41 Illustration shows the repositioning of the mobilized malar complex vertically **(A,B)** and horizontally **(C)** in a coronal-based approach to reduction malarplasty.

inferior to the frontozygomatic suture, carefully preserving the integrity of the lateral orbital wall along the entire length. A retractor positioned deep to the oscillating saw can preserve the soft tissue below. A proclivity to execute the medial cut too far laterally so as to protect the globe should be resisted, as this is both unnecessary (if the instrument is beveled away from the globe) and detrimental in that an unnatural step-off deformity may be created and limited reduction effected. Entry with the osteotome into the maxillary sinus usually does not bear any adverse outcomes.

4. The lateral osteotomy is performed anterior to the zygomatic tubercle, with the blade angled obliquely in the posterior to anterior direction. The freely mobile malar bone is repositioned vertically and/or horizontally to effect a favorable reduction and then secured with miniplate or wire fixation (Fig. **12–41A–C**).

5. The coronal flap is returned to its native position and reapproximated with deep absorbable sutures and skin staples.

6. A pressure dressing kept intact for 2 days should minimize hematoma and seroma accumulation.

Unexpected outcomes parallel those enumerated in mandibular-angle reduction surgery and can be avoided with deliberate adherence to proper surgical technique.

References

1. Chang EW, Lam SM, Karen M, Donlevy JL. Sliding genioplasty for correction of chin abnormalities. Arch Facial Plast Surg 2001;3:8–15

2. Baek SM, Oh KS, Baek RM. Skeletal aesthetic surgery: reductions. Facial Plast Surg Clin North Am 1996;4:145–175[x1]

3. Baek SM, Baek RM, Shin MS. Refinements in aesthetic contouring of the prominent mandibular angle. Aesthetic Plast Surg 1994;18:283–289

4. Onizuka T, Watanabe K, Takasu K, Keyama A. Reduction malar plasty. Aesthetic Plast Surg 1983;7:121–125

5. Whitaker LA. Aesthetic augmentation of the malar-midface structures. Plast Reconstr Surg 1987;80:337–346

6. Lee JS, Kang S, Kim YW. Endoscopically assisted malarplasty: one incision and two dissection planes. Plast Reconstr Surg 2003;111:461–467

7. Kim YH, Seul JH. Reduction malarplasty through an intraoral incision: a new method. Plast Reconstr Surg 2000;106:1514–1519

8. Sumiya N, Kondo S, Ito Y, Ozumi K, Otani K, Wako M. Reduction malarplasty. Plast Reconstr Surg 1997;100:461–467

9. Baek SM, Chung YD, Kim SS. Reduction malarplasty. Plast Reconstr Surg 1991;88:53–61

13

Ancillary Procedures for the Asian Face

◆ General and Anatomic Considerations

The first edition of this book covered the subject of miscellaneous cosmetic surgical procedures in a single, cursory chapter. The original chapter discussed both minor operative procedures and various resurfacing techniques that were suitable for the Asian face. Since publication of that edition, the field of facial plastic surgery has undergone a veritable explosion. Surgical advances have been made that enable the patient to undergo a more natural surgical rejuvenation or modification with less recovery time. As part of this movement toward minimally invasive surgery, a byzantine array of minor techniques, soft-tissue augmentation materials, and paralytic agents have arisen to meet the demand of the "quick fix" mindset. Furthermore, resurfacing techniques have now embraced both newer modalities (laser ablation, coblation, nonablation) and more traditional methods (dermabrasion and chemical peels).

What constitutes an ancillary procedure is an ill-defined entity and reflects this author's construct of this proposed subject. This chapter will endeavor to cover disparate, minor procedures that can be performed in the office setting without sedation, that is, botulinum toxin (Botox, Allergan, Irvine, CA), soft-tissue fillers, lip reduction, dimple fabrication, and micropigmentation, particularly for the Asian patient, excluding implants and resurfacing, which have their own dedicated chapters. As mentioned, many different techniques and materials have expanded the surgeon's armamentarium to address a host of minor aesthetic flaws in the office setting. Among these soft-tissue fillers and chemical agents, only a few have met approval by the Food and Drug Administration for use in the United States, where both authors practice. Therefore, the experimental and foreign ancillary materials will not be addressed in this chapter.

The characteristic anatomy of the Asian face and the particular aging process that the Asian face undergoes have been covered in detail elsewhere in this book. However, a few salient points that are applicable to the decision-making process necessary for the implementation of adjunctive procedures are reviewed here. The more pigmented Asian skin may be relatively recalcitrant to photoaging. Although rhytidosis is a less prevalent phenomenon, the more poorly defined skeletal structure, more substantial facial adipose accumulation, and thicker soft-tissue envelope predispose toward increased gravitational descent of the buccal region. Therefore, soft-tissue augmentation along the nasolabial and labiomandibular folds deserves special attention. In this chapter, proper use of various injectable soft-tissue fillers will be reviewed. Liquid injectables serve a particularly important role in the management of the Asian face, as implantation of solid materials that require discrete incisions may remain conspicuous for an unacceptably protracted time in the Asian skin that is predisposed toward erythema, hypertrophic scarring, and hyper- and hypopigmentation. Although fine panfacial rhytidosis may be less prevalent in Asian populations, periocular rhytids and brow ptosis, both amenable to botulinum toxin (BTX) in certain situations, are quite common and will also be discussed. A simplified algorithm for selection of BTX and injectable soft-tissue fillers as well as details in proper injection technique will be reviewed.

Another ancillary procedure that merits discussion concerns surgical lip reduction. As most Caucasians complain of hypoplastic lips, especially as maturity accentuates this deficiency, certain Asian populations (e.g., southern, Malaysian, and Polynesian ethnicities) exhibit a characteristic lip protuberance, which they at times perceive as an unbecoming attribute. Partly, motivation for surgical intervention may be derived from the inclination to soften this overly ethnic feature. Overall, Asian demand for this procedure falls far short of the frequency with which darker-complected individuals of African descent seek this form of surgery. Generally, the more conservative and common request is for only lower-lip modification, although this procedure paired with an upper-lip reduction is not altogether rare. Isolated upper-lip reduction has also been sought as an independent procedure.

Another procedure that is far more commonly requested in Asia is the fabrication of a dimple. Besides the aesthetic charm that this entity imparts, many Asians traditionally consider the dimple a sign of good fortune. In fact, dimples that fall in various regions around the mouth have unique appellations that correspond to the degree of good favor that a particular location on the face bestows. The surgical creation of one or more dimples is a relatively simple, straightforward endeavor that can be performed in the office setting and designed according to the patient's precise aesthetic criteria.

Finally, the prevalence of micropigmentation, or cosmetic tattooing, far exceeds that of Caucasian societies. Although this technique has been increasingly relegated to lay technicians, often justifiably so, the surgeon should comprehend the cultural dynamics and appreciate the technical aspects of the process to communicate more effectively with his or her Asian patients.

Generally, a reasonable treatment strategy for adjunctive procedures such as BTX and soft-tissue injectable fillers divides the face vertically into two halves via an imaginary horizontal line drawn through the base of the nose (Fig. **13–1**). BTX therapy is particularly well suited for early wrinkles present in animation above this line but may be less appropriate for wrinkles below this line. Perioral BTX therapy for an overactive depressor offers limited benefit with the attendant risk of oral incompetence. An exception to this rule that will be discussed in this chapter concerns the reduction of masseteric hypertrophy with BTX for lower facial contouring, an aesthetic objective that is more commonly sought in the Asian population. This unique application of BTX therapy has achieved particularly widespread implementation in Korea but was first reported in the British literature in 1994.[1] This use of BTX violates the horizontal line principle, as it concerns a distinct aesthetic pathology, masseteric hypertrophy, as opposed to its more conventional use of wrinkle effacement.

With the foregoing exception in mind, soft-tissue augmentation is the preferred method of addressing the lower half of the face rather than with BTX. A fundamental

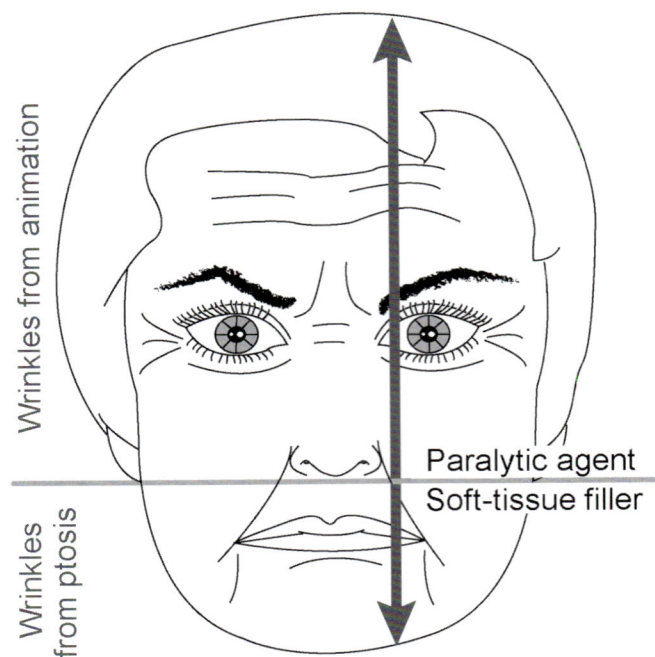

Figure 13–1 Illustration shows the benefit of adjunctive procedures based on an imaginary line drawn through the nasal base. Wrinkles above this line are typically attributed to animation, whereas, below this line, wrinkles develop principally due to tissue descent. Accordingly, botulinum toxin (BTX) is well suited to address incipient or early wrinkles above this horizontal line; and an appropriate soft-tissue filler is preferable to augment the ptotic tissues below the line. Although BTX has been successfully used below this line, and a filler, above this line, the author believes that the risk outweighs the benefits (refer to text for further details). (Adapted from Williams EF, Lam SM. Comprehensive Facial Rejuvenation: A Practical and Systematic Guide to Surgical Management of the Aging Face. Philadelphia: Lippincott, Williams & Wilkins; 2004; with permission.)

difference in wrinkle quality above versus below this line explains this author's rationale for the strategy. Wrinkles that form above this line are generally etched-in lines from repeated motion and benefit from either BTX therapy early (incipient lines) or resurfacing later (mature lines). Deeper glabellar lines may also be appropriately excised if very advanced. Solid or liquid soft-tissue augmentation in the periocular region cannot readily and evenly efface the fine, etched-in lines in this region. Although the glabella tolerates this type of augmentation, many liquid fillers are contraindicated due to skin necrosis and retrograde thrombosis and blindness; and solid augmentation may not be the best modality to treat this area (consider either resurfacing or excision as better alternatives).

Below this horizontal axis, the lines that develop (e.g., the nasolabial and labiomandibular folds) usually do so due to gravitational ptosis. These folds, rather than wrinkles, are more amenable to soft-tissue augmentation with either liquid or solid fillers than BTX therapy. The one exception to this rule is the perioral rhagades, or smoker's lines. These fine crevices around the mouth are more akin to the fine lines that circumscribe the eye. Therefore, solid or liquid augmentation of these lines is not as effective but still possible for some limited improvement (a limitation that the patient should well comprehend beforehand). Unlike the periocular rhytids, however, the perioral rhagades are not as amenable to BTX (which may be an apparent caveat) but should be treated with laser ablation, coblation, or dermabrasion. Hypoplastic lips, in contrast, may be appropriately treated with soft-tissue augmentation materials like the other areas described below this horizontal axis, but augmentation is less often requested in the far Southeast Asian patient for the previously enumerated reasons. Besides the anatomic differences between the Asian and Caucasian faces, BTX and soft-tissue filler injection techniques differ little but should be well understood to ensure maximal aesthetic benefit and minimal risk of adverse outcome.

◆ Botulinum Exotoxin A (Botox)

This section on use of botulinum toxin is divided into two principal parts: management of facial wrinkles and management of masseteric hypertrophy. Although treatment of facial rhytidosis represents a common indication for BTX therapy, this chapter endeavors to present a systematic approach that has been clinically useful irrespective of race and ethnicity. The latter technique of masseteric reduction may also be applied to Caucasians and other races who should desire this type of intervention, but generally it is reserved for Asian patients who request this procedure.

The first step that is required before BTX can be used is reconstitution of the lyophilized concentrate. Typically 2 to 2.5 cc of saline is recommended for each bottle of 100 U of BTX. This dilution yields an approximate concentration of 5 units per 0.1 cc. The authors recommend a double-dilution method of 4 cc of saline for each bottle of BTX to yield a concentration of 5 units per 0.2 cc. This dilution permits a more even distribution of toxin across the intended muscle, particularly in the forehead region. Furthermore, maximal yield of toxin is more easily obtained with this greater dilution, as minor, inadvertent toxin spillage during administration and recovery of remaining toxin from the bottle are less problematic with this more dilute concentration. The reader is cautioned that further dilution of toxin has two potential drawbacks (and is not advised): unintended migration of toxin to adjacent muscles due to higher injected volume amounts and loss of toxin activity (with a fourfold or greater dilution). The side effect of using this decreased concentration (and therefore higher volume) is the potential increased postinjection edema and ecchymosis from the volume effect. Nevertheless, appropriate application of

ice packs prior to injection and local pressure after injection minimize the likelihood of this sequela significantly. One further comment is warranted: the amount of BTX needed for masseteric reduction (25 to 30 units per side, which equals 1 to 1.2 cc of volume based on the double-dilution method) may lead to slightly more edema postinjection with the less concentrated BTX than would be encountered with the conventional concentration. Accordingly, if an entire bottle will be dedicated for use of masseteric reduction, then the single-dilution method may be justified. The reader is advised to use his or her own discretion when deciding the appropriate dilution.

Reconstitution of the dehydrated solid may be a relatively straightforward affair, but a few remarks will be made as to optimal technique so as to minimize potential waste and to enhance ease of use. A 5 cc syringe outfitted with an 18-gauge needle should be used to withdraw 4 cc of saline, which in turn is injected into the BTX bottle. The reconstituted BTX solution should be gently swirled, as shaking the bottle can deactivate toxin activity. A 1 cc syringe with an 18-gauge needle can be used to draw up the solution for clinical use. After the solution has been drawn into the syringe, the bottle should be turned back upright, the hub of the syringe drawn back slightly until the fluid is completely withdrawn from the needle into the syringe, and the syringe is then detached from the needle (with the needle remaining in the top of the bottle to load the next syringe). A $\frac{1}{2}$ inch, 30-gauge needle can then be placed onto the syringe for injection. Use of separate syringes drawn up with the appropriate amount of toxin for each particular area of injection (e.g., glabellar and forehead) facilitates an easy method to keep track of how much toxin should be injected into each muscle area.

A few general principles of BTX therapy will also be elaborated before a detailed discussion of clinical application. First, the intended area of treatment should receive 3 to 5 minutes of direct ice-pack application immediately prior to injection to anesthetize the area, decrease postinjection edema, and enhance vasoconstriction and thereby limit postinjection ecchymosis. An alcohol preparatory pad should not be used, as the alcohol can serve to render the toxin inactive. If used, the alcohol should be entirely evaporated before toxin injection. After injection, local pressure should be applied steadily without interruption for 7 to 10 minutes with a gauze pad, especially in the periocular region, which is predisposed toward greater ecchymosis than the forehead and the glabella. After injection, the patient should remain upright for a minimum of 1 to 2 hours and should not massage or manipulate the area to avoid spreading the toxin to unintended areas. Minimizing exercise and alcohol intake for the first few hours has also been reported to avoid the likelihood of a complication.

New evidence supports the finding that the toxin binds to the target muscle in less than 90 minutes, making these behavioral modifications theoretically unnecessary beyond this short time period. The patient should be advised that BTX requires a full 7 days to witness its complete therapeutic effect but may begin to be evident as early as 3 days postinjection. The patient is routinely called 7 days after injection to increase rapport and to ensure that the BTX has taken effect to the patient's satisfaction. Preoperative photographs are also advised to document improvement if the patient testifies to the contrary.

Botulinum Toxin Therapy for Management of Rhytidosis

This section will present a systematic method of BTX injection for the upper half of the face. The upper facial area is divided into three principal zones: zone I, the glabella; zone II, the forehead; and zone III, the periocular region (Fig. **13–2**; Table **13–1**).[2] Each of these zones will be discussed separately in terms of clinical indications, recommended toxin amount, injection method, and avoidance of danger zones.

Zone I represents the cluster of depressor muscles located in the glabellar region. The corrugator muscle extends over the medial eyebrow and merges medially in the central glabellar region, with overactivity of this muscle leading to vertical rhytids in this area. The procerus muscle that runs more medially in a vertical direction contributes to the lower horizontal rhytids. Patients who suffer from this type of rhytidosis typically appear angry or tired and often strike this pose out of habit. BTX therapy can arrest this behavior by blocking this unwanted expression. Accordingly, even though BTX is unequivocally temporary in its effect, repeated treatments may serve to break the cycle of unintended (or intended) frowning, and the patient may ultimately forget about engaging in the habit of frowning. Therefore, the benefit of BTX in this area may at times be considered "permanent" for this facial zone, so long as what that means exactly is conveyed to the patient.

A total of 15 to 20 units (0.6 to 0.8 cc) is required to efface the wrinkles of animation in this area. The patient should be asked to squint and frown to reproduce the target wrinkles prior to injection. Care must be taken to avoid toxin spread over the orbital rim, which might lead to blepharoptosis. Accordingly, all injections should be aimed superiorly (from inferomedial to superolateral) so that toxin migration will be away from the orbital rim (Fig. **13–2**). Because the corrugators lie deep adjacent to the bone, a deeper injection is warranted for more definitive paralysis. Using the nondominant hand, the supraorbital notch is depressed during the injection, and the corrugator is pinched between the forefinger and thumb for several reasons. First, digital pressure along the orbital rim will serve as a physical barrier for toxin migration toward the levator muscle. Second, the supraorbital nerve can be depressed and the muscle belly

Table 13–1 Summary of Botulinum Toxin Technique and Precautions

	Zone I	Zone II	Zone IIIA	Zone IIIB	Zone IIIC
Area	Glabella	Forehead	Upper lateral periocular region	Middle lateral periocular region	Lower lateral periocular region
Muscles targeted	Corrugator and procerus	Frontalis	Upper lateral orbicularis oculi	Middle lateral orbicularis oculi	Lower lateral orbicularis oculi
Objective	Eliminate medial depressor rhytidosis	Attenuate forehead rhytidosis	Effect chemical browlift	Eliminate lateral rhytids, or crow's-feet	Eliminate lower-lid hypertrophic roll of orbicularis oculi and lower-lid rhytidosis
# units	15–20 units	15–20 units	5–7 units*	5–7 units*	5–7 units*
Volume	0.6–0.8 cc**	0.6–0.8 cc**	0.2–0.3 cc†	0.2–0.3 cc†	0.2–0.3 cc†
Technique	Fanning	Percutaneous	Percutaneous	Percutaneous	Percutaneous
Cautions	Eye opening and closing dysfunction, ptosis	Brow ptosis	Brow ptosis, eye opening and closing dysfunction, ptosis, ecchymosis‡	Eye opening and closing dysfunction, ptosis, ecchymosis‡	Ectropion, ecchymosis‡

Modified from Williams EF, Lam SM. Comprehensive Facial Rejuvenation: A Practical and Systematic Guide to Surgical Management of the Aging Face. Philadephia: Lippincott, Williams & Wilkins; 2004; with permission.
* 5–7 units per side.
†Volume calculated based on the double-dilutional method (0.2 cc = 5 units).
‡Direct digital pressure should be applied for a sustained 7 to 9 minutes using a 4 × 4 gauze pad immediately after injection to minimize ecchymosis.

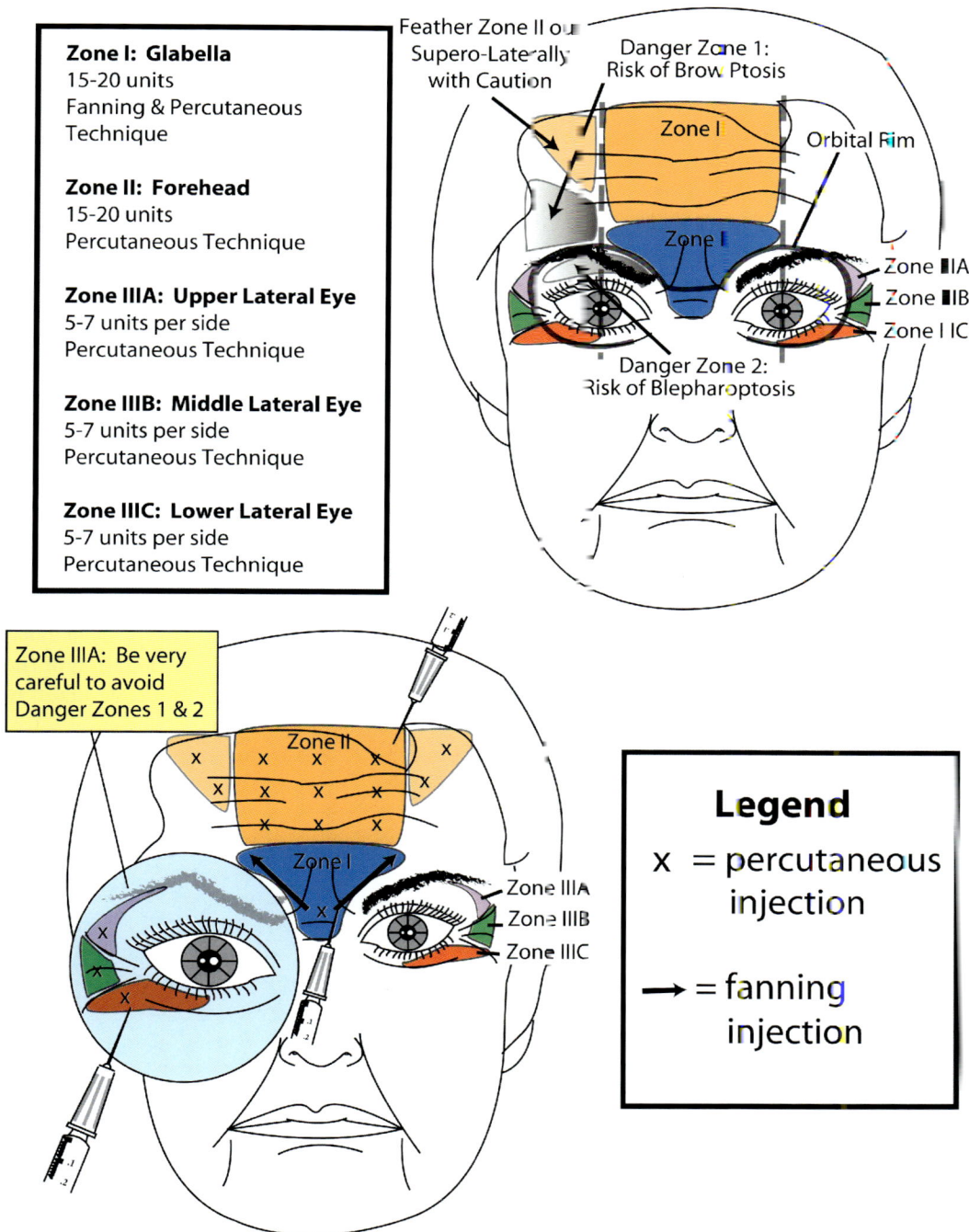

Zone I: Glabella
15-20 units
Fanning & Percutaneous
Technique

Zone II: Forehead
15-20 units
Percutaneous Technique

Zone IIIA: Upper Lateral Eye
5-7 units per side
Percutaneous Technique

Zone IIIB: Middle Lateral Eye
5-7 units per side
Percutaneous Technique

Zone IIIC: Lower Lateral Eye
5-7 units per side
Percutaneous Technique

Zone IIIA: Be very careful to avoid Danger Zones 1 & 2

Legend

x = percutaneous injection

→ = fanning injection

Figure 13–2 Illustration shows the three zones for BTX injection. Zone I is defined as the glabellar region; zone II is the forehead; and zone III refers to the lateral-canthal region, which in turn is subdivided into vertical thirds (zones III A, B, C). The two danger zones to be avoided are the upper-eyelid region (which can lead to blepharoptosis) and the lateral-brow region (which can lead to brow ptosis). Zone II should be feathered carefully superolaterally to avoid the risk of brow ptosis. Preferred injection amounts and techniques are also shown. (Adapted from Williams EF, Lam SM. Comprehensive Facial Rejuvenation: A Practical and Systematic Guide to Surgical Management of the Aging Face. Philadelphia: Lippincott, Williams & Wilkins; 2004; with permission.)

pinched between the forefinger and thumb (as a form of distraction) to help alleviate the discomfort associated with the deeper injection. Third, pinching the muscle belly facilitates a deeper injection. The toxin is injected during needle withdrawal. Additional toxin can be placed percutaneously in the midline to improve the procerus muscle, depending on the extent of horizontal rhytidosis

Zone II refers to the frontalis muscle that spans across the central forehead. Injection should be uniform and remain principally medial to the midpupil to avoid the risk of lateral brow ptosis (danger zone 1). However, injection can fan superolaterally toward the lateral brow extent with caution, remaining at a minimum of one or two fingerbreadths above the orbital rim. Very little toxin should be placed lateral to the midpupillary line during the initial BTX session to avoid the risk of brow ptosis that may occur, particularly in older individuals with a weak frontalis muscle laterally or in women who cannot tolerate any degree of brow descent or in those who desire some brow elevation.* A careful history that delves into the patient's prior BTX experience will gain useful insight into the precise distribution and amount of toxin that will provide safe and efficacious therapy. Because the muscle extends over a large expanse of territory, the fanning technique is an ineffective method of covering the entire central forehead. Accordingly, the percutaneous technique (Fig. **13–2**) should be used in a symmetrical fashion. As the patient is asked to elevate his or her forehead, the areas of concentrated muscle activity should be addressed with the injection. Typically, 15 to 20 units (0.6 to 0.8 cc) are required to address the forehead wrinkles. A broader forehead may require proportionately more BTX, and a diminutive forehead, less. In the preoperative setting, the patient is informed that the inferolateral wrinkles will not be ameliorated so as to avoid the risk of brow ptosis.

For the forehead, a marking pen may be a helpful tool to delineate all of the points to be injected to ensure symmetry and precision. A Sharpie permanent marker is preferred to gentian violet, as it can be easily erased after the treatment session with alcohol. Use of a marking pen also helps the physician establish dialogue with the patient about the intended areas for injection. Injection superior and inferior to a particular rhytid rather than directly over one has the theoretical advantage of more completely targeting the particular muscle responsible for the rhytid, but excellent results are still attainable by injecting over the wrinkle itself.

Zone III is divided in turn into three subzones: zone IIIA, the upper lateral periocular region; zone IIIB, the middle lateral periocular region; and zone IIIC, the lower lateral periocular region. Each of these subzones can be treated with 5 to 7 units (0.2 to 0.3 cc) per side to effect maximal benefit. However, 5 to 7 units can also be distributed more widely if less rhytidosis is present.

Zone IIIA extends just inferior to the hairy eyebrow and just along the orbital rim that corresponds to the superolateral aspect of the orbicularis oculi muscle. Injection of this area with BTX effects a chemical brow lift by partially blocking the depressor function of the orbicularis oculi muscle to permit unopposed brow elevation of the frontalis muscle (Fig. **13–3A,B**). Care should be taken to

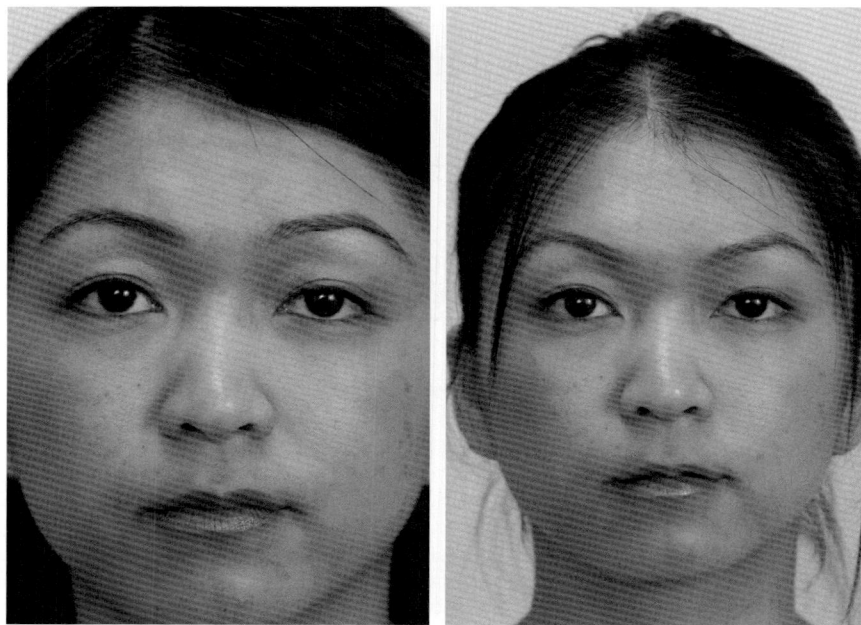

A   **B**

Figure 13–3   (A,B) This 23-year-old Vietnamese woman shows a congenitally heavy brow that imparts a tired expression to her face. She also exhibits a corrugated appearance to her forehead region that is attributable to an overactive frontalis muscle. She had BTX therapy performed in zone II alone by another physician in the past and subsequently developed significant brow ptosis. Most likely, injection technique was correct, but her entire brow was drawn downward due to a very strong depressor muscle complex. She underwent injection of zones I, II, and IIIA and is shown 2 weeks after injection with notable improvement in her forehead muscle activity and maintenance of her brow position. She also appears more awake due to the chemical brow lift imparted by injection of zone IIIA. Of note, she required additional injection of toxin farther laterally in zone I because her corrugator muscle extended over a wider distance than typically encountered, resulting in some residual rhytidosis upon frowning.

---

*Men may tolerate some minimal brow ptosis, as heaviness is a characteristic of the male brow. Nevertheless, a careful consultation with the patient will help dictate what would be the most favorable course of action. Women tend not to tolerate any brow ptosis due to the resultant, unfavorable aesthetic look as well as the greater difficulty in applying makeup over a descended supraorbital crease.

avoid too medial or inferior an injection that could predispose toward onset of blepharoptosis or too superior an injection that could lead to brow ptosis; this narrow isthmus must be cautiously navigated. The patient also should be advised in advance that a chemical brow lift may not be effective in every patient, particularly the older individual who has a less vigorous frontalis muscle to lift the brow upwards. If the patient is fully cognizant of this potential limitation, then BTX therapy can proceed. Also, if the patient has an asymmetric brow, BTX can be injected more superiorly in the lateral tail of the eyebrow on the descended side in an attempt to raise this side to match the more superiorly positioned contralateral side.

The reader is reminded that the periocular region is a highly vascular zone and not only should be thoroughly iced before injection but also should be managed with constant pressure for a sustained 7 to 9 minutes after injection to limit postinjection ecchymosis. Injection of toxin only into the subcutaneous tissue can also help reduce injection discomfort and contribute to less postinjection ecchymosis without loss of efficacy: subcutaneous injection can be performed in all zones but is most beneficial in zones IIIA, B, and C. Raising a subcutaneous wheal may create more visible swelling temporarily (for a few hours) but is justified, given the reduced likelihood for discomfort and bruising associated with a deeper injection.

Zone IIIB represents the midlateral extent of the orbicularis oculi that is evident as crow's-feet in this area during smiling. When these wrinkles extend down to the lower-lid and upper-cheek region, then zone IIIC is also

affected. Proper amount of BTX must be administered (5 to 7 units per side per subzone) to achieve complete ablation of these wrinkles. A hypertrophic orbicularis oculi roll that is evident along the lower lid (also part of zone IIIC) can be addressed with injection over the preseptal and pretarsal orbicularis muscle. Care should be taken to avoid injection along the lower-lid/upper-cheek region when two conditions should exist. First, a relatively lax lower lid may result in scleral show or frank ectropion if injected with BTX. Second, malar bags that are present due to a weakened orbicularis oculi can be exacerbated when injected with BTX. Furthermore, injection too far laterally or inferiorly can paralyze the zygomaticus muscle and compromise the patient's smile. The patient should understand these limitations and relative contraindications before injection can be safely performed.

Botulinum Toxin Therapy for Management of Masseteric Hypertrophy

Discussion of BTX use for the lower half of the face will be restricted to treatment of benign masseteric hypertrophy, which contributes to the unaesthetic appearance of a wide, square jaw. The ideal shape for the Asian face, particularly for the female, is an oval configuration (Figs. **13–4A,B, 13–5A,B**). A prominent jawline is associated with an overly masculine and aggressive appearance that is often considered an unbecoming feature. However, men also seek reduction of a prominent jawline when this attribute appears to render the face wider and flatter in aspect. In general, the Asian face tends to

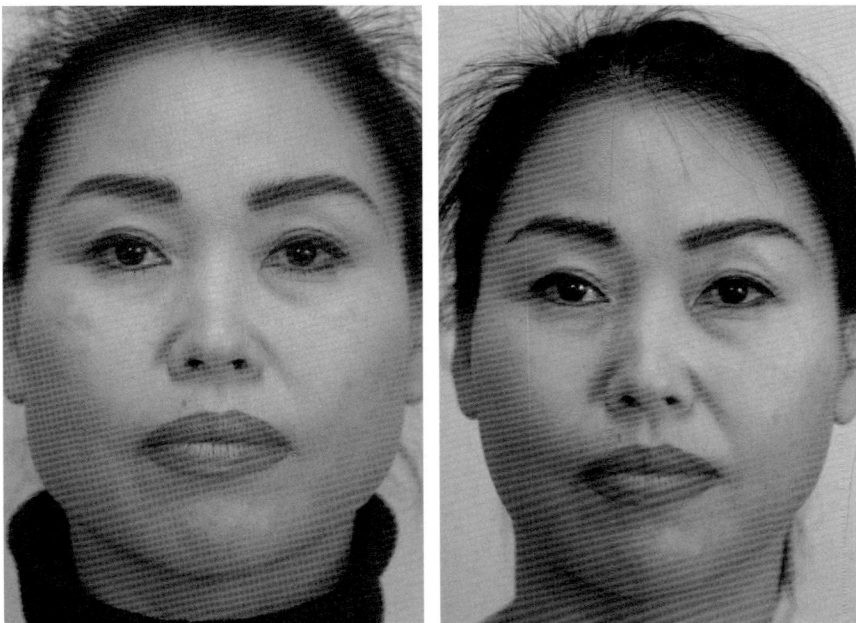

Figure 13–4 (A,B) This 44-year-old Korean woman underwent 50 units of BTX and is shown 3 months after injection with good improvement in the contour of her jawline.

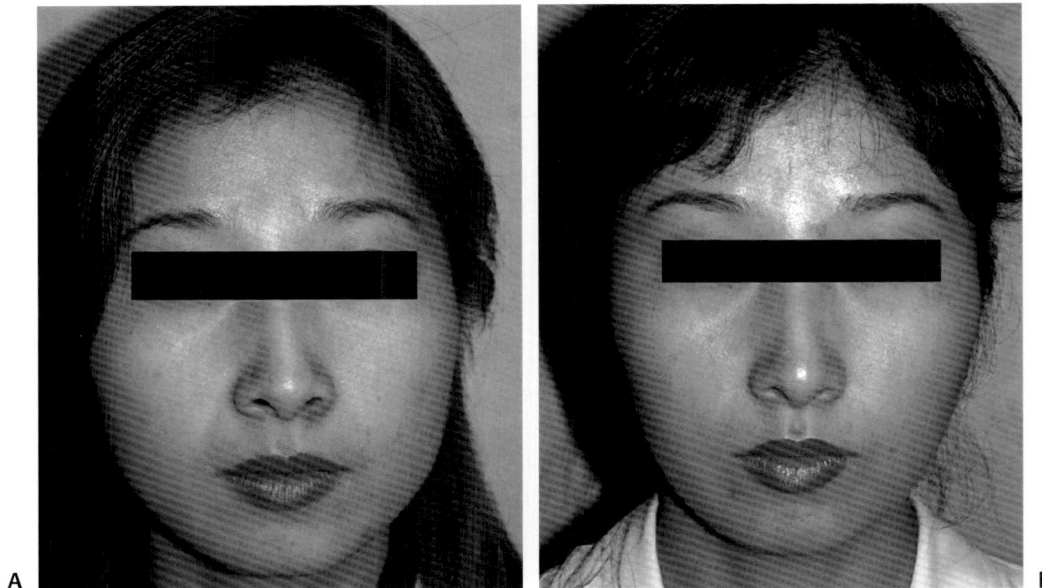

Figure 13–5   (A,B) This 28-year-old Korean woman underwent one injection session with 50 units of BTX to reduce the square appearance of her jaw and is shown 10 months after one treatment with maintenance of her result. (From Park MY, Ahn KY, Jung DS. Botulinum toxin type A treatment for contouring of the lower face. Dermatol Surg 2003;29:477–483; with permission.)

be flatter and wider than the Caucasian model, and some Asians seek to reduce this ethnic appearance by softening the jawline and thereby reducing the effective girth of the face.

To determine the proper candidate for this technique, a relevant history and targeted physical examination should be performed prior to electing to proceed. A patient should be asked how long this feature has been present and whether it is related to any dental or temporomandibular joint problem (pain, clicking, etc.). A history of bruxism may also be elicited. These dental/orthodontic/orthognathic considerations may suggest that the patient be better served with a formal dental evaluation and consultation rather than or prior to BTX therapy. Chewing gum or the curious habit of cuttlefish chewing in Asia may also be contributing factors and can be curtailed to effect a change without BTX therapy. On physical examination, the anteroposterior view assumes the most important perspective. The patient should be evaluated with and without clenching the teeth, during which time the examiner carefully palpates the degree of masseteric activity. If the examiner feels a significant contribution of the masseter, the patient can be asked to palpate the examiner's masseter as a point of comparison. The prominence of the bony angle should also be inspected both visually and by palpation. Based on this examination, the physician should decide on the relative contribution of the muscle and bone to the overall appearance of the jawline. The

physician can then guide the patient regarding the relative benefit or lack thereof that BTX therapy will yield. If the patient requires more invasive skeletal reduction, then an osteotomy may be the preferred treatment of choice (refer to Chapter 12).

Before undertaking BTX injection, the patient should be informed of the potential benefit and drawbacks of this technique. Clearly, the benefit would be a reduction of the masseter muscle, which will contribute to a softer oval contour of the mandibular angle. Also, unlike traditional BTX therapy, reports have indicated that the effect of this type of therapy may endure considerably longer, upwards of a year, compared with the 3 to 6 month window observed with conventional BTX administration.[3,4] Injection in this area may also lead to potential side effects that include masticatory difficulty, speech disturbance, muscle ache, a relatively prominent zygoma, facial asymmetry, and facial nerve paresis. Although these complications are unlikely, they must be detailed to the patient in the preoperative setting. Along with these more serious problems, the patient should be informed as per routine that ecchymosis, swelling, and lack of efficacy could be observed.

Prior to injection, the patient should be iced down thoroughly with an ice pack to minimize ecchymosis and edema after injection and to anesthetize the area prior to injection. A total of 25 to 30 units of toxin should be injected into each side of the face along five

Masseter

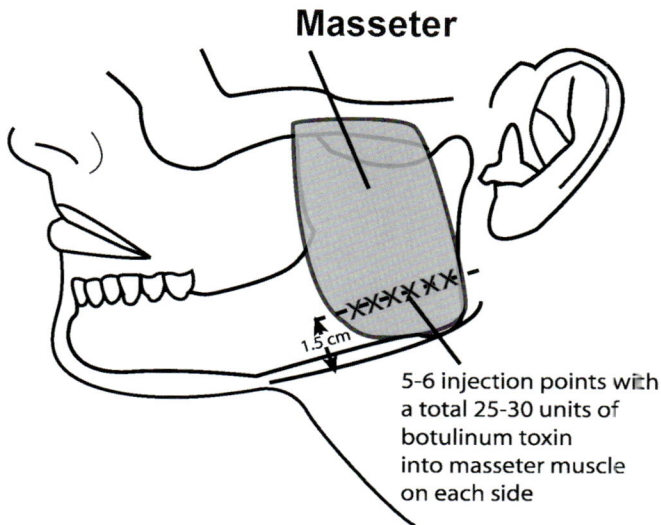

5-6 injection points with
a total 25-30 units of
botulinum toxin
into masseter muscle
on each side

1.5 cm

Figure 13–6 Illustration shows proper injection technique of BTX for masseteric reduction. A total of 25 to 30 units of toxin should be injected into each side of the face along five or six injection points that span horizontally across the muscle at a level ~1.5 cm above the jawline.

or six injection points that span horizontally across the muscle at a level ~1.5 cm above the jawline (Fig. **13–6**). A standard 1 cc syringe outfitted with a 1/2 inch, 30-gauge needle can be used to perform this procedure. The patient should be asked to clench the jaw firmly throughout the procedure so that the muscle can be more readily identified and therefore targeted. It is safer to inject deeper into the muscle than superficially which could potentially affect the facial nerve branch Pressure application should be maintained for 5 to 10 minutes after injection to minimize swelling after injection.

The patient should be followed 1 week after surgery to determine that no complications have arisen. The physician can palpate the muscle at that time and feel that its strength has been attenuated somewhat. However, the aesthetic benefit will typically not be evident for 6 weeks. Park et al's study found that the masseter continued to undergo atrophy on computed tomography (CT) scan for 3 months and on ultrasound for the first 1 month, and they further observed the persistence of the aesthetic benefit to endure in some patients for 10 months.[4] The reason for the greater length of effect with this type of BTX injection remains speculative at this time.

◆ Hyaluronic Acid

Restylane was approved by the U.S. Food and Drug Administration as a soft-tissue filler for cosmetic usage in December 2003. Prior to that time, bovine collagen was long considered the purported gold standard. Bovine collagen, however, has numerous drawbacks, including the relatively short timeframe of enhancement, lasting ~3 to 4 months in duration, as well as its immunogenicity, that is, its ability to stimulate an unfavorable allergic reaction. A skin test prior to the first treatment session with bovine collagen is also required to minimize the risk of an adverse reaction. This 30-day delay between skin test and treatment does not appeal to the mindset of the individual wanting to have a quick fix. Furthermore, collagen is derived from an animal source, which harbors the theoretical risk of transmitted disease.

Restylane offers many advantages over bovine collagen, including no need for a skin test, twice the longevity (lasting ~5 to 7 months), and greater biocompatibility. Restylane consists of hyaluronic acid, which, despite its name, actually physiologically exists as a neutral salt, sodium hyaluronate, and not an acid. However, the proposal for a less menacing sounding term, hyaluronan, has not entirely caught on. What makes hyaluronic acid special is that it has the exact same molecular structure across all species (varying only in its degree of polymerization), making it much more biocompatible. Nevertheless, hyaluronic acid that is extracted from animal tissue (e.g., Hylaform, Inamed, Irvine, CA), in this case, from rooster's combs, may still retain some immunogenicity, owing to impurities during the extraction process. Restylane, however, is completely bioengineered and is not derived from an animal source. This fact improves Restylane's biocompatibility profile and longevity. Hyaluronic acid in its native state has a short half-life of several days and must be stabilized by disaccharide cross-linkage to lengthen its duration of action. Minimizing cross-linkage, however, is important to limit the body's reaction to the injected material. Restylane is stabilized only by 1% cross-linkage to maintain a high degree of biocompatibility without compromising clinical longevity. Animal-derived hyaluronic acid oftentimes requires various methods of stabilization that may affect overall biocompatibility and longevity.

Restylane is used for injection in the middermal plane to augment soft-tissue depressions and for lip augmentation. A serial puncture and threading technique are both acceptable for clinical use. Given the longer duration of action of Radiesse (see below), the author prefers to use Restylane in those patients who cannot afford the relatively higher initial expense of Radiesse (but which will pay for itself due to the greater longevity and the convenience of less frequent injections) and for lip augmentation due to a lower incidence of postinjection nodularity with Restylane.

◆ Calcium Hydroxylapatite (Radiesse FN)

Currently, calcium hydroxylapatite (CaHA), marketed as Radiesse FN* (Bioform, Inc., Franksville, WI), represents an off-label use in the United States for soft-tissue augmentation. It has been safely used for over 8 years in the United States as an on-label injectable agent for urologic purposes, as a radiopaque marker, and as an augmentation material for cranial defects and for medialization of a paralyzed vocal cord. The implant can be stored at room temperature for up to 2 years and can be reused for the same patient simply by recapping the syringe. Since 2002, CaHA has been used reliably in over 10,000 aesthetic cases, and the clinical experience in Italy has borne out a safe record over the past 4 years. The longevity of the implant ranges from a year to several years, with the implant remaining radiopaque past 5 years, a fact that the patient should be aware of prior to injection.

Unlike many long-term fillers, CaHA is completely biocompatible, as it is found naturally in human bone and teeth. Therefore, hypersensitivity has not been reported, and no skin test is required. Besides biocompatibility, the implant is biodegradable, which may be considered an important safety feature. Previous animal studies have found that the implant does not migrate, ossify, or engender any local tissue response.[5–7] One study found no migration, inflammation, or heterotopic bone formation after subcutaneous injection of CaHA following 1 year in rats and 6 years in dogs.[5] CaHA is suspended in a matrix of water, glycerin, and carboxymethylcellulose gel, which is gradually resorbed over 3 to 4 months of time and is replaced by tissue ingrowth at a 1:1 ratio. Soft-tissue augmentation also occurs at a 1:1 ratio of correction, and the injection plane is in the immediate subcutaneous level below the deep dermis. The implant can be molded up to 2 weeks after implantation with decreasing ease over this period. The implant comes packaged in 1 cc syringes, which is equivalent to 2.5 cc of Zyplast collagen in terms of augmentation benefit. The implant may remain palpable for several months until all of the matrix is resorbed and replaced with native soft-tissue ingrowth.

CaHA is ideal for correction of deep lines and wrinkles as well as of other facial soft-tissue defects, for example, non-ice-pick acne scarring, traumatic defects, lipodystrophy, and other discrete soft-tissue depressions (Figs. **13–7**, **13–8A,B**). It is not intended for use in superficial wrinkles (e.g., in the periocular crow's-feet). Use of CaHA for lip augmentation should be used with discretion and experience, as nodularity may arise

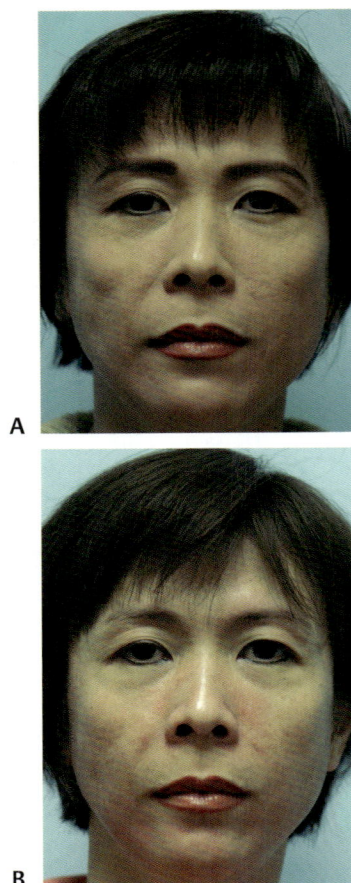

Figure 13–7   This 43-year-old Vietnamese woman is unhappy with the submalar depression that renders her face bony in appearance. She is shown after an injection of 0.5 cc of Radiesse along each submalar depression, with notable improvement in her appearance.

in ~30% of the cases. However, only ~4% require intervention, and experience and proper technique will reduce the likelihood of nodularity in the lip. The potential for nodularity is attributed to the cohesive quality of the implant (which also limits unfavorable postinjection migration) and the action of the orbicularis oris muscle, which may serve to aggregate the implant. If nodularity arises, an 18-gauge needle can be used to break up the aggregated accumulation, or, if more significant nodularity is encountered, the nodule can be openly excised and curettaged. Triamcinolone (40 mg/cc) can also be directly injected into the site. Generally speaking, most cases of nodularity will resolve without intervention in several months' time, but many patients may demand earlier intervention to expedite resolution. Nodularity is not encountered outside the lip area.

Many different injection techniques are acceptable. A 25-, 27-, or 30-gauge needle can be used for injection. Generally, a threading or fanning technique can be used reliably for augmentation. The author relies principally on the threading technique with a 27-gauge needle for

*FN stands for "fine needle" and refers to the preparation of Radiesse designated for aesthetic augmentation of soft tissue.

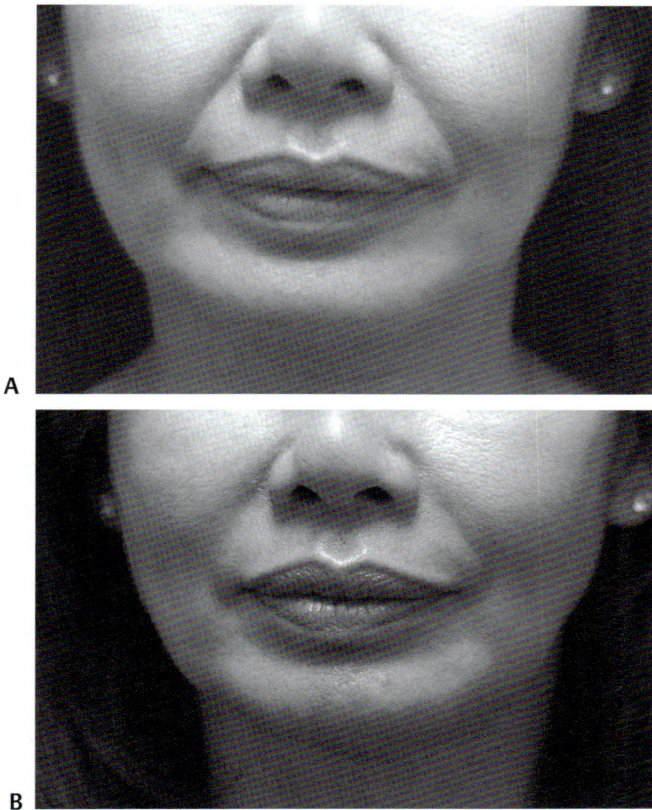

A

B

Figure 13–8   (A,B) This 59-year-old Chinese woman, who exhibits a deep nasolabial fold and only minimal jowling, desired softening of her appearance. She was told that augmentation of her nasolabial folds would be more beneficial for her than a traditional face lift, as her neckline appeared to be quite youthful and that a face lift would not improve her smile lines. She is shown after injection of 1 cc of calcium hydroxylapatite into her smile lines.

should progress in an orderly fashion, completing augmentation in each area before moving on to the next because the rise of edema will prevent the physician from accurate assessment of how much more injection is required. For injection, the full length of the needle is inserted in the immediate subcutaneous plane, and steady pressure on the syringe is applied as the needle is withdrawn. After the area is augmented to the desired level, digital pressure can be applied and the area massaged until the desired appearance is attained. If the area appears to be augmented uniformly, massage may be unnecessary and only serve to displace the implant from its intended site and thereby diminish the cosmetic effect. As the augmented area can continue to be shaped somewhat over the next 2 weeks, the patient is instructed to do so for any perceived contour irregularities that persist.

As mentioned earlier in this chapter, incisions in the central aspect of the Asian face require a long time to disappear completely. Accordingly, non-incision-based augmentation with the use of an injectable agent may offer a valuable method to correct deep smile lines or other facial soft-tissue defects with minimal recovery period. Use of permanent injectable agents may not be the best option, as injection of foreign material may engender an unfavorable tissue response even years after implantation. CaHA may offer a long-term solution that is biocompatible and ultimately biodegradable.

augmentation of linear defects, e.g., the nasolabial folds and a fanning technique for broader soft-tissue defects (e.g., rolling-type acne scarring defects).[†] For anesthesia, a regional block with 2% plain lidocaine is administered through the intraoral route for nasolabial fold augmentation and lip enhancement. Prior to implant injection, the intended area for augmentation should be delineated with a marking pen so that when edema arises, the precise area for injection can still be readily discerned.[‡] As some slight edema will arise, the physician

◆ Reduction Cheiloplasty

As mentioned in the introduction of this chapter, reduction cheiloplasty is a more common request from South and Malaysian Asians than their central Asian counterparts, as the former tend to exhibit more protuberance of the lips. This racial predilection for Asian inhabitants of more southern latitudes parallels the characteristic facial features that dominate the southern latitudes of the West, namely Africans. Dr. Nabil Fanous has notably remarked on the ethnic differences between Asians based on a latitudinal distribution (refer to Chapter 14).[8] To reiterate a valuable point, lower-lip protuberance is a more defining ethnic attribute and is the most common lip requested for reduction cheiloplasty.

Surgical Technique

1. Proper preoperative marking is the key to successful reduction cheiloplasty. The anterior mark is typically placed at the "wet line" delineating the area of lip seal on oral closure; this location maximizes the potential for an imperceptible scar. However,

---

[†] The reader is reminded that CaHA is not preferred for ice-pick type-acne scarring and that a saline test may be advisable prior to the first injection. Because acne scars may exhibit tethering of the dermis to the underlying fascia, injection of material may pass circumferentially around the scar and thereby exacerbate the condition (the so-called donut effect). Accordingly, infiltration of saline can be used as a test to ensure that soft-tissue augmentation will be beneficial for the patient. If the donut effect is present, an 18-gauge needle can be used to break up the dermal-fascial adhesions by fanning the needle under the skin before proceeding with injection.

[‡] As explained in the section on BTX, use of a Sharpie permanent marker is preferable to gentian violet, as the former is readily erasable with alcohol after the treatment session.

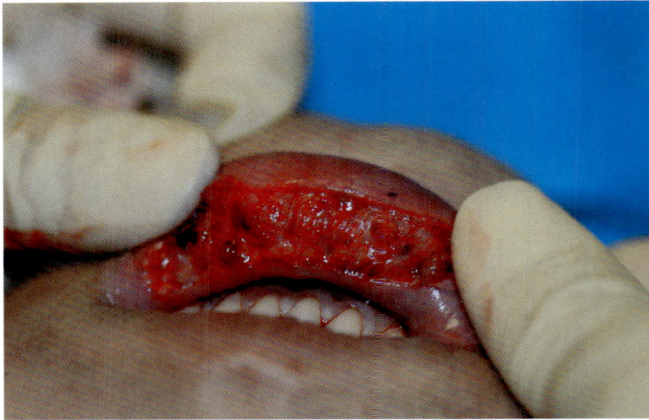

Figure 13–9 The anterior mark is placed on the dry red lip to remove some of the excess vertical height and anterior protrusion of the lip that is comprised, in this case, of the dry red portion of the vermilion. The extent and location of resection is determined on an individual basis, experienced surgeons often noting that a more conservative tissue excision than initially appears to be required generally yields an excellent result. However, experience will guide the proper amount of excision.

oftentimes a very full, dry red lip must be reduced by removing a judicious amount of dry red lip as well (Fig. **13–9**). The posterior incision is marked on the oral mucosa (a tenacious material such as gentian violet minimizes the possibility of disappearance of the mark following anesthetic infiltration). The extent of resection is determined on an individual basis, experienced surgeons often noting that a more conservative tissue excision than initially appears to be required generally yields an excellent result.

2. The procedure is performed under local anesthesia. A regional nerve block should be performed first. Injection of local anesthesia directly into the lip mucosa may be quite painful, and injection of a large amount of anesthetic into the lip mucosa may distort the tissue and affect the surgeon's ability to discern accurately the amount of tissue excision necessary. When the patient's lip is properly anesthetized by the regional block, a small amount of additional anesthetic (with epinephrine) should be infiltrated directly into the submucosa to minimize hemorrhage.

3. Tissue excision should encompass mucosa and submucosa to the level of the orbicularis oris muscle, which is left intact. Care must be taken to ensure that the resulting scar does not cross the commissure so that a constricting scar band does not form.

4. Three to four key sutures (4–0 or 5–0 chromic) are placed initially to facilitate proper alignment (Fig. **13–10A**).

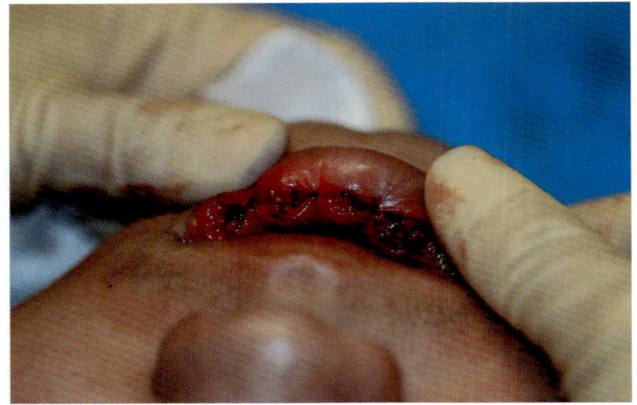

A

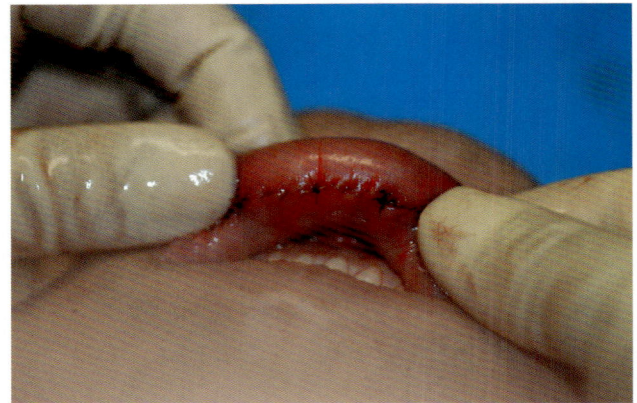

B

Figure 13–10 **(A)** Three to four key sutures (4–0 chromic) are placed initially to facilitate proper tissue alignment. **(B)** The wound is closed with a running, nonlocking suture of 4–0 chromic.

5. The wound is closed with a running, nonlocking suture of 4–0 (or 5–0) chromic (Fig. **13–10B**).

Patients are treated preoperatively with dexamethasone (4 mg IM) in an attempt to minimize postoperative edema that in many cases can be marked following reduction cheiloplasty, particularly if upper and lower lip reduction is performed simultaneously. Head elevation for 48 to 72 hours and local application of ice also are of value in minimizing edema.

A full liquid diet is recommended for 48 hours, after which normal eating habits may be resumed. Patients generally are able to resume work and/or social activities in ~1 week, although they are carefully counseled that the final result of surgery may not be apparent for at least 6 to 12 weeks postoperatively (Fig. **13–11**).

◆ Dimple Fabrication

As indicated earlier, the presence of a dimple may signify good fortune, beauty, and fertility for the bearer in Asian culture. According to Asian folklore, the dimpled

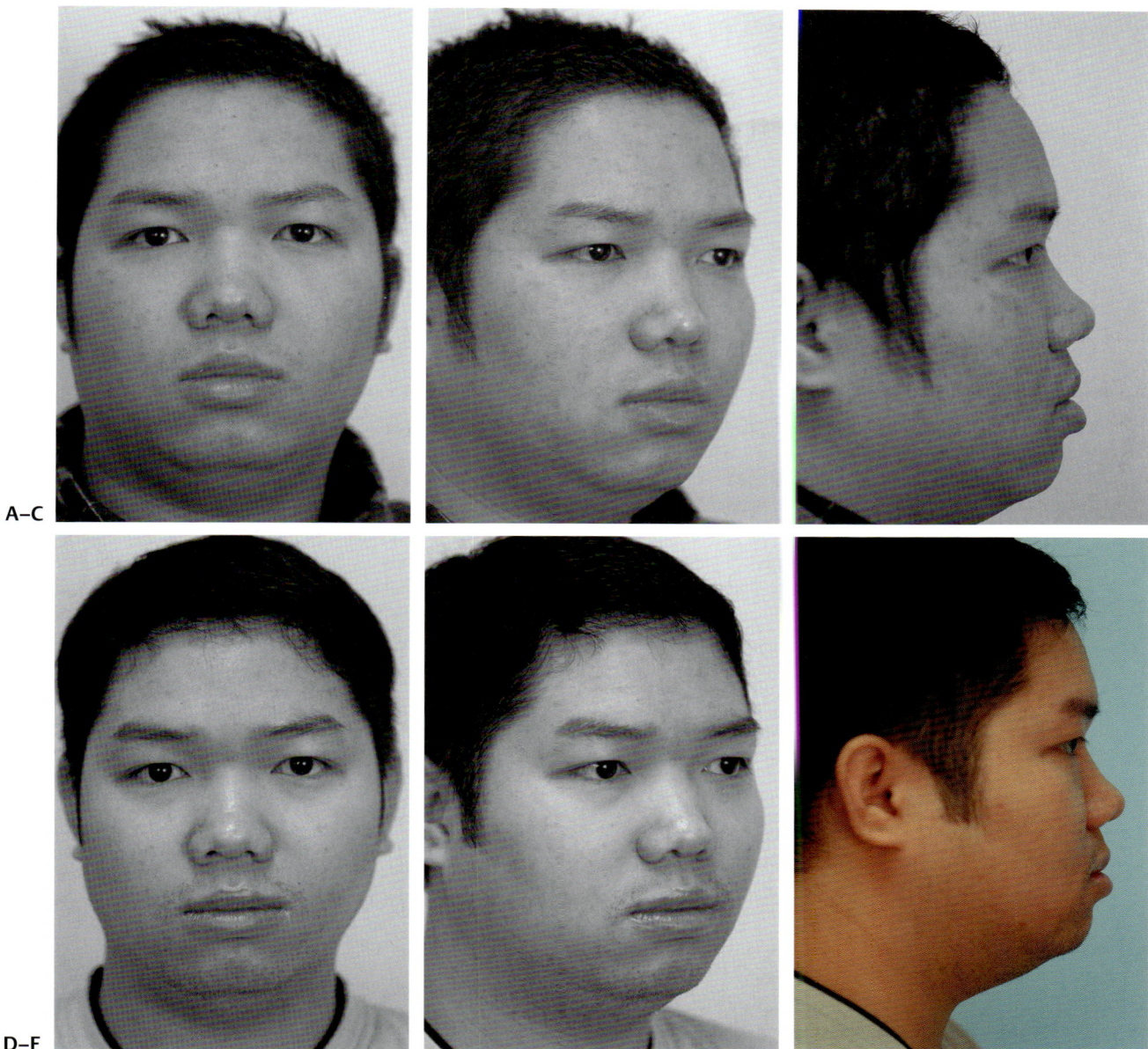

A–C

D–F

Figure 13–11 **(A–C)** This 23-year-old Vietnamese man is shown preoperatively with an ethnic appearing, protuberant lower lip. **(D–F)** Patient shown 2 weeks after surgery with persistent edema of his lower lip but with improvement already noted in the vertical and horizontal dimensions of his lip.

individual will be granted lifelong conjugal bliss. Based on cultural or aesthetic values, the Asian patient may be more inclined to request this surgical procedure, as t remains relatively unheard of in the West.

The consultation should begin with how many, what size, what shape, what depth, and what location(s) the patient desires to have the dimple(s) placed. Typical locations for dimples are near the oral commissure (above, below, and at the same level) or farther laterally (and slightly superiorly), as indicated by the illustration of the proposed sites (Fig. **13–12**). *Of note, the patient should be encouraged to have only one dimple fabricated,* *as bilateral or multiple placement is often encumbered by likely asymmetry.* Once these aesthetic attributes have been clearly established, the patient should understand the nature of the procedure and attendant risks and benefits. The procedure is undertaken in an outpatient office setting under local anesthesia in which the patient is fully awake. Not only does this simplify the anesthetic delivery, but it also permits the patient to interact with the physician to confirm that the dimple has been appropriately established to his or her aesthetic specifications. The most ominous risk of this procedure is clearly facial nerve injury, which can be devastating

Proposed Dimple Sites

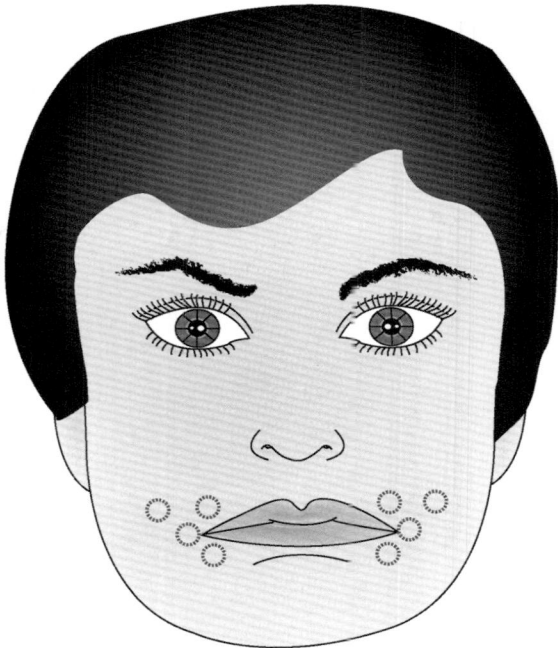

Figure 13–12 The illustration shows the proposed dimple sites that are commonly desired by patients. Typical locations for dimples are near the oral commissure (above, below, and at the same level) or farther laterally (and slightly superiorly).

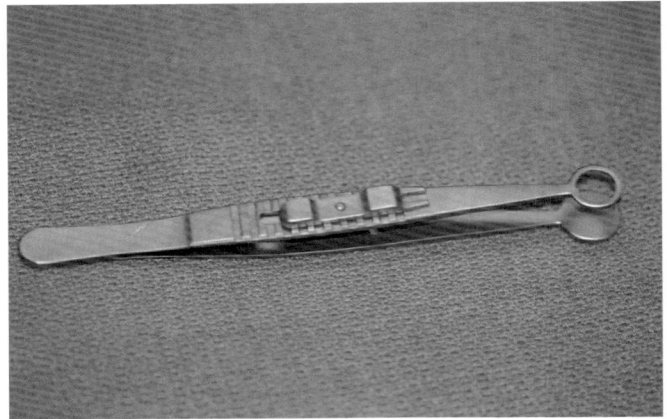

Figure 13–13 This special instrument is designed to facilitate dimple fabrication by fixating the tissue during the initial punch biopsy of the mucosa and muscle.

but has not been encountered. A technique will be elaborated that will minimize the chance of this complication in the forthcoming section,[9] but the patient should be cognizant of this potential risk at the time of the informed consent. In addition, placement of a dimple too far laterally (beyond the lateral canthus of the eye) may predispose toward facial nerve injury. The dimple remains as a permanent, omnipresent entity (with or without facial animation) for a 6 to 12 week period until which time the dimple only becomes apparent when the patient should smile or be expressive. The patient should also be fully aware of this fact.

Surgical Technique

1. The surgery begins with the area(s) that the patient desires to have the dimple placed clearly and precisely marked with a surgical marking pen. Symmetry is confirmed visually and with ruler measurements. The patient is then brought to the operating suite and placed in the supine position.

2. A 1 cc syringe with a 27-gauge needle is used to infiltrate 0.8 to 1 cc of local anesthesia consisting of 1% lidocaine with 1:100,000 epinephrine. After

anesthetic placement, the patient is asked to purse his or her lips to ensure that the facial nerve does not lie in the direct path of dissection. Accordingly, a long-acting anesthetic (e.g., bupivicaine) should not be used, as neuronal anesthesia will persist for 12 or more hours, making further work on this side of the face hazardous until the anesthetic effect has completely dissipated. After 10 minutes have elapsed, the patient's neural function is reconfirmed before proceeding.

3. The specialized dimple-retaining instrument is centered over the proposed dimple site and locked into position (Fig. **13–13**). The buccal mucosa is then everted, and a punch biopsy instrument is used to core out the mucosa and muscle to the level of the buccal fat (Figs. **13–14, 13–15A,B**). (In lieu of the specialized dimple clamp, a needle can be passed from the outside skin at the desired point through to the buccal side and the punch biopsy instrument placed over the guide needle.) The cuff of mucosa and muscle are then excised and discarded. Generally speaking, a 5 mm punch biopsy is standard, but a 4 or 6 mm biopsy instrument can be used according to the patient's size preference.

4. The dimple-retaining instrument is then unlocked and placed closer to the oral commissure so that an unobstructed passage of the needle through the biopsy site can be afforded.

5. A 5–0 nylon suture with a sufficiently large needle is passed through the biopsy site, catching muscle and fat before exiting through the skin.

6. The needle is passed back through the epidermis in the precise exit location, being careful not to sever the suture upon reentry.

Dimple Fabrication

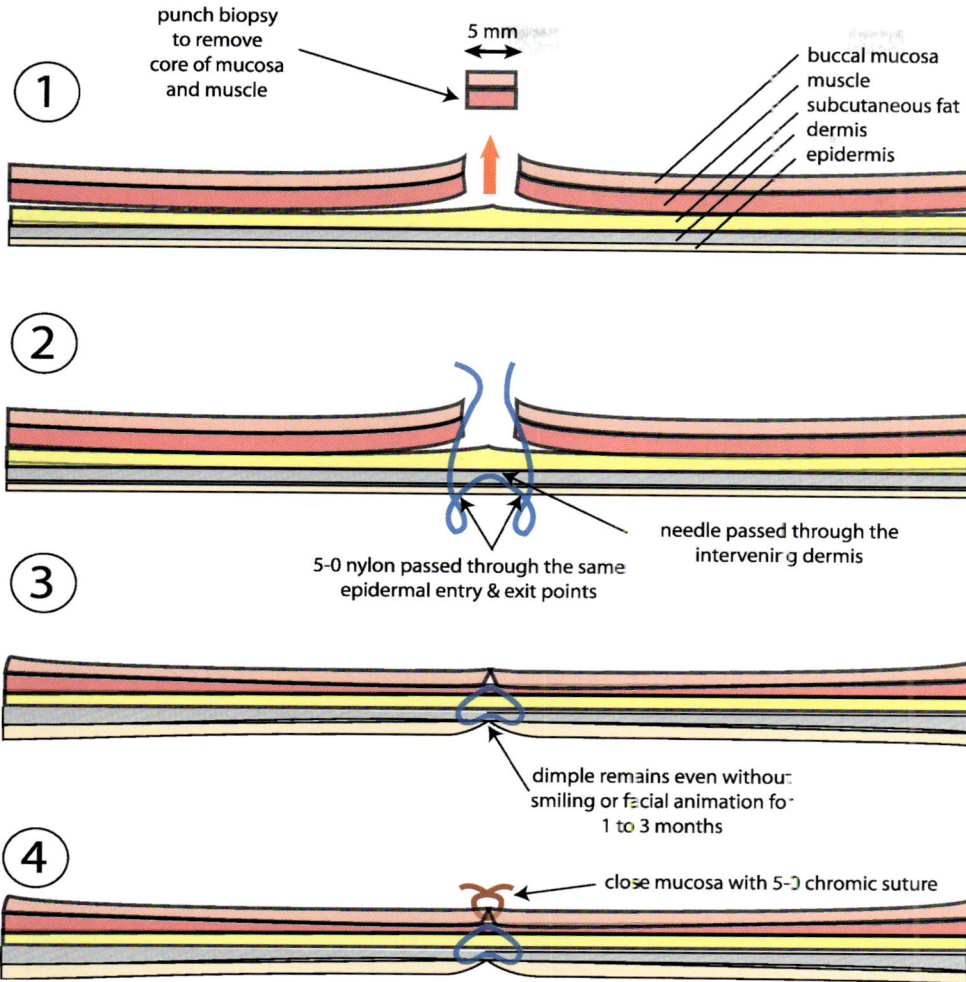

Figure 13–14 The illustration shows the stepwise surgical approach to dimple fabrication: (1) A 5 mm (or alternate size) round punch biopsy is undertaken through the buccal mucosa, and the core of mucosa and muscle are excised. (2) A 5–0 nylon suture is passed through the defect from buccal mucosa to skin, catching muscle only before passing through to the skin. The needle is then passed back through the skin in the exact same exit point through which the needle just passed and continued through the dermis for a variable distance (2–3 mm). The needle is then passed back through the exact same exit point toward the buccal side, catching only muscle before exiting through the buccal-side defect. (3) The suture is tied down until a visible depression is noted on the skin side that meets the patient's expectations of the dimple depth. (4) The buccal mucosa is closed with simple, interrupted 5–0 chromic sutures.

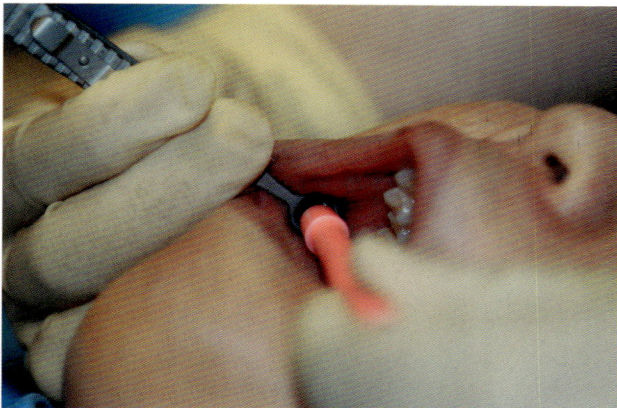

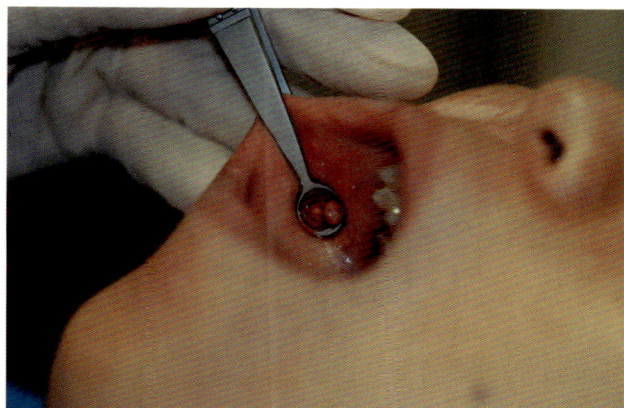

Figure 13–15 *Dimple Fabrication, Step 1:* **(A)** A 5 mm punch biopsy instrument is used to core out the mucosa and muscle with the aid of the dimple instrument that holds the tissue in fixation. The dimple instrument is centered on the skin side with the proposed dimple site. **(B)** The photograph shows the core of mucosa and muscle prior to excision.

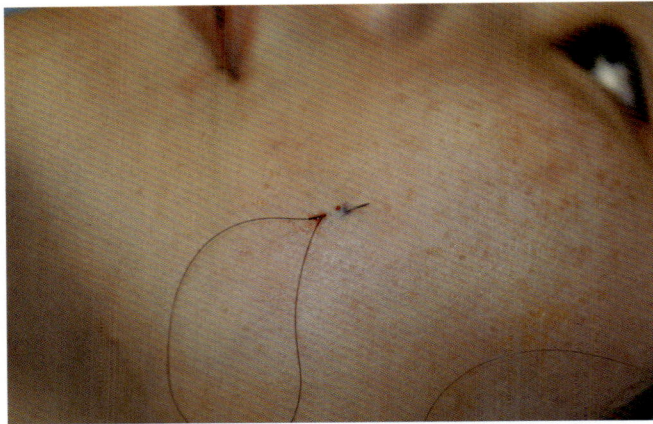

Figure 13–16   *Dimple Fabrication, Step 2:* A 5–0 nylon suture is passed from the buccal side through to the skin side, catching a good bite of muscle on the way through to the skin side. The photograph shows the same needle passed back through the same skin exit point and passed 3 mm through the dermis to a separate skin exit point.

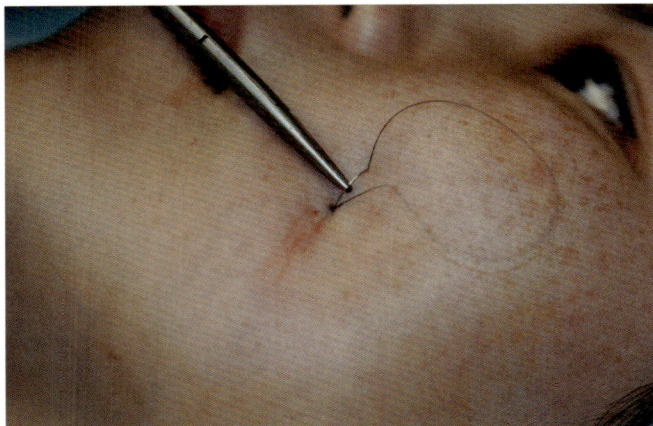

Figure 13–18   *Dimple Fabrication, Step 4:* The suture tails are tied down, and the patient confirms that the shape and depth of the dimple approximate his or her expectations. The photograph shows the suture tails passing through the buccal defect.

7. The needle is passed a short distance, typically 2 to 3 mm, under the dermis and back out through a different exit point (Fig. **13–16**). This distance will define the shape and size of the dimple. A longer distance that the needle traverses through the dermis will produce a more oval and larger dimple as opposed to a smaller, rounder dimple. If a more oval shape is preferred, the direction that the needle should be passed is vertical, as an oval shape appears more natural when oriented with its long axis in a vertical plane.

8. The needle is passed again precisely through this second exit point to the buccal side (Fig. **13–17**), carefully ensuring that the needle catches some underlying muscle and still exits through the biopsy-site defect.

9. The suture is then tied down, and the depth of the dimple is confirmed to the patient's satisfaction before fully securing the knot (Fig. **13–18**).

10. Both tails of the nylon suture are trimmed and buried into the biopsy defect, and the overlying mucosal edges are reapproximated with 5–0 chromic suture in an interrupted fashion.

The patient is advised that the area will most likely swell in the ensuing 7 to 10 days and that ice packs are warranted for the first 2 postoperative days. Although the patient can resume a normal diet, he or she should be advised to restrict excessive facial animation to expedite resolution of edema. As mentioned, the dimple will appear at rest and in animation for 6 to 8 weeks, then gradually disappear and only present itself thereafter naturally during facial expression (Fig. **13–19A,B,C**). If the dimple entirely disappears, this complication is a result of a failed knot and can be corrected with an additional surgical procedure. The knot may also predispose the patient to a foreign-body reaction, which will present as a nodule followed by drainage. This problem can be handled by knot removal through a slit incision.

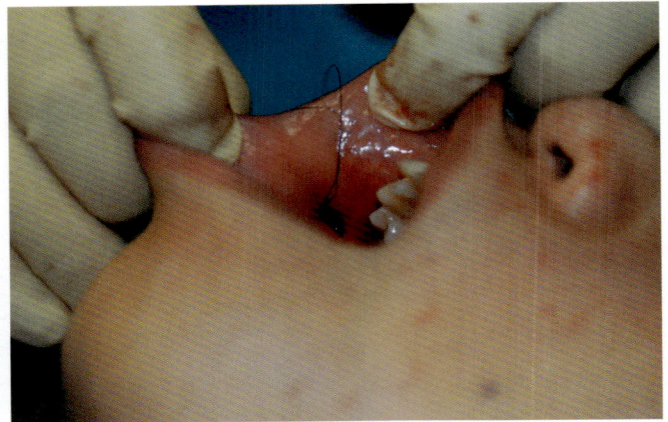

Figure 13–17   *Dimple Fabrication, Step 3:* The needle is then driven back through the same, second skin exit point to the buccal side, carefully purchasing a substantive bite of muscle before exiting through the created buccal defect.

◆ Micropigmentation

Micropigmentation, or permanent cosmetic tattooing, is a common service that many Asians request to enhance their eyebrow, eyelids, and lips.[10] Like cosmetic surgery, micropigmentation is subject to the aesthetic judgment and technical proficiency of the technician, cosmetologist, aesthetician, physician, or surgeon performing the

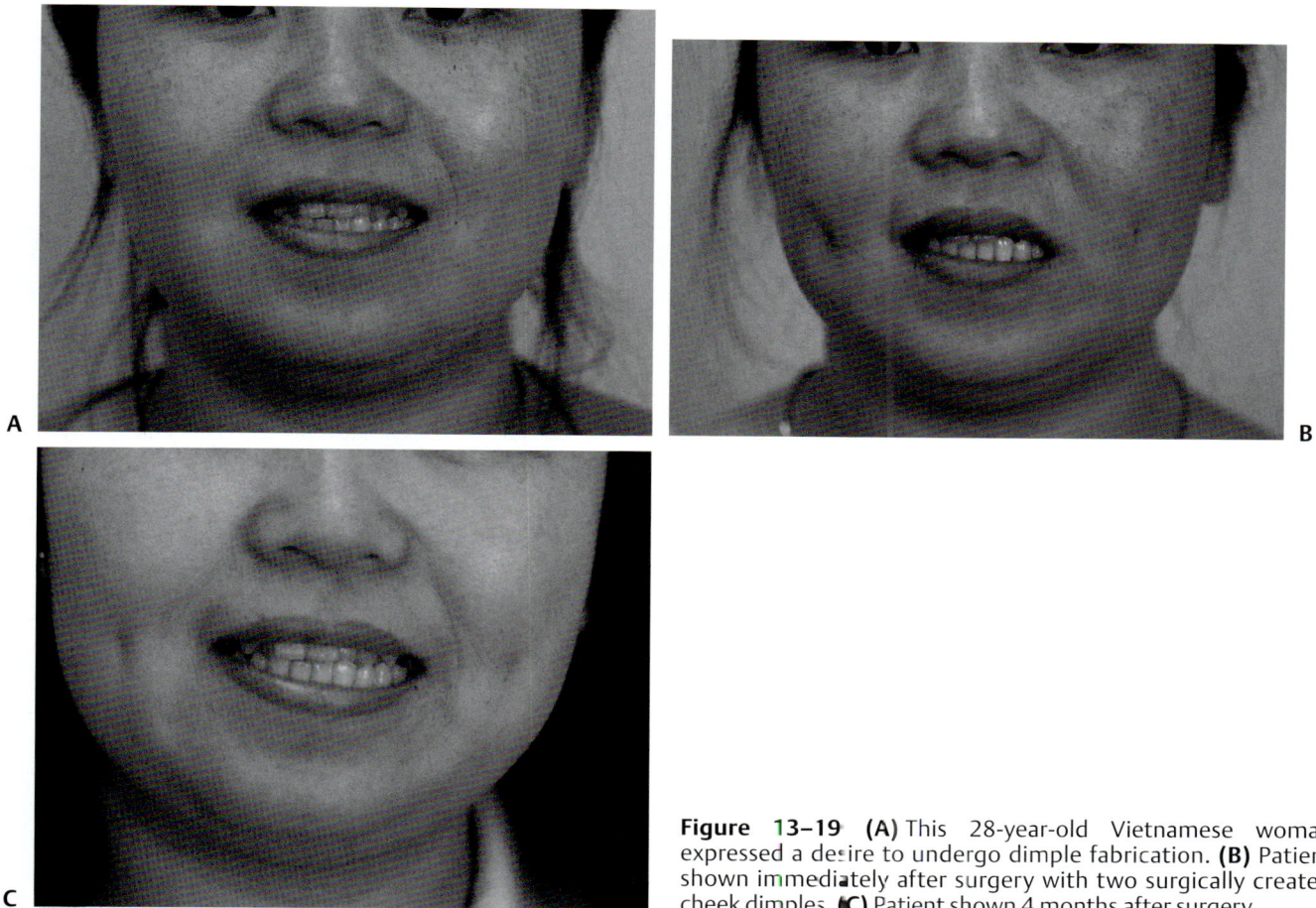

Figure 13–19 (A) This 28-year-old Vietnamese woman expressed a desire to undergo dimple fabrication. **(B)** Patient shown immediately after surgery with two surgically created cheek dimples. **(C)** Patient shown 4 months after surgery.

procedure. Done poorly, the tattooed area may appear unnatural and unaesthetic, but executed well, it can save the patient invaluable time and energy in makeup application and serve to enhance a surgical result (e.g., brow or eyelid surgery). However, tattooing should be deferred until after any eyelid or brow surgery so that the ultimate transposition of soft tissue may dictate permanent cosmetic application. Micropigmentation has increasingly entered the exclusive preserve of para-medical personnel (e.g., aestheticians or technicians), who are dedicated to this practice and who can offer the patient a more cost-effective service than that which the physician or surgeon is capable.

Preoperative Considerations

Basic Principles

Micropigmentation offers the individual an expedient solution to daily makeup application. Like superior cosmetic surgery, first-rate micropigmentation is predicated upon a natural enhancement of one's beauty and should not appear overly done or artificial in nature (Fig. 13–20A–J). Gone are the days when the heavy Groucho

Marx–style eyebrows dominated the industry and frightened the prospective customer away. The principle "Less is more' should be the mantra in the art of micropigmentation. Judicious use of micropigmentation can exceed the natural appearance of routine cosmetic application: the shiny, patent leather luster of the immediate tattoo gives way to a dull leather patina of worn shoes, as the pigment penetrates fully and resides solely in the dermis. This faded quality of the permanent tattoo that evolves over time may impart a more natural look than cosmetic products that rest exclusively on the skin's surface. Proper patient selection, thorough understanding of color theory and pigment application, combined with technically precise execution offer the patient the hope for a superb result that will endure.

Choice of Pigment

Deciding which pigment is appropriate for a particular patient requires skill, artistry, and experience. Typically, the technician will select from six to eight color shades for a specific clinical application (e.g., eyebrow

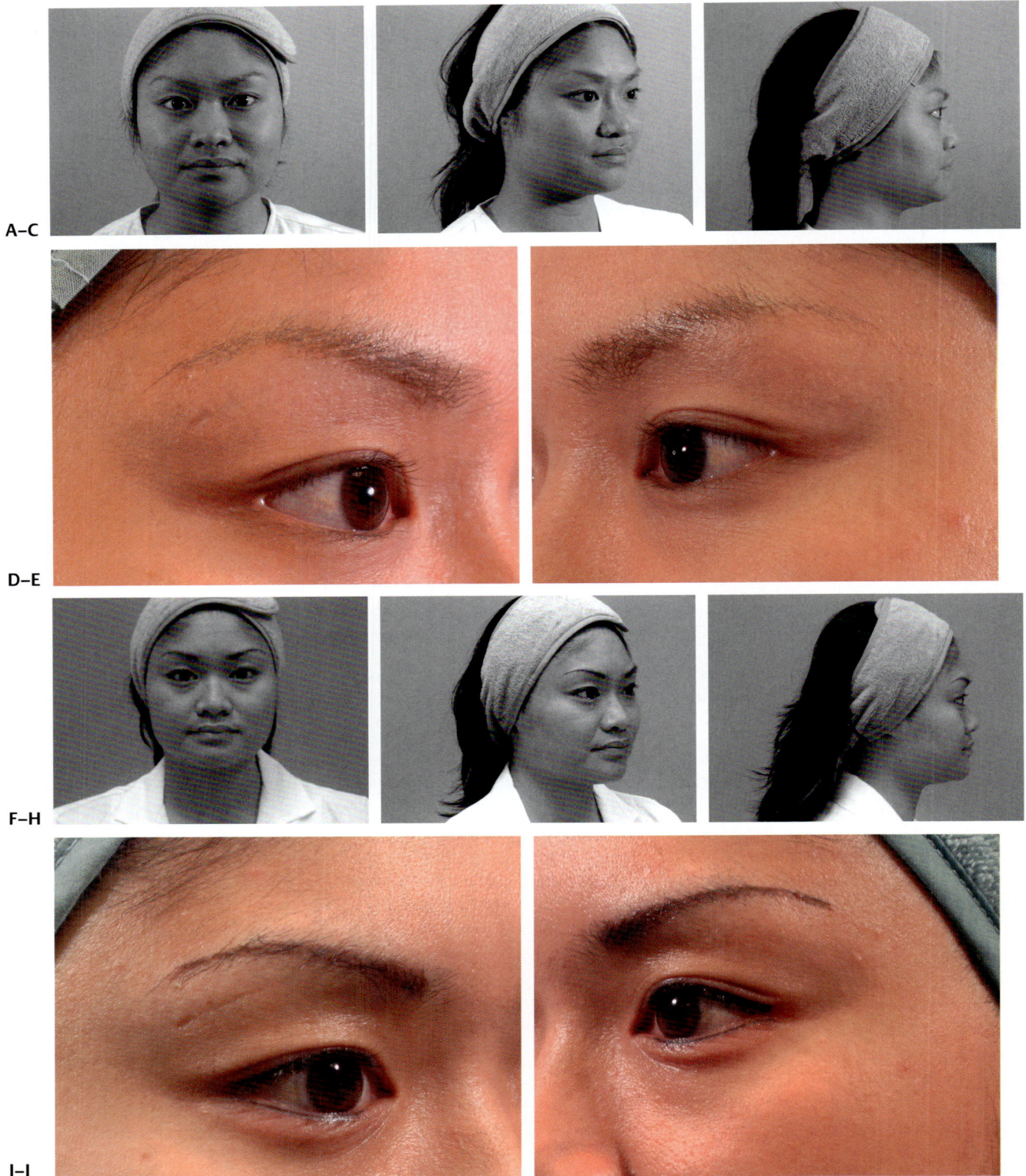

Figure 13–20   **(A–E)** This 25-year-old Taiwanese woman desired permanent enhancement of her eyebrows and eyeliner with micropigmentation. **(F–J)** She is shown 3 days after her micropigmentation session.

enhancement). The technician can refine that selection by mixing designated pigments that can lighten or darken a particular shade. By grouping shades of color by clinical indication, the technician can simplify selection of color when approaching a patient. The lighter the patient's skin, the more color choices may be available for the patient and the greater likelihood that a technician will have to mix an existing color shade to achieve the precise match of skin with pigment. The opposite is true: a darker-complected patient will require a darker shade of color so that the pigment will stand out against the native skin; therefore, fewer color choices are available. For dark African skin, only the darkest pigments will be suitable for application. Accordingly, skin color is an important consideration when selecting a suitable pigment. When deciding on a pigment for a dark-haired, light-skinned patient, the technician should not evaluate the hair color alone but consider the fairness of the skin as well: a dark pigment selected for the eyebrow may stand out against the background of light skin like the classic Groucho Marx look. As a rule, the chosen pigment should not exceed three or four shades darker than the native skin color.

When discussing color choice with a patient, several other considerations must be entertained. First of all, the chosen pigment will often change after application and may not resemble the bottled color after several weeks to months. In fact, color change may occur differently for various parts of the body (e.g., on the face, on the areola, or on the extremities), as each body part has a different skin thickness, sebaceous quality, and pigmentation that affect pigment absorption, retention, and expression. If the technician is uncertain as to the potential color shift, a small test spot can be performed and evaluated over a 12-week period to ensure that the color stays true. After the first 12 weeks, color changes will be subtler but may still evolve somewhat thereafter. For example, application of black color to the eyebrows rarely should be performed today, as black pigment is inherently unstable and will give way to lighter, unnatural blue hues. Therefore, despite an Asian patient's strong wishes to have black pigment applied as eyeliner or for eyebrow enhancement, the technician should resist the urge to comply. Instead, darker shades of brown are preferable that appear less harsh and more natural and also remain more steadfast in color over time. Alternatively, black pigment can be mixed with a corrective color (e.g., orange), which can mask the blue undertones that may manifest over time. Mixing orange and black will yield a rich, dark chocolate color that is a popular color choice in the eyelid and eyebrow regions for many Asian patients. Orange pigment can also be applied at a later date to correct the blue cast that develops from the improper use of black pigment only.

Another practical example of untoward color transformation is the rise of an unsightly purple from the mixture of white to lighten darker shades of brown. Typically, a fair-haired, light-skinned individual will benefit from lighter shades of brown for enhancement of her eyelids and eyebrows. To achieve this mix, white may be combined with a darker brown pigment. However, the titanium dioxide that comprises the white pigment may alter the combination over time to an eerie purple hue. Use of yellow can help restore the original brown color. Even brown shades may change over time to a light pink if green is not added to the initial mix because brown is a secondary color composed of red and black, the latter of which may dissipate over time, as previously mentioned.

Permanent lip liners may undergo a color change over time that can be quite devastating to the patient. A lustrous burgundy red will often give way to a dark blue over time that will appear frighteningly unnatural around the lip region. Differential pigment retention accounts for this unsightly occurrence: the blue undertone is retained to a greater extent than the other mixed pigments. Accordingly, a permanent lip liner should *never* include any blue at all to avoid this undesirable outcome. If the technician encounters a patient with this problem, orange can be added to ameliorate this condition but may also fade with time to reveal the blue undertone once again. Laser tattoo removal with a Q-switched Nd:YAG machine may be the only option that remains for the discouraged patient.

Finally, permanent lip liners should be used with great caution in darker complected patients. The tendency toward hyperpigmentation should not be underestimated: a black ring that permanently circumscribes the lips is a devastating outcome. In contrast, if the eyebrow or eyeliner undergoes hyperpigmentation, the result can actually enhance the look, especially in very dark individuals whose initially dark tattoo may otherwise fade to the same hue as the native skin color and effectively disappear. Hyperpigmentation that develops after cosmetic tattooing differs from routine post-inflammatory hyperpigmentation, the latter of which is almost uniformly temporary in nature. However, hyperpigmentation that arises from micropigmentation is more recalcitrant, as the hyperpigmentation persists as a tattoo in the dermis. At times, hyperpigmentation may be a favorable advantage for the technician, especially in very dark-complected patients who desire eyelid or eyebrow enhancement; the hyperpigmentation that develops helps maintain the darker contrast to the already dark surrounding background skin, as alluded to earlier.

Lip shading denotes micropigmentation of the entire dry red lip with color that replaces conventional lipstick application. Lip shading is not preferable for Asians or darker-complected patients who have significant vermilion coloration that tends to make color retention difficult and also serve to obscure the result. Fuller, ethnic lips are harder to fill, given the increased surface area, and fuller lips are also inherently more vascular, leading to greater ecchymosis, edema, and discomfort. Generally speaking, lip liners and shaders are more easily applied to a mature woman's attenuated lips, and the result can be stunningly dramatic.

This section on pigment choices is intended to provide concrete examples of commonly encountered clinical scenarios that can enhance or compromise the aesthetic result in micropigmentation. A detailed review of color theory and color correction lies beyond the scope of this text, and a professional micropigmentation course is advised for a more systematic appraisal of the subject.

Preoperative Consultation & Evaluation

If the eyebrow or eyelid region is to be treated, the individual who is to perform the procedure must comprehend the intricacies of ethnic variations of the Asian eye, namely, epicanthal fullness, presence of a single or double eyelid, intercanthal distance, and size and shape of palpebral fissure. All these factors can influence judgment as to the configuration, length, and position of the eyeliner or eyebrow shadowing. For instance, widely spaced eyes, either due to a prominent epicanthal fold or telecanthic distance, may be compensated with more medial extension of the eyebrow. Conversely, more closely spaced eyes can be offset with eyebrows that commence just lateral to the medial aspect of the eye. Similarly, a poorly defined or attenuated lip appearance may be accentuated with micropigmentation that matches skin and vermilion color and does not appear injudiciously overly exaggerated.

Besides a carefully and mutually agreed upon objective between patient and technician, the technician must entertain other preoperative considerations. Skin type is a very important indicator of how well applied pigment will be ultimately retained. Asian skin tends to have a natural propensity toward a uniform absorption of pigmentary material. More sebaceous skin, characteristic of many eyebrow regions, retains pigment better than thinner, less oily skin. In contrast, thinner, less oily skin fails to accept pigment well initially, but with repeated application, it does exceptionally well. The risk of hyperpigmentation should be carefully elaborated for the patient, especially if lip enhancement is entertained. Color change and color loss must also be well understood by the patient. The longevity of the tattoo is predicated upon many factors but will endure longer for the darker-skinned patient, especially in the eyeliner region as compared with that of the eyebrow. For lighter-skinned patients, a touch-up may be required after 5 to 7 years.

As per routine for any operative procedure, a detailed medical history, standardized before-and-after photos, and informed consent should be undertaken for every patient. The history should focus on any previous scarring, wound healing problems (e.g., due to diabetes, HIV disease, etc.), and previous perioral herpetic outbreaks. Any history of prior herpes or cold sores should warrant perioperative, prophylactic oral antiviral medication: valcyclovir can be instituted 2 days prior to the procedure and continued for a 7-day period. If an eruption develops, the dose can be doubled and the patient carefully followed for symptom resolution. If the patient objects to treatment, this refusal should be meticulously documented in the medical chart, and the adverse outcomes that include potential scarring, uneven pigment absorption, and rapid loss of pigment, recorded. Besides a practical discussion of pricing and scheduling, the patient should be advised as to whether touch-ups will be included in the initial price and for what period that this courtesy will be extended. For instance, a patient returning for a 4-week follow-up with an uneven or imperfect result may deserve a complimentary touch-up, whereas a patient returning 1 year later should probably be charged for further treatment. Policy is guided by individual preference but should be implemented in a standardized fashion.

Equipment

Before the digital era, two principal devices were enlisted for micropigmentation: a reciprocating two-coil machine, which relies on rapidly oscillating needles, and a rotary device in which the needles rotate in a circular fashion. These machines are still in widespread use today and are acceptable in experienced hands. However, computerized digital models (e.g., Nouveau Contour Digital 600 [Nouveau Contour BV, Weert, Netherlands]) have provided both the novice and the seasoned technician a reliable, reproducible, rapid, and safe method of micropigmentation (Fig. **13–21**). Digital technology facilitates penetration of pigment to the intended dermal layer in a more uniform manner and reduces operator fatigue and inaccuracy. The safety margin has been greatly enhanced, and scarring and uneven results are far less likely with these advanced models. Accordingly, the number of touch-up sessions can be dramatically reduced. The longer treatment sessions that were routine with noncomputerized machines often elicited operator hand and eye fatigue. In the past, the reciprocating machines were frequently preferred because color retention was superior to the less invasive rotary-style versions. However, digital machines feature a rotary-style delivery with better pigment retention than even the older reciprocating, hand-controlled devices could offer.

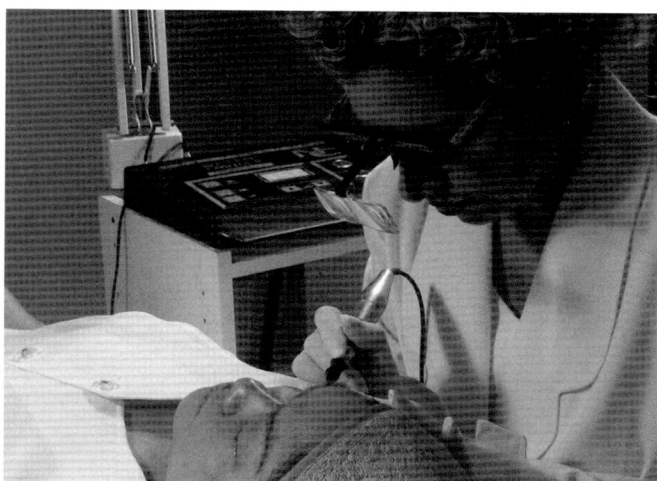

Figure 13–21   The technician, wearing 5X loupe magnification to perform the procedure, is situated to the right of the patient, as the technician is right-handed. The Nouveau Contour Digital 600 model is seen in the background.

The tattoo pigment is delivered to the dermis via a variety of clustered needle configurations, depending on the intended clinical objective and technician preference. The needles are made of stainless steel, which are disposable. The individual needles are fixed to a rigid bar in two configuration patterns: round and flat. The bar in turn is affixed to the tattoo machine. A round type of needle configuration consists of a round cluster of needles designed for creation of linear details (e.g., for an eyeliner, lip liner, or eyebrow follicle simulator), while beveling the angle of the instrument to permit a single needle contact can be used for even greater precision. The standard sizes include one, three, five, and seven round needle clusters. [§] The no. 3 size is also available with a configuration consisting of finer needle calibers and denoted accordingly, as no. 3 fine. The flat type is configured to fill in larger areas that require pigmentary enhancement and typically comes in two sizes: 4 flat and 9 magnum, with the former consisting of a linear row of four needles and the latter consisting of two, parallel rows of four and five needles. The artistry of the technician will determine what combination of needle patterns will best serve the envisioned aesthetic goal. The following section on technique will highlight particular needle configurations suitable for designated clinical scenarios.

Anesthesia

Patient comfort is clearly a preeminent concern and will reap dividends in patient compliance for ease of application and in patient satisfaction for return visits and referrals. Injectable anesthesia is often unnecessary

and can lead to excessive edema that can obscure the topography of the area to be treated. Furthermore, as physician supervision or performance of micropigmentation may often be lacking, injectable local anesthesia may be an unavailable option. Topical anesthesia (e.g., EMLA, ELA-Max, etc.) is indispensable for every micropigmentation session. The most uncomfortable area is typically the eyebrow region, which should be well anesthetized before commencing and reapplied with additional anesthetic as needed. Application of topical anesthesia can be performed early in the consultation to permit the anesthesia to work. Nevertheless, topical anesthesia applied to intact skin only anesthetizes the epidermis, and dermal penetration of the tattoo is fundamental to uniform and lasting pigment retention. Furthermore, dermal entry elicits a large proportion of patient discomfort. Accordingly, a single, light pass of micropigmentation application should be performed and additional topical anesthesia immediately applied that permits penetration of the anesthetic agent to the dermal layer, where it can appreciably affect patient comfort. Additional anesthesia and delay for the anesthetic to work may be required to achieve maximal comfort and compliance during the treatment session.

Technique

Although this text elaborates a detailed, stepwise strategy for micropigmentation, professional, supervised course work with a reputable school and ongoing clinical experience are integral to a successful and safe practice of micropigmentation. As a general rule, haste makes waste: a careful, deliberate technique will ensure uniform results and obviate the need for repeated touch-up sessions. Use of 5X loupe magnification greatly enhances accuracy and reduces eye fatigue and should be considered an obligatory accessory for superior performance (Fig. **13–21**).

Application of pigment at a uniform depth is key to ensuring an even result and color retention. With the skin under stretched tension with the nondominant hand, the dominant hand controls the needle depth by feeling the resistance of the skin as the needle enters the dermis. If no resistance is felt, the needle most likely is too superficial and has only penetrated the epidermis, which will contribute to early loss of color. If the skin is not held under tension, the needle may snag on the skin, which will feel like excessive skin resistance and also elicit significant patient discomfort. Therefore, the role of the nondominant hand in skin stretch is vital, and the precise method of skin stretch differs for each clinical application, which will be elaborated further.

Finally, technician positioning vis-à-vis the patient is a critical factor for successful tattoo delivery. For a

---

[§]Needle size configurations differ by manufacturer. The needle sizes mentioned refer to those used for the Nouveau Contour Digital 600 model.

right-handed technician, the technician should be seated to the right side of the patient for all procedures (Fig. **13–21**). Similarly, a left-handed technician must always be stationed to the left of the patient. This kind of seating arrangement will facilitate perfect alignment of the machine and the patient such that the instruments will not be oriented in an oblique angle, which would lead to an imprecise, thickened tattoo line to be applied. For the right-handed technician, the head can be rotated toward the operator as needed to facilitate easy access to the left side of the face. The converse is true for the left-handed operator.

Principles of Eyebrow Application

The thick, blocked-in Groucho Marx eyebrow has been replaced with gentle, curvilinear painted strokes that mimic naturally growing eyebrow follicles. This newer technique provides a more natural appearance and reduces the painted-on look of yesteryear. The technician should attempt to match the same length, shape, and density of the patient's own eyebrow hairs to achieve the most natural look.

As mentioned, the eyebrow region is the most sensitive for the patient, and adequate anesthesia is imperative for patient comfort and compliance: it has been observed that the younger patient may encounter substantially more discomfort than the more mature individual. Also, some bleeding is typically encountered, and a liberal supply of moistened towelettes should be readily at hand to keep the operative field free of visual distraction: 4 × 4 gauze tends to be too abrasive to the skin and should not be used. Finally, the type of skin stretch differs from that used for the lower eyelid: the skin is stretched along the direction of the hair follicles (a two-direction rather than a three-direction stretch). If the skin is stretched perpendicular to the hair follicles (i.e., vertically), the needles can transect the skin like a knife blade. Generally, a low number of 20 and a high number of 50 to 70 tattooed strokes are necessary per side to achieve adequate density to meet the intended aesthetic objective.

Technique for Eyebrow Application

1. During the consultation, the patient has already had the topical anesthetic placed on the skin to allow time for it to work.

2. When the time comes for the procedure, the anesthetic is wiped away, and an eyebrow pencil is used to shape the eyebrow in the manner pleasing to the patient and technician (Fig. **13–22**).

3. A gentian violet marking pen with a fine point is used to outline the penciled area (Fig. **13–23**), and

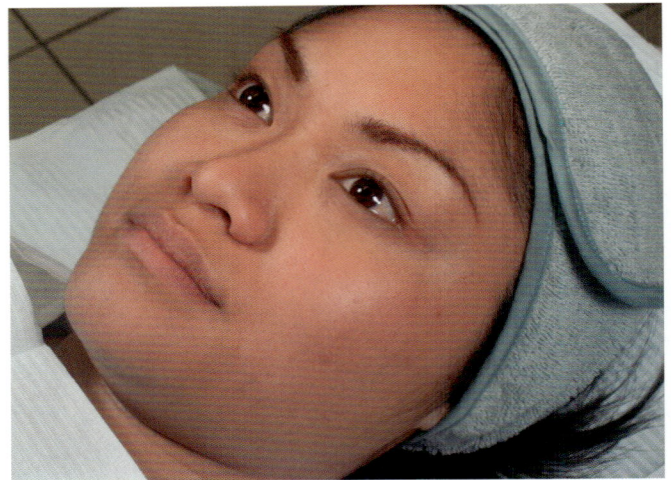

Figure 13–22   *Eyebrow Micropigmentation, Step 1*: The eyebrow pencil is used to design the shape of the eyebrow in the configuration that is pleasing to both the patient and the technician and that will serve as a guide for micropigmentation.

the applied eyebrow pencil is removed to leave only the gentian violet outline behind. It is important to use gentian violet because the constant wiping away of blood and pigment during the procedure will quickly erase the outline if a less tenacious material is used.

4. As for the eyeliner, an initial, lighter pass should be performed for all of the individual eyebrow strokes so that a second application of topical anesthetic can be more readily delivered to the dermis (Fig. **13–24**). The needle configuration for eyebrow application is either a round no. 1 or a round no. 3 fine. As mentioned, the strokes should mimic natural eyebrow hairs in direction, curvilinear design, and

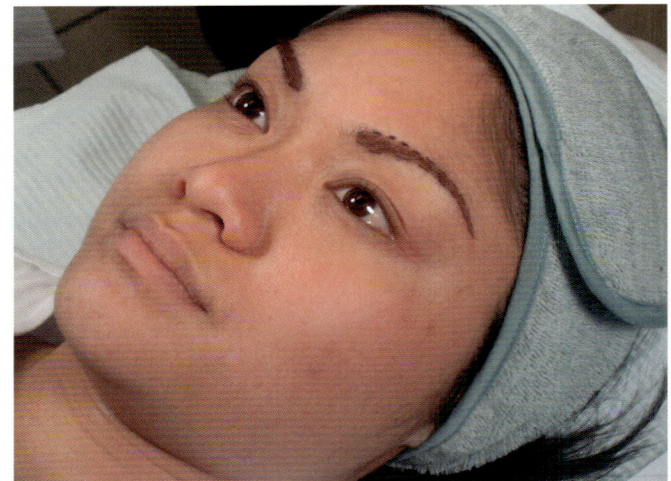

Figure 13–23   *Eyebrow Micropigmentation, Step 2*: A gentian violet marking pen is used to outline the area intended for micropigmentation.

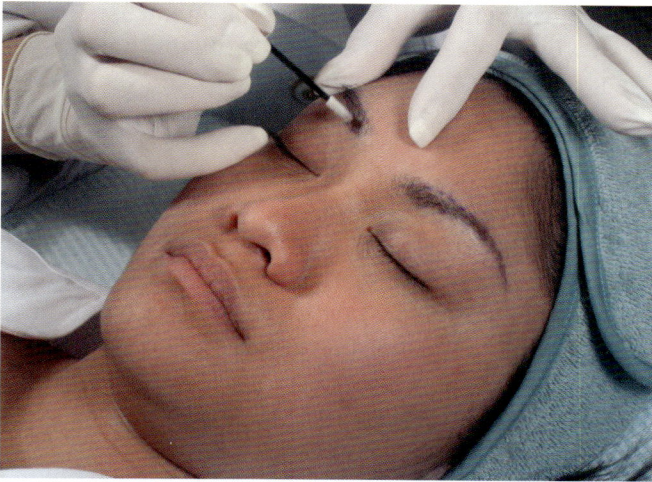

Figure 13–24 *Eyebrow Micropigmentation, Step 3*: After the initial pass with the tattoo machine, topical anesthetic is reapplied to the skin so that the anesthetic can readily pass into the dermal layer, where it can provide maximal benefit to the patient.

relative density (Fig. **13–25A,B**). Care should be taken to remain entirely within the gentian violet border and not trespass even directly over the marked outline.

Principles of Eyeliner Application

Application of the tattoo should fall at the lash line in continuity with the eyelashes to make it appear that the eyelashes are fuller and longer and also to enhance the eye shape. An abbreviated tail that curves in the opposite direction to the principal eyeliner and extends farther laterally from the lateral end of the eyeliner can be

added to enhance the almond-shaped Asian eye. Care should be taken not to overdo this feature, as it may look overly dramatic, like an Egyptian painted eyelid, and also look odd when the person exits a swimming pool without any other makeup enhancement.

Generally speaking, the eyeliner is applied slightly wider in dimension on the Asian patient, as the naturally dark eyelashes may render the eyeliner less visible than if applied adjacent to lighter-toned eyelashes and skin. The upper eyeliner is applied even wider than the lower eyeliner because the skin that folds downward when the eye is open narrows the appearance of the eyeliner: a no. 3 round needle configuration is preferred for the lower eyeliner, and a no. 5 or no. 7 round is optimal for an upper eyeliner. When an Asian patient does not have a "double-eyelid" crease, the upper eyeliner should not be made too wide, which can look unaesthetic.

Technique for Lower-eyeliner Application

1. After topical anesthesia has been applied to the intact skin and allowed to work (Fig. **13–26**), the first light pass may be performed so that the second application of anesthetic can penetrate to the dermal layer. The patient should rest in a supine position with her eyes gently closed. A three-direction stretch is performed with the nondominant hand's index and middle finger retracting laterally and the dominant hand's fourth (ring) and/or fifth fingers retracting inferiorly to provide an even surface for micropigmentation application. The first pass is initiated 4 to 5 mm medial to the lateral canthus along the eyelash line and continued medially until the

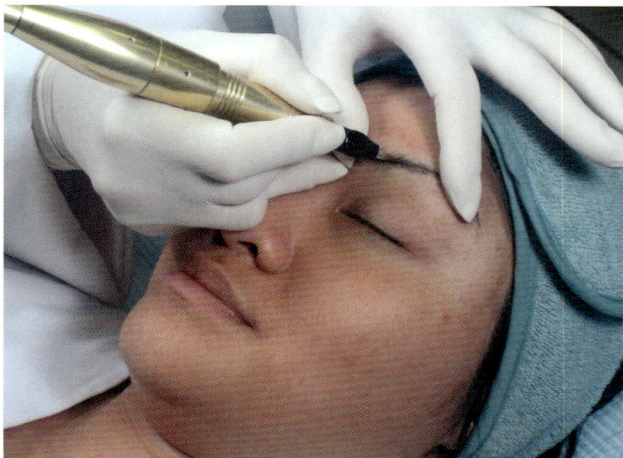

A

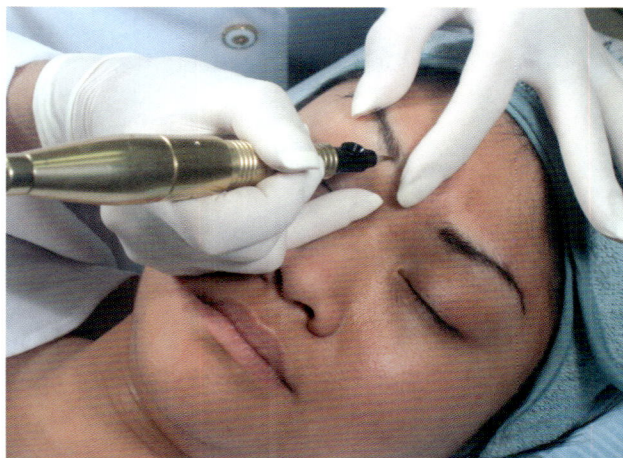

B

Figure 13–25 **(A,B)** *Eyebrow Micropigmentation, Step 4*: The stroke should follow a curvilinear design that follows the natural thickness, shape, density, length, and direction of the patient's existing hair follicles. The nondominant hand should provide

even, two-direction stretch in the direction of the applied stroke, as shown. The needle configuration preferred is a round no. 1 or round no. 3 fine.

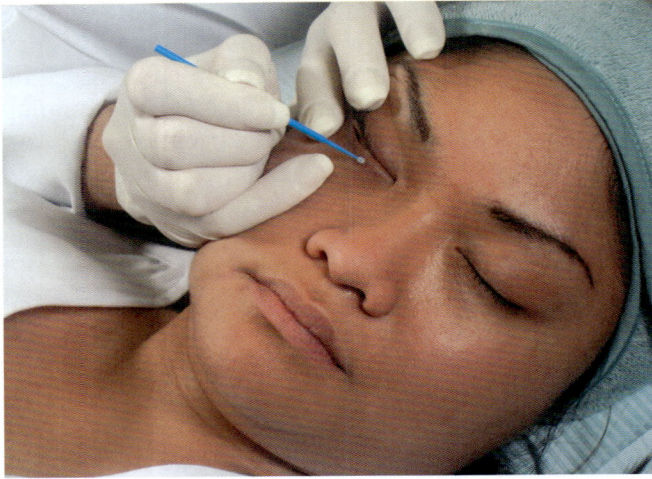

Figure 13–26 *Lower Eyeliner Micropigmentation, Step 1*: Topical anesthetic is applied along the ciliary margin prior to the first light pass with the micropigmentation device. After the first light pass is completed, a second application of anesthetic is undertaken to permit dermal penetration of the anesthetic.

medial canthus is met. The lateral canthal region is avoided because the pigment tends to bleed in this area.

2. Generally, two to four passes are needed to attain a good result but fewer or more passes can be applied as needed (Fig. **13–27A**). However, a greater number of passes only causes additional trauma and edema. With experience, the ideal goal is to complete the tattoo delivery within four passes. A no. 3 round needle configuration is preferred and is used for all passes.

3. If the patient desires a tail on the lateral extent, this feature can be added after the principal line is completed. The tail should only be undertaken at the end to improve the likelihood of a symmetric and even tattoo application.

4. The contralateral side is approached in the same fashion: lateral to medial direction, starting 4 to 5 mm medial to the lateral canthus (Fig. **13–27B**). The reader is reminded that the technician should remain on the same side of the patient for the entire session, as explained previously.

Technique for Upper-Eyeliner Application

1. The technique for upper eyeliner application follows the same guidelines as for the lower eyelid (Figs. **13–28, 13–29A,B**). However, a no. 5 or 7 needle size is preferred to achieve a broader stroke. As mentioned, the upper eyeliner will appear too thick because the eye is closed during application. Even after the session is completed, the eyeliner may still appear too wide due to the initial intensity of the tattooed color that will fade over the following few weeks.

2. The three-direction stretch is undertaken in precisely the same manner as described for the lower eyeliner but is particularly difficult for the upper eyelid because the skin is more mobile over the globe than the relatively taut lower eyelid. Accordingly, greater care should be paid to maintain proper tension during tattoo delivery to avoid uneven application of pigment.

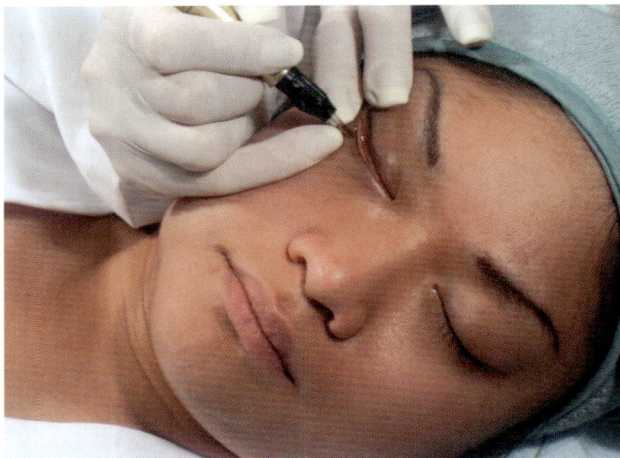

A

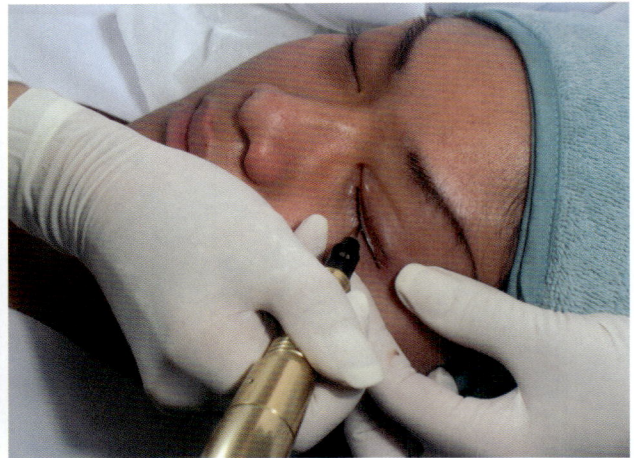

B

Figure 13–27 **(A,B)** *Lower Eyeliner Micropigmentation, Step 2*: The lower eyeliner is started 4 to 5 mm medial to the lateral canthus and delivered from a lateral to a medial direction at the ciliary margin. The photographs also demonstrate the three-direction stretch in which the nondominant index and middle fingers retract the upper and lower eyelids laterally, and the fourth and/or fifth finger of the dominant hand retracts the lower eyelid inferiorly. The technician always remains on one side of the patient when applying all micropigmentation: in this case, a right-handed technician is always situated on the right side of the patient.

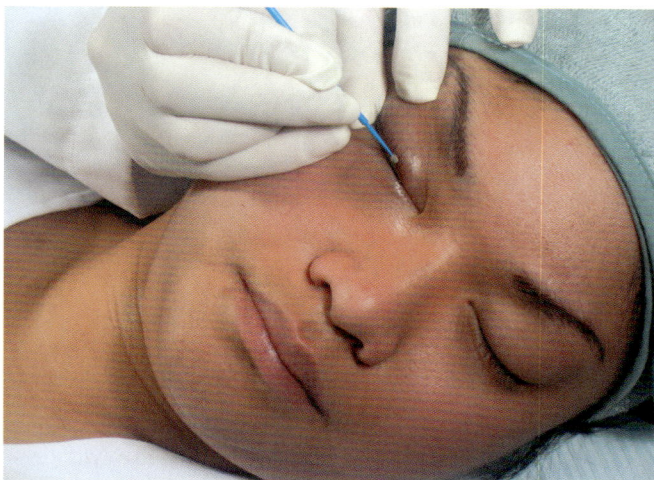

Figure 13–28 *Upper Eyeliner Micropigmentation, Step 1*: Topical anesthetic is applied in the manner prescribed previously for the lower eyeliner and eyebrow areas.

Principles for Lip-Liner Application

It is worth briefly reiterating the caveat of applying lip liner in darker-skinned patients who may risk permanent hyperpigmentation. Also, the use of any blue pigment in the original color mix should be avoided so that a blue line will not develop over time as other colors fade away. Stretching the lip in the direction of the tattoo (i.e., in line with the lip border) follows the same principle as outlined for eyebrow application. The most important aspect of applying lip liner is to follow a medial to a lateral direction for all four quadrants of the lips to ensure symmetry. The edema that ensues from application mandates that the lip be approached in this

sequential fashion to avoid the risk of an uneven, clown-like mouth. The vascular, pigmented nature of the Asian lip proves to be particularly onerous for the technician in the lower lip because of its relatively greater dimension. As the patient matures, the thinner, less vascular lips experience less edema and discomfort during treatment; and transformation of these aged lips may also be more striking.

Technique for Lip-Liner Application

1. The topical anesthetic should be applied with adequate time for it to work.

2. When the time comes for the procedure, the anesthetic is removed, and a lip-liner pencil is applied to match the thickness and color that the patient desires.

3. The lip is outlined with the initial, light pass using a round no. 3, 5, or 7 needle configuration, depending on the thickness of the desired line, so that a second coat of anesthetic can be applied to penetrate into the dermis. More commonly, a no. 5 or 7 needle is preferred to construct the tattooed lip line. The tattooed line should follow the vermilion border and remain principally over the white roll but lie in continuity (if not slightly overlap) with the red vermilion. The principle of following a medial to lateral direction for tattoo application, as outlined above, should be performed to ensure symmetry. Precise symmetry is hardest to achieve with lip-liner tattooing when compared with the relative ease for eyebrow and eyeliner application. Therefore, meticulous attention to systematic application is

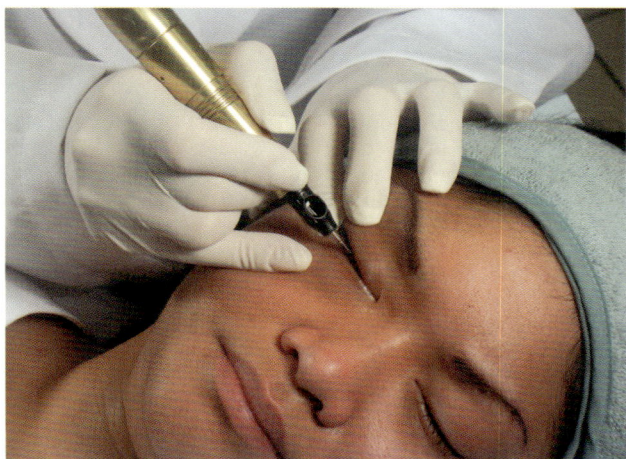

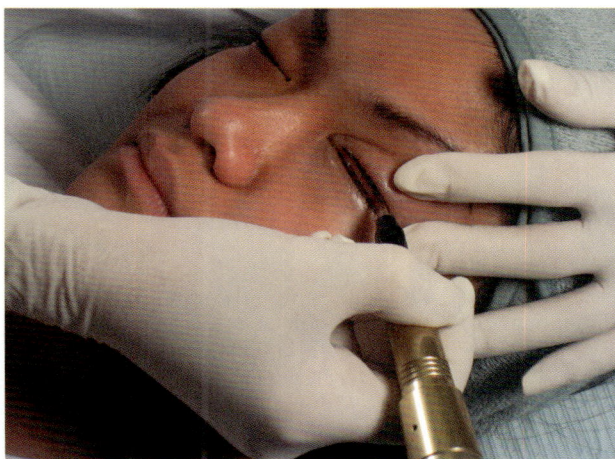

Figure 13–29 **(A,B)** *Upper Eyeliner Micropigmentation, Step 2*: The same technique is used to apply the upper eyeliner as is used for the lower eyeliner. The three-way stretch is also the same for the upper and lower eyeliner. However, the upper-eyelid skin is more mobile over the globe, and care must be taken to ensure that the

skin stretch remains even and taut throughout the procedure. The more mobile skin that folds over itself when the eye is open renders the tattooed line overly narrow in appearance. Accordingly, a wider no. 5 or 7 needle is preferred to achieve this broader stroke, as compared with the no. 3 needle used for the lower eyeliner.

mandatory. It is advisable to divide both the upper and lower lips into thirds: the central third of the upper lip extends from one peak to the other peak of Cupid's bow, and the remaining thirds occupy the distance from the peak to the oral commissure; for the lower lip, the central full pout is less well defined but can be thought of as occupying the central third of the lower lip (Fig. **13–30**). The tattoo stroke should progress in the following manner:

1. Complete the central third of the upper lip.
2. Complete one side of the lateral third of the upper lip, progressing medially to laterally.
3. Complete the other side of the lateral third of the upper lip, progressing medially to laterally.
4. Complete the central third of the lower lip.
5. Complete one side of the lateral third of the lower lip, progressing medially to laterally.
6. Complete the other side of the lateral third of the lower lip, progressing medially to laterally.

Like eyebrow and eyeliner application, two to four passes are generally required to achieve the uniformity and color depth that are desired. The technician should complete one light pass across the entire lip, then apply the anesthetic. After the initial light pass, two to four passes are carefully undertaken for each third of the lip before advancing to the next third. Following this method will enhance symmetry and consistency in application.

Postoperative Considerations

Postoperative care is relatively limited. A balm of rose hips, aloe vera, and vitamin E or, alternatively, an antibiotic

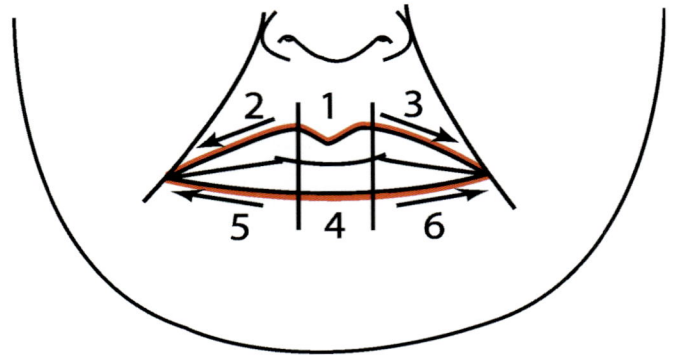

Figure 13–30 The illustration shows the sequential order of lip-liner application by dividing the upper and lower lips roughly into thirds. Following this method will improve symmetry and consistency, which is more difficult to achieve than with eyebrow and eyeliner application.

ointment can be applied for the first several days after the micropigmentation session. Keeping the treated areas liberally moistened with the above ointments facilitates healing. Sun exposure should be limited for the first 6 weeks to minimize the risk of hyperpigmentation; and gentle cleansing of the treated areas should be encouraged and aggressive scrubbing avoided. Routine showering can be resumed immediately, but excessively hot water exposure on the treated area should be restricted during the first 3 to 4 weeks post-treatment, as hot water can be dehydrating. Follow-up visits can be scheduled at 4 and 8 weeks afterwards to ensure that pigment retention has been maintained evenly and that the original, applied color has been preserved. A touch-up session should be performed no sooner than 4 weeks after treatment to permit adequate time to elapse for an accurate assessment.

References

1. Moore AP, Wood GD. The medical management of masseteric hypertrophy with botulinum toxin type A. Br J Oral Maxillofac Surg 1994;32:26–28
2. Williams EF, Lam SM. Comprehensive Facial Rejuvenation: A Practical and Systematic Guide to Surgical Management of the Aging face. Philadelphia: Lippincott, Williams & Wilkins; 2004.
3. To EW, Ahuja AT, Ho WS, et al. A prospective study of the effect of botulinum toxin A on masseteric muscle hypertrophy with ultrasonographic and electromyographic measurement. Br J Plast Surg 2001;54:197–200
4. Park MY, Ahn KY, Jung DS. Botulinum toxin type A treatment for contouring of the lower face. Dermatol Surg 2003;29:477–483
5. Drobeck HP, Rothstein SS, Gumaer KI, et al. Histologic observation of soft tissue responses to implanted, multifaceted particles and discs of hydroxylapatite. J Oral Maxillofac Surg 1984;42:143–149
6. Misiek DJ, Kent JN, Carr RF. Soft tissue responses to hydroxylapatite particles of different shapes. J Oral Maxillofac Surg 1984;42:150–160
7. Pettis GY, Kaban LB, Glowacki J. Tissue response to composite ceramic hydroxyapatite/demineralized bone implants. J Oral Maxillofac Surg 1990;48:1068–1074
8. Fanous N. TCA peel for Asians: a new classification and a modified approach. Fac Plast Surg Clin North Am 1996;4:195–200[x1]
9. Koire B. Cosmetic dimples and clefts. Fac Plast Surg Clin North Am 1996;4:187–194[x2]
10. Carmichael MJ, DeLorean D, Goldstein N. Micropigmentation of the Oriental face. Dermapigmentation. Fac Plast Surg Clin North Am 1996;4:211–218[x3]

14

Management of the Asian Skin

◆ General and Anatomic Considerations

The past decade has marked an exciting period for management of the Asian skin. With the rise of nonablative laser and light therapy, a host of skin ailments that afflicted Asian skin can now be addressed without the burden of a protracted recovery period traditionally observed in the postresurfaced Asian skin. Use of ablative modalities, for example, carbon dioxide (CO_2) laser resurfacing, medium to deep chemical peeling, and mechanical dermabrasion, led to an unacceptably long recovery in most Asian patients, who suffered from postinflammatory hyperpigmentation, hypopigmentation, lingering erythema, and potential scarring.[1] Judicious and conservative use of these ablative treatment modalities still play an important adjunctive role when nonablative therapy is inappropriate or ineffective. The CO_2 laser is a particularly poor tool for the Asian skin, which can face a recovery time that approaches a year and can lead to permanent pigmentary loss. Lighter chemical peels (15 to 35% tricholoroacetic acid [TCA] with or without Jessner's solution or Jessner's solution alone) can be used in combination or separately from nonablative therapy to effect maximal improvement in cutaneous dyschromias and wrinkles. Asian skin stands in marked distinction to that of Caucasian. The fine to deep wrinkles that characterize mature Caucasian skin are less prevalent in Asian skin partly due to the photoprotective effect of the darker complexion and to the thicker dermal structure. Asians are instead plagued by superficial dyschromias, including solar lentigines, melanocytic nevi, ephelides (freckles), nevi of Ota, and melasma. Although these conditions exist in the Caucasian, they tend to be less common, and Caucasians better tolerate ablative removal of these lesions than Asians. Although freckles may be deemed charming in Western culture, Asians from the Far East may consider any skin discoloration to fall short of the unblemished complexion idealized in the Orient. Understanding this cultural difference may help Western physicians in their treatment objectives with the Asian patient.

A new paradigm has been proposed that may facilitate a more systematic appraisal for the complexities that define the disparate Asian populations and their related skin types. Dr. Nabil Fanous has recently delineated a racially based skin classification system that divides the globe into latitudinal zones (Fig. **14–1**).[2] His taxonomy envisions the West as subdivided into Nordic, European, Mediterranean, Indo-Paki, and African as the latitudes are traversed from northernmost to southernmost. Accordingly, the finer features and fairer complexion (Nordic) in the far northern climes give way to increasingly darker and coarser attributes (African) of the southern reaches. In the East, Fanous argues that Asians may also be classified according to the same methodology as their Occidental counterparts. However, the geographic span of the Asian world roughly parallels the corresponding latitudes of the Mediterranean to the African. Therefore, despite a milky-white complexion, northern Koreans who occupy the northernmost Asian latitude will have a similar response to ablative resurfacing as Mediterranean skin. Likewise, the Polynesian skin of the southernmost zone will be more akin to the Western equivalent of African skin. Actual skin color (Fitzpatrick grading) becomes only one variable in the overall racially defined (features and skin type) classification scheme.

As far as the West is concerned, Fanous argues that the European skin type is most suitable for resurfacing. The Nordic race has very thin skin that is more susceptible

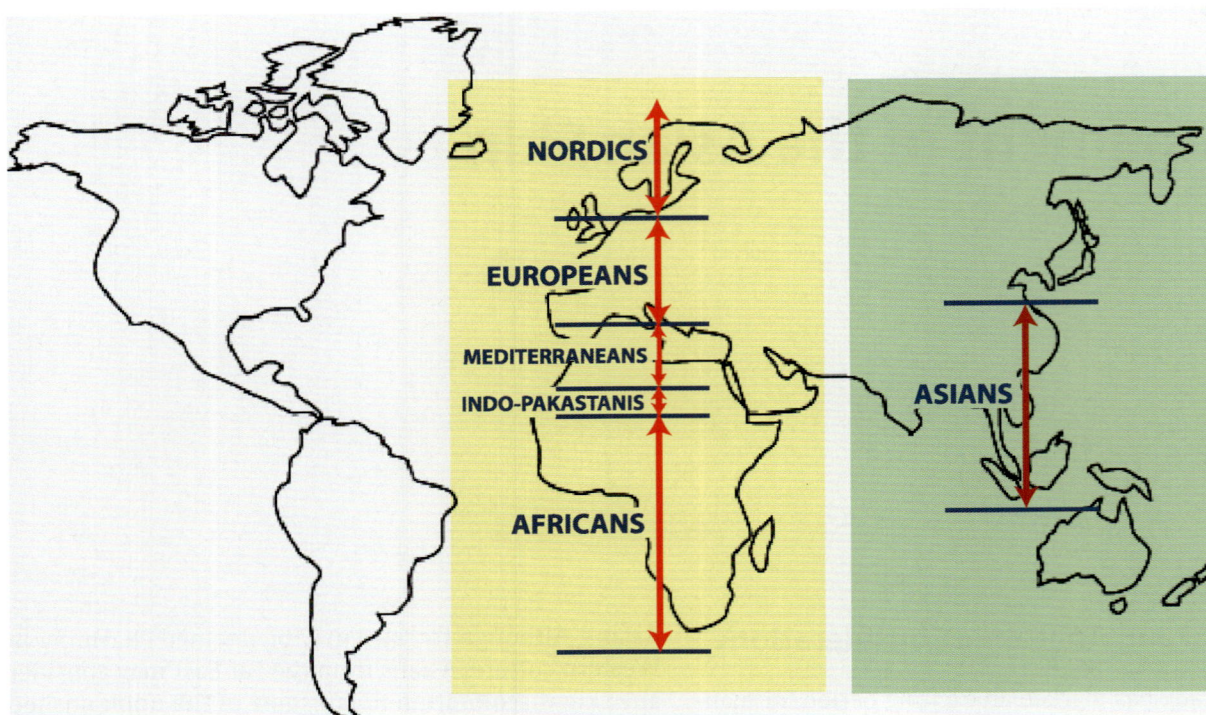

Figure 14–1 A new racially based skin classification system divides the globe into latitudinal zones. The West is divided into the Nordic, European, Mediterranean, Indo-Paki, and African zones, in which both skin color and facial features change from lighter and finer to darker and coarser from north to south. A similar zonal distribution is paralleled in Asia that roughly corresponds to the Mediterranean and African zones in the West. These corresponding latitudes serve to define skin response to therapy.

to atrophic scarring and telangiectasia. Conversely, the Indo-Paki and African skin types have a greater propensity to hypertrophic scarring and pigmentary abnormalities, ranging from transient hyperpigmentation to more irreversible hypopigmentation. Therefore, the extremes of skin color and type represent the most precarious recipients of resurfacing. The intermediate skin types, the European followed by the Mediterranean, constitute the most favorable skin types for resurfacing. Similarly, as mentioned, the Asian hemisphere falls along latitudinal lines that parallel the Mediterranean to the mid-African zones but oftentimes behaves more like the European to the African in terms of response to resurfacing. Therefore, perspicacious attention to these factors that delineate different Asian skin types will help to navigate a safe course for the physician about to embark on a resurfacing plan for the Asian patient.

Beyond all the dissimilarities that flourish between Asian populations, definite anatomic traits unify these apparently disparate groups. Overall, Asian dermis tends to be thicker and more sebaceous in quality, a characteristic that is independent of skin color. Even the fairer-complected northern Asian races exhibit this skin quality, which informs their response to peeling as well as their postoperative course. Most Asians, except the darker Malay or South Asians, tend to be suitable candidates for resurfacing if the proper risks and limitations

are grasped by surgeon and patient alike. The most troublesome sequela or complication that arises concerns pigmentary problems, including prolonged erythema, hyperpigmentation, and hypopigmentation. It is unclear whether a rigorous preoperative course of tretinoin and/or hydroquinone can circumvent this outcome. West and Alster's prospective, blinded and controlled study of their patients (who were primarily Caucasian) proved that intensive preoperative regimens failed to suppress postoperative melanin production. Their theory holds that the superficial melanocytes that have been curbed by the topical agents are eventually removed by the peel anyway and that the deeper melanocytes remain undisturbed by the preoperative treatment.[3]

◆ **Nonablative Therapy**

Nonablative skin therapy refers to laser and light therapies that do not efface the epidermis but instead target a specific chromophore in the skin (e.g., melanin pigment or a red vascular lesion), based on the principle of selective photothermolysis expounded by Anderson and Parrish.[4] Each type of laser possesses a certain characteristic wavelength that may be better suited to address a lesion of a particular color. Nonablative lasers and

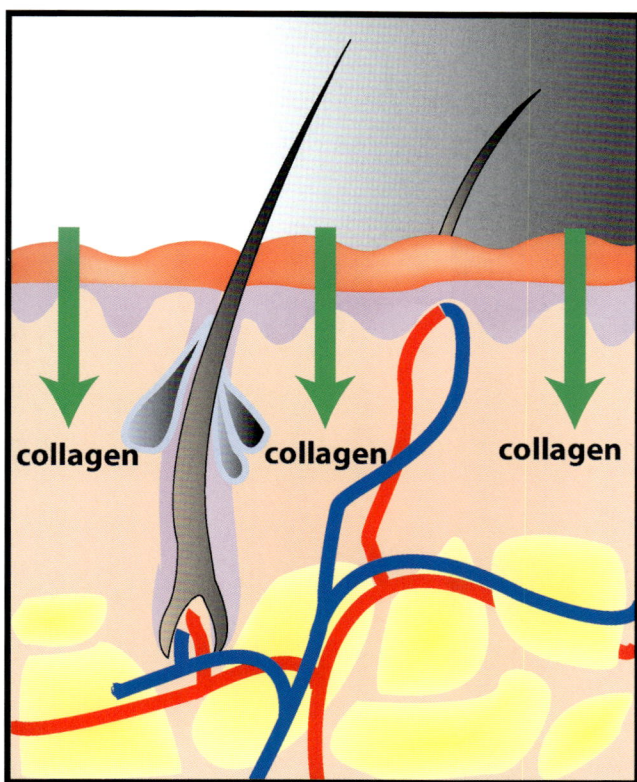

Figure 14–2 Illustration shows the nonablative laser or light beam (*green arrow*) passing into the dermal layer of the skin to effect collagen stimulation by thermal injury without any epidermal damage.

broadband light devices can also rejuvenate the skin by increasing collagen in the dermal layer via nonselective thermal stimulation (Fig. **14–2**).[5] Wrinkle reduction and treatment of acne scarring have been addressed with variable success using nonablative therapy. To overstate the impact that nonablative therapy has on wrinkles and scarring would be fallacious, as this technology provides only subtle but definite improvement. When significant rhytidosis or scarring is present, then traditional ablative techniques may be used instead or in combination with nonablative therapy. Similarly, recalcitrant pigmentation may be best addressed with both ablative chemical peeling and nonablative laser therapy. This section is not intended to be exhaustive in nature but reflects the author's clinical experience as well as reviews techniques that have been effective in the Orient for Asian skin.

532 nm KTP Nd:YAG Laser

Q-switched (QS) lasers customarily have been thought to have the greatest utility with effacing pigmented cutaneous lesions. Q-switching permits a short burst of intense energy that leads to a temperature gradient between the target and neighboring tissue. As the temperature difference falls, local shockwaves are emitted that cause tissue fragmentation and thereby melanasomal injury. QS lasers that have been used successfully for pigmentary ablation in Asian patients include the QS neodymium: yttrium aluminum garnet (Nd:YAG) (potassium-titanyl-phosphate (KTP)) 532 nm laser, the QS ruby laser, and the QS alexandrite laser.[6,7]

One prospective, randomized study evaluated the efficacy of the Medlite QS 532 nm Nd:YAG laser, the Versapulse QS 532 nm Nd:YAG laser, and the Versapulse long-pulsed 532 nm Nd:YAG laser in 34 Chinese patients who had their hemifaces treated with the respective laser types.[8] A visual analog questionnaire given to the patients and two blinded observers found that the long-pulsed laser was significantly better than the Versapulse QS 532 nm Nd:YAG laser but comparable to the Medlite QS 532 nm Nd:YAG laser in terms of efficacy for pigmentary clearing and associated complications of hyperpigmentation, hypopigmentation, and erythema. A long-pulsed laser can be safely and effectively used for the Asian skin as long as the pulse duration is kept shorter than the thermal relaxation time of 10 msec given an epidermal thickness of 100 mm. This shorter pulse duration theoretically limits the thermal diffusion from the epidermis to the dermis, which could in turn engender scarring. However, when the principal pathology resides in the dermis, targeting vascular ectasias and the local blood supply to various lesions (verrucae, sebaceous hyperplasia, etc.), the pulse duration may be intentionally lengthened to penetrate to the intended depth.

The author has the most experience with the long-pulse 532 nm (KTP) Nd:YAG laser to address a host of cutaneous disorders in Asian patients, including unwanted pigmentation, vascular lesions, fine wrinkles, sebaceous hyperplasia, and verrucae (Figs. **14–3A–D, 14–4A,B**). The patient who desires treatment of unwanted pigmentation should be carefully evaluated first for any suspicion of neoplasia before electing to proceed with aesthetic removal. The patient should also be fully cognizant that treatment of aberrant pigmentation may take several sessions, depending on the type of skin pathology, and should be combined with topical agents for maximal benefit. The patient may be started on 4% hydroquinone or alternative lightening regimen (e.g., kojic acid or azelaic acid) throughout the treatment period as well as a sunblock containing SPF 30 or 35. Proper avoidance of sun exposure is the key to success and to maintain the longevity of the result. Because abnormal pigmentation is a result of chronic sun exposure, the patient should also be made aware that ongoing sun exposure would predispose toward an early recurrence of solar lentigines and ephelides. Use of a lightening agent and sunblock are particularly important in the peritreatment period to minimize the risk of unwanted

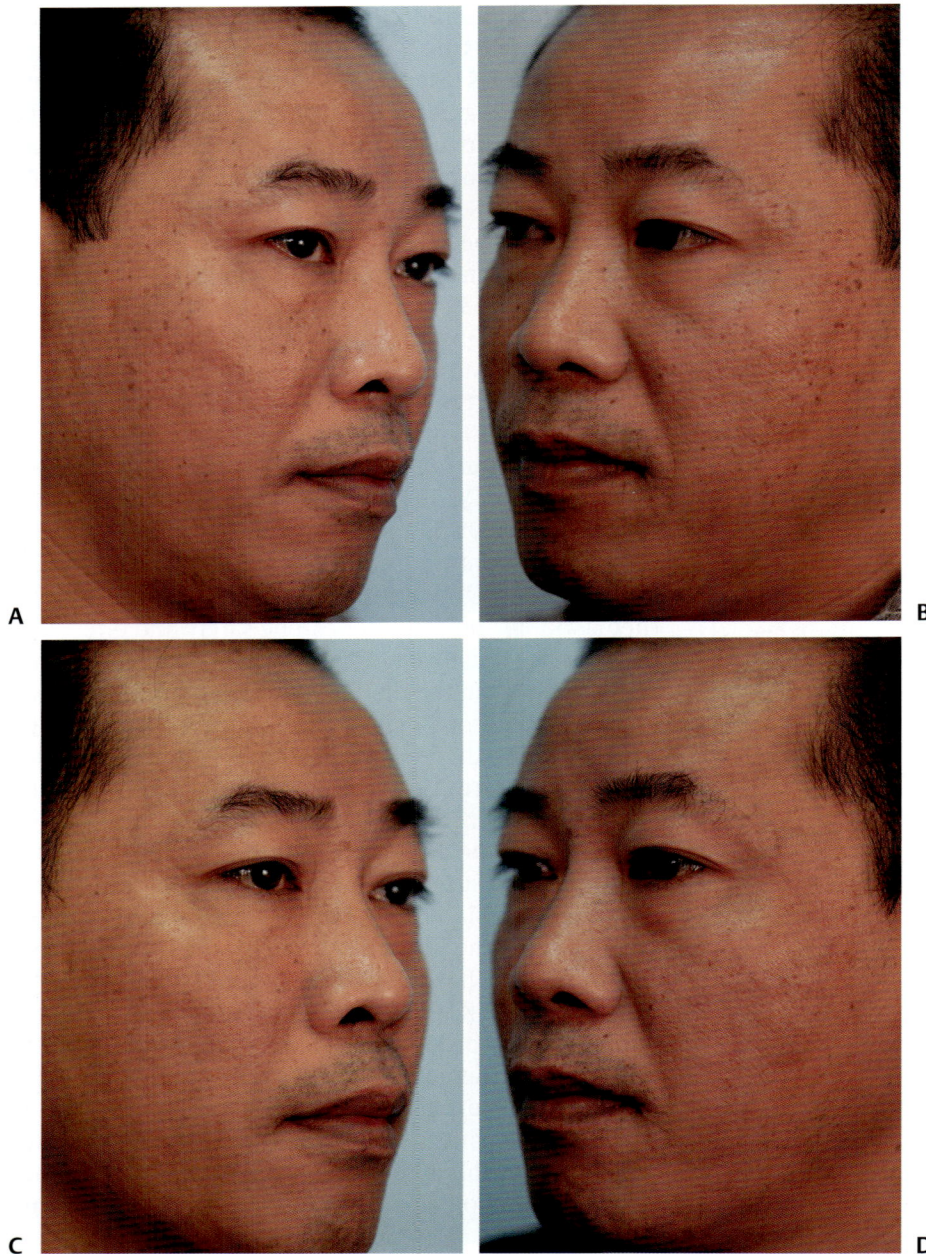

Figure 14–3   **(A,B)** This 39-year-old Vietnamese man had multiple pigmented lesions on both cheeks. **(C,D)** Patient shown 2 weeks after one treatment with the 532 nm KTP laser. The settings used were 7 J/cm^2, 8 msec pulse duration, and two passes per lesion.

postinflammatory hyperpigmentation, which is a common sequela in the Asian patient. The sensitive patient may be prescribed a topical anesthetic cream, for example, EMLA (Astra Pharmaceuticals, Westborough, MA) or ELA-Max (Ferndale Laboratories, Ferndale MI), to be applied to all proposed treatment areas at least 1 hour before laser therapy.

After informed consent is obtained, the patient is brought to the treatment room, which should comply with proper laser precautions. The room door should be closed (preferably locked), a laser warning sign should be posted on the door, and the patient and physician should don wavelength-specific protective eyewear

(Fig. **14–5**). Generally, freckles can be treated in one setting, but melasma and deeper (dermal) pigmentation may require 5 to 10 sessions, with an interval of 4 to 6 weeks between treatment sessions. Depending on the lesion size, a 1, 2, or 4 mm handpiece is employed. Generally speaking, a 2 mm spot size is preferred to address the majority of dyschromias, as the 1 mm size is often too small, and the 4 mm size may cause too much deep thermal injury. A fluence of 7 to 10 J/cm^2 set at a 7 to 10 msec pulse duration can be used, depending on the amount of observed pigmentation, with a higher fluence used for light-colored lesions and a lower fluence for more pigmented lesions. A lower fluence can be

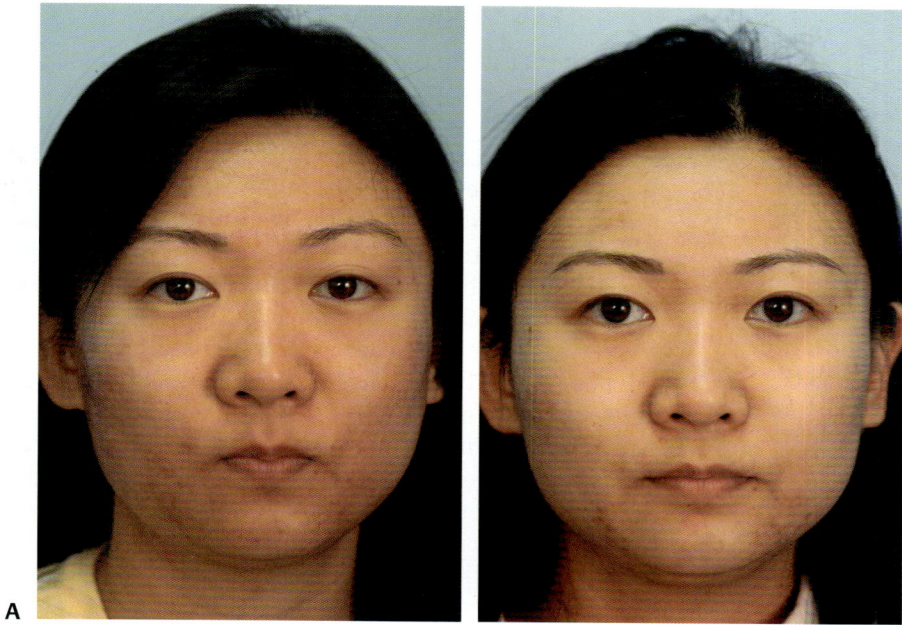

Figure 14–4 **(A)** This 30-year-old Chinese woman shows large areas of post-inflammatory hyperpigmentation on her cheeks and smaller, discrete areas across the remainder of her face due to acne flare-ups. **(B)** She is shown 1 month after one treatment with the 532 nm KTP laser, with notable improvement in areas of hyperpigmentation. She now shows some new areas of hyperpigmentation from new acne flare-ups. She was treated with 6 J/cm², 8 msec, and two pulses and was retreated for the new areas of hyperpigmentation. She also underwent topical therapy for her acne.

used for darker lesions because the more pigmented lesion readily absorbs the wavelength-specific energy of the laser than a comparable lighter lesion. The color end point of treatment should be an ashen gray without discernible purpura. The lowest fluence that can bring about this color change should be used to minimize adverse effects. Patients may benefit from a test patch with the fluence and other laser parameters recorded to

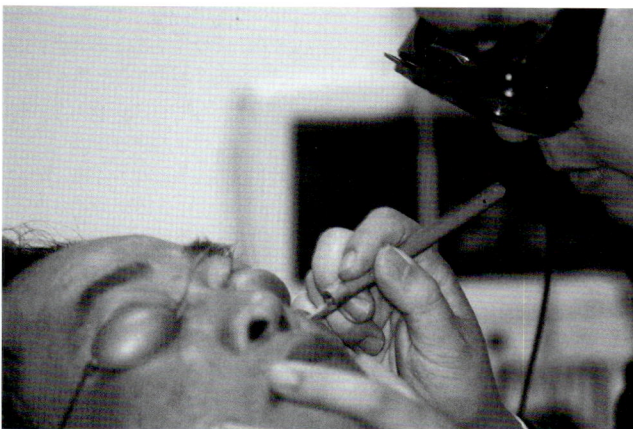

Figure 14–5 A patient undergoing treatment for pigmented lesions with a long-pulsed 532 nm laser. The physician wears wavelength-specific protective goggles, and the patient also wears protective eyeshields and is further instructed to keep his eyes closed during the entire treatment session. In accordance with laser precautionary measures, a danger sign warning that a laser is in use is posted outside the door, and the room door is locked from entry. The 2 mm handpiece is used to treat these superficial dyschromias set at 7 J/cm² and 8 msec pulse duration for this particular patient with two passes per lesion to achieve an ashen gray color end point.

determine the efficacy and likelihood for postinflammatory hyperpigmentation. Even patients who do not report tanning after sunbathing can develop hyperpigmentation and therefore should be assessed for this development with a test patch.

For pigmented lesions, the author prefers to begin in a less conspicuous area away from the central aspect of the face for the test spot. As mentioned, the 2 mm handpiece is used unless the lesions appear to be very small and would be amenable to the 1 mm handpiece. The starting laser parameter preferred for pigmented lesions is 7 to 8 J/cm², at 8 to 10 msec pulse duration set at two pulses per second. Unlike vascular lesions, the pigmented lesions should generally be hit with two consecutive pulses until the lesion appears ashen gray. Oftentimes, an audible snap sound may be heard after the second pulse that confirms that the pigment has been properly ablated. If the fluence is insufficient to achieve the desired color end point, the laser is adjusted higher. Use of cooling spray or gel may actually make determination of color change more difficult. The lowest fluence that will achieve this color change should be used to avoid unnecessary overtreatment and risk of thermal injury with resultant blistering and potential scarring.

This laser can also be used to address vascular lesions, particularly those that are red in color and more superficial in distribution. Although cutaneous lesions of a vascular nature are more common in the fairer-skinned Caucasian patient, telangiectasia, angiomata, and rosacea can also afflict the Asian patient. The size of the handpiece should be 2 mm for both telangiectasia and angiomata, whereas a scanning 1 mm handpiece or a 4 mm handpiece is more appropriate for rosacea. For telangiectasia, the 2 mm handpiece is preferred even though the caliber of the vessel may be only 1 mm in diameter, because the wider beam width will ensure that the vessel is entirely circumscribed and vaporized. With this type of laser, no purpura should be encountered. Unlike treatment of superficial pigmented lesions, only one pass of the laser is used to ablate vascular lesions at a higher fluence. Typically, a setting of 13 to 16 J/cm^2 with a pulse duration of 16 to 20 msec is used for vascular lesions, but lower fluences should always be tried first to ensure that the lowest, safe fluence for therapy is used. In addition, a cooling apparatus is favored to minimize epidermal damage and to minimize discomfort. Of note, use of a cooling apparatus obviates the need for pretreatment topical anesthesia. In addition, ultrasound gel will facilitate easy passage of the cooling head over the skin.

For sebaceous hyperplasia, a 1 mm handpiece is used at a higher fluence (25 to 35 J/cm^2) and longer pulse duration (30 msec) to attenuate the blood supply to the lesion and thereby effect involution. For verrucae, similar parameters are used (30 to 40 J/cm^2 and 30 to 40 msec), but the tissue is ablated with multiple stacked hits (typically five or six pulses) until the tissue evaporates. The charred tissue is wiped away with a moistened 4 × 4 gauze, and the process is continued until the wart is brought level with the surrounding tissue or pain is encountered, which signifies arrival at normal tissue. For photorejuvenation of aged Asian skin, a low fluence (6 to 7 J/cm^2), a long pulse duration (30 to 40 msec), and a larger handpiece (4 mm) are used with a cooling device and chilled gel and passed over the skin evenly two or three times. Repeat treatment sessions for photorejuvenation may be undertaken every 4 to 6 weeks. The same settings can be used to treat rosacea.

After treatment, the patient can apply a light coating of bacitracin or Aquaphor ointment, which can be particularly beneficial in the healing process when a microcrust forms. The patient should be advised not to abrade or manipulate the area during the first week after treatment. The application of hydroquinone and sunblock should be resumed unless the patient reports significant irritation with these topical agents during the healing phase. Blistering after therapy may rarely occur and signifies overtreatment. Any blisters should be reported to the physician immediately for close scrutiny and follow-up. The blistered areas should be treated with bacitracin or Aquaphor until full epithelialization is encountered, and the patient should be sternly advised not to scratch, pick, or manipulate the areas to minimize the risk of scarring. Temporary hypo- or hyperpigmentation may occur, which typically resolves if the proper laser parameters described above are followed. The reader is advised to consult the manufacturer of his or her laser device for specific recommendations as to the proper settings for that particular laser model.

Intense Pulsed Light (IPL)

As an alternative to the 532 nm laser (or other comparable laser), intense pulsed light (IPL) has been used successfully in Asian skin for a wide spectrum of skin ailments. IPL can be used for dark spots, vascular lesions, and photorejuvenation of fine wrinkles. It is a noncoherent, broadband (500 to 1200 nm) light device in which selective cut-off filters can be employed to block specific shorter wavelengths (e.g., 515, 550, 570, 590, 615, 645, 695, 715, 755 nm). Accordingly, it is not a true laser. Pulse width varies from 0.5 to 25 msec, and fluence ranges from 3 to 90 J/cm^2. The fluence can be delivered from one to three separate emissions with a 1 to 300 msec interval between individual pulses. Three spot sizes can be selected: 8 × 8 mm, 8 × 15 mm, and 8 × 35 mm. Epidermal protection is afforded by a cooling gel applied topically and by a built-in thermoelectrically cooled crystal filter and a physical spacer to maintain the requisite 2 mm distance from the skin. The literature has reported effective use of this technology to address solar lentigines, ephelides, telangiectasia, and wrinkles in the Asian patient.[9–12]

Compared with targeted laser systems, IPL can still address dyschromias effectively but may require more treatment sessions to demonstrate the same benefit. Ultraviolet (UV) photography may also enhance the visibility of epidermal melanocytic hyperpigmentation. The IPL may be associated with less chance of postlaser hyperpigmentation and can be used for those patients who are more predisposed to this outcome. Generally, a total fluence of 23 to 32 J/cm^2 in a double-pulse mode of 2.5 to 4.0/4.0 to 5.0 msec pulse durations and an interval of 20.0/40.0 msec between pulses may be used safely for Asian skin. Typically, a topical anesthetic is not required but can be used for more sensitive patients. The color end point should be a slight erythema immediately after light exposure and a slight increase in pigmentation in the treated dark spots. If the patient experiences significant discomfort after light application, a superficial burn may have occurred, and the fluence should be appropriately reduced. The upper eyelids should always be spared as well as the beard distribution in men. Typically, a minimum of three treatment sessions is required, but a benefit may be more noticeable after only five sessions, depending on the type of cutaneous pathology being treated.

Safety with IPL is of paramount importance to avoid burn injury (Figs. **14–6, 14–7**). Consistency of therapy will be attained with clinical experience. However, certain protective measures may be followed to minimize the risk of burn injury, which may be more likely in the Asian patient, given the darker skin that more readily absorbs the light energy. Use of cooling gel is important for epidermal protection, and the handpiece should be

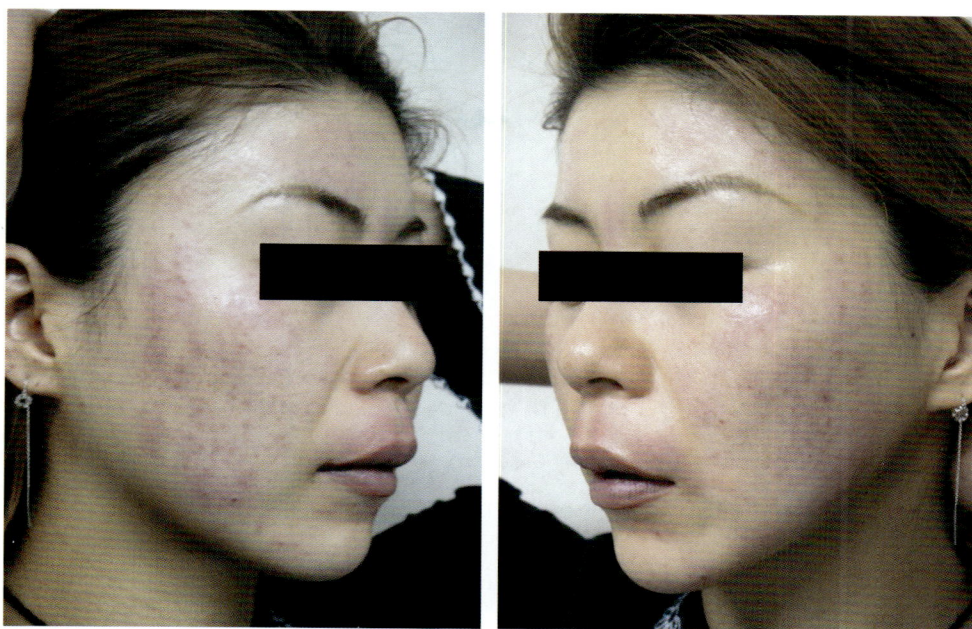

Figure 14–6 This 27-year-old Japanese woman underwent six intense pulsed light (IPL) treatments and experienced a burn injury on the sixth session. Her first treatment was undertaken at 24 J/cm^2; the second, at 25 J/cm^2; the third, at 26 J/cm^2, the fourth, at 27 J/cm^2; and the fifth, at 28 J/cm^2. The sixth session was started at 28 J/cm^2 initially when the patient complained of some discomfort, so the fluence was reduced to 27 J/cm^2, after which she was noted to have a burn injury. Upon recognition of the burn, the patient was treated with topical application of steroid cream (0.12% betamethasone valerate) for a 1-week period, and her condition resolved without any scarring. (Courtesy of Tomoyuki Takahashi, M.D.)

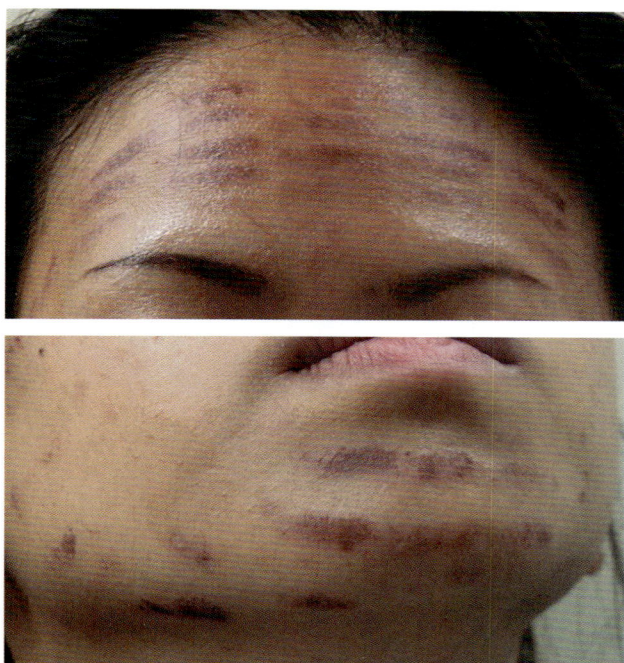

Figure 14–7 This 29-year-old Japanese woman experienced a burn injury on the third treatment session at 26 J/cm^2, the same setting that was successfully used during the second treatment session. The patient's burn was treated with steroid cream application with successful resolution without scarring. (Courtesy of Tomoyuki Takahashi, M.D.)

at a uniform distance of ~2 mm from the skin, with the intervening gel serving as the interface. Maintaining this 2 mm distance uniformly is perhaps the most difficult aspect in light therapy and may predispose toward burn injury (Fig. **14–8**). When the trigger switch is initially

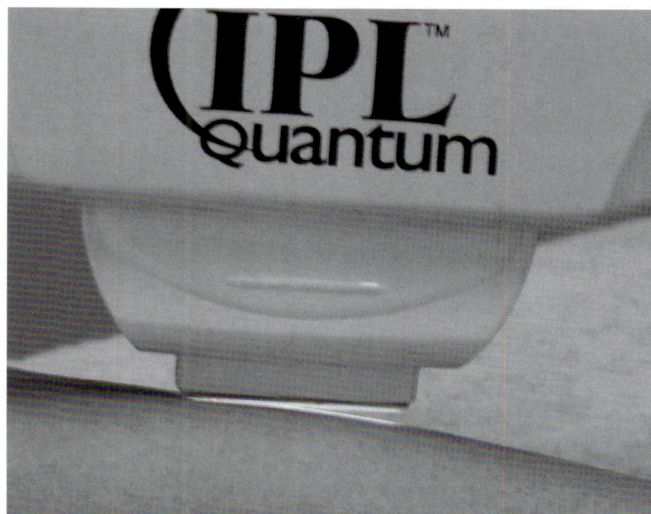

Figure 14–8 Given the broad configuration of the light-emitting head, the ability for the entire surface area to maintain a uniform distance from the skin may be difficult. (Courtesy of Tomoyuki Takahashi, M.D.)

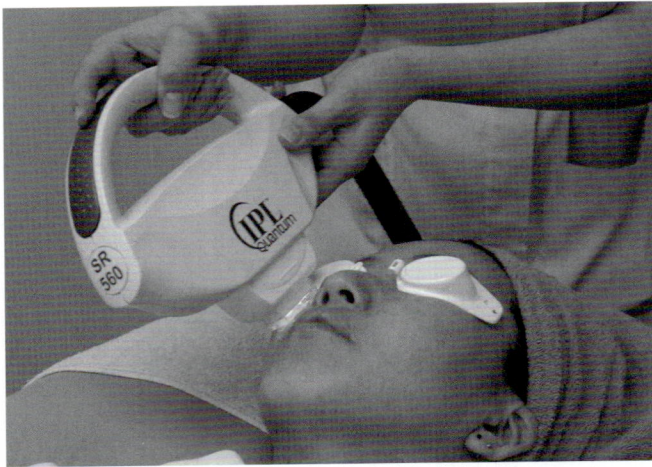

Figure 14–9   Maintaining a uniform distance to the skin is particularly difficult when the trigger button is depressed, as the light head tends to move closer to the skin, predisposing to burn injury. (Courtesy of Tomoyuki Takahashi, M.D.)

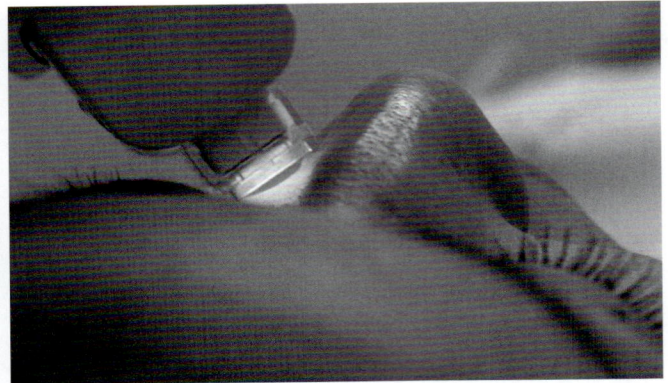

Figure 14–10   Maintaining a uniform distance from the skin is quite difficult when passing over areas that have depressed and/or raised contours, predisposing to burn injury in areas that are approached too closely with the light-emitting head. (Courtesy of Tomoyuki Takahashi, M.D.)

turned on, depressing the button on the handpiece often moves the device too close to the skin, predisposing toward burn injury (Fig. **14–9**). Also, passage of the IPL over raised or depressed contours of the face makes maintenance of a uniform distance from the skin demanding

(Fig. **14–10**), especially because the light-emitting head is broadly configured in a relatively large rectangular block. A physical spacer device that extends from the light-emitting head will help maintain the prescribed 2 mm distance more easily (Fig. **14–11A**). Dr. Takahashi has developed a grid-shaped spacer that has proven to be invaluable in achieving the most uniform distance

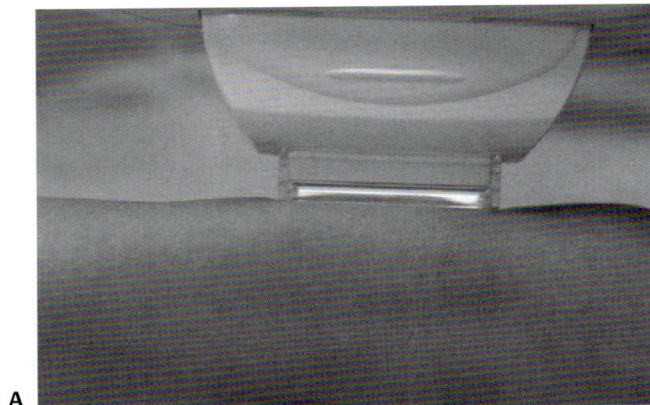

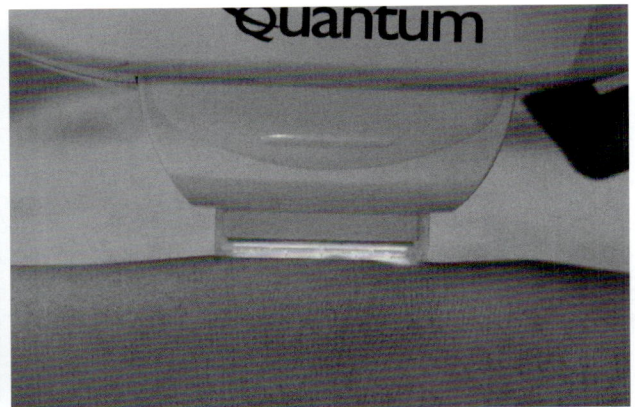

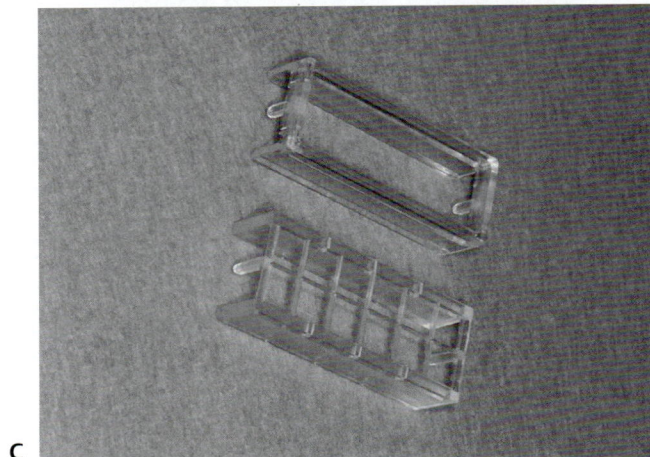

Figure 14–11   **(A)** The manufacturer's spacer device has a hollow center, which allows the skin to bulge inward, closer to the light-emitting head, which may predispose to burn injury. The more pressure that is applied to the handle, the closer that the skin in the center of the spacer bulges toward the light-emitting head. **(B)** The grid-spacer modification is entirely enclosed plastic that prevents the laser head from approaching the skin any closer than a 2 mm distance. **(C)** Photograph of the manufacturer's spacer (above) and the grid-spacer (below) unattached from the light-emitting head. (Courtesy of Tomoyuki Takahashi, M.D.)

from the skin for the novice to the experienced technician (**Fig. 14–11B**).* The standard spacer is hollow in the center, allowing the skin to bulge closer to the light-emitting head, especially with slight pressure. The modified grid shape is chosen over a completely flat contour to enhance skin cooling but not overly cool the skin that would arise with the latter design. Cooling gel should still be applied, as it permits ease of gliding over the skin surface and provides additional thermal protection. Careful administration of IPL can result in excellent clinical results, but caution should always be heeded when approaching the darker-complected patient.

◆ Ablative Therapy

Traditionally, skin resurfacing has been relegated to ablative therapy, in which the epidermis and part of the dermis are removed to effect the desired improvement. Broadly speaking, ablative techniques can be classified into chemical, laser, and mechanical. As mentioned, ablative laser therapy (e.g., CO_2 laser) is associated with a remarkably long recovery period in Asian skin and risks permanent hypopigmentation and scarring. Although the CO_2 laser may engender too much of a recovery period for the Asian patient, spot treatment of small superficial lesions (e.g., ephelides) may be safely and easily performed for the Asian patient but is less ideal than a chromophore-specific, nonablative laser. As an economical method for selective destruction of superficial lesions, an electrocautery device can be used instead. Again, these nonselective, destructive modalities stand as inferior options compared with a wavelength-specific, nonablative laser device.

Chemical peeling may be a gentler method of ablative skin therapy in the Asian patient. However, medium-depth chemical peeling still inflicts a relatively substantial recovery period that may last 6 to 12 weeks until all postinflammatory hyperpigmentation resolves. Deep chemical peeling like phenol is relatively unsafe in Asian skin no matter what the pigmentation of the patient is. Like the laser, higher-strength, medium-depth chemical concentrations, for example, 35% trichloroacetic acid (TCA), can be used as a spot treatment on superficial freckles with minimal downtime. The sharp point of a broken cotton-tipped applicator or toothpick can be used to apply the peel solution in a

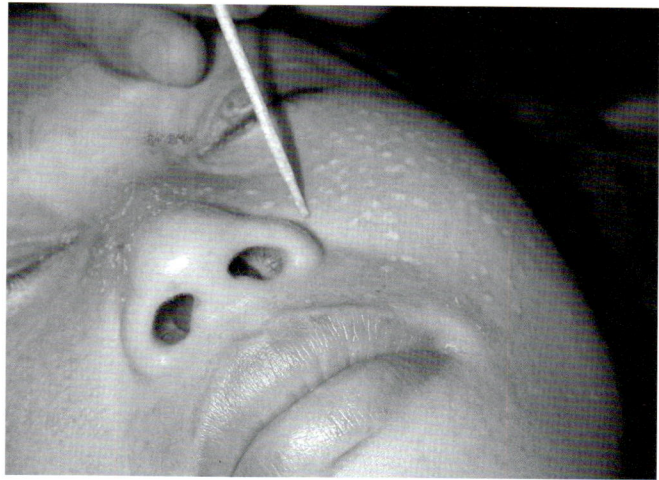

Figure 14–12 Intraoperative photograph shows spot treatment of freckles with 35% trichloroacetic acid (TCA) using the sharpened point of a wooden applicator. (Courtesy of Young-Kyoon Kim, M.D.)

selective fashion (Fig. **14–12**). Very high concentrations of 80 to 100% TCA can also be used selectively as well in depressed acne scars as spot treatments over multiple treatment sessions to stimulate collagen synthesis in these hypotrophic areas.[13] Clearly, these very high concentrations are unsafe when applied uniformly to the skin in any race. For patients who would like mild rejuvenation of their skin or who want to control their acne, a Jessner's solution or glycolic peels can be used with almost no discernible downtime[14] (Figs. **14–13, 14–14, 14–15, 14–16**). For fine rhytids and pigmentary lesions, a deeper chemical peel will be required, ranging from 20 to 35% TCA. If only selective areas of the face are to be treated (e.g., the lower-eyelid region), the peel should be feathered in a circumferential fashion, with fewer passes of peel or with a lighter concentration of peel toward the periphery. This technique is especially relevant for the darker-complected Asian patient.

Mechanical dermabrasion can be safely used if feathered with chemical peeling or used without aggressive application to minimize pigmentary loss and to shorten the recovery period. Dermabrasion is indicated for patients with uneven skin contour (e.g., acne scarring), in which chemical peeling alone cannot achieve the intended result. Mechanical dermabrasion effectively lowers the raised segments of the skin in a differential fashion to achieve a more uniform contour that is unachievable with conventional chemical peeling.

Newer techniques are used today to stimulate collagen in the depressed areas with targeted chemical peeling (as previously mentioned) or with nonablative laser/light therapy rather than lowering the raised areas with dermabrasion. These techniques require serial

---

*Dr. Tomoyuki Takahashi has developed and manufactured this unique grid spacer for his own professional use and does not receive any profit or compensation for the device. He has not manufactured the device for widespread commercial distribution. He performs over 2000 cases of IPL therapy with 20 machines per month in his four clinics.

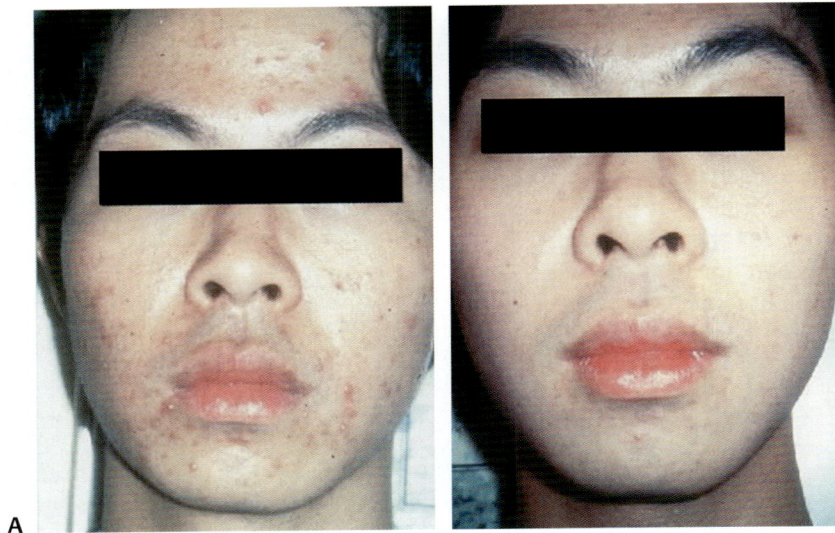

Figure 14–13 **(A)** This Chinese male in his late teenage years shows significant active acne with pustules, papules, and comedones. **(B)** He underwent a series of six glycolic acid treatments ranging from 30 to 50% every week and is shown after his final treatment, with considerable improvement in his acne. (Courtesy of Constance Yam, M.D.)

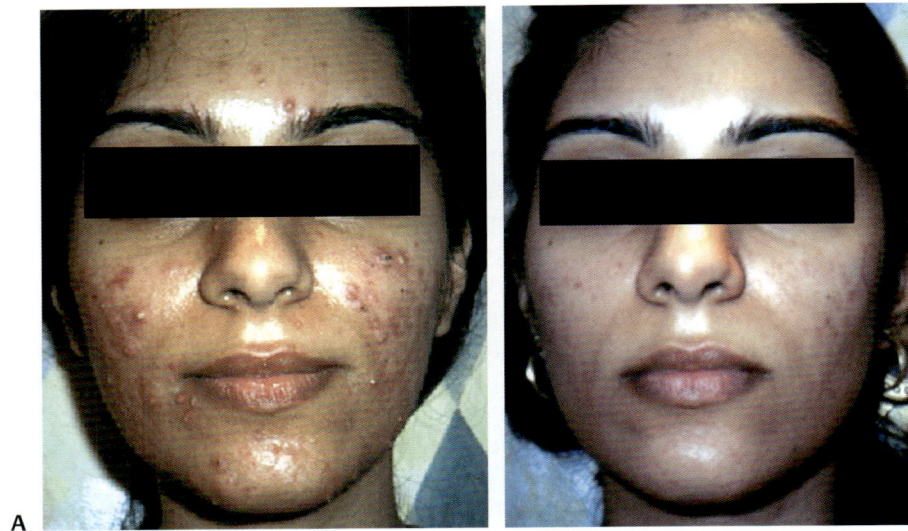

Figure 14–14 **(A)** This 20-year-old Indian woman exhibits a very oily complexion and active acne, with many pustular eruptions. **(B)** She received a total of six chemical peels (two 30% glycolic acid peels and four Jessner's peels) at weekly intervals. The patient shows good improvement in her active acne, and her residual postinflammatory hyperpigmentation resolved within several months. (Courtesy of Constance Yam, M.D.)

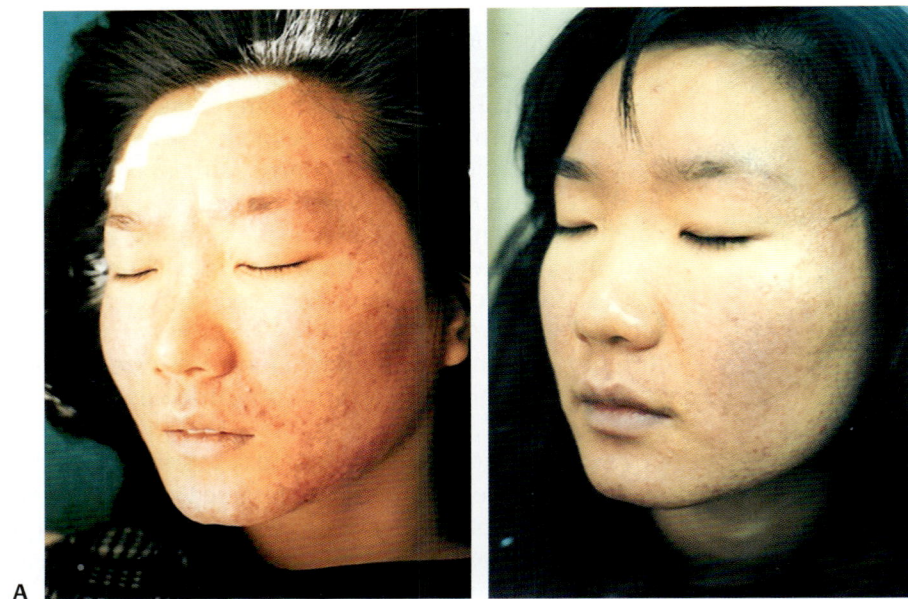

Figure 14–15 This 24-year-old Korean woman exhibits active acne and underwent a single application of Jessner's solution and is shown with noticeable improvement 2 weeks afterwards. (Courtesy of Young-Kyoon Kim, M.D.)

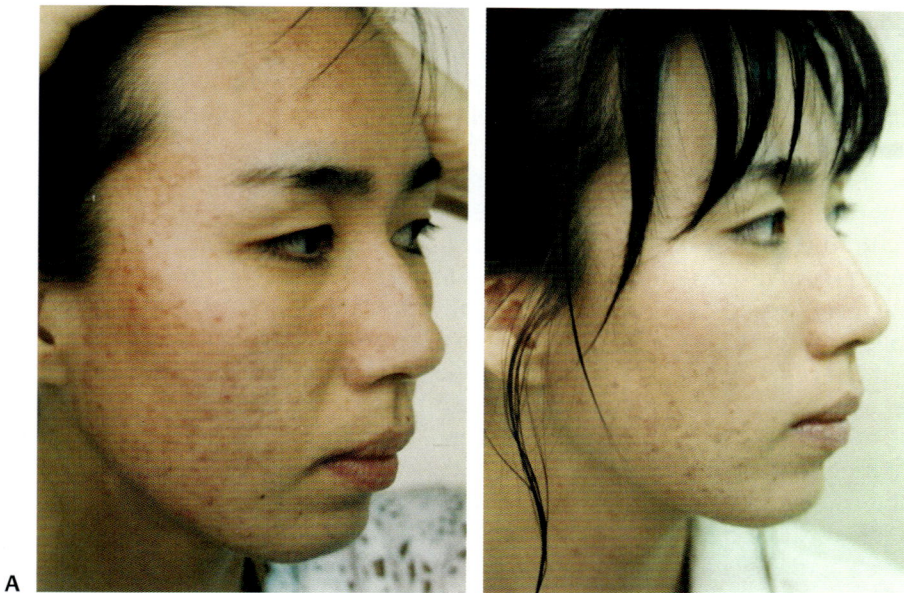

Figure 14–16 This 26-year-old Korean woman exhibits active acne and underwent a single application of Jessner's solution and is shown with improvement 2 weeks later. (Courtesy of Young-Kyoon Kim, M.D.)

treatment to obtain optimal improvement, but the recovery period is less intensive, and pigmentation problems and scarring are also minimized. Another category of ablative resurfacing is entitled "coblation," which refers to a type of radio-frequency ablation of the skin (refer to Chapter 7). These conventional and unconventional techniques will be covered in a systematic fashion that is applicable for Asian skin.

General Preoperative Considerations for Ablative Therapy

After the surgeon has carefully elucidated what the patient's aesthetic goals are and further has tempered those desires with realistic expectations, the surgeon should endeavor to conduct a proper history that would be relevant to resurfacing. Salient historical points that should be determined include whether, when, and by what method the patient had any prior resurfacing and also if any complications arose. Prior flap-type surgery (e.g., face lift) may slightly predispose the patient indefinitely to increased scarring due to compromised vascularity. Any recent undermining of the skin within 6 weeks would prove to be a relatively strong contraindication to resurfacing. Although keloid formation on the body may be instructive, the face (which excludes the ears, neck, and scalp) tends to be relatively immune from frank keloid production. However, facial hypertrophic scarring can arise and frequently does in Asian patients and should be duly noted. Poor wound healing that may arise due to diabetes mellitus and cigarette smoking should alert the physician to possible

delayed healing, whereas prior irradiation and cutaneous burns may constitute more significant contraindications to ablative resurfacing. Active acne that has not been quiescent for at least 9 months should be considered an unsuitable risk factor; more importantly, recent isotretinoin usage (Accutane) within the past year is an absolute contraindication to ablative resurfacing. If the patient stands in good measure after all these factors have been properly identified, then the surgeon may elect to proceed with resurfacing. As part of the preoperative regimen, the surgeon may elect to give a perioperative course (typically 5 days) of antibiotics that will cover skin flora, but this policy has not been conclusively proven beneficial through scientific studies. Finally, an antiviral medication (e.g., valacyclovir or famciclovir) should be initiated either immediately before or after the resurfacing procedure for a period of 10 days if resurfacing is planned in the perioral region. If a herpetic outbreak manifests during the postoperative period, then the dosage should be doubled and the patient's symptomatology carefully followed.

Chemical Peeling

Although chemical peeling may appear to be a worrisome resurfacing modality for the Asian race, it has been used with great success for rejuvenation of mild to moderate rhytidosis and superficial dyschromias. Although melasma tends to be a recalcitrant entity, many physicians have successfully treated this condition with chemical peeling, but recurrence has proven to be the rule rather than the exception. Uneven pigmentation or spot areas of hyperpigmentation may be addressed with this resurfacing technique, as long as the patient is cognizant of the risk of postoperative hyperpigmentation and is vigilant in sun-protective measures and postpeel lightening regimens. The depth of the pathology should dictate the appropriate penetration of the peel. For instance, melasma that presents with well-demarcated borders typically signifies an epidermal origin for the hypermelanosis. Conversely, poorly circumscribed lesions suggest a deeper dermal etiology that may require a deeper peel. Often, a medium-deep peel (uniform but medium white frost) should be targeted but can be varied, depending on surgeon preference, experience, and objective. As postinflammatory hyperpigmentation is the norm rather than the exception, the patient should be fully aware of this sequela, the length of recovery, and the appropriate topical agents that are required to shorten its course. In lieu of chemical peeling, a wavelength-specific, nonablative laser (as described previously) may be preferable to address melasma, but the patient should understand that the treatment course will require multiple sessions and may not entirely eradicate the abnormal pigmentation.

Jessner's Solution*

Unquestionably, vigorous and thorough cleansing of the skin with 100% acetone is a critical first step to ensure that an even peel will be attained. The acetone solution should be applied with a 4 × 4 gauze pad, which more effectively abrades the skin than a cotton ball or a cotton-tipped applicator. The purpose of the acetone is twofold: remove the outer layer of oil and function as a keratolytic of the stratum corneum, both of which may serve as physical barriers to attain a deep and uniform peel. The patient should be informed that the application of acetone might be somewhat unpleasant due to the noxious odors and the vigorous application.

Jessner's solution, which is comprised principally of alpha-hydroxy acids acts to complete the keratolytic process. Jessner's solution may be applied with relative impunity as the liberal application usually penetrates just into the outer epidermal layer. Often, a light frost may be evident, but it indicates only a reversible salt deposition rather than the irreversible blanching that ensues due to protein coagulation when the actual TCA peel is applied. Unlike the TCA peel, no visual change of the skin color is targeted, as the superficial nature of Jessner's solution usually does not impart any color change. The patient does not require any sedation for this part of the procedure, as Jessner's solution usually engenders a mild tingling sensation and only rarely frank discomfort.

Like application of TCA, the subunit principle is followed with application of Jessner's solution. First, attention is paid to the lower eyelid/periocular region in the same fashion as will be described for the TCA peel. The patient is placed in an upright position, inclined ~60 degrees from the horizontal. This semi-inclined orientation minimizes inadvertent entry of solution into the eyes during application over the lower-eyelid region while maintaining patient comfort. The assistant gently holds cotton-tipped applicators at both the lateral and medial canthi to prevent tears from unevenly diluting the peeled area and, more importantly, to minimize peel solution from entering the eye via capillary conduction. A bottle of balanced-saline solution (BSS) should always be on the tableside should the patient report any ocular irritation or burning. (If the patient does complain of ocular discomfort, the surgeon should recline the patient to a supine position and gently flush the eyes with BSS, with the stream targeted at the medial canthus. This method minimizes reflexive closure of the eye that would impair proper ocular irrigation.) Jessner's solution is applied with a cotton-tipped applicator in the lower-eyelid region and with a cotton ball for the remainder of the face. It is important that the cotton ball be squeezed semidry before applying the solution to avoid unintentional trickle of solution onto the neck. Furthermore, the used cotton-tipped swabs and cotton balls should be promptly discarded into the waste bin so that confusion does not arise as to which cotton ball was used for which peel solution.

After each lower-eyelid/periocular region has been treated, the physician should advance in a systematic fashion by subunit from forehead/temple region, right cheek region, left cheek region, the upper lip/lower lip/chin region, and the nasal region. The order is not important, but it is recommended that the physician proceed in the same order every time to ensure that no area is repeeled or missed. The nasal and upper-lid areas are relatively recalcitrant to significant rejuvenation with a peeling agent but are treated nonetheless to achieve a complete and uniform peel. However, the upper-lid area is treated very superficially, given the attenuated skin in this area and the attendant risk of scarring. Also, the cheek and chin subunits should be gently feathered for about ~1 cm onto the neck to curtail an abrupt transition. If a lifting procedure is entertained concurrently or independently, the transposition of ptotic tissues upward may result in the unpeeled area of the neck also moving upward into the facial region. After the peel has remained on the skin for 1 to 5 minutes, the chemical can be diluted to abort further reaction with cold saline compresses.[15]

---

*Resorcinol 14 g, salicylic acid 14 g, lactic acid 14 cc, QS ethanol 100 cc.

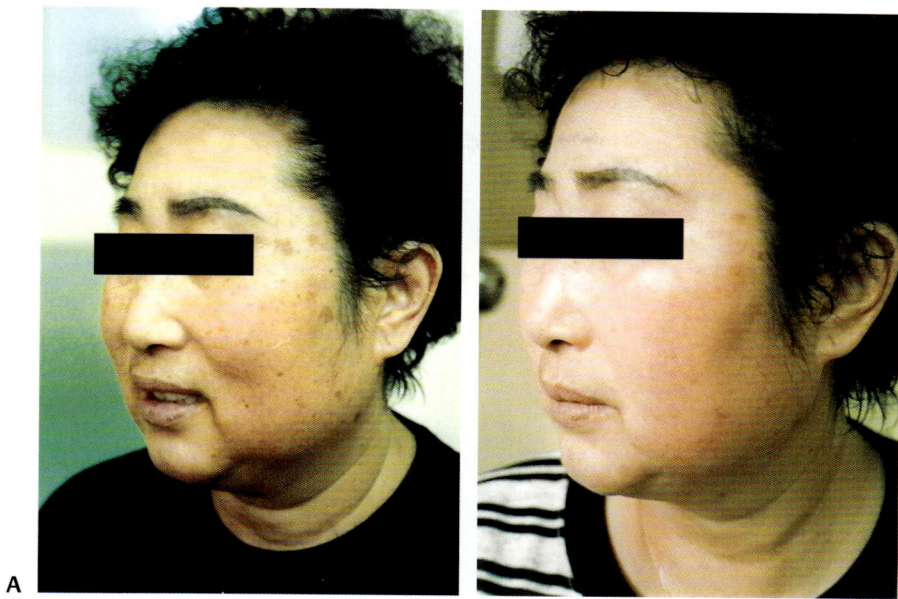

Figure 14–17 This 56-year-old Korean woman exhibits seborrheic keratosis and underwent treatment with Jessner's solution to the entire face, followed by focal application of 30% TCA to the areas of seborrheic keratosis. She is shown 4 weeks after treatment. (Courtesy of Young-Kyoon Kim, M.D.)

As mentioned, Jessner's solution can be applied independently or as a preparatory peel to the TCA. Jessner's solution alone is intended to treat active acne as well as to improve skin tone in a gentle way. If the patient is suffering from open acne lesions, the resorcinol component should be removed to lessen systemic absorption and thus hepatic toxicity. Recovery time after a Jessner's peel is minimal and typically persists 1 to 2 days with some slight erythema or no reaction at all, depending on the degree of skin peeling. The number of passes of Jessner's solution and the time that the peel remains on the skin prior to neutralization (1 minute) will dictate the extent of observed peeling. During the first few days, the patient should apply a nonirritating moisturizer like Cetaphil lotion and clean his or her skin with a similarly innocuous cleanser like Cetaphil cleanser.[ω] The patient should remain out of direct sun exposure and begin to resume an SPF 30 to 35 sunblock after any evidence of skin peeling has been completed, which can be safely done in 1 to 2 days after the peel. Serial treatments can be undertaken every 2 to 4 weeks, depending on the patient's motivation and tolerance.

Trichloroacetic Acid Peel (15–35%[Φ])

Jessner's solution serves as the standard preparatory peel immediately prior to a TCA peel to achieve a

deeper and more uniform TCA chemical exfoliation. Another important consideration is that the depth of the chemical peel is not solely dependent upon the concentration but more importantly derived from the number of layers applied and the ultimate color end point of the skin at the end of treatment. The Asian patient tends to exhibit discrete fine rhytidosis in the periocular region and may benefit from a selective chemical peel in this area. If a deeper 35% TCA peel is used in this subunit, then fewer passes or shorter "leave on" time should be performed in the periphery to soften the transition between treated and untreated skin. This technique should be used in any case of selective chemical peeling in the Asian face. The author typically uses 35% TCA for more entrenched rhytidosis or deeper pigmentary lesions and 20% TCA for lesser pathologies. The 20% TCA has also been used to feather the periphery of areas treated more aggressively with 35% TCA. Various strengths of TCA can be used focally to treat different cutaneous pathologies (Figs. **14–17, 14–18, 14–19, 14–20, 14–21, 14–22**).

After the Jessner's peel has been completed, the TCA may be immediately applied. First, the patient is marked out along subunits with a surgical marking pen, as the application of TCA must rigorously conform to the subunit principle to avoid over-, under-, or retreatment of areas. If the patient is marked out before the application of Jessner's solution, the marked areas will be lost or markedly diminished by the Jessner's peel. The lower-eyelid area is again treated first with the same technique and patient positioning described above for the Jessner's application

---

[ω]Product names are listed only for the reader's convenience and do not imply that the author has any affiliation with any stated manufacturer. The author would like to disavow direct or indirect financial reimbursement or gain from any listed manufacturer.

[Φ]When TCA is ordered from the pharmacist, the percentage of the concentration should be requested on a per weight basis.

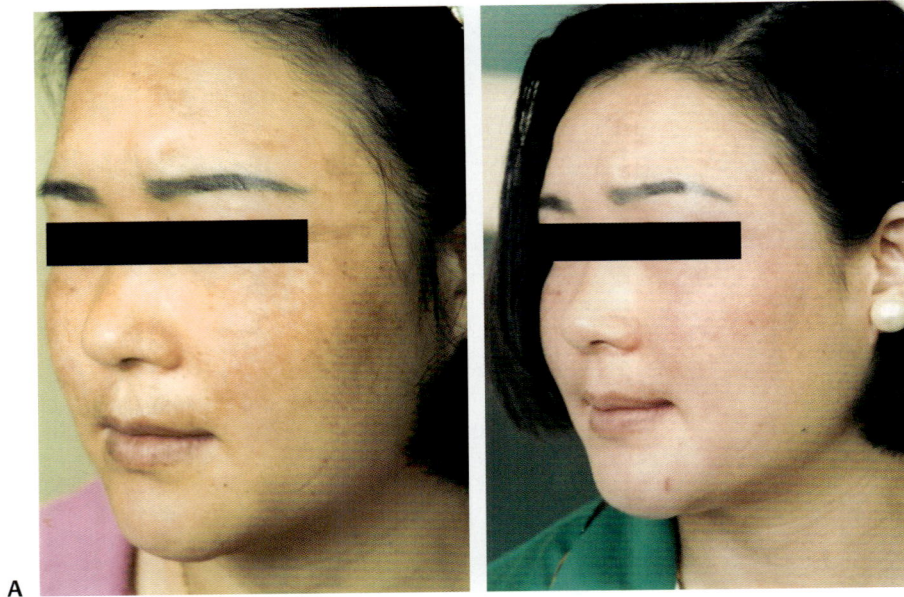

Figure 14–18 This 35-year-old Korean woman exhibits melasma and underwent application of Jessner's solution, followed by 2 passes of 15% TCA, and is shown 3 weeks after treatment. (Courtesy of Young-Kyoon Kim, M.D.)

(Figs. 14–23, 14–24, 14–25, 14–26). Although the patient will experience noteworthy burning discomfort, the lower-eyelid application must be undertaken with the patient fully awake or only minimally sedated, so that he or she may report any ocular burning due to entry of peeling solution into the eyes. To offset the burning sensation, a cooling fan is held by the second assistant at the level of the patient's waist and aimed tangentially upward toward the face, as a more direct gust may cause undesirable tearing and reflexive blinking. Furthermore, Jessner's peel can be undertaken without any sedation, but TCA peeling requires some form of intravenous sedation or deeper anesthesia to be tolerable. A dosage of 10 mg of oral Valium can provide some comfort for the patient but falls short of the aforementioned methods of anesthetic delivery. It remains uncertain whether topical anesthetic creams (e.g., EMLA or ELA-Max) adversely affect chemical peeling.[16,17]

Unlike with the Jessner's application, the blanched appearance of the skin is a critical factor in determining when the desired end point is achieved. The skin first assumes a mild erythema as the papillary dermis is entered, then a light frost, that finally a more complete, that opaque white. After a few minutes, the skin may

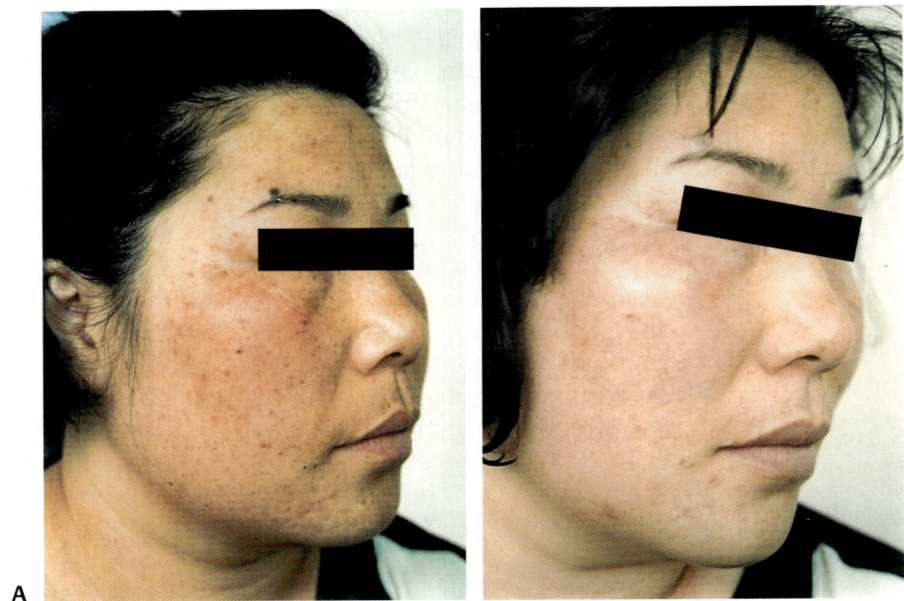

Figure 14–19 This 34-year-old Korean woman exhibits solar lentigines and underwent treatment with Jessner's solution to the entire face, followed by focal application of 30% TCA to the areas of lentigines. She is shown 4 weeks after treatment. (Courtesy of Young-Kyoon Kim, M.D.)

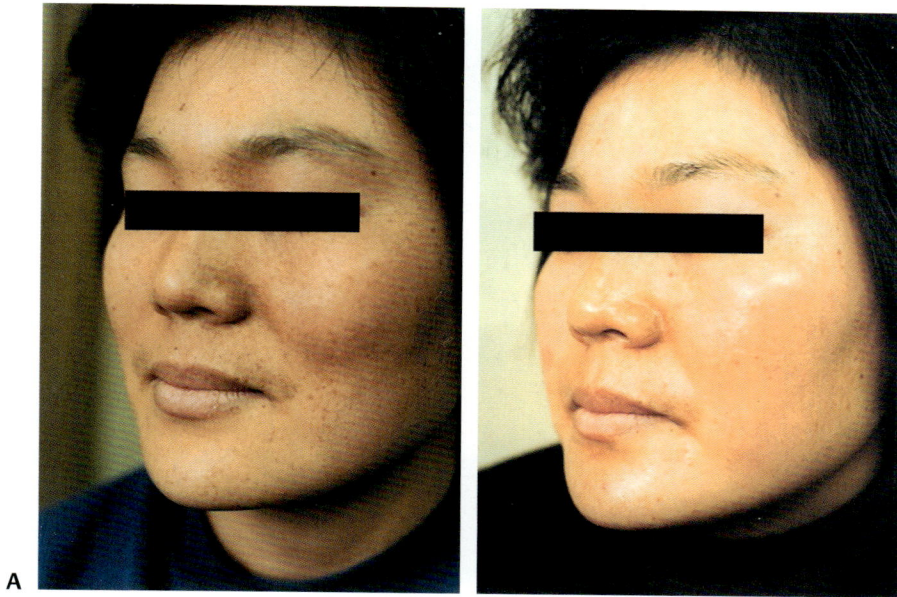

Figure 14–20 This 35-year-old Korean woman exhibits many ephelides (freckles) across her face. She underwent treatment with Jessner's solution over the entire face, with focal application of 30% TCA, and is shown 2 weeks after treatment. (Courtesy of Young-Kyoon Kim, M.D.)

begin to regress back to a light erythema, fooling the physician into thinking that the area is undertreated. The return to erythema is a major reason that the subunit principle should be adhered to to avoid retreatment of areas known to be treated already. Generally, the end point should be a completely uniform frost but not excessively opaque, which may risk scarring. Experience will dictate proper depth of the peel. Lesser depths of peel are satisfactory in the Asian patient and may be preferable to the standard uniform white peel. An ashen gray color is generally too deep for Asian skin but may be suitable for deeper wrinkles in the Caucasian skin. As

mentioned, the upper eyelids should be only lightly treated (light frost), as this particular area exhibits much thinner skin. The nose and forehead tend to withstand a deeper peel, but a deeper peel is not generally effective for the former area in any case. If the peeled area appears to have been overtreated, immediate application of gauze impregnated with water should be undertaken to dilute the peel solution and retard the action of the peel.

The neck or décolletage may be treated with a lighter TCA peel (e.g., 15–25%). However, the reader is cautioned that aggressive and repeated application of a

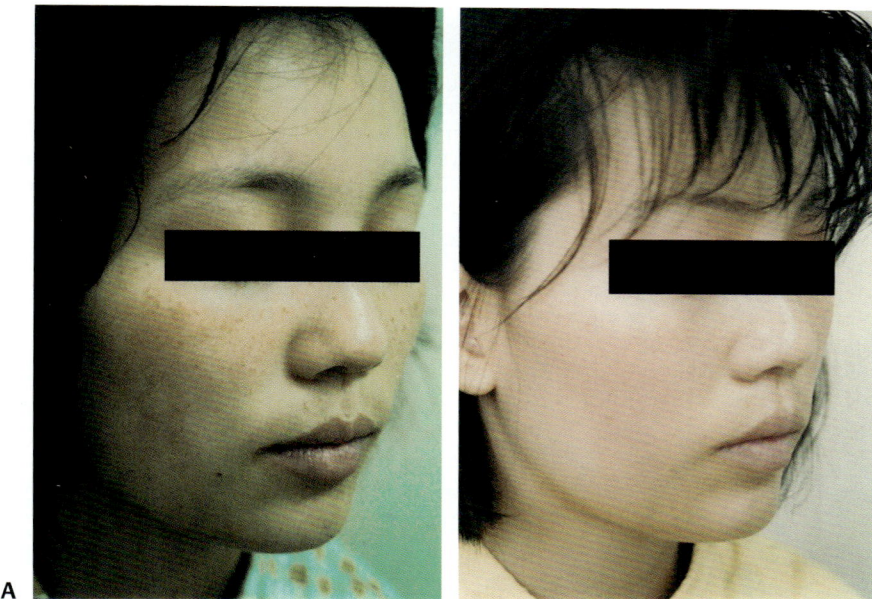

Figure 14–21 This 21-year-old Korean woman exhibits numerous ephelides (freckles) on her face. She underwent treatment with Jessner's solution over the entire face, with focal application of 30% TCA, and is shown 4 weeks after treatment. (Courtesy of Young-Kyoon Kim, M.D.)

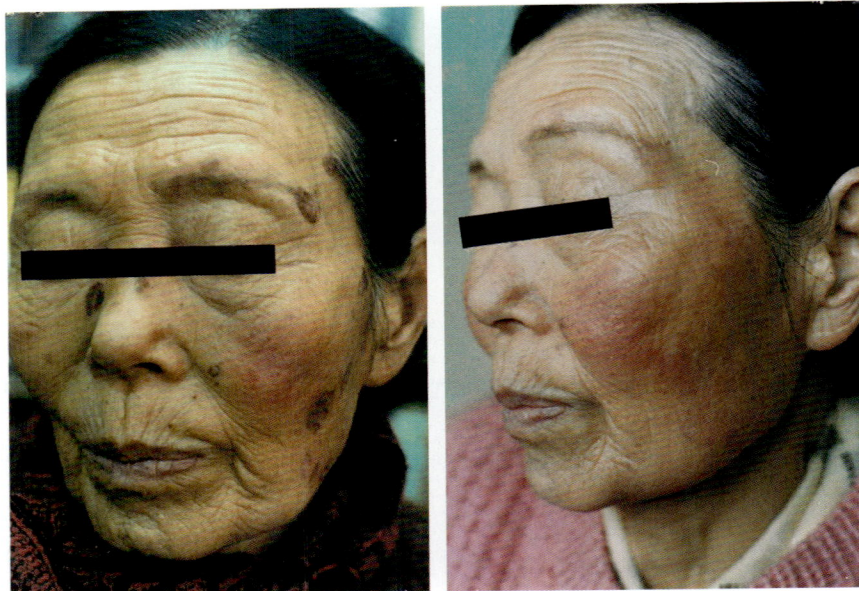

A

B

Figure 14–22 This 65-year-old Korean woman exhibits multiple seborrheic keratoses, for which she underwent treatment with Jessner's solution to the entire face, followed by focal application of 30% TCA. She is shown 2 months after treatment. (Courtesy of Young-Kyoon Kim, M.D.)

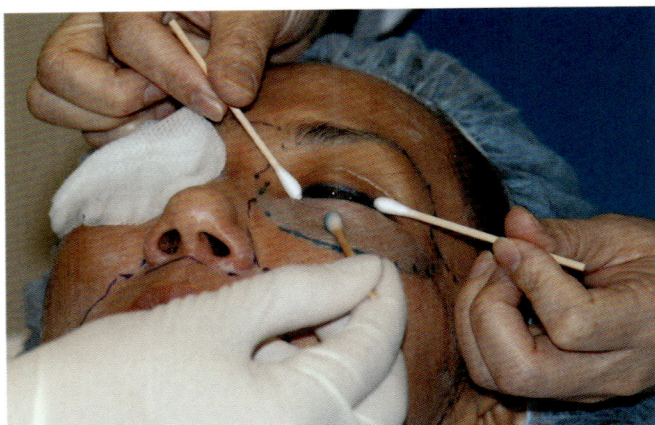

Figure 14–23 *TCA Chemical Peel, Step 1:* The patient is positioned at ~60 degrees upright and is shown with all of the facial subunits marked out. Before the patient is overly sedated, the lower eyelid region is treated first, so that the patient can report if any of the chemical solution should pass onto the globe. Balanced saline solution is always ready nearby to irrigate the globe if this problem should arise. The assistant gently holds cotton-tipped applicators on the medial and lateral canthi to collect any tearing from diluting the peeled areas unevenly and to prevent capillary action in which the peel is drawn back onto the globe. The patient is asked to look upward and fix his or her attention on a defined area so that the lower lid surface remains taut. The chemical peel is applied with even coats until a white frost is encountered. After a particular subunit is treated, cold, saline-soaked eye pads or 4 × 4 gauze is immediately applied to retard any further depth of the peel.

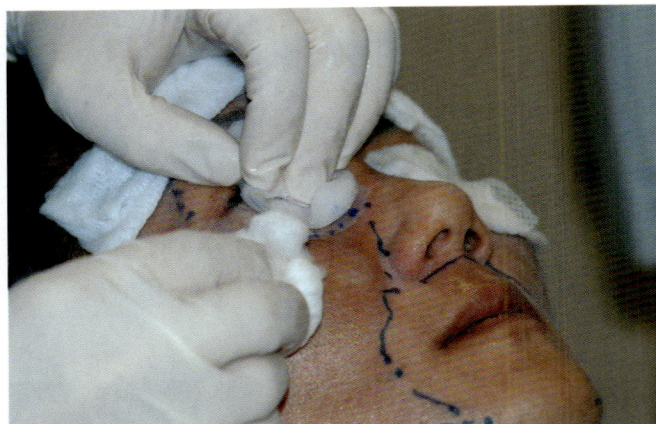

Figure 14–24 *TCA Chemical Peel, Step 2:* The physician should then progress in an orderly fashion from subunit to subunit until the entire face has been treated. By advancing in this fashion, overtreatment can be avoided, as the blanched peel color begins to regress toward a light erythema and should not be treated again. For the remainder of the face, cotton balls soaked (and wrung out) with TCA are used to apply the peel solution to the face in a systematic fashion. The color end point should be achieved uniformly for each area. The photograph shows the eyelid and forehead areas already treated and covered with cold saline pads and the right cheek currently being addressed with a cotton ball.

lighter-strength TCA will eventually equal that of a higher concentration. The desired color change should be a light and semitranslucent white and not assume a completely opaque appearance.

After the peeling is complete, Aquaphor ointment is generously applied over all peeled areas of the face with a tongue depressor. As the epidermis remains intact for several days, no occlusive dressing is required.

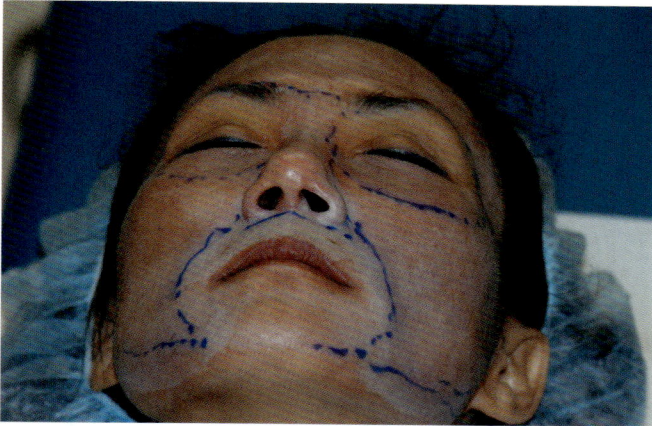

Figure 14–25 *TCA Chemical Peel, Step 3:* The photograph shows the patient having completed a TCA peel to the entire face. Note that the forehead and eyelid color have already regressed from a frosted appearance, as these areas were treated early on; the cheeks are fading back to a normal color somewhat as well. The perioral region shows a more opaque color, as this area was treated last.

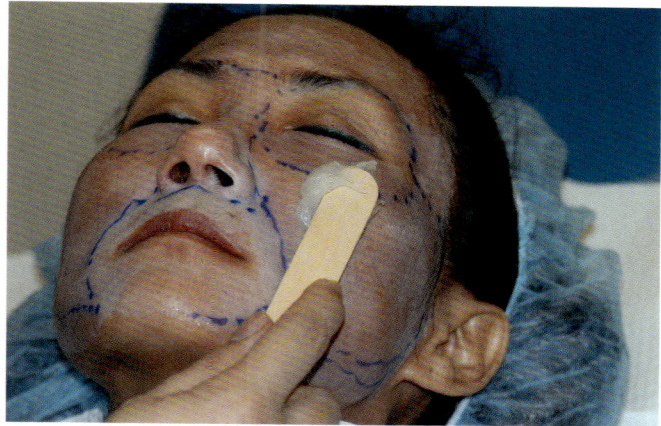

Figure 14–26 *TCA Chemical Peel, Step 4:* After treatment of all subunits, a liberal amount of Aquaphor ointment is applied to the patient's face, and the patient is instructed on the proper postpeel regimen, as described in the text.

100% TCA: Chemical Reconstruction of Skin Scars (CROSS) Method

Method of Jung Bock Lee

Traditional dermabrasion of acne scarring may engender too long a recovery period for the Asian patient. Instead, focal application of high concentrations of unbuffered trichloroacetic acid may provide a favorable solution for the darker-complected patient (Figs. **14–27A,B, 14–28**). This method is ideal for atrophic acne scars that are discrete in nature: ice-pick scars; small, localized depressions; and enlarged pores. A 100% TCA treatment would otherwise not be safe for large areas of skin due to the real risk of scarring. Instead, focal application in areas that are depressed will permit the surrounding adnexa to regenerate the localized peeled skin. Furthermore, the high concentration of TCA will stimulate collagen production and raise the depressed acne scar or enlarged pore (Fig. **14–29**). Serial treatment

sessions are needed to achieve a noticeable aesthetic improvement in the depressed scars. Generally, a minimum of three treatments is needed before any improvement may be discerned. A total of four or five treatments is typically needed to attain a favorable result. Sessions should be spaced at 4 to 6 week intervals.

The patient thoroughly cleanses his or her face with soap, and the physician then wipes the areas to be treated with alcohol. The depressed acne scar is addressed by pressing a toothpick or back of a wooden applicator dipped into 100% TCA firmly into the depression until a frosted appearance of the skin is achieved (Fig. **14–30**). Typically, less than 10 seconds of exposure time to TCA is required to arrive at this color end point. The back of a wooden applicator or the sharp end of a toothpick should be used, depending on the size of the acne scar. When removing the toothpick or wooden applicator from the 100% TCA container, the toothpick/applicator should be tapped on the side of the rim to remove excess chemical, thereby avoiding dripping or dispersion when the TCA is applied to the skin. With this technique, no anesthesia is required, as focal treatment

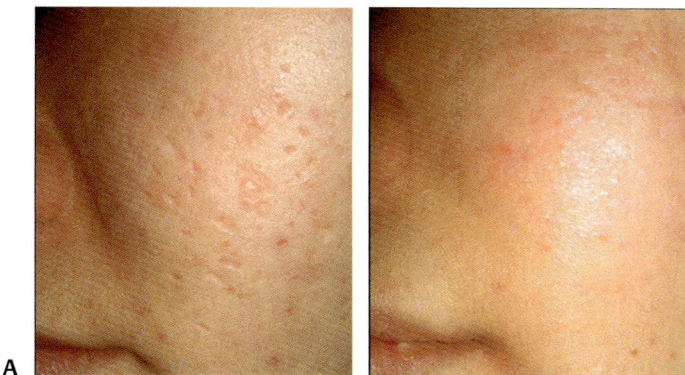

A   B

Figure 14–27 **(A,B)** This 37-year-old Korean woman exhibits acne scarring, for which she underwent focal application with 100% TCA according to the CROSS method, for a total of nine treatment sessions. The patient shows noticeable aesthetic improvement. (Courtesy of Jung Bock Lee, M.D.)

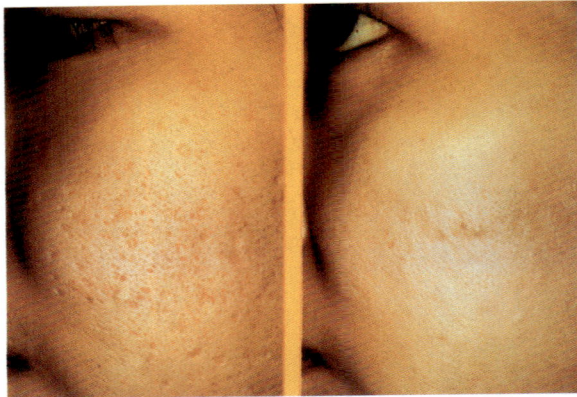

Figure 14–28   This 26-year-old Korean woman exhibits acne scarring, for which she underwent focal application with 100% TCA according to the CROSS method, for a total of six treatment sessions. The patient shows noticeable aesthetic improvement. (Courtesy of Jung Bock Lee, M.D.)

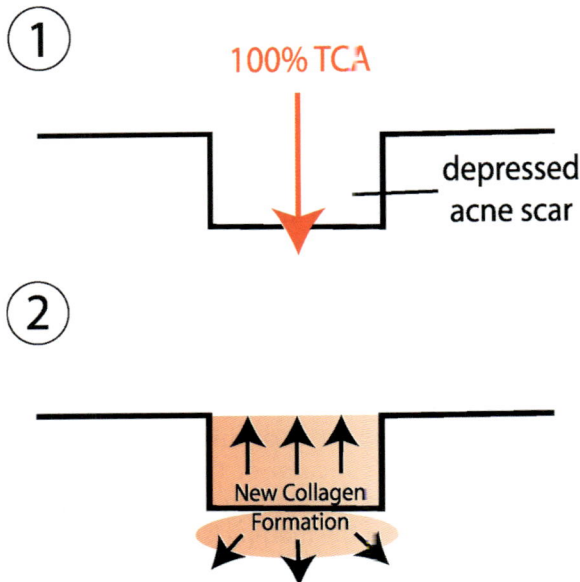

Figure 14–29   Illustration shows focal application of 100% TCA using the CROSS method, which leads to new collagen synthesis and elevation of the scarred depression.

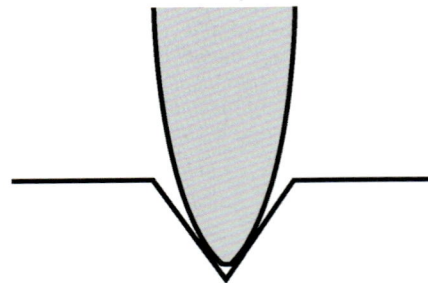

Figure 14–30   Illustration shows use of the back of a wooden applicator for wider depressed acne scars and a toothpick for smaller depressions or enlarged pores when applying 100% TCA as part of the CROSS method.

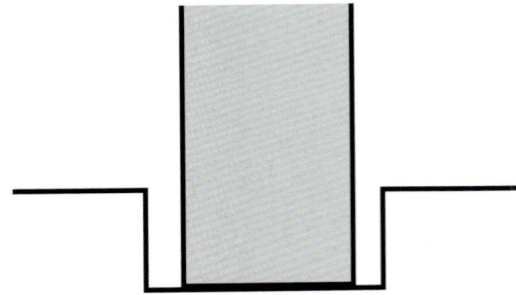

generally does not elicit much discomfort. After treatment of all affected areas, Aquaphor ointment is applied liberally, and the standard postpeel regimen is followed, as delineated in Table **14–1**.

◆ Dermabrasion

The most established resurfacing technique is mechanical dermabrasion. Dermabrasion has been successfully employed in the Asian patient to address a host of contour and pigmentary irregularities. Most commonly, dermabrasion is used to manage acne scarring but

has also been reported to efface melasma.[18] Selective mechanical abrasion with a dermabrader permits reduction of only the raised portion of a contour deformity to achieve a more uniform cutaneous surface. A chemical peel, in contrast, treats the entire skin surface indiscriminately and is less beneficial for strict contour deformities. However, high concentrations of targeted chemical peel application to depressed areas are used to stimulate collagen and to raise these areas to the height of the surrounding tissue (as described in the previous section), which is the converse objective of mechanical dermabrasion.

Despite its reported successes, the recovery period after dermabrasion can be considerable and extend over a timeframe of several months because of Asian skin's predilection to prolonged hyperpigmentation, hypopigmentation, erythema, and scarring. During the postdermabrasion period, the patient will often need to be managed with lightening creams for hyperpigmentation, topical steroid creams for dermatitis and prolonged erythema, and injectable steroid solutions for any incipient scarring. After complete epithelialization, sunblock and sun avoidance should also be followed to limit postinflammatory hyperpigmentation. If the patient understands these potential postoperative sequelae, then the surgeon can elect to proceed. Furthermore, treating

Table 14–1 Postoperative Care for the Ablative Patient*

Postoperative Days	Ointment Regimen	Cleaning Regimen	Makeup Regimen
1 to 5	Aquaphor	Vinegar and water** bid for the first postoperative day, then QID thereafter	None
5 to 10	Aquaphor (until epithelialization is complete)	Cetaphil cleanser (without sunscreen)	None
10 to 30	Cetaphil lotion	Cetaphil cleanser (without sunscreen)	Natural, powder-based makeup with titanium dioxide or zinc oxide sunblock (when epithelialization is complete)

bid = twice a day; qid four times a day
*The dermabraded-treated patient follows the same regimen, except he or she has an occlusive dressing for the first 2 postoperative days. Accordingly, the patient cannot clean the skin during this period when the occlusive dressing is applied.
**One-half tablespoon of vinegar mixed with 1 cup of distilled water, then rinsed off with distilled water and dried with a cotton-tipped applicator. Patients may begin showering on postoperative day 3 as tolerated.

the Asian skin with the same vigor as Caucasian skin will prove to be problematic for the physician and patient alike. If dermabrasion is planned for discrete areas of the face (as it almost always is used in this limited context), then a chemical peel (20–35% TCA) should be combined with dermabrasion to soften the transition between treated and untreated areas.[19] *A chemical peel should always precede mechanical dermabrasion*, as peeling intact skin is mandatory to avoid an uncontrolled cutaneous burn.

As mentioned, a chemical peel should be planned immediately before dermabrasion to soften the transition between dermabraded and nondermabraded areas. The same methodology outlined above in the chemical peel section should be followed.

Mechanical dermabrasion may be best performed under general anesthesia, when a significant area must be resurfaced for several reasons. First, use of local anesthesia may be limited to minimize tissue distortion that may interfere with correct identification of tissue depth. Second, patient movement is reduced, which is critical to safe and successful dermabrasion. Third, a curious phenomenon of unconscious, reflexive patient quivering, which is witnessed when dermabrasion is performed under sedation, is avoided. However, limited dermabrasion should be conducted under the minimum anesthesia that would aid in patient comfort and secure patient compliance.

When dermabrasion is performed near the lip, the surgeon should ensure that the rotation of the dermabrader head should be toward the lip edge to lessen the chance that the lip should be caught in the dermabrader. Similarly, 4 × 4 gauze pads used to wipe the blood from the resurfaced area should maintain a distance from the dermabrader head to minimize ensnarement. Dermabrasion should be performed with a firm hand and a gentle touch. The full weight of the instrument should not rest on the skin surface but only the lightest contact established. The surgeon should observe the microlaceration of the skin and the bleeding that ensues as the papillary dermis is violated. After the initial pass of the dermabrader has been completed, the surgeon should then rotate the direction of the dermabrader head perpendicular to the first pass to achieve uniform resurfacing and laceration of the dermis (Fig. **14–31A,B**). The depth of dermabrasion is dependent on the depth of the pathology but should generally not greatly exceed the level of initial bleeding observed at the level of the papillary dermis. At the end of the procedure, all dermabraded areas are dressed with a petroleum-based ointment and an occlusive dressing (e.g., N-terface, Winfield Laboratories, Richardson, TX) may be beneficial to minimize discomfort for the first 2 or 3 postoperative days.

◆ Postoperative Care

Postoperative care differs for the nonablative versus the ablative-resurfaced patient, with almost no care necessary for the former and a labor-intensive regimen for the latter.[20] The patient who has undergone nonablative laser therapy need only protect the skin from sun exposure to minimize the chance of hyperpigmentation. Furthermore, any microcrusts that form should be left undisturbed until they resolve in a few days' time. Sunblock, sun avoidance, and a lightening cream constitute the tripartite protocol for both the nonablative and ablative patient, with the former able to initiate topical

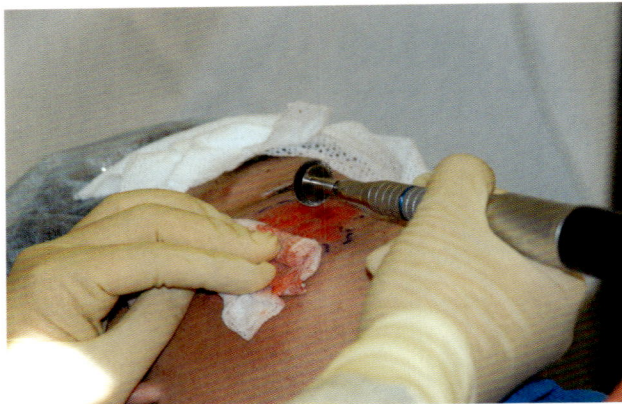

Figure 14–31 (A,B) Dermabrasion of the cheek for acne scarring is undertaken in perpendicular directions to achieve uniform resurfacing and maximal dermal laceration. Punctate bleeding indicates that the papillary dermis has been entered, and care should be taken not to be heavy handed with the dermabrader to avoid potential scarring.

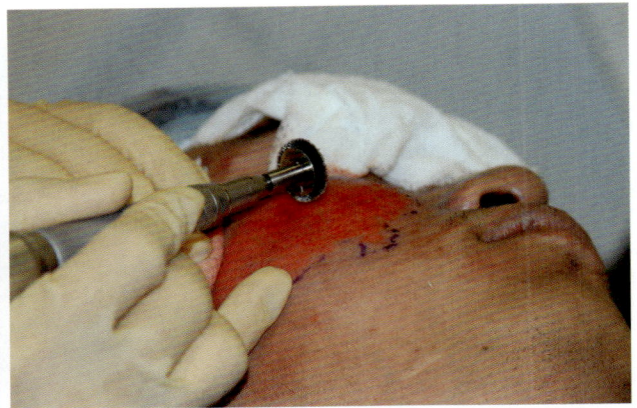

therapy immediately, whereas the latter must wait for a period after complete epithelialization has occurred before it is safe to commence irritating topical agents (as will be discussed).

For the ablative-treated patient, a complete epithelial layer and a partial dermal layer have been removed. The typical period of time for complete epithelialization is ~7 to 10 days but may extend for a variable period longer, depending on the patient's proclivity to heal that may be compromised by smoking, diabetes, and other factors. During this period of time, the denuded skin should be treated with a generous coating of petroleum-based ointment (e.g., Aquaphor ointment) to ensure even epithelialization and to avoid scar formation. The patient who has undergone a chemical peel typically undergoes several phases of healing. The first 2 or 3 days is marked by a change from the white frost that is seen at the time of chemical peeling to a dark brown transformation of the peeled overlying epithelium. During the initial few days, the brown epithelial layer falls away in a piecemeal fashion, revealing a fresh pink color that represents unepithelialized, dermal-exposed skin. Subsequently, the pink color will begin to be replaced with a new epithelial layer. When the pink, denuded skin has been completely replaced with a new skin layer, the petroleum dressing can be ceased, and a more cosmetically acceptable lotion is applied (e.g., Cetaphil lotion). Unlike the chemically peeled patient, the dermabraded patient will exhibit the denuded, pink color immediately after the procedure, as the epithelium has already been abraded away. Recovery time toward complete epithelialization is similar to chemical peeling but may persist for a longer period if dermabraded areas were treated more aggressively.

The cleaning regimen after ablative therapy is also quite involved (Table **14–1**). The patient should clean the skin with vinegar and water for the first 5 days, in which $\frac{1}{2}$ tablespoon of vinegar is mixed with 1 cup of distilled water and applied gently to the face with a cotton pad to remove the petroleum ointment. The skin is then washed with distilled water before reapplying the petroleum ointment. This is done twice the first day and then four times a day for the following 4 days. The denuded skin exhibits a higher likelihood of infection, and vinegar and water cleansing prevents this complication. After the first 5 days, Cetaphil cleanser is used instead of vinegar and water and should be continued for the first 30 days. After complete epithelialization is observed, Cetaphil lotion can be used to replace Aquaphor as a more cosmetically acceptable means of moisturization.

The first 30 days after ablative therapy represents a very sensitive time for the newly resurfaced skin. Even after complete epithelialization, the new skin is prone to dermatitis and irritation by noxious chemicals. Soaps, perfumes, and other topical agents that were applied without consequence prior to ablative therapy may engender a reaction of dermatitis during the first 30 days, as the new skin is considerably more sensitive in this period.

◆ Complications

Postinflammatory Hyperpigmentation

Asian skin has a natural proclivity to hyperpigmentation, which can involve a prolonged and diligent treatment program to correct. As previously mentioned, a preoperative course of hydroquinone fails to address the deeper melanocytes that persist after a resurfacing procedure. Instead, hyperpigmentation commonly develops after 3 to 5 weeks postprocedure and should be treated with hydroquinone, or an alternative lightening agent.

Prophylactic usage of hydroquinone prior to 3 week postablative resurfacing should be discouraged, as this agent tends to be quite irritative to the new skin. However, prophylactic 4% hydroquinone at 3 weeks, starting every other day at bedtime for 1 to 2 weeks followed by daily application, should be recommended in Asian patients who exhibit a Fitzpatrick III or higher skin grade to abort or curtail the rise of hyperpigmentation. Fortunately, hyperpigmentation is quite readily reversible but may require a protracted course given the tenacity of Asian skin to persist in a hyperpigmented state. If hydroquinone fails to resolve the problem on a timely basis, other adjunctive measures may be used to expedite recovery, namely, azelaic acid, tretinoin, and kojic acid. These agents can be combined with hydroquinone in the diligent patient interested in the most expeditious recovery and used as alternatives when the skin is overly sensitive to hydroquinone. All of these medications have proven useful in the management of postinflammatory hyperpigmentation.

The patient can also be started on a daily regimen of 10% glycolic acid in addition to 4% hydroquinone to effect a cure. Some reports suggest that higher-strength glycolic acid peels (30–70%) can be used in conjunction with the daily glycolic acid regimen to enhance resolution of hyperpigmentation, even in very dark Fitzpatrick VI skin without untoward hyper- or hypopigmentation. This treatment modality is recommended only in the patient who is at a minimum of 6 weeks after initial chemical peel to avoid overpeeling.

Hypopigmentation

Unlike postinflammatory hyperpigmentation, which is reversible, hypopigmentation proves to be a more recalcitrant entity. Hyperpigmentation typically occurs several weeks after resurfacing, whereas hypopigmentation arises after several months to years postprocedure. Hypopigmentation rarely occurs after a medium-depth chemical peel, such as with Jessner's solution followed by 35% TCA. However, phenol peels may be more prone to develop hypopigmentation (the so-called porcelain mask appearance), particularly if the croton oil component is increased, and are generally not recommended for Asian skin. Hypopigmentation may improve over time if full melanocyte destruction has not occurred. Accordingly, hypopigmentation should be distinguished from frank depigmentation when no chance of recovery is possible.

Erythema/Dermatitis

Prolonged erythema is a known phenomenon in Asian skin. Erythema may even be observed along an incision line after surgery or in any traumatized area (e.g., after collagen injection). Typically, erythema that persists in the Caucasian skin may be indicative of incipient dermatitis; and based on symptomatology, it should be treated to avoid the onset of recalcitrant dermatitis and eventual scarring. *The continuum of erythema, dermatitis, and scarring must be carefully understood by the physician so that aggressive management may be employed to abort this chain of events.* Because erythema is such a common observance in the postoperative/postpeeling setting in Asian skin, it may be unjustly overlooked in its significance. Also, because scarring is much more common in Asian skin, prolonged erythema should not be ignored. When observed with any other signs and symptoms consistent with dermatitis, erythema should be managed early. Dermatitis typically manifests as a bright red coloration with possible raised, bumpy areas associated with burning and/or pruritus. A careful history should also be taken to investigate any offending topical agents that may be eliciting the dermatitis. Even innocuous topical creams (e.g., Aquaphor and Cetaphil) have been known to cause an allergic cutaneous reaction and should be stopped if suspected of inciting the condition. Management should begin with a topical steroid cream, for example, desonide (DesOwen, Galderma), that can be applied twice daily. Flurandrenolide tape (Cordran tape, Oclassen Pharmaceuticals, Corona, CA), which contains a potent steroid, can be applied to the area in question at night and left in place until the morning, when showering can loosen the adhesive for easy removal. The patient should be followed clinically to ensure improvement and resolution of the problem. If the skin appears to be unresponsive or is worsening and showing signs of dermal thickening (scarring), an injectable steroid (e.g., triamcinolone 10 mg/cc) can be used to abort the reaction more vigorously. Supplemental oral steroids (e.g., a Medrol dose pack) can be initiated as an ancillary measure.

◆ Basic Skin Care

The patient is encouraged to begin a routine daily regimen of proper skin care after any type of ablative or nonablative resurfacing to maintain the longevity of the result. Patients often ask whether the "dark spots will come back" or proffer a similar query regarding the durability of the dermatologic benefit. During the initial consultation, the author always cautions that poor skin care and behavior after any kind of resurfacing will circumvent the permanence of the aesthetic result. Similar to a patient who has undergone liposuction who then returns to a grossly unhealthy diet, the longevity of the result is undoubtedly thwarted. The patient is made to understand that skin diseases reflect a pathologic process that should be kept under control with proper skin care. Besides skin care with topical agents, the patient should be advised to subscribe to a good diet, adequate sleep, stress reduction, abstinence from smoking and excessive alcohol intake, and routine exercise. Avoidance of sun exposure, especially during the hours between 10:00 AM and 4:00 PM, should also be practiced. Routine sunblock and a wide-brimmed hat are also important prescriptive elements in overall skin care. Basic skin care does not differ significantly across racial divides except for therapeutic ingredients that target hyperpigmentation that may be more beneficial for the Asian skin.

Many different skin care product lines abound and offer the patient a dizzying array of choices. The following text is not meant to advocate any particular product but to offer the physician a basic review of ingredients essential in a good skin care strategy. The first step that is critical is a suitable cleanser. Most over-the-counter soaps are overly alkaline and strip the skin of essential oils, making dry skin drier and oily skin oilier. Aggressive removal of natural oils will stimulate sebaceous gland activity, which encourages additional cleansing, leading to a vicious cycle. Instead, a gentle pH-balanced cleanser can offer proper cleaning without undue oil gland stimulation. Also, this cleanser should be used only once (and most twice) daily to avoid local irritation to the skin. Additional cleansing can be performed with water only unless excessive dirt accumulation has been encountered that day.

Toners can be used after cleansing but may not be a critical component to daily skin care. They serve to further pH balance the skin and remove any residual debris and can be helpful for makeup removal after cleansing. Toners that contain salicylic acid may help minimize acne flare-ups, but the salicylic acid may have been incorporated into the cleanser or the moisturizer instead. Toners with a high alcohol content should be avoided to minimize excessive drying and irritation of the skin.

A good moisturizer is an important aspect of basic care for both dry and oily skin. Albeit at first glance counterintuitive, a moisturizer can help reduce the tendency for oily skin to produce oil and thereby keep the oiliness of the skin in check. A sunblock can be incorporated into a moisturizer and should be applied daily to combat even transient exposure to indirect sunrays. An SPF 15 is generally sufficient for daily protection, but an SPF 30 to 35 is recommended for prolonged, direct exposure and for Asians who aim to minimize exacerbation of cutaneous hyperpigmentation. The sunscreen should contain both chemical (octyl methoxy cinnamate) and physical (titanium dioxide and zinc oxide) blocking agents for maximal effectiveness. If the same moisturizer is used at night, the individual should ensure that no sunblock ingredients are present, which can irritate the skin with prolonged contact. At night when the patient is asleep, the skin is in its most restorative mode and should be treated during this critical period. Vitamins and lipids can provide nutritive supply to the skin and may be beneficial ingredients for optimal skin health. Vitamin C, in particular, can provide a valuable aid to combat aging and to minimize the tendency toward hyperpigmentation. Similarly, alpha-hydroxy acids can be incorporated in the cleanser or in the moisturizer and be used to address hyperpigmentation, acne, and signs of aging.

◆ Conclusion

This chapter was not intended as an exhaustive review of every treatment modality possible to manage Asian skin. Instead, remarks have been based principally on clinical experience and have been supplemented with recent literature review and personal communication with experts on Asian skin. Asian skin exhibits different cutaneous pathologies than Caucasian skin and responds very differently to resurfacing. Today, conservative combination of nonablative and ablative resurfacing techniques have provided the optimal therapy while minimizing recovery period and potential complications in the sensitive Asian skin.

References

1. Peterson RL, Chrisman BC. Dermabrasion in Oriental patients. Facial Plast Surg Clin North Am 1996;4:201–209
2. Fanous N. A new patient classification for laser resurfacing and peels: predicting responses, risks, and results. Aesthetic Plast Surg 2002;26:99–104
3. West TB, Alster TS. Effect of pretreatment on the incidence of hyperpigmentation following cutaneous CO_2 laser resurfacing. Dermatol Surg 1999;25:15–17
4. Anderson RR, Parrish JA. Selective photothermolysis: precise microsurgery by selective absorption of pulsed radiation. Science 1983;220:524–527
5. Dahiya R, Lam SM, Williams EF. A systematic histologic analysis of the pulsed-dye laser in a porcine model. Arch Facial Plast Surg 2003;5:218–223
6. Jang KA, Chung EC, Choi JH, Sung KJ, Moon KC, Koh JK. Successful removal of freckles in Asian skin with a Q-switched Alexandrite laser. Dermatol Surg 2000;26:231–234
7. Chan HH, Leung RSC, Ying SY, et al. A retrospective analysis of complications in the treatment of nevus of Ota with the Q-switched Alexandrite and Q-switched Nd:YAG lasers. Dermatol Surg 2000;26:1000–1006

8. Chan HH, Fung WKK, Ying SY, Kono T. An in vivo trial comparing the use of different types of 532 nm Nd:YAG lasers in the treatment of facial lentigines in Oriental patients. Dermatol Surg 2000;26:743–749

9. Negishi K, Tezuka Y, Kushikata N, Wakamatsu S. Photorejuvenation for Asian skin by intense pulsed light. Dermatol Surg 2001;27:627–632

10. Negishi K, Wakamatsu S, Kushikata N, Tezuka Y, Kotani Y, Shiba K. Full-face photorejuvenation of photodamaged skin by intense pulsed light with integrated contact cooling: initial experiences in Asian patients. Lasers Surg Med 2002;30:298–305

11. Ho WS, Chan HH, Ying SY, Chan PC, Burd A, King WWK. Prospective study on the treatment of postburn hyperpigmentation by intense pulsed light. Lasers Surg Med 2003;32:42–45

12. Huang YL, Liao YL, Lee SH, Hong HS. Intense pulsed light for the treatment of facial freckles in Asian skin. Dermatol Surg 2002;28:1007–1012

13. Lee JB, Chung WG. Kwahck H, Lee KH. Focal treatment of acne scars with tricholoroacetic acid: chemical reconstruction of skin scars method. Dermatol Surg 2002;28:1017–1021

14. Wang CM, Huang CL, Sindy Hu CT, Chan HL. The effect of glycolic acid on the treatment of acne in Asian skin. Dermatol Surg 1997;23:23–29

15. Williams EF III, Lam SM. Comprehensive Facial Rejuvenation: A Practical and Systematic Guide to Surgical Management of the Aging Face. Philadephia: Lippincott, Williams, & Wilkins; 2003

16. Rubin MG. The efficacy of a topical lidocaine/prilocaine anesthetic gel in 35% trichloracetic acid peels. Dermatol Surg 1995;21:223–225

17. Koppel RA, Coleman KM, Coleman WP. The efficacy of EMLA versus ELA-Max for pain relief in medium-depth chemical peeling: a clinical and histopathologic evaluation. Dermatol Surg 2000;26:61–64

18. Kunachak S, Leelaudomlipi P, Wongwaisayawan S. Dermabrasion: a curative treatment for melasma. Aesthetic Plast Surg 2001;25:114–117

19. Williams EF, Lam SM. Combined resurfacing techniques: a systematic approach. Int J Cosm Surg Aesthetic Dermatol 2002;4:88–91

20. Lam SM, Sullivan SE, Williams EF. Management of the postpeel and laser resurfaced patient: a ten-year experience. Int J Cosm Surg Aesthetic Dermatol 2002;4:189–199

Index

Page numbers followed by f or t denote figures or tables, respectively.